ARTERIAL SURGERY

MANAGEMENT OF CHALLENGING PROBLEMS

Edited by

James S.T. Yao, MD, PhD
Magerstadt Professor of Surgery
Division of Vascular Surgery
Department of Surgery
Northwestern University Medical School
Chief, Division of Vascular Surgery
Northwestern Memorial Hospital
Chicago, Illinois

William H. Pearce, MD
Professor of Surgery
Division of Vascular Surgery
Department of Surgery
Northwestern University Medical School
Chicago, Illinois

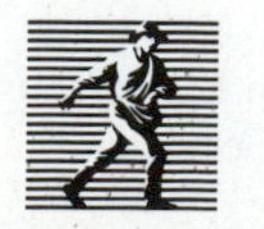

APPLETON & LANGE
Stamford, Connecticut

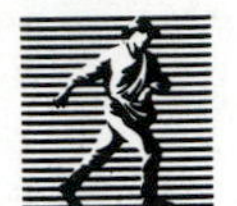

96 97 98 99 00 / 10 9 8 7 6 5 4 3 2 1

Prentice Hall International (UK) Limited, *London*
Prentice Hall of Australia Pty. Limited, *Sydney*
Prentice Hall Canada, Inc., *Toronto*
Prentice Hall Hispanoamericana, S.A., *Mexico*
Prentice Hall of India Private Limited, *New Delhi*
Prentice Hall of Japan, Inc., *Tokyo*
Simon & Schuster Asia Pte. Ltd., *Singapore*
Editora Prentice Hall do Brasil Ltda., *Rio de Janeiro*
Prentice Hall, *Upper Saddle River, New Jersey*

Library of Congress Cataloging-in-Publication Data

Arterial surgery : management of challenging problems / edited by
James S.T. Yao, William H. Pearce.
p. cm.
Includes bibliographical references.
ISBN 0-8385-0338-1 (case : alk. paper)
1. Arteries—Surgery. I. Yao, James S.T. II. Pearce, William
H.
[DNLM: 1. Arteries—surgery. 2. Vascular Surgery—methods.
3. Vascular Diseases—surgery. WG 170 A78545 1996]
RD598.A78 1996
617.4' 13—dc20
DNLM/DLC
for Library of Congress

95-43212
CIP

Managing Editor, Development: Kathleen McCullough
Production Service: Spectrum Publisher Services
Designer: Janice Barsevich Bielawa

PRINTED IN THE UNITED STATES OF AMERICA

Contents

Contributors

Mark A. Adelman, MD
Assistant Professor of Surgery
New York University Medical School
Attending Surgeon
New York University Medical Center
New York, New York

Robert C. Allen, MD
Assistant Professor of Medical Education
Department of Surgery
Baylor University Medical Center
Baylor University
Dallas, Texas

George Andros, MD
Medical Director
Vascular Laboratory
St. Joseph Medical Center
Burbank, California

Amine Bahnini, MD
Staff Surgeon
Pitié-Salpêtrière University Hospital
Paris, France

William H. Baker, MD
Professor of Surgery
Stritch School of Medicine
Loyola University Medical School
Chief, Division of Peripheral Vascular Surgery
Foster G. McGaw Hospital, Loyola University Medical Center
Maywood, Illinois

Aires A.B. Barros D'Sa, MD, FRCS, FRCS (Ed)
Honorary Lecturer in Surgery
The Queen's University of Belfast
Consultant Vascular Surgeon, Vascular Surgery Unit
Royal Victoria Hospital
Belfast, United Kingdom

Ramon Berguer, MD, PhD
Professor of Surgery
Wayne State University School of Medicine
Chief, Division of Vascular Surgery
Harper Hospital
Detroit, Michigan

Victor M. Bernhard, MD
EndoVascular Technologies, Inc.
Menlo Park, California

Eugene F. Bernstein, MD, PhD†
Clinical Professor of Surgery
University of California, San Diego
San Diego, California
Senior Consultant
Scripps Clinic
La Jolla, California

F. William Blaisdell, MD
Professor of Surgery
Chair, Department of Surgery
University of California, Davis
Sacramento, California

† Deceased.

Thomas C. Bower, MD
Associate Professor
Mayo Medical School
Consultant, Division of Vascular Surgery
Mayo Clinic
Rochester, Minnesota

David C. Brewster, MD
Clinical Professor of Surgery
Harvard Medical School and
Massachusetts General Hospital
Boston, Massachusetts

Linda G. Canton, RN, BSN
Physician Extender
Division of Vascular Surgery
Mayo Clinic
Rochester, Minnesota

Sandra C. Carr, MD
Fellow in Vascular Surgery
Northwestern University Medical School
Northwestern Memorial Hospital
Chicago, Illinois

Kenneth J. Cherry, Jr., MD
Professor of Surgery
Mayo Medical School
Chair, Division of Vascular Surgery
Mayo Clinic
Rochester, Minnesota

Richard W. Chitwood, MD
Clinical Vascular Fellow
Division of Vascular Surgery
Henry Ford Hospital
Detroit, Michigan

G. Patrick Clagett, MD
Professor
University of Texas
Head, Vascular Surgery Section
University of Texas Southwestern
Medical Center
Dallas, Texas

Alexander W. Clowes, MD
Professor of Surgery and Vice Chairman
University of Washington School of
Medicine
Seattle, Washington

Michael D. Colburn, MD
Clinical Instructor in Surgery
Vascular Fellow
UCLA Medical Center
Los Angeles, California

Joseph S. Coselli, MD
Associate Professor of Surgery
Baylor College of Medicine
Attending Surgeon
The Methodist Hospital
Houston, Texas

Enrique Criado, MD, FACS
Assistant Professor of Surgery
Division of Vascular Surgery
University of North Carolina at
Chapel Hill
Chapel Hill, North Carolina

Michael D. Dake, MD
Assistant Professor of Radiology and
Medicine
Stanford University
Chief, Cardiovascular and Interventional
Radiology
Stanford University Hospital
Stanford, California

Richard H. Dean, MD
Professor of Surgery
Director, Division of Surgical Sciences
The Bowman Gray School of Medicine at
Wake Forest University
Chairman, Department of Surgery
North Carolina Baptist Hospital
Winston-Salem, North Carolina

James A. DeWeese, MD
Professor of Surgery
Chair Emeritis, Cardiothoracic and
Vascular Surgery
University of Rochester
Rochester, New York

Calvin B. Ernst, MD
Clinical Professor of Surgery
University of Michigan Medical School
Head, Division of Vascular Surgery
Henry Ford Hospital
Detroit, Michigan

Joseph H. Frankhouse, MD
Resident, Surgery
Los Angeles County and University of Southern California Medical Center
Los Angeles, California

Stanley B. Fuller, MD
Bradshaw Fellow of Surgical Research
The Bowman Gray School of Medicine at Wake Forest University
Winston-Salem, North Carolina

Spencer Galt, MD
Assistant Professor of Surgery
University of Utah School of Medicine
Staff Surgeon
University of Utah Hospital and Salt Lake City VA Hospital
Salt Lake City, Utah

Bruce L. Gewertz, MD
Dallas B. Phemister Professor
University of Chicago Pritzker School of Medicine
Chair, Department of Surgery
University of Chicago Hospitals and Clinics
Chicago, Illinois

Jean W. Gillon, MD
Assistant Professor of Surgery
University of California, San Francisco
San Francisco, California

Peter Gloviczki, MD
Professor of Surgery
Mayo Medical School
Vice-Chair, Division of Vascular Surgery
Mayo Clinic
Rochester, Minnesota

Jerry Goldstone, MD
Professor of Surgery
University of California, San Francisco
San Francisco, California

Richard M. Green, MD
Associate Professor of Surgery
University of Rochester
Chief, Section of Vascular Surgery
Strong Memorial Hospital
Rochester, New York

John W. Hallett, Jr., MD
Associate Professor of Surgery
Mayo Medical School
Mayo Clinic
Rochester, Minnesota

John Preston Harris, MS, FRACS, FACS
Vascular Surgeon
Department of Surgery
University of Sydney
Royal Prince Alfred Hospital
Sydney, NSW, Australia

Asher Hirshberg, MD
Adjunct Associate Professor of Surgery
Baylor College of Medicine
Houston, Texas
Lecturer in Surgery
The Sackler Medical School
Tel Aviv University
Ramat Aviv, Israel
Co-Director of Trauma Service and Staff Surgeon
The Chaim Sheba Medical Center
Tel Hoshomer, Israel

Robert W. Hobson II, MD
Professor of Surgery
UMDNJ—New Jersey Medical School
Chief, Section of Vascular Surgery
UMDNJ—University Hospital
Newark, New Jersey

C. Michael Johnson, MD
Assistant Professor of Radiology
Mayo Medical School
Mayo Clinic
Rochester, Minnesota

Blair A. Keagy, MD
Professor of Surgery
Chief, Division of Vascular Surgery
University of North Carolina at Chapel Hill
Chapel Hill, North Carolina

Edouard Kieffer, MD
Professor of Surgery
Pitié-Salpêtrière University Medical School
Chief, Department of Vascular Surgery
Pitié-Salpêtrière University Hospital
Paris, France

Fabien Koskas, MD
Staff Surgeon
Pitié-Salpêtrière University Hospital
Paris, France

Patrick J. Lamparello, MD
Associate Professor of Surgery
New York University
Associate Attending in Surgery
New York University Medical Center
New York, New York

Sandro Lepidi, MD
Senior Vascular Research Fellow
Department of Surgery
University of Washington School of Medicine
University of Washington
Seattle, Washington

Alan B. Lumsden, MD
Assistant Professor of Surgery
Department of Surgery
Emory University School of Medicine
Atlanta, Georgia

Michael L. Marin, MD
Assistant Professor of Surgery
Albert Einstein College of Medicine
Assistant Attending in Surgery
Montefiore Medical Center
New York, New York

Kenneth L. Mattox, MD
Professor and Vice Chairman
Department of Surgery
Baylor College of Medicine
Chief of Staff and Chief of Surgery
Ben Taub General Hospital
Houston, Texas

James May, MS, MRACS, FACS
Bosch Professor of Surgery
University of Sydney
Vascular Surgeon
Royal Prince Alfred Hospital
Sydney, NSW, Australia

Walter McCarthy, MD
Associate Professor of Surgery
Northwestern University Medical School, Northwestern Memorial Hospital, and Lakeside VA Hospital
Chicago, Illinois

Timothy J. McGahan, FRACS (Vasc)
Vascular Surgeon
Princess Alexandra Hospital
Brisbane, QLD, Australia

William D. McMillan, MD
Surgical Resident
Division of Vascular Surgery
Northwestern University Medical School
Chicago, Illinois

Louis M. Messina, MD
Chief, Vascular Surgery
University of California, San Francisco
San Francisco, California

D. Craig Miller, MD
Professor of Cardiovascular Surgery
Stanford University School of Medicine
Stanford University Hospital
Stanford, California

Wesley S. Moore, MD
Professor of Surgery
UCLA School of Medicine
Chief, Section of Vascular Surgery
UCLA Medical Center
Los Angeles, California

Andrew C. Novick, MD
Chairman, Department of Urology
Cleveland Clinic Foundation
Cleveland, Ohio

John L. Ochsner, MD
Chief, Cardiovascular Surgery Section
Ochsner Clinic and Alton Ochsner Medical Foundation
New Orleans, Louisiana

Charles S. O'Mara, MD
Clinical Assistant Professor of Surgery
University Medical Center
Staff Surgeon
Mississippi Baptist Medical Center
St. Dominic-Jackson Memorial Hospital
Jackson, Mississippi

Frank T. Padberg, Jr., MD
Professor of Surgery
Department of Surgery
UMDNJ—New Jersey Medical School
Newark, New Jersey

Marc Passman, MD
Research Fellow
Division of Vascular Surgery
Oregon Health Sciences University
Portland, Oregon

William H. Pearce, MD
Professor of Surgery
Division of Vascular Surgery
Department of Surgery
Northwestern University Medical School
Chicago, Illinois

John M. Porter, MD
Professor of Surgery
Head, Division of Vascular Surgery
Oregon Health Sciences University
Portland, Oregon

Martin R. Prince, MD, PhD
Assistant Professor
University of Michigan Medical Center
Co-Director of Magnetic Resonance Imaging
University Hospital
Ann Arbor, Michigan

Robert Y. Rhee, MD
Assistant Professor of Surgery
University of Pittsburgh School of Medicine
Attending Surgeon, Division of Vascular Surgery
University of Pittsburgh Medical Center
Pittsburgh, Pennsylvania

Thomas S. Riles, MD
Professor of Surgery
New York University School of Medicine
Director, Division of Vascular Surgery
New York University Medical Center
New York, New York

Christopher M. Rose, MD
Department of Radiation Therapy
St. Joseph Medical Center
Burbank, California

Carlo Ruotolo, MD
Staff Surgeon
Pitié-Salpêtrière University Hospital
Paris, France

Eric J. Russell, MD
Professor of Radiology
Northwestern University Medical School
Director of Neuroradiology
Northwestern Memorial Hospital
Chicago, Illinois

Robert B. Rutherford, MD
Chief, Vascular Surgery
University Hospital
Professor of Surgery
University of Colorado Health Sciences Center
Denver, Colorado

Jean Sabatier, MD
Staff Surgeon
Pitié-Salpêtrière University Hospital
Paris, France

Steven M. Santilli, MD, PhD
Assistant Professor
University of Minnesota
Department of Surgery
VA Medical Center
Minneapolis, Minnesota

Mark W. Sebastian, MD
Department of Surgery
Duke University Medical Center
Durham, North Carolina

Suzanne M. Slonim, MD
Fellow
Cardiovascular and Interventional Radiology
Stanford University Hospital
Stanford, California

Robert B. Smith III, MD
Professor of Surgery
Head, Division of Vascular Surgery
Department of Surgery
Emory University School of Medicine
Atlanta, Georgia

James C. Stanley, MD
Professor of Surgery
University of Michigan Medical School
Head, Section of Vascular Surgery
University Hospital
Ann Arbor, Michigan

Michael S. Stephen, FRACS
Department of Surgery
University of Sydney
Vascular Surgeon
Royal Prince Alfred Hospital
Camperdown, NSW, Australia

Ronald J. Stoney, MD
Professor of Surgery
University of California, San Francisco
San Francisco, California

Lloyd Taylor, Jr., MD
Professor of Surgery
Director, Vascular Laboratory
Oregon Health Sciences University
Portland, Oregon

Jonathan B. Towne, MD
Professor, Vascular Surgery
Department of Surgery
Medical College of Wisconsin
Chairman, Vascular Surgery
Milwaukee County Medical Complex
Milwaukee, Wisconsin

William D. Turnipseed, MD
Professor, Department of Surgery
University Medical School
Chief, Vascular Surgery Section
University of Wisconsin Hospital and Clinics
Madison, Wisconsin

Frank J. Veith, MD
Professor of Surgery
Albert Einstein College of Medicine
Director of Vascular Surgical Services
Montefiore Medical Center
New York, New York

Robert L. Vogelzang, MD
Professor of Radiology
Northwestern University Medical School
Chief of Vascular Surgery and Interventional Radiology
Northwestern Memorial Hospital
Chicago, Illinois

Matthew J. Wall, Jr., MD
Assistant Professor of Surgery
Baylor College of Medicine
Chief of General Surgery and Director of the Trauma/Critical Care Center
Ben Taub General Hospital
Houston, Texas

Richard Waugh, FRACR
Staff Specialist, Radiology
Department of Radiology
Royal Prince Alfred Hospital
Camperdown, NSW, Australia

Fred A. Weaver, MD, FACS
Associate Professor of Surgery
University of Southern California School of Medicine
Chief, Vascular Surgery Service
Los Angeles County and University of Southern California School of Medicine
Los Angeles, California

Geoffrey H. White, FRACS
Clinical Associate Professor of Surgery
University of Sydney
Vascular Surgeon
Royal Prince Alfred Hospital
Sydney, NSW, Australia

Walter G. Wolfe, MD
Professor of Surgery
Department of Surgery
Duke University Medical Center
Durham, North Carolina

Wayne F. Yakes, MD
Director, Interventional Neuroradiology and Interventional Radiology
Colorado Neurological Institute
Swedish Medical Center
Englewood, Colorado

James S.T. Yao, MD, PhD
Magerstadt Professor of Surgery
Division of Vascular Surgery
Department of Surgery
Northwestern University Medical School
Chief, Division of Vascular Surgery
Northwestern Memorial Hospital
Chicago, Illinois

Albert E. Yellin, MD, FACS
Professor of Surgery
Chief, Division of Vascular Surgery
University of Southern California School of Medicine
Medical Director, Surgical Services
Los Angeles County and University of Southern California Medical Center
Los Angeles, California

Weiyun Yu, BSc (Med), MB, BS
Endovascular Research Fellow
Department of Surgery
University of Sydney
Royal Prince Alfred Hospital
Sydney, NSW, Australia

R. Eugene Zierler, MD
Associate Professor of Surgery
Division of Vascular Surgery
Department of Surgery
University of Washington School of Medicine
Seattle, Washington

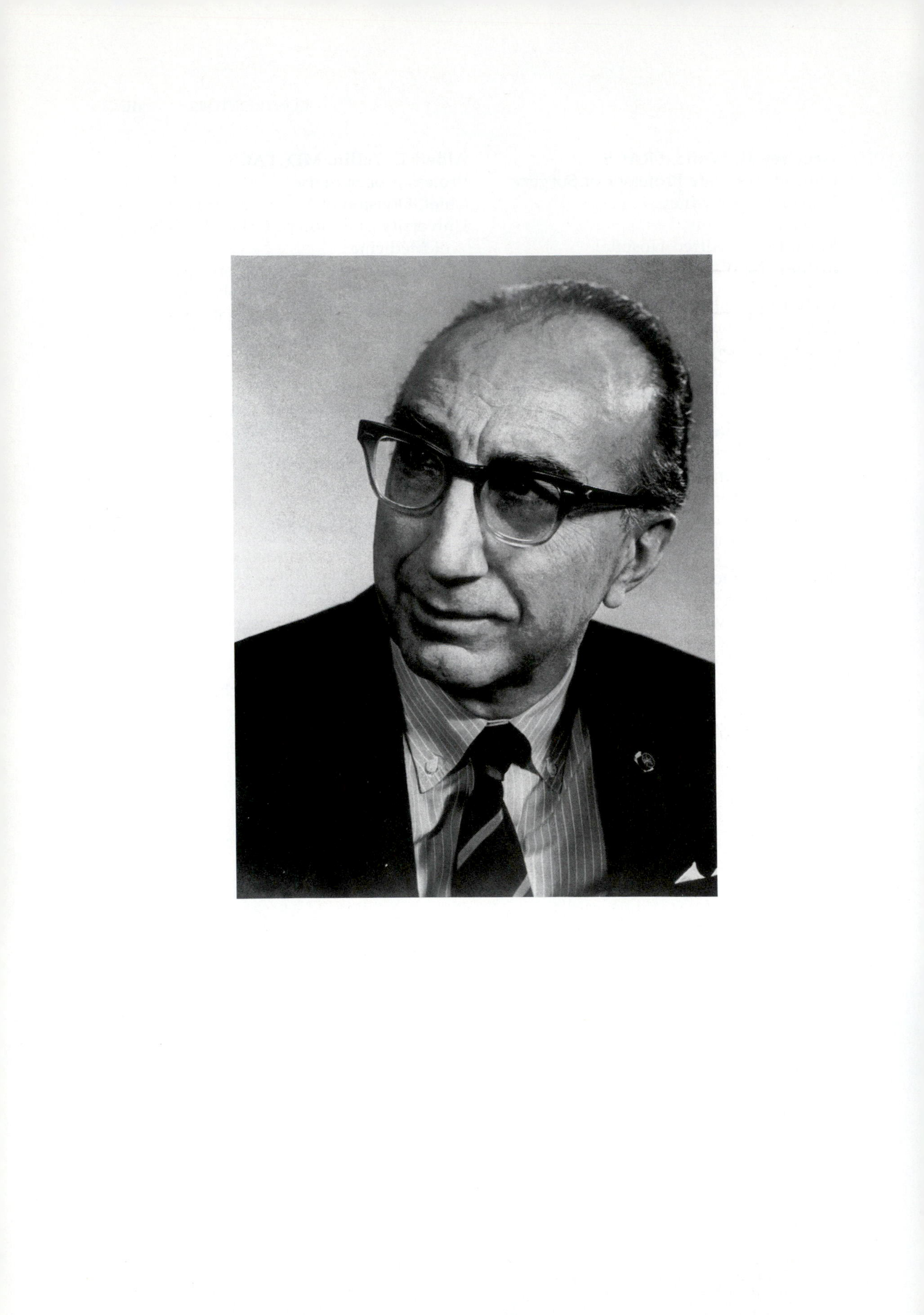

Dedication—Michael E. DeBakey, MD

A Surgeon for All Seasons

Despite advances in technique in arterial surgery, surgeons continue to face challenging and different clinical problems in the management of arterial occlusive disease. It is hoped that this symposium provides useful guidance for surgeons who may encounter some of these challenges in their practice. All invited contributors are experts of their own fields. Like us, most surgeons are in awe of the contributions of Dr. Michael DeBakey in the field of vascular surgery. We thank the participants, as well as the invited contributors, for joining us for the celebration of this truly remarkable surgeon.

We dedicate this symposium to honor the many accomplishments of Dr. Michael E. DeBakey. Nearly all the operations listed here have been touched by Dr. DeBakey during his earlier years. His contributions to surgery, and in particular, to vascular surgery, are so numerous that there is not enough space to cite all of them. To state it simply, Dr. DeBakey presided over the debut of vascular surgery and is a surgeon's surgeon.

PERSONAL BACKGROUND

Michael Ellis DeBakey was born in Lake Charles, Louisiana. Dr. DeBakey received his bachelor's degree and Doctor of Medicine degree from Tulane University in New Orleans. He completed his internship at Charity Hospital in New Orleans and his residency in surgery at Charity Hospital, at the University of Strasbourg, France, under Professor René Leriche, and also at the University of Heidelberg, Germany, under Professor Martin Kirschner.

Success in any field requires character, courage, and hard work. His character was first recognized by his mentor, Dr. Alton Ochsner. DeBakey, 12 years younger than Ochsner, was a sophomore at the Tulane Medical School when he first came to Ochsner's attention. Ochsner was immediately impressed with this shy student "who seemed to have a great deal of intelligence and who was a very hard worker." Ochsner also recalled, "DeBakey loved to write and loved to do research."[1] True to Dr. Ochsner's observation, the working habits of Dr. DeBakey are legendary. His days began as early as 5:30 A.M. By 7:00 A.M., he was in the hospital and by 7:30 A.M. in the operating room. His sleep patterns have been flexible, and he can go for days on as little as 4 hours of sleep per night, rarely needing more than 5 or 6. In fact, he believes that sleep deprived him of time to enjoy himself in surgery.

From Tulane to Baylor College of Medicine in a span of more than 60 years, Dr. DeBakey has contributed to every facet of the medical profession. The following is a synopsis of his professional background; contributions to medical science and vascular surgery; and honors, awards, and many accomplishments.

PROFESSIONAL BACKGROUND

1937 Faculty of Tulane University

1942 Director of the surgical consultant's division in the Surgeon General's Office
Colonel, Army of the United States (Reserve)

1945	Legion of Merit Award
	Development of mobile army surgical hospitals (MASHs)
	Committee on Veterans Medical Problems of the National Research Council
	Medical Research Program, Veterans Administration
1948	Chairman, Department of Surgery, Baylor College of Medicine, Houston, Texas
1969	President, Baylor College of Medicine
1979	Chancellor, Baylor College of Medicine

SCIENTIFIC ACCOMPLISHMENTS

There have been many "firsts" accomplished by Dr. DeBakey. The following is the chronology of the first attempts initiated by this remarkable surgeon:

1930s–1940s	Roller pump-heart-lung machine
1950	Segmental nature of vascular disease
1953	Dacron and Dacron-velour arterial grafts
	Graft replacement for thoracic aortic aneurysm
	Carotid endarterectomy
1954	Graft replacement—distal aortic arch and descending thoracic aorta, aneurysm of the ascending aorta
1955	Graft replacement—thoracoabdominal aorta
1958	Patch-graft angioplasty
1963	Standards for surgical treatment for arterial occlusive disease
	Aortocoronary artery bypass
1966	Artificial heart
1968	Heart transplantation
	Cardiovascular research and training center
1975	First National Heart and Blood Vessel Research and Demonstration Center, National Institutes of Health
1983	Cytomegalovirus and atherosclerosis
1987	Analysis of risk factors in atherosclerosis in 1,400 patients

MEDICAL WRITINGS

As Dr. Ochsner rightly observed, Dr. DeBakey loves to write. Indeed, he is a prolific writer with a publication record of 1,400 scientific articles. In addition to scientific articles, he also has authored and/or edited 26 books, some of which are listed in the following:

The Blood Bank and Technique and Therapeutics of Transfusions
Battle Casualties: Incidence, Mortality and Logistic Considerations
Vascular Surgery in World War II
Christopher's Minor Surgery
Cold Injury
Buerger's Disease: A Follow-Up Study of World War II Army Cases
A Report to the President: A National Program to Conquer Heart Disease, Cancer and Stroke

Advances in Cardiac Valves
Factors Influencing the Course of Myocardial Ischemia
A Surgeon's Diary of a Visit to China
The Living Heart
The Living Heart Diet
The Living Heart Brand Name Shopper's Guide
The Living Heart Guide to Eating Out

He also has served as Editor for the following journals:

Founding Editor, *Journal of Vascular Surgery*
Year Book of General Surgery, 14 years
Annals of Surgery
Surgery
Journal of Cardiovascular Surgery
Postgraduate Medicine
Contemporary Surgery
Comprehensive Therapy
Evaluation and the Health Professions
Family Circle
The DeBakey Health Letter

HONORS, AWARDS, AND ACCOMPLISHMENTS

Dr. DeBakey has received more than 40 honorary degrees from prestigious colleges and universities, as well as innumerable awards from educational institutions, professional and civic organizations, and governments throughout the world. In 1969, President Lyndon B. Johnson bestowed on him the highest honor a U.S. citizen can receive: the Presidential Medal of Freedom with Distinction. In 1987, President Ronald Reagan awarded him the National Medal of Science. Other major awards are selectively listed as follows:

1945	Legion of Merit, U.S. Army
1954 and 1970	American Medical Association Hektoen Gold Medal
1954	Rudolph Matas Award in Vascular Surgery
1958 and 1959	International Society of Surgery Distinguished Service Award and Leriche Award
1963	Albert Lasker Award for Clinical Research
1968	American Heart Association Gold Heart Award
1981	American Surgical Association Distinguished Service Award

Dr. DeBakey is a member of numerous distinguished medical societies. He has been named an honorary member of many foreign medical societies, including the Royal Societies of England, Ireland, and Scotland.

In the United States, he served on the Task Force on Medical Services of the Hoover Commission on Organization of the Executive Branch of the Government in 1949. In 1964, he served on President Lyndon B. Johnson's Commission on Heart Disease, Cancer and Stroke, as well as serving three terms on the Advisory Council of the National Heart, Lung, and Blood Institute of the National Institutes of Health.

CONTRIBUTIONS IN VASCULAR SURGERY

Dr. DeBakey was a founding member of the Society for Vascular Surgery in 1946. He served as President of the Society for Vascular Surgery in 1954 and as President of the International Society for Cardiovascular Surgery in 1964. In 1984, he founded the *Journal of Vascular Surgery* and served as the founding editor. Together with Dr. Emerick Szilagyi and Dr. Jesse Thompson, he guided the journal to emerge as a leading journal in surgery. Although he is well known for his contributions to arterial surgery, he also is interested in many other aspects of vascular disease. His first article, which appeared in 1933, was on the subject of blood transfusion. In 1935, he and Dr. Alton Ochsner discussed scalenus anticus syndrome (*Am J Surgery*. 1935;28:669–693). He showed an interest in small artery disease and published an article on scleroderma with Professor Rene Leriche (*Surgery*. 1937;1:6–24). An article he co-authored with Dr. Ochsner, "The rational consideration of peripheral vascular disease: Based on physiologic principles," represents his early entry into the field of arterial surgery (*JAMA*. 1939;112:230–236). In the ensuing years, he became interested in venous problems and has published extensively on thrombophlebitis (*Proc Soc Exp Biol Med*. 1939;41:585–590), venous pressure on venous pulsation (*Proc Soc Exp Biol Med*. 1939;42:858–861), treatment of venous thrombosis (*Arch Surg*. 1940;40:208–231; *N Engl J Med*. 1941;225:207–227), primary thrombosis of the axillary vein (*New Orleans M & S J*. 1942;95:62–70), anticoagulant therapy (*Surgery*. 1943;13:456–459), postphlebitic sequelae (*JAMA*. 1949;139:423–429), venous gangrene (*Surgery*. 1949;26:16–29), and venous thromboembolism (*Ann Surg*. 1950;132:158–160). World War II brought experience in treating arterial injury, and he has published key articles on this subject (*Ann Surg*. 1946;123:534–579; *N Engl J Med*. 1947;236:341–350). In the late 1940s and early 1950s, Dr. DeBakey expressed interest in hemodynamic phenomena in arterial disease (*Ann Surg*. 1947;126:850–865) and also in sympathectomy (*JAMA*. 1950;144:1227–1231).

As direct surgery in arteries was being introduced in the 1950s and 1960s, Dr. DeBakey became the leader in shaping the practice of vascular surgery. Many of his journal contributions in this period are landmark articles. These include surgical considerations of intrathoracic aneurysms of the aorta and great vessels (*Ann Surg*. 1952;135:660–680); graft replacement of aneurysms of the thoracic aorta (*JAMA*. 1953;152:673–676); the use of homograft for abdominal aortic aneurysms (*Surg Gynecol Obstet*. 1953;97:257–266); treatment of aortic occlusive disease (*Postgrad Med*. 1954;15:120–127); peripheral aneurysms (*Arch Surg*. 1959;78:226–238); arterial bypass below the knee (*Surg Gynecol Obstet*. 1959;108:321–332); innominate, subclavian, and vertebral arteries (*Ann Surg*. 1959;149:690–710); and distal aortic arch replacement (*JAMA*. 1954;155:1398–1403). He transformed Baylor College of Medicine into a premier center for vascular surgery. Dr. DeBakey performed the first carotid endarterectomy, a technique that is now a standard surgical procedure to prevent stroke (*JAMA*. 1975;233:1083–1085) and also the first patch angioplasty in segmental occlusion of an artery (*J Cardiovasc Surg*. 1962;3:106–141). He perfected and popularized the use of Dacron graft as a bypass procedure (*Ann Surg*. 1955;142:836–843; *Arch Surg*. 1958;77:713–724; *Surgery*. 1969;65:70–77). Perhaps the greatest contribution is his observation that atherosclerotic lesion is often segmental in nature (*Chicago Med Soc Bull*. 1960;63:487–490; *Ann Surg*. 1985;201:115–131). This concept paves the way for vascular surgeons to perform arterial bypass surgery. In his early years, Dr. DeBakey was an active participant in the Surgical Forum on various vascular problems. In the 1970s and 1980s, Dr. DeBakey and the Baylor group of surgeons (Drs. Cooley, Crawford,

Morris, and Beall) continued to expand the boundaries of arterial surgery to mesenteric, renal, and other vascular beds and also to treat vascular injuries. Even with his busy surgical practice, he maintains an interest in the role of cholesterol in vascular disease and has co-authored with Dr. Antonio Grotto several classic articles on this subject. In recent years, he reported on the role of cytomegalovirus in atherosclerosis (*Lancet.* 1987;2:291–293). As a true leader in surgery, he also spoke out on important issues such as the use of animals in research, high technology, and, most recently, on health care reform and academic centers, and telemedicine.

Dr. DeBakey is a legend of his time and truly a surgeon for all seasons. In the subsequent writings, four former trainees provide personal insights on Dr. DeBakey as an investigator (Dr. F. William Blaisdell), as a surgeon (Dr. Victor M. Bernhard), as an educator (Dr. Kenneth L. Mattox), and as a leader (Dr. John L. Ochsner).

James S.T. Yao
William H. Pearce

REFERENCE

1. Wilds, J, Harkey, I. *Alton Ochsner: Surgeon of the South.* Baton Rouge: Louisiana State University Press; 1990.

The Investigator

The publication list of Michael E. DeBakey, MD, consists of nearly 1,400 articles, which requires 150 pages to list. Therefore, it seems both practical and of interest to concentrate on his academic career prior to his massive breakthrough in cardiovascular surgery. Also, Dr. DeBakey's later cardiovascular contributions, from 1960 to the present, are well known, as he established the specialties of vascular and cardiac surgery on solid foundations.

His early career was extremely active from an investigational point of view, and many of his contributions are less well known to the present-day surgical community. His initial publications at Tulane University were released during his residency, which was based at Charity Hospital.

In reviewing Dr. DeBakey's publications, it is apparent that his initial academic interest was in transfusion. His first publication in 1933 was on a new method of syringe transfusion.[1] Subsequent publications in 1934 were related to developing a means of rapid blood transfer from donor to recipient.[2] The end product of this investigation was the development of a "continuous-flow blood transfusion instrument" (Fig. D–1). Known as the roller pump, this instrument is almost identical to the pump that is used today except that it was operated by a hand crank. There also were a number of minor

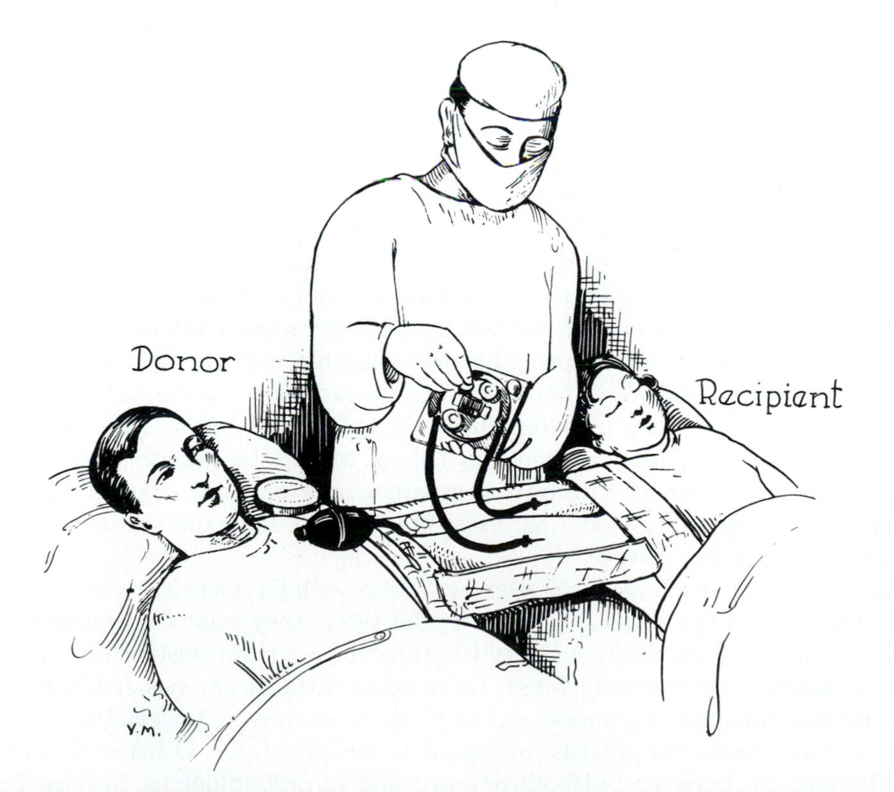

Figure D–1. Drawing illustrating DeBakey's method of continuous flow transfusion and showing how the instrument is held in the hand like a palette. *(From DeBakey ME. A simple continuous flow blood transfusion instrument. New Orleans Med Surg J. 1934;87:386–389.)*

subsequent modifications made to the pump, including the addition of special tubing to prevent slippage within the machine. This pump was used and credited by Gibbon in the first cardiopulmonary bypass machine and has remained the primary pump for all cardiac and vascular bypass operations.

To facilitate transfusion, Dr. DeBakey developed a new needle, and outlined techniques for the introduction of the needle into the vein and for the management of the transfusion tubing and pump so as to prevent clotting in the tubing (note: no anticoagulant was available in the 1930s). His work on transfusion culminated in the joint publication of a monograph with Robert Killduffe in 1942 entitled *The Blood Bank and Technique and Therapeutics of Transfusions.*

Dr. DeBakey's thesis, upon completing his residency in 1935, was on the protective effect of alkaline juice on peptic ulcers. His early years show a continuing interest in this subject, and he published additional articles in the 1930s and 1940s on the pathophysiology of peptic ulcers, perforated gastric ulcers, and duodenal ulcers.[3] In 1953, he demonstrated the advantages of immediate gastrectomy for the treatment of perforated ulcers. He continued to publish regularly on peptic ulcers, with publications appearing as late as 1959.[4]

In 1935, also while still in his residency, he initiated with his mentor, Dr. Alton Ochsner, a series of classic articles on various surgical subjects. The names Ochsner and DeBakey on a paper inevitably meant that this was the definitive article on that subject. Their initial articles in the 1930s were on hepatic and perihepatic infections. Their classic review of amebiasis in 1938 covered a collected series of 28,634 cases,[5] discussing the management of intestinal and extraintestinal amebiasis and of pleuroperitoneal complications. A definitive article on amebic liver abscesses emphasized the differentiation of amebic abscesses from hepatic abscesses and the importance of closed rather than open drainage. This led to other articles on pygenic liver abscesses and included a classic review of 3,608 cases of subphrenic abscesses.[6] In this latter review, Dr. Ochsner and Dr. DeBakey established the value of retroserous, rather than transperitoneal, drainage and emphasized the value of the posterior retroperitoneal approach. Multiple publications by these two authors on this subject appeared between 1935 and 1943, with additional major publications as late as 1949.

In the 1930s and 1940s, direct surgery of blood vessels was essentially nonexistent. Ligation was the only treatment for aneurysms. Vascular occlusive disease was treated by methods designed to increase collateral flow. Dr. DeBakey's initial interest in sympathectomy and vascular spasm came during his preceptorship with Dr. René Leriche in 1936. Upon returning from Europe in 1937, he joined the faculty at Tulane. Dr. DeBakey published nearly a dozen articles on sympathectomy for venous and arterial vascular disease from 1937, when he joined the faculty at Tulane, to 1952. He described technical approaches to upper and lower extremity sympathectomy and investigated its use in thrombophlebitis, angina, scleroderma, Buerger's disease, Raynaud's disease, and peripheral arterial occlusive disease.

Another major area of interest Dr. DeBakey shared with Dr. Ochsner was venous thrombosis. Throughout the 1940s and well into the 1950s, they published numerous articles differentiating silent thrombosis (phlebothrombosis) from obstructive or inflammatory thrombosis (thrombophlebitis). These classic articles emphasized prevention and treatment. Adequate hydration and early ambulation were believed to be the keys to preventing venous thrombosis. In regard to treatment, Dr. Ochsner and Dr. DeBakey differentiated between phlebothrombosis and thrombophlebitis. Specific investigations by Dr. DeBakey related specifically to the role of "spasm" in the pain, swelling, and compromised arterial flow associated with venous thrombosis. "Heat tents" and sympathectomy were the primary treatments utilized with resultant prompt improvement in symptoms.

In addition, Dr. Ochsner and Dr. DeBakey described phlegmasia cerulea dolens, venous occlusion associated with massive swelling and gangrene, and outlined the requirements for its management. Dr. DeBakey performed parallel laboratory investigations that demonstrated the relationship of elevated venous pressure to depressed arterial pulse volume. Both Dr. DeBakey and Dr. Ochsner also established criteria for intervention in septic iliofemoral thrombophlebitis. They investigated the role of sympathectomy in postphlebitic syndrome and found it to be beneficial in 50% of the cases in which it was used. Articles on the subject of venous thromboembolic disease totaled more than 35 between 1939 and 1959.

Just before World War II and especially immediately thereafter, thoracic surgery developed rapidly. Dr. DeBakey and Dr. Ochsner had a major interest in pulmonary and esophageal surgery. The first of their classic articles on lung resection for carcinoma was published in 1939. They reported 79 collected cases and 7 personal cases.[7] In this study, they connected the increasing incidence of lung cancer to smoking: "In our opinion, the increase in smoking with the universal custom of inhaling is probably a responsible factor, as the inhaled smoke, constantly repeated over a long period of time, undoubtedly is a source of chronic irritation to the bronchial mucosa."

Beginning in 1948, their articles on thoracic surgery also involved esophageal disease, particularly esophageal carcinoma. In 1949, Dr. DeBakey and Dr. Ochsner reported outstanding results in the surgical treatment of bronchiectasis.[8] In this study, they analyzed 96 cases and described the indications for surgery, and they also reported on 92 consecutive operations without mortality.[9] As a result, New Orleans became a major center for lung surgery. Between 1945 and 1949, Dr. DeBakey authored 20 publications on thoracic surgery.

With the beginning of World War II, Dr. DeBakey joined the Surgeon General's Office. He had just published in *Surgery, Gynecology, and Obstetrics* in 1942, a definitive work on the management of chest wounds, which pointed out how military wounds differ from civilian wounds.[10] In addition, his extensive monograph with Killdufte on blood transfusion was published during that same year. Starting in 1942 and continuing through 1956, he contributed actively to the military, publishing *Vascular Surgery in World War II*, a treatise that provided the background for the definitive treatment of vascular injuries in Korea. In fact, he published a review article in 1949 immediately before the Korean War began, describing the advantages of vascular repair and outlining the technique and indications for arterial substitutes.[11] In particular, he stressed the importance of prompt repair, emphasizing repair within 6 to 8 hours of injury as the optimal time for best results. Assisted by co-author Gilbert Beebe, Dr. DeBakey wrote a definitive book entitled *Battle Casualties: Incidence, Mortality and Logistic Considerations.* Other publications that resulted from World War II included articles on shock, transfusion, antibiotics, and plasma substitutes.

It was after his move to Baylor College of Medicine that Dr. DeBakey's interest in arterial disease blossomed. Until 1950, he averaged one publication per year on arterial disease. Starting in 1951, his publications on abdominal and thoracic vascular disease rapidly escalated with the development of operations to treat abdominal, and then thoracic, aneurysmal disease.

The development of cardiovascular surgery subsequently needs no further comment except that the challenge in this era was to develop an adequate vascular graft. Many of Dr. DeBakey's publications between 1954 and 1958 were written on arterial substitutes. He reported on the preparation of, the structural changes in, and the fate of arterial homografts in three publications in 1954. Additional publications in 1955 related to problems of healing and graft degeneration. In 1957, Dr. DeBakey reported on his experience with plastic prostheses, including nylon, ivalon, orlon, and Dacron. He prepared a number of these grafts, including the initial Dacron graft, on his wife's sewing machine. By 1958, it was apparent that Dacron was the material of choice, and he was able to convince the Philadelphia College of Textiles and Science to manufacture the graft on their special knitting machine. Now for the first time, there was a satisfactory arterial substitute. This, more than any other factor, made modern reconstructive vascular surgery possible.

As the reader analyzes the remainder of his career, it is apparent that Dr. DeBakey has never lost interest in the artificial heart.[12] Starting in 1957, he had a major interest in developing an implantable heart. In recent years, he has developed an outstanding research team directed toward solving the problem that has occupied so much of his career. He is now collaborating with the National Aeronautics and Space Administration on the development of an axial flow ventricular assist device that can pump 5.1 L/min against a pressure of 100 mm Hg and requires less than 10 W of power.[13] This device is now being tested in large animals. Hopefully, the realization of this dream is not far away.

In summary, it is interesting to review the cycles of Dr. DeBakey's early academic interests (Fig. D–2). His research career began with an interest in transfusion and devices for its successful accomplishment. This was followed by an interest in hepatic

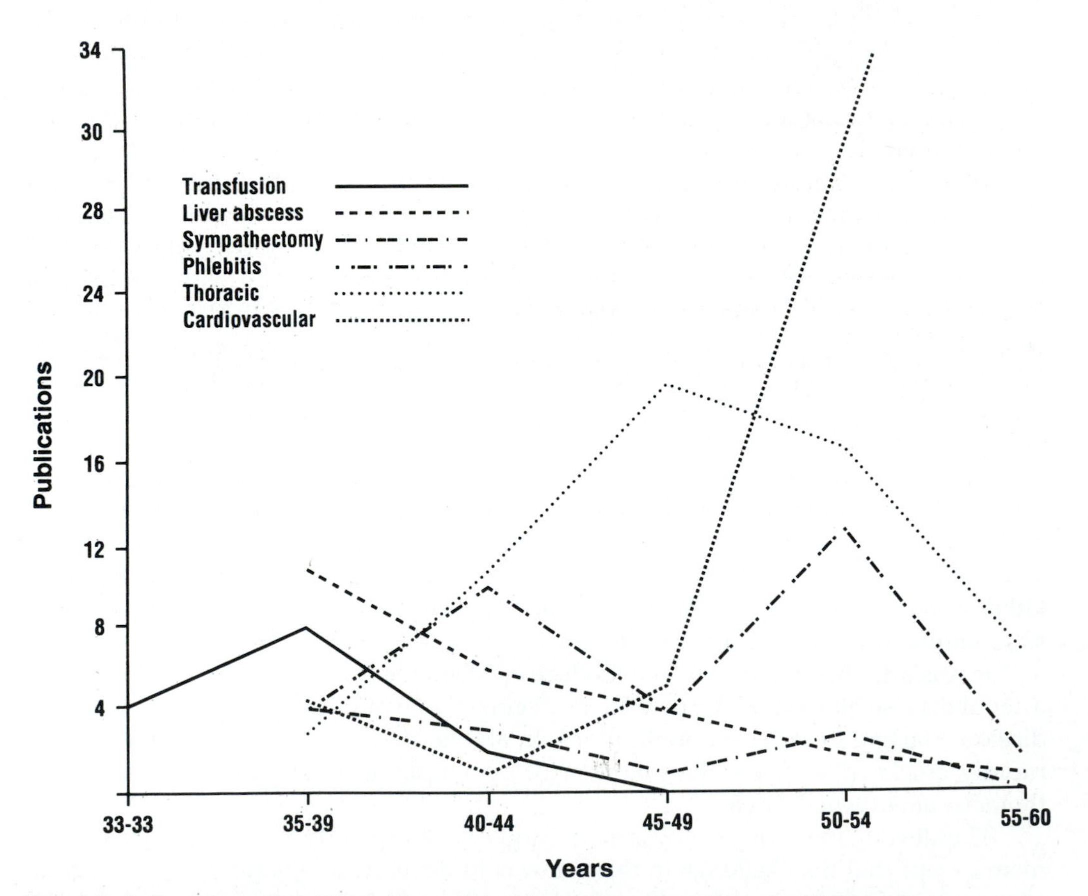

Figure D–2. Graphic representation of the cycles of the early academic interests of Michael E. DeBakey, MD.

and perihepatic abscesses. In parallel came the application of sympathectomy to treat vasospastic disorders and the treatment of venous thrombosis and its sequelae. Thoracic surgery, in particular lung carcinoma, occupied Dr. DeBakey's major attention in the late 1940s and early 1950s. With his move to Houston, cardiovascular surgery became supreme, starting with the treatment of aneurysms and culminating with the development of the Dacron graft, which placed reconstructive vascular surgery on a firm base. The artificial heart, his first love, has emerged as the final problem Dr. DeBakey has yet to solve.

F. William Blaisdell

REFERENCES

1. Gillentine WH, DeBakey ME. New method of syringe transfusion. *New Orleans Med Surg J.* 1933;86:100–102.
2. DeBakey ME. A simple continuous-flow blood transfusion instrument. *New Orleans Med Surg J.* 1934;87:386–389.
3. DeBakey ME. The physiology of peptic ulcer. *Surgery.* 1937;2:653–674.
4. DeBakey ME. Acute perforated gastric duodenal ulceration. *Surgery.* 1940;8:852–884.
5. Ochsner A, DeBakey ME. Diagnosis and treatment of amebic abscess of the liver (Study based on 4,484 collected and personal cases). *Am J Digest Dis Nutr.* 1935;2:47–51.
6. Ochsner A, DeBakey ME. Subphrenic abscess: collective review and an analysis of 3,608 collected and personal cases. *Int Abstr Surg.* 1938;66:426–438.
7. Ochsner A, DeBakey M. Primary pulmonary malignancy: treatment by total pneumonectomy: analysis of 79 collected cases and presentation of 7 personal cases. *Surg Gynecol Obstet.* 1939;68:435–451.
8. DeBakey ME, Ochsner A. Subtotal esophagectomy and esophagogastrostomy for high intrathoracic esophageal lesions. *Surgery.* 1948;23:935–951.
9. Ochsner A, DeBakey ME, Decamp PT. Bronchiectasis: its curative treatment by pulmonary resection: an analysis of ninety-six cases. *Surgery.* 1949;25:518–532.
10. DeBakey ME. The management of chest wounds: collective review. *Surg Gynecol Obstet.* 1942;74:203–237.
11. DeBakey ME, Amspacher WH. Acute arterial injuries. *Surg Clin North Am.* 1949;29:1513–1522.
12. Takatani S, Shiono M, Sasaki T, Orime Y, Sakuma I, Noon G, Nos Y, DeBakey ME. Left and right pump output control in one-piece electromechanical total artificial heart. *Artif Organs.* 1993;17:176–184.
13. Damm G, Mizuguchi K, Bozeman R, Akkerman J, Aber G, Svejkovsky P, Takatani S, Nos Y, Noon GP, DeBakey ME. In vitro performance of the Baylor/NASA axial flow pump. *Artif Organs.* 1993;17:609–613.

The Surgeon

A dictionary definition of surgery simply states that it is the "medical diagnosis and treatment of injury, deformity, and disease by manual and instrumental operations" and a surgeon is one who specializes in "surgery." This vague description offers little insight into the underlying characteristics required of the individual who accepts the role of surgeon and only minimally suggests the complexities of the daily activities and the life-long devotion required. These are left to the imagination and experience of the beholder. Drawing on 45 years in this arena, 1 year of which was spent as Dr. DeBakey's fellow and 30 years as a maturing pupil, I attempt to flesh out these sterile definitions as they apply to a most significant mentor in my career.

I met Dr. DeBakey for the first time in May 1964, when he came to Milwaukee as the Eberbach Visiting Professor at Marquette School of Medicine. The department chairman, Dr. Ed Ellison, offered me the privilege of being our guest's companion and chauffeur. It had already been arranged that I would go to Houston for a fellowship in vascular surgery the following January, and this would provide me with the opportunity to become acquainted with my new chief. I was expected to meet him for breakfast at 7 A.M. When I arrived 10 minutes early, he was standing in the lobby of the University Club, finishing the morning paper and anxious to be off to the Milwaukee County Hospital to begin his professorial duties in the operating room. He was scheduled to perform an aneurysm resection and a carotid endarterectomy with our residents on patients he had examined during rounds the prior evening. The abdominal incision was made at 8 A.M. and the last closing skin suture in the neck was placed at 10:15 A.M. I called Dr. Ellison to inform him that the myth of Dr. DeBakey's surgical proficiency was indeed a reality in spite of the impediments imposed by an unfamiliar environment and assistants who were minimally acquainted with vascular surgery. The remainder of the day was filled with a visit with our chairman, a rocking chair conference with the house staff and students, teaching rounds, and a lecture that evening. The list of events for the next day was similar and included both a femoropopliteal and a carotid–subclavian bypass, which were accomplished with a similar degree of skill and alacrity. I was ecstatic with the prospect that I was about to spend the next year of my career in one of the world's most exciting surgical clinics, participating in a daily regimen of activities similar to that which I had just observed.

In the ensuing years, I have often reflected on these and many other personal experiences with Dr. DeBakey in order to better define a concept of the "complete surgeon." It is axiomatic that a profound understanding of disease processes and the underlying basic sciences is fundamental to the craft of the surgeon. In the early days of vascular and cardiac surgery, this essential body of knowledge, although apparently voluminous, often failed to cast light on newly recognized problems. The available data were frequently inadequate, sometimes incorrect, and usually in need of repackaging. The surgical arena provides an intense stimulus for refining our understanding of these fundamental concepts. When there are no other options, new problems presenting in the operating theater require immediate and bold address to resolve life- and limb-threatening dilemmas. Dr. DeBakey's surgical skills were most evident in these difficult circumstances. The insights derived from his responses as a surgical innovator who met these challenges is faithfully documented in his ever-expanding list of publications. This record of the details of his massive experience has significantly advanced our knowledge of the basic sciences of a territory in which he is a pioneer.

Surgery is an art intimately related to the anxieties, fears, and misapprehensions of our patients. It requires both human understanding and a willingness to become personally involved with those individuals who require our skills. Those of us who worked with Dr. DeBakey remember well his insistence on visiting his patients at least twice daily to recognize and relieve their concerns as he became acquainted with their illnesses. His rounds often occurred at inconvenient hours to meet the exigencies of an extensive and complex surgical and administrative schedule, but were delegated to others only when the requirements of academic travel interfered with this important routine.

The craft of the surgeon requires exquisite manual dexterity in order to accomplish subtle tissue manipulations and reliable reconstructions in an expeditious manner. Those of us who have had the opportunity to scrub with Dr. DeBakey were delighted and encouraged by the skillful, direct, and effective approach that marked him as a master technician. At times, an assistant would become so entranced by his elegant management of a complex problem that he or she would stand transfixed, his or her supporting role momentarily forgotten. This might prompt Dr. DeBakey's professorial admonition against becoming "mesmerized" or his reminder that effective function at the operating table required that "your fingers needed to be connected to your brain."

The hallmark of a great surgical leader is his or her ability to identify and surround him- or herself with talented associates. They are essential for the support and advancement of his or her vision of a constantly progressing and creative environment in which patient services must be of the highest quality. To sustain this group of talented individuals and ensure their productivity over an extended period requires that the chief strongly encourage his or her associates to rise to the full height of their capacities and requires a perception on their part that the leader is delighted with their mounting success. There is a long list of productive surgeons who derived an important share of their surgical development from Dr. DeBakey and who have become recognized for their skills and contributions, both in Houston and in celebrated venues throughout the world. This is strong testimony that he has fulfilled this most important obligation as a surgical mentor.

Starting before World War II, where he made significant contributions, and continuing to the present, Dr. DeBakey remains a role model for those who aspire to a career in surgery. He has been an innovator, investigator, teacher, mentor, humanitarian, skilled operator, leader, and councilor, a list of accomplishments that marks him as one of the world's "grandes chirurgiens."

Victor M. Bernhard

The Educator

In the lobby of The Methodist Hospital in Houston's Texas Medical Center stands a bronze statue of Dr. Michael E. DeBakey, presented by King Leopold and Princess Lilian of Belgium in 1978. On its base, the inscription reads: "Michael E. DeBakey, M.D., Surgeon, Educator, Medical Statesman. In recognition of one who served so many." Although Dr. DeBakey is a legend, an international treasure, an innovator, a master surgeon, a writer, and a diplomat, this chapter focuses on his role as an educator—a "master teacher."

THE EARLY STUDENT

The son of a pharmacist in Lake Charles, Louisiana, Michael DeBakey was scholarly in grade school and high school and began teaching at an early age. As a junior high school student, during a summer vacation to Lebanon, Dr. DeBakey taught his hometown about the Middle East by sending daily letters about the family's travels to the editor of the local newspaper to be published.

In high school, he was acknowledged as a superior saxophone player, and upon entering Tulane University in New Orleans, he wanted to play in the school orchestra. When told on a Friday that a clarinet player, not a saxophone player, was needed, he replied that he would return on Tuesday to vie for the available position. Having never before played the clarinet, he borrowed one over the weekend and by Tuesday was proficient enough to gain a seat in the marching band. It seems Dr. DeBakey could teach himself as well as others, even before he began college. Years later, I overheard Dr. DeBakey and trumpeter Al Hirt discussing the wind and reed instruments played by both of them in New Orleans.

Arising early to read and study in the library, Michael DeBakey would walk to school or to the streetcar stop by 4:00 A.M. Rudolph Matas, New Orleans surgeon and professor at Tulane, also rose very early and noticed the student walking with his books. Eventually the young medical student was provided regular rides to the Tulane campus by Dr. Matas. Dr. Matas and Dr. DeBakey became life-long friends, and Dr. Matas eventually loaned the young student many of the books and obscure journals that were stored on virtually every wall of his home. Dr. DeBakey's insatiable appetite for reading and beginning his day at an early hour became life-long habits. Undoubtedly, these habits contributed significantly to his knowledge base, as well as his ability to impart this knowledge to others.

Dr. Alton Ochsner learned of the eager young medical student from Dr. Matas. By Dr. DeBakey's second year in medical school, he and Dr. Ochsner were working on research together, and Dr. Ochsner was convinced this able student would become a surgeon. Indeed, Dr. DeBakey's formal training as a surgeon was strongly supported by Dr. Ochsner. In fact, after Dr. DeBakey became Chair of Surgery at Baylor College of Medicine, Houston, he taught two of Dr. Ochsner's sons the art and science of surgery.

Near the end of Dr. DeBakey's formal surgical training at Tulane, Dr. Ochsner sent him to many of the major surgical centers and research laboratories of Europe. Dr. DeBakey worked with Dr. René Leriche for several months and was a visiting surgical professor at many major medical centers in Europe.

WORLD WAR II YEARS

Stimulated by research in vascular surgery in Europe and recognizing the fortuitous simultaneous availability of new vascular imaging (angiography), synthetic material, and advancing suture technology, Dr. DeBakey returned to teach these concepts to the faculty at Tulane. His teaching activities at Tulane were temporarily interrupted while he served as the Surgical Consultant to the U.S. Army Surgeon General during World War II. He taught the army medical corps via the "Surgeon General's Memorandum," addressing mandatory colostomy for colon wounds, a dictum that is still a part of military medical doctrine. It was also during this assignment that Dr. DeBakey began to edit surgical volumes of the U.S. Army's World War II medical experiences. This many-volume compendium remains the most complete documentation of wartime military medicine in existence. Also, Dr. DeBakey and Dr. Fiorindo Simione reported the results of the vascular wounds from the war. They pointed out that more than 90% of the wartime vascular wounds at that time were in the extremities, and options other than ligation and amputation were limited.

BAYLOR COLLEGE OF MEDICINE

Dr. DeBakey returned to Tulane following his military assignments and was selected to be the chairman of the newly formed Department of Surgery at the Baylor University College of Medicine in Houston, Texas, in 1948. As there were no Baylor-affiliated hospitals, he was made "chief of the teaching surgical service" at Hermann Hospital, but had no beds or patients of his own. He met with Mr. Ben Taub, the Chairman of the City/County Hospital Board that oversaw the Jefferson Davis Hospital, and requested that this hospital serve as Baylor's "teaching hospital." It became not only Baylor University College of Medicine's first affiliated hospital in Houston, but it also became the site for many surgical "firsts" introduced by Dr. DeBakey, giving him yet another arena in which to develop his role as a teacher. He made rounds on every patient in the hospital each Sunday morning, and he moderated the surgical mortality and morbidity conference each week. In 1949, he established the nation's first trauma research center, using a grant from the U.S. Army. It was at the Jefferson Davis Hospital in 1957 that he performed the first abdominal aortic aneurysm replacement in the United States and the first heart valve replacement in Houston. Both of these "firsts" were observed by numerous trainees, and in subsequent years as the number of affiliated hospitals grew, so did the number of aspiring surgeons who were taught by Dr. DeBakey and his faculty. In 1979, these trainees formed the core of the Michael E. DeBakey International Surgical Society. This organization continues today with more than 600 members from around the world, all of whom readily acknowledge the significant role Dr. DeBakey played in their surgical education. At Baylor, he developed the teaching faculty who would work with him for the next 45 years and who would train even more surgeons.

CASUAL CONVERSATION WITH DR. GIBBON

While Dr. DeBakey was a medical student, it was the medical student's task to perform direct person-to-person blood transfusions. Both an inventor and an innovator, Dr. DeBakey had learned of a roller pump principle, as well as the problem of tube creep associated with this principle. He developed a crimped tubing and a roller pump (initially hand turned) to move the blood more effectively, and also introduced a calibrated counter to precisely determine the volume of blood being transfused. Newly developed plastics technology allowed for the introduction of a flanged tube, which prevented the tube creep. With the development of blood banking, this invention lay dormant for many years.

In 1953, as Dr. DeBakey sat beside Dr. John Gibbon at the American Surgical Association meeting, Dr. Gibbon talked about a new oxygenator that held promise for the treatment of pulmonary embolism and possibly open heart surgery, if the existing pump mechanisms could be modified to provide adequate and rapid perfusion support. Always the teacher, Dr. DeBakey explained his earlier invention and how it might be applicable to the new oxygenator. Dr. Gibbon added the roller pump to his oxygenator and introduced the prototype that is still the standard for cardiopulmonary bypass surgery.

MY FIRST LESSONS

I first encountered Dr. DeBakey (at a distance) in 1960 when I enrolled in Baylor College of Medicine as a freshman medical student. I absorbed his early lectures and watched his many movies on developing techniques in cardiac and vascular surgery. However, it was while on his service during a student rotation in 1963 that I personally experienced many of his special tactics in teaching. Although the thousands of "DeBakey stories" that are embellished with each retelling could (and undoubtedly will) fill a book, one special intraoperative "lesson" is particularly memorable to me. After repeatedly being admonished about my inability to follow suture, use the sucker, stay out of the light, and cut suture correctly, the biggest retractors I had ever seen were placed in my hands. It was immediately evident that I did not know how to hold retractors either, as Dr. DeBakey repositioned my right hand, palm up, to "hold the retractor as it was designed." Not one to be caught at a same mistake twice, I subtly duplicated the left-hand positioning to match the right. Although my hand movement might have been subtle, its effect was not. The maneuver resulted in loss of aortic exposure, and my left hand was firmly repositioned to have the palm down, complete with a lecture about appropriate and intelligent retraction. Neither retractor slipped a millimeter during the remainder of the operation. Indelibly imprinted in my mind was the knowledge that even in retraction, every detail requires focused attention.

TEACHING ON ROUNDS

Two years later I was an intern, and one of my first rotations was on Dr. DeBakey's service. He made lightning, albeit quite thorough, rounds on all of his patients each day, led by the "floor" resident or intern. A well-worn "bed and guide book" was passed from resident to resident, so that even last-minute bed changes would not catch the resident by surprise. Dr. DeBakey would visit both pre- and postoperative patients, taking pulses, listening to hearts, mentioning referring physicians, and saying hello to families. The names, diagnoses, operations, laboratory data, and bed assignments *had* to match and *had* to be correct. On one memorable day, he taught me a special lesson in observation and perception. The senior resident and junior faculty working with Dr. DeBakey were in the operating room, and it was left to just the two of us to blitzkrieg through more than 150 in-house patients. He said his hellos, took my word for the pulse status, and told me who to pre-op for the following day. He must have been in a hurry to make an airplane, because he touched only the last patient. As we approached the patient, I felt that I had "made it" for that day, when Dr. DeBakey, for the first time, pulled back the sheets to discover a cyanotic arm beneath a still-in-place tourniquet, which had been placed by a phlebotomist during our rounds in other parts of the hospital. Seeing us coming the phlebotomist had retreated, leaving her equipment behind for Dr. DeBakey to have an opportunity to teach me about attention to detail, being precise, and preventing unnecessary patient pain. To this day, I do not know how he managed to single out this particular patient to examine, especially when the "evidence" was safely tucked underneath the sheets. Also, I still believe that observation and attention to detail are among the most valuable principles and guiding philosophies ever taught to me. That I learned them from Dr. DeBakey meant that they would be a part of my character forever. He lives what he teaches. No detail of a patient's condition or care ever escapes him, and as his student, resident, or colleague, no less is expected and demanded from you.

TEACHING IN THE OPERATING ROOM

The operating room has always been Dr. DeBakey's prime lecture hall. He continuously teaches by example, by direct instruction, by discussing historical development, by development of innovative instrumentation, and by always demonstrating a "passion for excellence." He worked longer hours than any of his associates. His times were the fastest. He seemed to know what everyone in the operating room was doing, even though the anesthesiologists were behind the ether screen and the perfusionist was behind him. He arranged the operative team and the various instruments, tables, monitors, and people as a coach would prepare for a championship game or a conductor would prepare for a command symphony performance. He continually designed and redesigned instruments, operative tables, and monitors.

Foremost, his lessons are legend. Space does not permit recounting the countless lessons learned in this forum. The classic surgical principles related to the choice of incision, exposure, and appropriate instruments; the techniques of assisting, retracting, holding the suture ("without any looping or bombing"), and positioning the suction tip; and detailed knowledge of anatomy were continually taught, sometimes in a manner that, at the time, evoked some discomfort for the student, but always in such a manner that invaluable knowledge would be gained and retained.

TEACHING DURING OFFICE CHART REVIEW

Daily, in the inner sanctum of his office, the associates, residents, students, and consultants would gather around a huge bank of x-ray view boxes and the preoperative list would be reviewed in detail. The office charts would methodically be stacked and ready for completion (with Dr. DeBakey's own red and black pencils), as the consultants, laboratory results, and angiograms were integrated simultaneously. It was like clockwork: No motion was lost and no extra words were allowed to deter from this production. The art of teaching, organization, precision, and patient care, and the integration of all aspects of a disease or condition, were fine tuned to an art in this forum. Textbook chapters were conceived from the thousands of arteriograms and office charts. New research projects were envisioned. Five decades and three generations of surgeons have learned practice precision from these office chart reviews. These lessons were entirely different from those learned on rounds and in the operating room. None should or could be missed.

TEACHING IN THE LECTURE ROOM

I have heard Dr. DeBakey present formal and informal lectures in the lecture hall. His slide productions of drawings beside radiographs are internationally recognized as being his own signature. Whether serving as a visiting professor to surgical residents, lecturing to a group of medical students at the Uniformed Services University for the Health Sciences (where he was one of the original board members), or standing before a huge room of medical professionals at a national/international meeting, he has always commanded the respect and awe of those who seek the pearls of his wisdom and experience. His lectures and published papers contain the most researched and detailed references of any I have ever read. Reviewing some of his classic lectures and articles from the 1930s and 1940s, not only hundreds, but thousands of appropriate and correctly positioned citations are found in the bibliographies. Such detail, integration, and understanding of international medical knowledge was always presented with unwavering confidence, but, at the same time, with unassuming humility. What a lesson!

TEACHING IN THE SURGICAL FACULTY MEETING

Closed surgical faculty meetings are times to review the finances, student programs, research, resident performance and promotion, new programs, and other administrative duties. Dr. DeBakey, as chairman of the department, ran these meetings, the attendance of which included such recognized leaders in the field of surgery as E. Stanley Crawford, George L. Jordan, Jr., George Morris, Arthur Beall, George Noon, Jimmy Howell, Paul Jordan, and many others. Dr. DeBakey conducted these faculty meetings with the combined insight, sensitivity, and skill of an army general, a King Solomon, a Wall Street broker, a Germanic professor, a visionary politician, and an ecclesiastical clergyman.

One memorable event demonstrates Dr. DeBakey's special ability to teach, even in this environment. In the late 1970s, a shift from the presentation of predominantly clinical and procedural papers at the national vascular meetings to the introduction of basic science papers relating to vascular surgery occurred. Following one such meeting, when it seemed that "all" of the papers were nonclinical and nonprocedural, the clinical-oriented surgical faculty assembled for a departmental meeting and, before the formal agenda was introduced, began expressing skepticism and dismay at this change in focus, especially with regard to prostaglandins and prostacyclins. Dr. DeBakey let the conversation "heat up" for more than 10 minutes, allowing each member of the faculty to "vent." He then, in an almost imperceptible voice, said, "Gentlemen, I think all of you need to understand the ramifications of these molecular changes." All heads turned in surprise. Dr. DeBakey, the epitome of a clinical researcher, had never before indicated an interest in this area. He then, however, proceeded to cite the entire intermediary metabolism for arachidonic acid, progressing to each of the prostaglandins and their metabolites. At each point, he cited how these families of compounds had an impact on surgery, cardiac and vascular surgery in particular. He cited effects on the ductus arteriosus, the endothelium, clotting cascade, and cardiopulmonary dynamics. Just when I thought the field of prostaglandins was exhausted, Dr. DeBakey reminded us of the interactions of these metabolic pathways and the emerging field of "complement" understanding. He projected that cells communicate, react, and are affected by these "modifiers." (He did not use the word "mediators" as it had not been introduced into our medical vocabulary at that point.) Dr. DeBakey then returned to the prepared agenda as we silently contemplated our individual lack of knowledge application, as well as this great teacher's amazing ability to always stay far ahead of us and most of the surgical community in all areas; his ability to not only accept change but also to understand, adapt, and integrate new knowledge with existing tenets; and last, but most important to his faculty and trainees, his ability to take new knowledge and convey it in such a manner that it guided and inspired, rather than overwhelmed. This particular incident is but one of many where I have been awed by Dr. DeBakey's seemingly unbounded knowledge base. I have never been present at any professional or social gathering when a topic arose that he could not only comment on, but also offer additional insightful information.

TEACHING IN THE COMMITTEE AND BOARD ROOM

In the committee or board room, Dr. DeBakey teaches the principles of organization, management, fund raising, and group dynamics. His leadership in this forum and his insightful questions leave no doubt that he is aware of innumerable ramifications to the many sides of the corporate discussions. He listens attentively, seeming to immediately absorb new information and integrate it with past history and current corporate cultural needs. His silence subtly implies consent. His advice and probing, directed questions suggest areas of concern and needed resolution. An early pointed comment becomes either a "show stopper" or reorganizes the agenda. A comment late in the discussion of an agenda item consolidates the discussion and summarizes the salient points of the issue. Dr. DeBakey is as masterful a teacher and technician in the committee room as he is in the operating room and research laboratory. Unfortunately, many of his students do not have the opportunity to observe and learn from his surgical precision and thought processes in this setting.

TEACHING AT NATIONAL MEETINGS

Dr. DeBakey attends many national and international meetings. His "pew" is usually in the center or left section. He sits near the front, often surrounded by other national teachers of repute. He listens attentively to each paper, discussing only those that need his input, although the presenters always are aware of his presence and wonder if his special probing questions will be asked. Actually, his discussions have always been gracefully submitted, usually to the surprise of younger academicians who want desperately to have their work acknowledged by Dr. DeBakey but are almost paralyzed with fear at the thought of such recognition actually occurring. When Dr. DeBakey is the presenter of a paper, the details amaze the listener. When he is the discussant, he amplifies the research of the scientist, rather than citing his own case work. Again, in this arena his teaching style assumes yet another face.

SPECIAL LESSONS

Dr. DeBakey selected associates who, in turn, taught his philosophies and visions while developing their own styles and images. Dr. DeBakey is a master at selecting motivated people and then giving them enough time, authority, and resources to accomplish their programs, all the while maintaining parental, supervisory, "arms-length" control. During the majority of my medical education and development, Dr. DeBakey was my chairman—the conscience that gave the surgical program at Baylor College of Medicine its breadth and direction. He was and continues to be my master teacher, and I know that thousands of surgeons around the world believe just as I do. All of us, when confronted with a surgical dilemma or complex problem, begin our approach by asking, "What would Dr. DeBakey do?"

Kenneth L. Mattox

The Leader

Man and woman can lead others in many fashions and to various degrees. The route and distance depend on the talent of the leader. I truthfully believe that Dr. DeBakey has led more individuals along different paths to reach a rightful goal than any other person. He has demonstrated an extraordinary ability to lead as an academician, a scientist, and as a medical spokesman and statesman.

As an academician, his rise through the ranks of academia will probably never be equalled. He has led the Baylor College of Medicine from near obscurity to one of the preeminent medical institutions of the world. Dr. DeBakey was appointed professor of surgery at Baylor College of Medicine in 1948, and 48 years later he still holds this position. In 1948, he was also named chairman of the Department of Surgery, and his leadership is emphasized by progressive authority conferred upon him by this institution. In 1968, he was named the distinguished professor of surgery, and that same year he was made vice president. One year later, he was elected president, a position he held for 9 years. In 1978, he was named chancellor. His progressive rise in titles did not come about because of his mere presence, but because he demonstrated such strong leadership capabilities that he was able to fill multiple positions simultaneously. I am sure, had it been appropriate, that Baylor College of Medicine would have made him a czar, king, or emperor.

While performing his usual heraldic positions, Dr. DeBakey built within the university the National Heart and Blood Vessel Research Demonstration Center and the Cardiovascular Research and Training Center, which became the DeBakey Heart Center in 1985. He served as director of both and also formed the DeBakey Medical Foundation, of which he is president. Through Dr. DeBakey's leadership, Baylor College of Medicine has been among the top 10 institutions receiving grants from the National Institutes of Health.

The rest of the medical community thought so much of Dr. DeBakey that they made sure to tap his tremendous resources by selecting him as Clinical Professor of Surgery at the University of Texas Dental Branch, the Distinguished Professor of Surgery of Texas A&M University, Surgeon-in-Chief of the Ben Taub General Hospital, and consultant in surgery to the Methodist Hospital, the VA Hospital, the M.D. Anderson Cancer Center, the St. Luke Episcopal Hospital, the Texas Heart Hospital, the Texas Institute for Rehabilitation and Research, and the Brook General Hospital.

As a scientist, Dr. DeBakey's innovative ability was the principal mover in the development of cardiovascular surgery. As a young man working in the research laboratory under my father, Dr. Alton Ochsner, at Tulane University, he developed the roller pump in 1932, which eventually became the pumping system for open-heart surgery around the world. In that same period, he developed a push-pull method of blood delivery for continuous transfusion through a syringe, and later he developed many vascular instruments that allowed surgeons to handle and clamp blood vessels in a nontraumatic fashion. In 1952, he developed the first Dacron vascular prosthesis and actually made the initial graft at home, borrowing his wife's sewing machine. As a surgeon, he is best known for the development of surgical techniques and led the profession by being the first to perform many operations. These "firsts" are listed in chronologic order: 1953, graft replacement of the thoracic aorta and carotid endarterectomy; 1954, correction of dissecting aneurysm of the thoracic aorta; 1955, graft replacement of the thoracoabdominal aorta; 1956, graft replacement of the ascending aorta; 1957, graft replacement of the aortic arch; 1958, patch-graft angioplasty; 1964, coronary artery bypass graft; and 1966, left ventricular assist device. Never in history has one man pioneered so many different operations that have given the rest of us an opportunity to learn from his experience. I know his achievements were not without trial and tribulation, for as a resident under Dr. DeBakey's tutelage, I witnessed his strength in obtaining these advances during a most trying time when, the state of the art was so undeveloped that failures were inevitable. Coping with those failures required a great deal of fortitude. He was able to learn from the unfortunate experiences and persevere until success was achieved. Where lesser men would have folded, the challenge stimulated Dr. DeBakey to work even harder.

For 60 years, Dr. DeBakey has been an educator and teacher. He has taught thousands of students and his great love has been the training of general and thoracic residents, of which he has trained more than a thousand. However, in reality Dr. DeBakey has trained practically every vascular surgeon in the United States, possibly even in the world. I know this for a fact, for I had the opportunity to witness the thousands of doctors from all over the world who came to observe the exciting new development of vascular surgery in the 1950s and early 1960s. It was not uncommon to have 30 observers in the operating room, standing in tiered levels, behind the maestro as he performed these new and innovative procedures. Likewise, rounds on patients following surgery were like a tribe being led by a chieftain, and it was amusing to watch the visitors try to keep up with Dr. DeBakey as he ran up and down stairwells. Most of the time, by the end of the rounds, we had lost at least half of them because they could not match the stamina of Dr. DeBakey.

In those early days, surgeons around the world attempted to duplicate Dr. DeBakey's surgical achievements, but most to no avail. I vividly remember Dr. DeBakey's pleasure at being invited to the great Mayo Clinic to demonstrate how to perform an abdominal aortic aneurysmectomy. It was during this trip that he demonstrated to them the method of endoaneurysmorrhaphy to manage large aneurysms, allowing the Mayo Clinic to move forward in their normal progressive manner. There is no doubt that Dr. DeBakey ushered in and is known as the father of modern vascular surgery, making this a recognized specialty that has saved millions of lives, particularly through the surgical techniques he developed.

Dr. DeBakey has been a leader as a medical spokesman and statesman. Because of his wealth of knowledge and enviable reputation, Dr. DeBakey has been advisor to practically every president of the United States during the past 50 years. Both Democrats and Republicans respect him to the point of asking for advice to use in their platforms. He has also served as direct advisor to the president. President Lyndon B. Johnson appointed him chairman of the President's Commission on Heart Diseases, Cancer and Stroke. With this charge, Dr. DeBakey formulated plans for medical centers of excellence and recommended strategic geographic sites throughout the United States. He had an unprecedented 3-year term on the National Heart, Lung and Blood Advisory Council for the National Institutes of Health. As a member of the Task Force on Medical Services of the Hoover Commission on Organization of the Executive Branch of the Government, he was the prime mover in persuading Congress to establish the National Library of Medicine, which has become the largest and most prestigious depository of medical knowledge in the world. He served on the first Board of Regents of the National Library of Medicine.

I counted more than 150 advisory positions that Dr. DeBakey has been appointed to and the type of board varied from the Chinese-American Relations Society to the

U.S. Army. Not only has he been appointed to the advisory councils of many organizations, but he also has been a consultant around the world and has helped establish cardiovascular surgical programs in England, Germany, Spain, Belgium, Greece, Turkey, Italy, the CIC (former USSR), Yugoslavia, Egypt, Saudi Arabia, United Arab Emirates, Indonesia, Jordan, Morocco, Thailand, China, Japan, Australia, New Zealand, and countries throughout Central and South America.

The character and qualifications of a leader are reflected in those whom he develops and selects to be associated with him. As mentioned earlier, practically every cardiovascular surgeon in the 1950s and 1960s at one time or another toured to the mecca, Houston, to observe the greatness of Dr. DeBakey. Their pilgrimage witnessed both the large quantity and high quality of cardiovascular surgery as it was being developed. Likewise, the men and women who came to train with Dr. DeBakey were the same men and women who became the cornerstones in the development of vascular surgery as a specialty. In the group during my thoracic–cardiovascular training year, every man and woman eventually became chair of a department of surgery at a major medical institution. Dr. DeBakey's untiring efforts and his tremendous capacity for work were stimuli that drove these young doctors to achieve.

The staff that surrounded Dr. DeBakey rose to greatness, not only within his institution but also when they eventually left to take on new positions and challenges. Dr. DeBakey's tutelage instilled in his staff extreme devotion to work, the importance of scientific inquisitiveness, and a fearless attitude to strive to unfamiliar territories. The devotion of all who have trained and served under Dr. DeBakey as faculty members is emphasized by the fact that I have never heard any of these men or women, no matter how many years later, refer to him by his first name but always as Dr. DeBakey, or more commonly as "The Boss."

There are but a few physicians who are household words, recognized by the laity. Men such as Salk, Sabin, and Spock are known for a singular accomplishment. However, Dr. DeBakey, equally identified, is known for many attributes that have helped to serve and improve humankind. Dr. DeBakey's reason, calm judgment, endless energy, acute mind, and kind demeanor are the qualities that make him a special leader.

John Ochsner

Acknowledgments

We thank Beryl Dwight and Susan Parmentier for their editorial assistance. Without their help, the production of this book would not have been possible.

I

Basic Considerations

1

Pathogenesis of Restenosis

Sandro Lepidi, MD, and Alexander W. Clowes, MD

The development of new diagnostic and surgical techniques has improved the treatment of patients with atherosclerosis. At present, bypass grafting, endarterectomy, and percutaneous transluminal angioplasty (PTA) are the principal procedures to treat advanced symptomatic atherosclerotic lesions. Although often successful in alleviating ischemia, these interventions are susceptible to intimal hyperplasia and recurrent stenosis, a vascular response to the injury inherent in any form of vascular procedure.[1] The failure rate due to restenosis is extraordinarily high, ranging from 20% to 50%. Much of the current basic and clinical investigation is focused on defining the biologic mechanisms underlying the process of atherosclerosis, injury, and restenosis to find new pharmacologic ways to control the disease.

Several animal models of intimal hyperplasia have been developed in recent years, the most extensively studied of which has been the balloon angioplasty of normal rat carotid artery. Studies of this model have provided new insights into some of the processes underlying intimal hyperplasia. Certain drugs can block intimal hyperplasia, but these drugs have not been successful in reducing restenosis, and presumably intimal hyperplasia, in clinical trials.

Why have the animal studies failed to predict outcome in humans? There are many possible explanations. The animal experiments might not model the process in human vessels. The intimal hyperplasia we observe in humans has a different starting point and might have a different evolution. In the rat, for example, the starting point is a normal vessel while in humans it is a vessel with advanced atherosclerosis. Processes such as spasm, abrupt plaque rupture, and thrombotic occlusion occur in humans but rarely in animals. It is important to note that in human and animal atherosclerosis the usual response to an encroaching lesion is dilatation; only at the end of the disease process, when adaptive mechanisms have been exhausted, does stenosis develop. Recent studies show that all vessels have a mechanism for controlling lumen size in response to changes in pressure and flow. Apparently, this response is designed to provide the lumen calibre that is most appropriate for maintaining constant wall shear stress. This phenomenon is called *remodeling,* and failure of this mechanism may be responsible for luminal narrowing and restenosis.

CLINICAL IMPORTANCE OF INTIMAL HYPERPLASIA AND RESTENOSIS

As mentioned previously, all forms of vascular reconstruction are afflicted by recurrent narrowing of the vascular lumen. Restenosis may not be of great clinical importance in some circumstances (carotid endarterectomy); however, in others it is a significant cause of failure and loss of organ function (vein bypass grafting, coronary angioplasty). Although the starting point is quite different in each situation, the intimal lesion that forms is very much the same. These lesions form in diseased vessels treated with angioplasty, where little or no tissue is removed. They also form in endarterectomized arteries, where all of the plaque and two-thirds of the media are removed, and in vein grafts, which are normal vessels at the outset. The lesions develop typically within the first 3 to 6 months and at gross examination appear white, firm, and fibrous.[1] Histologicly, the lesions show accumulations of spindle-shaped smooth muscle cells (SMCs) and extracellular matrix.[2] At more than 2 years, the lesions resemble the primary atherosclerotic plaque.[1]

Since the mid-1970s, intimal hyperplasia has been considered the principal cause of restenosis. The basis for this hypothesis comes from animal experimentation (summarized as follows). Recently, the importance of intimal hyperplasia in the evolution of restenosis has been questioned and different theories have been developed.[3] We return to these theories later in this chapter when we describe the studies performed on human lesions in greater detail.

ANIMAL MODELS

Rat Carotid Model

The principal animal model of intimal hyperplasia is the balloon catheter-injured rat carotid artery. The passage of an inflated balloon Fogarty catheter along the artery removes the endothelium and damages the underlying media. Platelets adhere to the vessel wall and release the contents of their granules but do not form large thrombi on the damaged surface.[4] Immediately after injury, a number of genes are induced.[5] After 24 hours some smooth muscle cells (SMCs) begin to synthesize DNA. The thymidine labeling index of medial SMCs (a measure of proliferation) increases from 0.06% per day in normal arteries to 20% to 30% at 48 hours after injury.[4] At the same time, endothelial cells begin to regenerate a luminal surface. At approximately 4 days, migration of SMCs from the media to the intima can be detected. These migrating cells accumulate in the intima and replicate for several cycles. However, since not all migrating SMCs proliferate in the intima,[6] it is possible that migration and proliferation are regulated by different factors. Cellular accumulation in the intima reaches a maximum at 2 weeks, after which the intima is further thickened by the accumulation of extracellular matrix, including elastin, collagen, and proteoglycan (Fig. 1–1).[4] After 3 months, the fraction of intima occupied by matrix has reached a stable level of 80%. Endothelial regeneration proceeds from the ends of the traumatized arterial segment toward the middle and stops after about 1 cm, leaving the central portion of the balloon-injured carotid uncovered.[7] If a portion of the surface is without endothelial coverage for a long period of time, SMCs form a sort of nonthrombogenic pseudoendothelium.[8]

Vein and Synthetic Graft Models

Several different animal models have been utilized to study the processes involved in the healing of vascular grafts. Vascular grafts, like injured arteries, develop intimal

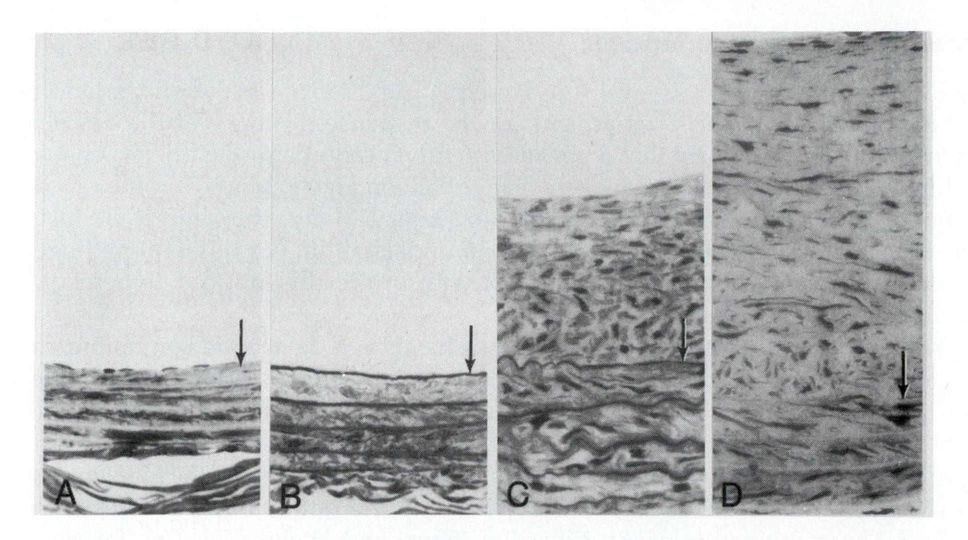

Figure 1–1. Histologic cross-sections of rat carotid arteries. **(A)** Normal vessel showing a single layer of endothelium in intima. **(B)** Denuded vessel at 2 days without endothelium. **(C)** Denuded vessel at 2 weeks showing a markedly thickened intima due to smooth muscle accumulation. **(D)** Denuded vessel at 12 weeks with a further intimal thickening due to smooth muscle cells and deposition of extracellular matrix. Arrows indicate internal elastic lamina. (*Reprinted with permission from Clowes AW, Reidy MA, Clowes MM. Kinetics of cellular proliferation after arterial injury. I. Smooth muscle growth in the absence of endothelium. J Clin Invest. 1983;49:329.*)

hyperplasia; however, some interesting differences exist. Veins transplanted into the arterial circulation undergo intimal hyperplasia and thickening of the media. The response is related to the degree of injury at the time of implantation (passage of a valvulotome, overdistension, clamp injury), and the structure of the vein seems to be regulated more by hemodynamic factors than by the degree of the initial injury. The wall of a vein graft begins to thicken in adaptation to the arterial circulation. In particular, arterial pressure increases wall stress. Smooth muscle cells in the wall respond to the increased stress by replicating and secreting extracellular matrix. The new vein structure might represent an attempt to reduce the value of the stress per cell to a more physiologic level. This phenomenon is reversible in some animal models.[9–11] When a vein graft adapted to the arterial circulation is reimplanted into the venous system, the vein thickening and intimal hyperplasia decrease.

In synthetic grafts, intimal thickening appears mainly at anastomoses, particularly at the distal end. Soon after implantation, the graft is invaded by cells from the adjacent artery and from the surrounding granulation tissue through the pores of the graft. The intimal thickening that develops comprises a monolayer of endothelium at the surface and an underlying neointima made of matrix and SMCs.[12] The neointima forms only where the endothelium is present, whereas intimal thickening develops in the absence of endothelium in injured arteries.

Hemodynamic factors are important in the regulation of intimal thickening in synthetic grafts. Under conditions of high flow, intimal thickening is decreased even though the structure resembles the neointima of grafts exposed to normal flow. To produce a high flow state, an arteriovenous fistula is constructed distal to the vascular grafts. If the fistula is closed several months after graft placement and normal flow restored, the intimal thickening increases rapidly (fivefold over the next month).[13] Similar observations also have been made in vein grafts and injured rat carotid arteries.[14]

Hypercholesterolemic Models

The rat carotid model has been of fundamental importance for the understanding of the biologic and molecular components of the response to injury of the vessel wall. However, it seems unlikely that a vessel with advanced atherosclerotic lesions would react in the same way as a healthy vessel after balloon injury. Moreover, the rat carotid artery does not normally develop stenosis after injury. Many other animal models have been utilized and are helpful in providing an understanding of different pathogenetic mechanisms. We focus on animal models with artificially induced hypercholesterolemia.

Rabbit models of complex human lesions have been developed combining cholesterol feeding with iliac arterial injury. The lesion that develops consists of a concentric foam cell infiltration of intima and media. After injury, there is the formation of a relatively acellular, lipid rich loose connective tissue that fills the dissection planes. In approximately half of the vessels, thrombus forms. Modifications of the high cholesterol diet composition and the degree of injury result in the formation of different types of lesions.[15] The combination of air dissection injury and cholesterol diet, for example, produce a fibrocellular plaque with a modest foam cell infiltrate, similar to the atherosclerotic plaques of young patients who die suddenly of acute myocardial infarction.[16] One of the major advantages of the rabbit injury hypercholesterolemic model is that it is possible to develop a stenosis and more easily a restenosis after a second injury. It is unfortunate that the characteristics of the lesion that forms are distinct from those of the human plaque.

Another interesting model of atherosclerotic lesions has been developed in nonhuman primates. In the monkey, hypercholesterolemia produces lesions that are very similar to human atherosclerotic lesions.[17–20] These observations show that there is a progression from fatty streak lesions to intermediate lesions, which are composed of layers of macrophages and SMCs. The intermediate lesions develop, in turn, into more advanced complex lesions with a lipid core covered by a dense cap of connective tissue containing SMCs. Atherosclerotic monkeys occasionally develop spontaneous lesions that are stenotic on angiography; attempts to produce stenotic lesions using both gentle endothelial denudation or balloon dilatation in normal and atherosclerotic monkeys have been unsuccessful (DD Heistad, personal communication, 1995).

The observations made in the hypercholesterolemic models have improved our understanding of the adaptive changes in arteries that develop an atherosclerotic lesion. As atheroma form, the arteries can adapt by dilating and thus preserving the size of the arterial lumen, a phenomenon called remodeling. Findings characteristic of remodeling were initially described in monkeys,[21] and then in human coronary and carotid arteries.[22] Recent studies suggest that these compensatory changes occur also following angioplasty in hypercholesterolemic rabbits. Vascular remodeling is able to limit the effects of intimal hyperplasia on lumen diameter, and the differences in the extent of vascular remodeling, not of intimal formation, determine whether restenosis occurs.[23] In normal femoral rabbit and in atherosclerotic Yucatan micropig iliac arteries, intimal thickening following balloon injury accounts for only one-third of the loss in angiographic lumen diameter.[24]

MOLECULAR MECHANISMS

Our understanding of the molecular components of the response to injury comes mainly from the studies of the response of normal arteries to injury. Growth factors and cytokines are the mediators that induce and regulate cell function involved in this process. There is a strong link between the degree of injury and the proliferative response of SMCs. A denuding injury that does not traumatize medial SMCs produces a much lower rate of smooth muscle replication than balloon catheter injury. The first wave of medial SMC proliferation is induced by basic fibroblast growth factor (bFGF). Injury causes release of bFGF, a protein with no signal sequence, from damaged vascular wall cells, and bFGF then stimulates the survivors in the media.[25] An antibody to bFGF prevents the initial SMC proliferation by 80% to 90%.[26] However, it has no effect on the subsequent intimal proliferation,[27] which may be maintained by other factors such as insulinlike growth factor 1 (IGF-1)[28] and angiotensin II.[29] Once platelets adhere to the denuded surface of the artery, they release the contents of their granules, among which is platelet-derived growth factor (PDGF). PDGF is also released from endothelial cells, macrophages, and SMCs.[30] *In vitro,* PDGF is a potent growth-promoting factor. However, its major role in intimal hyperplasia seems to be on SMC migration more than proliferation. Depletion of circulating platelets followed by balloon injury leads to a significant reduction in lesion size[31] but does not inhibit cell replication.[32] Administration of a blocking antibody to PDGF also inhibits intimal thickening without inhibiting SMC proliferation.[33] Infusion of PDGF stimulates SMC migration.[34]

Migration of cells from the media into the intima requires breakdown of the matrix surrounding the cells. Cellular proteases are involved in this process. Urokinaselike plasminogen activator (uPA) is activated within 2 to 3 hours after injury and tissue-type plasminogen activator (tPA) appears several days later. Plasmin activity is increased by day four, when migrating SMCs are first seen in the intima.[35] Another class of proteases linked with cell migration is the matrix metalloproteases (MMPs). This class of enzymes is able to digest many of the matrix components of the vessel wall. In the rat carotid artery, only gelatinase A (MMP2) and gelatinase B (MMP9) have been identified. Within hours after balloon injury, MMP9 expression increases and remains until day seven. MMP2 is present in normal arteries and is activated in the injured vessel.[36] The importance of matrix breakdown in lesion formation has been shown in experiments with selective inhibitors of these two different classes of proteases. When plasmin activity in the artery is blocked with tranexamic acid, SMC migration is significantly reduced.[35] The administration of a specific metalloproteinase inhibitor blocks the migration of SMCs and reduces the lesion size.[36]

Little is known about the regulation of SMCs once they have migrated into the intima. Expression of other growth factor genes, such as in insulinlike growth factor-1 (IGF-1) and transforming growth factor beta (TGF-β), has been detected in the vessel wall.[28,37] Transforming growth factor beta might stimulate intimal thickening,[37] even though *in vitro* it is a potent inhibitor of mitogenesis and a potent stimulator of connective tissue formation.[38]

Endothelial cells may play an important role in the regulation of intimal thickening. Endothelial cells have been considered the sensors of blood flow and shear, and they are able to express vasoactive and growth-modulating cytokines that act on the underlying SMCs. For example, they not only can express bFGF and PDGF, but also they can express inhibitors of SMC proliferation, including heparan sulphate and nitric oxide. Other cells can express inhibitors. Gamma interferon, an inhibitor of SMC growth, is secreted by activated T lymphocytes in the lesion.[39] The balance of the expression of positive and negative effectors of growth might have a significant impact on the extent to which vessels thicken during normal development and after injury (Fig. 1–2).

RESTENOSIS IN HUMAN ATHEROSCLEROTIC VESSELS

Intimal hyperplasia and SMC accumulation have been considered the pathogenetic basis of restenosis in human atherosclerotic vessels. This assumption derives from

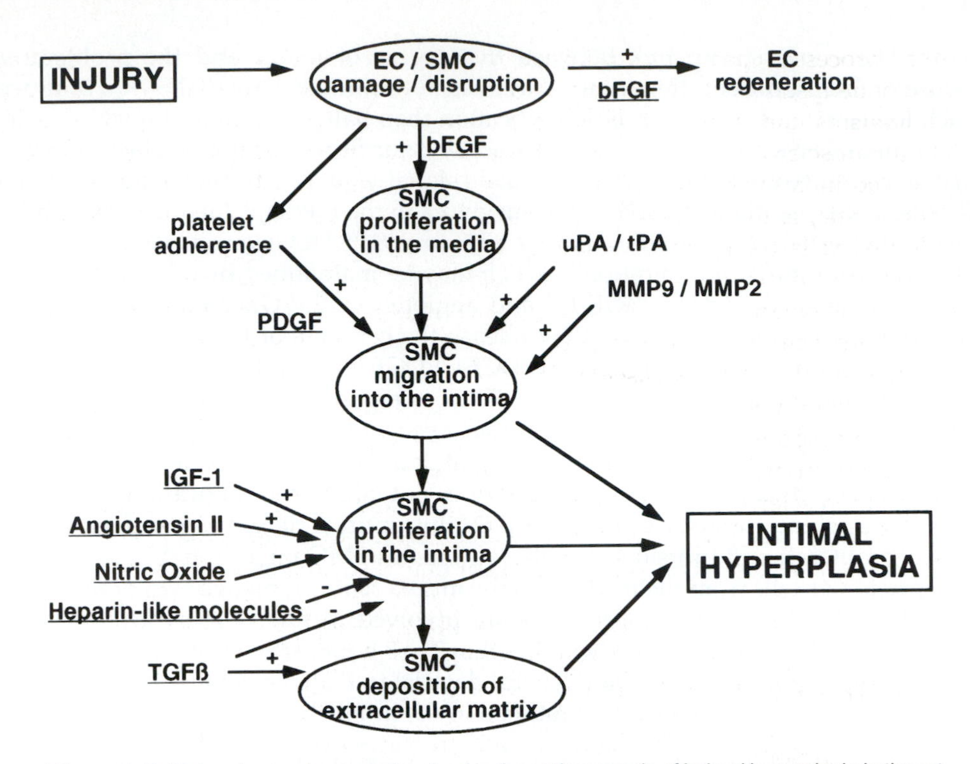

Figure 1–2. Molecular mechanisms involved in the pathogenesis of intimal hyperplasia in the rat carotid artery after balloon injury. The diagram suggests a relationship among injury to the artery, endothelial cell (EC) and smooth muscle cell (SMC) disruption, and release of regulatory molecules. bFGF, basic fibroblast growth factor; PDGF, platelet-derived growth factor; IGF-1, insulinlike growth factor-1; TGF-β, transforming growth factor beta; uPA, urokinaselike plasminogen activator; tPA, tissue-type plasminogen activator; MMP2, gelatinase A; MMP9, gelatinase B. (*Modified with permission from Clowes AW, Reidy MA. Prevention of stenosis after vascular reconstruction: pharmacologic control of intimal hyperplasia—a review. J Vasc Surg. 1991;13:888*).

necropsy examinations of dying patients at various intervals following different revascularization procedures or from atherectomy samples obtained after revascularization. Given the paucity of material, it has been difficult to define the biologic processes leading to restenosis after a vascular reconstruction. Also, some of the postmortem modifications of tone and structure and the artefactual shrinkage due to fixation and processing distort the observations. There has been no systematic effort to correlate the actual hyperplastic mass with angiographic lumen reduction.

The contribution of SMC proliferation to restenosis has been recently analyzed by examining cell cycle markers of proliferation, such as proliferating cell nuclear antigen (PCNA), in both primary and restenotic lesions obtained by a directional atherectomy device.[40] Immunohystochemical analyses showed that the proliferative index (percent of PCNA positive cells) was higher in restenotic (15.2 ± 13.6%) lesions than primary (3.6 ± 3.5%) lesions. Another study, using PCNA staining in atherectomy specimens obtained over a wide range of time following angioplasty, showed a lower proliferative index (<0.5%).[41] Recent studies using intravascular ultrasound to serially evaluate the acute and chronic response to percutaneous revascularization in patients showed that increase in mass accounts only for some cases of restenosis (GS Mintz, personal communication, 1993). These findings suggest that intimal hyperplasia is not a uniform response and may not be sufficient to explain restenosis in the majority of patients who develop it.

Other processes may play an important role in restenosis. Such processes may include plaque instability, which may lead to abrupt rupture, thrombosis, and spasm. The mechanisms underlying these processes are not well understood.

The atherosclerotic plaque contains a number of procoagulant factors normally not expressed in large amounts. The tissue factor activity, which is normally confined to the adventitia, is found in the intima of atherosclerotic vessels. It is expressed by mesenchymal cells (probably SMCs) and macrophages.[42] These lesions also contain large amounts of fibrinogen. Moreover, the natural inhibitor of plasminogen activator, plasminogen activator inhibitor type 1 (PAI-1), is expressed in excess.[43,44] Thus, there is increased procoagulant and antifibrinolytic activity, which may promote the tendency to generate thrombus after a vascular injury.

Animal experiments have shown that arteries have a mechanism for controlling lumen size in response to flow and pressure. This is probably to provide the lumen size most appropriate for minimizing wall shear stress. Moreover, arteries adapt to increasing atherosclerotic plaque by enlarging. Remodeling has been demonstrated in human coronary,[45] carotid,[46] and superficial femoral arteries and in abdominal and thoracic aortas. Aberrations of this mechanism may lead to stenosis or restenosis.

PHARMACOLOGIC CONTROL

More than 55 randomized clinical trials have been conducted and none have clearly shown efficacy, despite numerous positive animal studies.[47] A variety of different drugs has been tried, and extensive reviews have been published.[48,49] We examine the history of two of these agents, heparin and cilazapril, in order to outline some of the potential problems that will need to be resolved in the future.

Heparin was one of the first pharmacologic agents shown to inhibit intimal hyperplasia.[50] Endothelial cells and SMCs are able to express heparinlike molecules (heparan sulphate proteoglycan), which have inhibitory activity for SMC growth. Heparin effectively inhibits injury-induced intimal thickening in the rat by suppressing both migration and proliferation, when given within 24 hours after injury and continued for at least 3 to 7 days. The mechanism of this heparin action is not clear, although it has been shown to decrease the binding of several growth factors, including bFGF, PDGF, and TGF-β. It may also influence the activity of an important transacting factor, activator protein-1 (AP-1).[51] Heparin inhibits tPA and interstitial collagenase at the level of transcription and probably has a similar effect on gelatinase B and stromelysin.[52] Fractions of heparin depleted of anticoagulant activity by passage over an antithrombin III column still possess antiproliferative activity.[53] Preliminary trials using heparin in patients undergoing angioplasty have been negative,[54] although one trial of heparin in patients undergoing peripheral bypass showed an improvement in patency.[55] There are several reasons why the trials have failed. The dose of anticoagulant heparin that was used might have been reduced to avoid hemorrhagic complications and might have been too low; the length of time the heparin was administered might have been too short; and/or there might be intrinsic factors that limit heparin responsiveness since the cells of restenotic vein grafts are resistant to heparin.[56]

The angiotensin-converting enzyme (ACE) inhibitor cilazapril is a good inhibitor of intimal thickening after balloon injury in the rat carotid artery. Its effect is principally on cell migration.[57] Angiotensin-converting enzyme not only converts angiotensin I to angiotensin II, but it is also responsible for the degradation of bradykinin, a potential inhibitor of SMC migration.[58] A relative decrease in angiotensin II and an increase in bradykinin might be the consequence of ACE inhibitor treatment. Both mechanisms have been hypothesized to be important in the regulation of intimal hyperplasia. The results of ACE inhibitors have been confirmed in rabbits,[59] but not in pigs[60] and baboons.[61] Clinical trials conducted with the ACE inhibitor, cilazapril, have shown that the drug is ineffective in preventing restenosis after angioplasty.[62,63] The lack of effect in humans is likely to reflect not only the lower doses of cilazapril used, but also different reactions of atherosclerotic arteries to injury, interspecies differences in the healing response, and intrinsic differences in drug metabolism and in the activity of the fibrinolytic system. It is important to keep in mind that the basic hypothesis underlying all the clinical trials has been that restenosis is mainly the consequence of intimal hyperplasia. However, as previously discussed, other processes may play important roles in human atherosclerotic vessels. If vasospasm is a significant part of the stenotic process, then a weak inhibitory effect of the drug on intimal hyperplasia would be missed. Perhaps a better strategy would employ two or more drugs as a combined pharmacologic approach to treat vasocontraction as well as prevent intimal hyperplasia.

A new approach to the pharmacologic control of restenosis is the local delivery of therapeutic agents. Side effects or toxicity of some agents may limit their systemic administration to patients. This approach allows access to specific target sites with adequate concentrations of a therapeutic agent. Approaches for local, intravascular, site-specific delivery include (1) direct deposition of therapeutic agents into the vessel wall through an intravascular delivery system, (2) systemic administration of inactive agents followed by local activation, and (3) systemic administration of fusion toxins that have a specific affinity for proliferating SMCs at the angioplasty site. In addition to conventional drugs, new therapeutic agents based on molecular mechanisms, including recombinant genes and antisense oligonucleotides, are now under investigation.

Antisense oligonucleotides are designed to inhibit RNA transcripts.[64] Introduction of inhibitor genes stably or transiently expressed in vascular wall cells has been proposed as an innovative approach to limit the restenotic process. To this end, cultured vascular SMCs containing retrovirally introduced genes are a potential vehicle for gene replacement therapy.[65] Smooth muscle cells infected with replication-defective retrovirus expressing human adenosine deaminase or alkaline phosphatase were seeded in balloon-injured rat carotid arteries. After seeding, SMCs stop replicating but continue to express the introduced human genes over the long term.[66] Adenoviral vectors have also been used for the direct transfer of genetic material into the uninjured artery wall.[67] By using a highly efficient Sendai virus/liposome *in vivo* gene transfer technique, the introduction of cDNA encoding the endothelial cell nitric oxide synthase (ec NOS) was able to inhibit neointima formation in the rat carotid artery by 70% at day 14 after balloon injury.[68]

CONCLUSION

Restenosis is still the major limitation to long-term patency of vascular reconstructions. Despite progress in both experimental and clinical studies, the pathogenesis of restenosis remains unclear. Intimal hyperplasia may be important only in some cases of restenosis, and other mechanisms may play a more significant role. A better pharmacologic strategy may be to employ combinations of drugs, each of which blocks a particular component of restenosis. Recent developments in gene transfer techniques provide new and exciting therapeutic options for the management of this problem.

REFERENCES

1. Clowes AW, Reidy MA. Prevention of stenosis after vascular reconstruction: pharmacologic control of intimal hyperplasia—a review. *J Vasc Surg*. 1991;13:885–891.
2. Clagett GP, Robinowitz M, Youkey JR, et al. Morphogenesis and clinicopathologic characteristics of recurrent carotid disease. *J Vasc Surg*. 1986;3:10–23.
3. Schwartz RS, Holmes DRJ, Topol EJ. The restenosis paradigm revisited: an alternative proposal for cellular mechanisms. *J Am Coll Cardiol*. 1992;20:1284–1293.
4. Clowes AW, Reidy MA, Clowes MM. Kinetics of cellular proliferation after arterial injury. I. Smooth muscle growth in the absence of endothelium. *Lab Invest*. 1983;49:327–333.
5. Miano JM, Vlasic N, Tota RR, et al. Smooth muscle cell immediate-early gene and growth factor activation follows vascular injury. A putative in vivo mechanism for autocrine growth. *Arterioscler Thromb*. 1993;13:211–219.
6. Clowes AW, Schwartz SM. Significance of quiescent smooth muscle migration in the injured rat carotid artery. *Circ Res*. 1985;56:139–145.
7. Reidy MA, Clowes AW, Schwartz SM. Endothelial regeneration. V. Inhibition of endothelial regrowth in arteries of rat and rabbit. *Lab Invest*. 1983;49:569–575.
8. Clowes AW, Collazzo RE, Karnovsky MJ. A morphologic and permeability study of luminal smooth muscle cells after arterial injury in the rat. *Lab Invest*. 1978;39:141–150.
9. Morinaga K, Eguchi H, Miyazaki T, et al. Development and regression of intimal thickening of arterially transplanted autologous vein grafts in dogs. *J Vasc Surg*. 1987;5:719–730.
10. Davies MG, Klyachkin ML, Dalen H, et al. Regression of intimal hyperplasia with restoration of endothelium-dependent relaxing factor-mediated relaxation in experimental vein grafts. *Surgery*. 1993;114:258–271.
11. Lepidi S, Sterpetti AV, Cucina A, et al. bFGF release is dependent on flow conditions in experimental vein grafts. *Eur J Vasc Surg*. 1995;10.
12. Zacharias RK, Kirkman TR, Clowes SW. Mechanisms of healing in synthetic grafts. *J Vasc Surg*. 1987;6:429–436.
13. Kohler TR, Kirkman TR, Kraiss LW, et al. Increased blood flow inhibits neointimal hyperplasia in endothelialized vascular grafts. *Circ Res*. 1991;69:1557–1565.
14. Kohler TR, Jawien A. Flow affects development of intimal hyperplasia after arterial injury in rats. *Arterioscler Thromb*. 1992;12:963–971.
15. Sarembock IJ, LaVeau PJ, Sigal SL, et al. Influence of inflation pressure and balloon size on the development of intimal hyperplasia after balloon angioplasty. A study in the atherosclerotic rabbit. *Circulation*. 1989;80:1029–1040.
16. Kragel AH, Reddy SG, Wittes JT, et al. Morphometric analysis of the composition of atherosclerotic plaques in the four major epicardial coronary arteries in acute myocardial infarction and in sudden coronary death. *Circulation*. 1989;80:1747–1756.
17. Faggiotto A, Ross R, Harker L. Studies of hypercholesterolemia in the nonhuman primate. I. Changes that lead to fatty streak formation. *Arteriosclerosis*. 1984;4:323–340.
18. Faggiotto A, Ross R. Studies of hypercholesterolemia in the nonhuman primate. II. Fatty streak conversion to fibrous plaque. *Arteriosclerosis*. 1984;4:341–356.
19. Masuda J, Ross R. Atherogenesis during low level hypercholesterolemia in the nonhuman primate. I. Fatty streak formation. *Arteriosclerosis*. 1990;10:164–177.
20. Masuda J, Ross R. Atherogenesis during low level hypercholesterolemia in the nonhuman primate. II. Fatty streak conversion to fibrous plaque. *Arteriosclerosis*. 1990;10;178–187.
21. Bond MG, Adams MR, Bullock BC. Complicating factors in evaluating coronary artery atherosclerosis. *Artery*. 1981;9:21–29.
22. Glagov S, Weisenberg E, Zarins CK, et al. Compensatory enlargement of human atherosclerotic coronary arteries. *N Engl J Med*. 1987;316:1371–1375.
23. Kakuta T, Currier JW, Haudenschild CC, et al. Differences in compensatory vessel enlargement, not intimal formation, account for restenosis after angioplasty in the hypercholesterolemic rabbit model. *Circulation*. 1994;89:2809–2815.
24. Post MJ, Borst C, Kuntz RE. The relative importance of arterial remodeling compared with intimal hyperplasia in lumen renarrowing after balloon angioplasty. A study in the normal rabbit and the hypercholesterolemic Yucatan micropig. *Circulation*. 1994;89:2816–2821.

25. Lindner V, Olson NE, Clowes AW, et al. Inhibition of smooth muscle cell proliferation in injured rat arteries. Interaction of heparin with basic fibroblast growth factor. *J Clin Invest.* 1992;90:2044–2049.
26. Lindner V, Reidy MA. Proliferation of smooth muscle cells after vascular injury is inhibited by an antibody against fibroblast growth factor. *Proc Natl Acad Sci USA.* 1991;88:3739–3743.
27. Olson NE, Chao S, Lindner V, et al. Intimal smooth muscle cell proliferation after balloon catheter injury. The role of basic fibroblast growth factor. *Am J Pathol.* 1992;140:1017–1023.
28. Cercek B, Fishbein MC, Forrester JS, et al. Induction of insulin-like growth factor I messenger RNA in rat aorta after balloon denudation. *Circ Res.* 1990;66:1755–1760.
29. Rakugi H, Jacob HJ, Krieger JE, et al. Vascular injury induces angiotensinogen gene expression in the media and neointima. *Circulation.* 1993; 87:283–290.
30. Ross R, Bowen PDF, Raines EW. Platelet-derived growth factor and its role in health and disease. *Philos Trans R Soc Lond Biol.* 1990;327:155–169.
31. Friedman RJ, Stemerman MB, Wenz B, et al. The effect of thrombocytopenia on experimental arteriosclerotic lesion formation in rabbits. Smooth muscle cell proliferation and re-endothelialization. *J Clin Invest.* 1977;60:1191–1201.
32. Fingerle J, Johnson R, Clowes AW, et al. Role of platelets in smooth muscle cell proliferation and migration after vascular injury in rat carotid artery. *Proc Natl Acad Sci USA.* 1989;86: 8412–8416.
33. Ferns GA, Raines EW, Sprugel KH, et al. Inhibition of neointimal smooth muscle accumulation after angioplasty by an antibody to PDGF. *Science.* 1991;253:1129–1132.
34. Jawien A, Bowen PDF, Lindner V, et al. Platelet-derived growth factor promotes smooth muscle migration and intimal thickening in a rat model of balloon angioplasty. *J Clin Invest.* 1992;89:507–511.
35. Jackson CL, Raines EW, Ross R, et al. Role of endogenous platelet-derived growth factor in arterial smooth muscle cell migration after balloon catheter injury. *Arterioscler Thromb.* 1993;13:1218–1226.
36. Bendeck MP, Zempo N, Clowes AW, et al. Smooth muscle cell migration and matrix metalloproteinase expression after arterial injury in the rat. *Circ Res.* 1994;75:539–545.
37. Majesky MW, Lindner V, Twardzik DR, et al. Production of transforming growth factor beta 1 during repair of arterial injury. *J Clin Invest.* 1991;88:904–910.
38. Ross R. The pathogenesis of atherosclerosis: a perspective for the 1990s. *Nature.* 1993;362: 801–809.
39. Hansson GK, Jonasson L, Holm J, et al. Gamma-interferon regulates vascular smooth muscle proliferation and Ia antigen expression in vivo and in vitro. *Circ Res.* 1988;63:712–719.
40. Garratt KN, Edwards WD, Kaufmann UP, et al. Differential histopathology of primary atherosclerotic and restenotic lesions in coronary arteries and saphenous vein bypass grafts: analysis of tissue obtained from 73 patients by directional atherectomy. *J Am Coll Cardiol.* 1991;17:442–448.
41. O'Brien ER, Alpers CE, Stewart DK, et al. Proliferation in primary and restenotic coronary atherectomy tissue. Implications for antiproliferative therapy. *Circ Res.* 1993;73:223–231.
42. Wilcox JN, Smith KM, Schwartz SM, et al. Localization of tissue factor in the normal vessel wall and in the atherosclerotic plaque. *Proc Natl Acad Sci USA.* 1989;86:2839–2843.
43. Schneiderman J, Sawdey MS, Keeton MR, et al. Increased type 1 plasminogen activator inhibitor gene expression in atherosclerotic human arteries. *Proc Natl Acad Sci USA.* 1992;89:6998–7002.
44. Dawson S, Henney A. The status of PAI-1 as a risk factor for arterial and thrombotic disease: a review. *Atherosclerosis.* 1992;95:105–117.
45. Zarins CK, Weisenberg E, Kolettis G, et al. Differential enlargement of artery segments in response to enlarging atherosclerotic plaques. *J Vasc Surg.* 1988;7:386–394.
46. Masawa N, Glagov S, Zarins CK. Quantitative morphologic study of intimal thickening at the human carotid bifurcation: II. The compensatory enlargement response and the role of the intima in tensile support. *Atherosclerosis.* 1994;107:147–155.
47. Franklin SM, Faxon DP. Pharmacologic prevention of restenosis after coronary angioplasty: review of the randomized clinical trials. *Coron Artery Dis.* 1993;4:232–242.

48. Herrman JP, Hermans WR, Vos J, et al. Pharmacological approaches to the prevention of restenosis following angioplasty. The search for the Holy Grail? (Part I). *Drugs.* 1993;46:18–52.
49. Herrman JP, Hermans WR, Vos J, et al. Pharmacological approaches to the prevention of restenosis following angioplasty. The search for the Holy Grail? (Part II). *Drugs.* 1993;46: 249–262.
50. Au YP, Kenagy RD, Clowes MM, et al. Mechanisms of inhibition by heparin of vascular smooth muscle cell proliferation and migration. *Haemostasis.* 1993;23 (suppl 1):177–182.
51. Au YP, Dobrowolska G, Morris DR, et al. Heparin decreases activator protein-1 binding to DNA in part by posttranslational modification of Jun B. *Circ Res.* 1994;75:15–22.
52. Kenagy RD, Nikkari ST, Welgus HG, et al. Heparin inhibits the induction of three matrix metalloproteinases (stromelysin, 92-kD gelatinase, and collagenase) in primate arterial smooth muscle cells. *J Clin Invest.* 1994;93:1987–1993.
53. Pukac LA, Hirsch GM, Lormeau JC, et al. Antiproliferative effects of novel, nonanticoagulant heparin derivatives on vascular smooth muscle cells in vitro and in vivo. *Am J Pathol.* 1991;139:1501–1509.
54. Ellis SG, Roubin GS, Wilentz J, et al. Effect of 18- to 24-hour heparin administration for prevention of restenosis after uncomplicated coronary angioplasty. *Am Heart J.* 1989; 117:777–782.
55. Edmondson RA, Cohen AT, Das SK, et al. Low-molecular weight heparin versus aspirin and dipyridamole after femoropopliteal bypass grafting. *Lancet.* 1994;344:914–918.
56. Chan P, Patel M, Betteridge L, et al. Abnormal growth regulation of vascular smooth muscle cells by heparin in patients with restenosis. *Lancet.* 1993;341:341–342.
57. Prescott MF, Webb RL, Reidy MA. Angiotensin-converting enzyme inhibitor versus angiotensin II, AT1 receptor antagonist. Effects on smooth muscle cell migration and proliferation after balloon catheter injury. *Am J Pathol.* 1991;139:1291–1296.
58. Farhy RD, Carretero OA, Ho KL, et al. Role of kinins and nitric oxide in the effects of angiotensin converting enzyme inhibitors on neointima formation. *Circ Res.* 1993;72: 1202–1210.
59. O'Donohoe MK, Schwartz LB, Radic ZS, et al. Chronic ACE inhibition reduces intimal hyperplasia in experimental vein grafts. *Ann Surg.* 1991;214:727–732.
60. Huber KC, Schwartz RS, Edwards WD, et al. Effects of angiotensin converting enzyme inhibition on neointimal proliferation in a porcine coronary injury model. *Am Heart J.* 1993;125:695–701.
61. Hanson SR, Powell JS, Dodson T, et al. Effects of angiotensin converting enzyme inhibition with cilazapril on intimal hyperplasia in injured arteries and vascular grafts in the baboon. *Hypertension.* 1991;18 (suppl 4):1170–1176.
62. Multicenter European Research Trial with Cilazapril after Angioplasty to Prevent Transluminal Coronary Obstruction and Restenosis (MERCATOR) Study Group. Does the new angiotensin converting enzyme inhibitor cilazapril prevent restenosis after percutaneous transluminal coronary angioplasty? Results of the MERCATOR study: a multicenter, randomized, double-blind placebo-controlled trial. *Circulation.* 1992;86:100–110.
63. Heyndrickx GR. Angiotensin-converting enzyme inhibitor in a human model of restenosis. MERCATOR Study Group. *Basic Res Cardiol.* 1993;88 (suppl 1):169–182.
64. Simons M, Edelman ER, DeKeyser JL, et al. Antisense c-myb oligonucleotides inhibit intimal arterial smooth muscle cell accumulation in vivo. *Nature.* 1992;359:67–70.
65. Lynch CM, Clowes MM, Osborne WR, et al. Long-term expression of human adenosine deaminase in vascular smooth muscle cells of rats: a model for gene therapy. *Proc Natl Acad Sci USA.* 1992;89:1138–1142.
66. Clowes MM, Lynch CM, Miller AD, et al. Long-term biological response of injured rat carotid artery seeded with smooth muscle cells expressing retrovirally introduced human genes. *J Clin Invest.* 1994;93:644–651.
67. Lemarchand P, Jones M, Yamada I, et al. In vivo gene transfer and expression in normal uninjured blood vessels using replication-deficient recombinant adenovirus vectors. *Circ Res.* 1993;72:1132–1138.
68. Von Der Leyen HE, Gibbons GH, Morishita R, et al. Gene therapy inhibiting neointimal vascular lesion: in vivo transfer of endothelial cell nitric oxide synthase gene. *Proc Natl Acad Sci USA.* 1995;92:1137–1141.

2

Pharmacologic Management of Intimal Hyperplasia

Michael D. Colburn, MD, and Wesley S. Moore, MD

Technological advances and better training have made an increasing variety of vascular procedures available. Today, few, if any, vascular problems are surgically inaccessible, and bypass grafts to the most distal segments of the arterial tree are routinely performed across the country. Yet, despite improvements in operative morbidity and mortality and impressive early success rates, the long-term durability of these procedures has been disappointing and many problems remain unsolved. Perhaps the most important of these problems, and an area which is currently undergoing intense research, is that of restenosis. While prosthetic graft infections remain devastating, they are rare. Aberrant healing of an anastomosis or endarterectomy site, however, is not only common but also probably occurs to some degree in every procedure performed. Furthermore, a significant percentage of these restenotic lesions become clinically important and frequently lead to graft or reconstruction failure.

Intimal hyperplasia is the most common cause of failures occurring between 2 to 3 years postoperatively. Since early graft failures related to technical errors can often be corrected (and should ultimately be preventable with continued technologic improvements), and because late graft failures are related to the nature of the systemic atherosclerotic process and factors external to the bypass graft, most research in this area has been directed toward the problem of intimal hyperplasia. Intimal thickening is formed by the migration of smooth muscle cells (SMCs) from the medial to the intimal layer of vessel wall following an endothelial injury. Subsequent proliferation of these cells, and the ensuing deposition of extracellular matrix material, produces thickening of the intimal layer, luminal narrowing, and eventual thrombosis of the affected vessel. This hyperplastic intimal response is a characteristic fibromuscular cellular response of the vascular system to injury and is a normal feature of vascular healing. In many instances, however, progression of this process ultimately leads to graft failure and is a significant clinical problem. In one series, 50% of late failures identified in 5,000 arterial reconstructions, including both endarterectomy and bypass operations, were due to this exuberant hyperplastic intimal process.[1]

Intimal hyperplasia is triggered by any form or degree of endothelial cell injury, and therefore all types of vascular interventions are affected. The 3-year primary patency rates for infrainguinal bypass grafts ranges from 40% to 60% with prosthetic conduits, and from 60% to 80% when an autologous graft is utilized. In other words, approximately 20% to 60% of all grafts have failed at this time interval. Furthermore, of those grafts that fail between 6 months and 2 years, most fail due to intimal hyperplasia. The durability of carotid reconstructions has also been a concern. The incidence of asymptomatic carotid restenoses ranges between 7% to 15%, and between 1% to 5% develop restenoses associated with recurrent symptoms. Results following percutaneous transluminal balloon angioplasty (PTA) in the arterial tree vary greatly depending on the location of the lesion. If one considers the results of PTA procedures on aortoiliac lesions as representative of the best case results, a review of the contemporary literature we reported recently found a long-term patency rate of 32% to 90% (mean 70%).[2] Results of PTA on more distal lesions, however, are not nearly as impressive. Some of these recurrences are probably due to either a progression of atherosclerosis or to other mechanisms such as intraplaque hemorrhage. The majority, however, are the result of intimal hyperplasia. Since intimal hyperplasia is the common culprit behind much of the poor long-term success rate following these procedures, it is easy to appreciate why investigations into methods to prevent or reverse this process are of great importance.

Recent advances have been made in pharmacologic therapy for hyperplastic intimal lesions. The ability of various agents to augment the growth of intimal hyperplastic lesions has been studied by many investigators. Clearly, if effective therapy to suppress the growth of intimal hyperplasia and to prevent the associated recurrent arterial stenoses could be developed, it would have a major impact on the durability of vascular procedures and lower their associated morbidity, mortality, and cost. It may also prove possible to reverse established hyperplastic lesions. This would be an alternative therapy for the patient with a failing vascular procedure and would represent a significant advance in the management of this highly morbid and potentially lethal complication of peripheral vascular surgery.

In this chapter we first summarize the current concepts regarding the pathophysiology of intimal hyperplasia. Once described, we use the molecular pathways, thought to be important in the formation of intimal hyperplasia, as a framework from which to survey the current pharmacologic approaches for inhibiting this lesion. Finally, we speculate on possible future directions for research.

PATHOLOGIC FEATURES OF INTIMAL HYPERPLASIA

As early as 1910, it was noted that "within a few days after the operation, the stitches placed in making the anastomosis became covered with a glistening substance similar in appearance to the normal endothelium."[3] This early account accurately describes the appearance of the homogeneous lesion that is seen when operations are performed for restenosis or graft failure. The thickened vessel wall is smooth, shiny, and appears subendothelial. It is now recognized that this process probably represents the normal response of an artery to injury. This healing process becomes abnormal, however, when it leads to the formation of a hemodynamicly significant flow-restricting lesion. When this occurs, the process is referred to as *intimal hyperplasia.* Clearly, these processes are difficult to separate and the point of progression from normal healing to intimal hyperplasia is hard to distinguish. If one considers normal arterial healing a result of the proliferation of cells and connective tissue elements that occurs at sites of endothelial injury, then intimal hyperplasia can be thought of as the result of the inability to control this normal regenerative process.

Histologic examination of intimal hyperplastic thickening consistently reveals certain features. Because of the generation of new cellular layers within the arterial intima, many investigators refer to the process as *neointimal hyperplasia*. Others perfer the term *myointimal hyperplasia* because, in fact, a true new intima does not form on the surface of the injured lumen but rather is formed by the migration and proliferation of medial SMCs. Microscopically, these lesions show features consisting of many stellate cells surrounded by a clear fibromyxomatous appearing stroma and connective tissue. Careful and extensive histologic examination of these stellate cells has revealed several cytological fingerprints that have conclusively identified them as SMCs. These include a characteristic morphology (external lamina, dense bodies, and myofilaments), positive immunocytologic staining for SMC-specific actin chains, and positive histochemical staining for sulfated glycosaminoglycans. It is currently believed that these cells originate in the media as differentiated SMCs. In response to injury, the SMCs undergo a series of distinct changes. The first is replication, followed by migration from the media across the internal elastic lamina and into the intima. Once in the lumen, the cells proliferate and begin to synthesize and secrete stored connective tissue elements. This cellular proliferation, as well as the deposition of extracellular matrix, forms the basis of the observed intimal changes in the lumen of a traumatized vessel.

PATHOPHYSIOLOGY OF INTIMAL HYPERPLASIA

In order to understand intimal hyperplasia, it is essential to first review the physiology of medial SMCs and their role in the normal healing response of a vascular injury. The normal arterial wall is comprised primarily of three layers: the intima, media, and adventitia. The intima is generally considered to consist of a single layer of endothelial cells on the lumenal surface and a thin basal lamina. The medial layer consists of a connective tissue mixture of collagen, elastin, and other extracellular matrix proteins. The cellular component of this layer is made of SMCs and possibly some fibroblasts. The SMCs are responsible for maintaining the configuration and tone of the vascular wall. The normal cellular kinetics of a healthy vessel wall are marked by a slow growth rate of both intimal endothelial cells and their underlying medial SMCs. One characteristic biologic feature indicating some degree of vascular injury is a transformation from this resting state to one of increased activity. Damage to the vascular endothelium somehow triggers a complex series of events by which these cells undergo activation. Once activated, the medial SMCs begin to migrate toward the intima and ultimately form intimal hyperplasia.

Although much is known about the histology of intimal hyperplasia, the precise pathophysiologic pathways leading to the development of these lesions have not been identified. Clearly, the initiating event is some form of damage to the vascular endothelium. The resulting exposure of the subendothelial arterial wall to abnormal hemodynamic forces, circulating cells and proteins, and local growth factors triggers a myriad of cellular and enzymatic events that ultimately lead to the migration and proliferation of medial SMCs. The result of this complex process is intimal thickening and a reduction of the lumenal diameter.

The medial SMC response to vascular injury can be divided into four distinct stages: (1) an initial medial proliferative response, (2) migration from the media across the external elastic lamina and into the intima, (3) subsequent proliferation within the intima, and (4) synthesis and deposition of extracellular matrix. Several theories have attempted to describe the precise mechanisms responsible for controlling each of these four stages. The following subsections provide a detailed description of each of the biologic pathways thought to be most important in the development of intimal hyperplasia. With this background, it is then possible to review pharmacologic approaches for preventing this lesion and to better understand the rationale behind these efforts.

Hemodynamic Factors

As discussed, the stimulus for intimal hyperplasia has been the subject of intense experimental investigation. One of the first factors—thought to play at least a contributory role—was hemodynamic changes and their associated mechanical forces. Early observations attributed intimal thickening in bypass grafts simply to the exposure of the conduits to arterial pressure. Currently a wide variety of more complicated hemodynamic forces, including high- and low-flow velocities, high and low wall shear stress, and mechanical compliance mismatch, have all been implicated.

The effects of flow velocity, on the subsequent development of intimal hyperplasia, has been studied in a variety of models. Significant intimal thickening has been noted in arteriovenous fistulas constructed for hemodialysis access. Similar intimal lesions have been documented by electron microscopic examination 3 months after formation of a high-flow renal artery to venacava anastomosis.[4] Other studies, however, have demonstrated conflicting results. For example, in a canine carotid vein interposition model it was found that segments with low-flow velocities developed significantly thicker intimal layers.[5] Furthermore, other researchers have found that 6 months after construction of an arteriovenous fistula in monkey iliac vessels, no increase in intimal thickening was seen on the experimental side.[6] In this study, while flow rate and velocity were found to be markedly increased on the side of the arteriovenous fistula, the calculated wall shear stress was equal on both sides. In summary, these findings support the idea that flow velocity may not be a major determinant of intimal hyperplasia. However, tangential or wall shear stress may be an important hemodynamic factor leading to the development of this lesion.

When blood flows through a straight segment of the normal human arterial tree, the flow pattern tends to be laminar. In this laminar flow pattern, the layer of fluid adjacent to the wall is known as the boundary layer and is usually a region of low shear stress. Sudden changes in the geometric configuration of this arterial tree, such as occur in an area of an anastomosis, cause the blood flow pattern to become turbulent. This stops or reverses the flow within the boundary layer and creates areas with complex flow patterns. These flow patterns lead to greater flow separation between the flowing blood and the vessel wall and ultimately lead to the generation of shear stress forces. Paradoxicly, it has been postulated that both high and low wall shear stress may contribute to the development of intimal hyperplasia. The mechanisms by which each end of the shear stress spectrum stimulates this response, however, are very different. Regions of high shear stress probably promote the development of intimal lesions by increasing the size and degree of the local endothelial injury. Conversely, regions of low wall shear stress probably increase intimal proliferation by increasing the exposure of the injured vessel wall to platelets, growth factors, and other SMC stimulants.

The way in which these shear stress forces may interact clinically has been elegantly described in a model that incorporates the effects of both high and low wall shear stress.[7] In this study, dye was injected into the central high-velocity flow-lines of the common carotid artery. Subsequently, it was noted that the dye traveled to the vessel wall near the bifurcation (a high shear stress region) and then, with loss of momentum, traversed circumferentially along the carotid sinus wall to enter the adjacent boundary layer area. This is a low shear stress area and corresponds to the region, across from the external carotid origin, where most atherosclerotic plaques are known to occur. It has been hypothesized that there may be platelet activation, from intimal damage, in the region of high shear stress and that these same activated platelets may then enter the area of boundary layer separation causing further intimal damage by virtue of the increased exposure time afforded by the low shear stress forces. This hypothesis is strongly supported by the spectral analysis of pulsed Doppler velocity waveforms in carotid artery bifurcations of young healthy individuals. These studies demonstrate similar zones of flow separation.[8]

Another important hemodynamic factor, also reported to be important for production of anastomotic intimal hyperplasia, is compliance mismatch. Compliance can be thought of as the amount of radial or luminal volume change per unit change in pressure. In other words, compliance is a measure of the distensibility of a vessel wall following changes in luminal pressure; and it is therefore a useful measurement of the amount of force that is being applied to the vessel wall. Several studies have attempted to establish a connection between changes in compliance and the formation of intimal hyperplasia. The results of these investigations, however, have been inconclusive. One obvious argument suggesting a significant role for compliance in the pathophysiology of this lesion is the fact that, although both autologous vein and prosthetic reconstructions develop intimal hyperplasia, the magnitude of this effect differs and seems to correlate with the compliance characteristics of each type of bypass graft. The compliance of a vein graft, at the time of implantation, is similar to a native artery and, according to the results of one study, the compliance values remain within the normal range for a median follow-up of 33 months.[9] Textile and fabric prostheses, however, are relatively noncompliant. Because it is well known that the longevity of autologous vein grafts is superior to that of prosthetic bypasses, it follows that compliance forces have been suggested as a possible mechanism for this difference. While experimental and clinical studies have shown that grafts with compliance values approaching the native artery demonstrate increased patency, most of these studies have not controlled for graft surface differences. In one study that did, bilateral femoropopliteal grafts were constructed from autografts made from carotid arteries.[10] The compliant graft was infused with 0.025% glutaraldehyde and externally bathed with saline solution for 30 minutes. The stiff graft was infused with a similar concentration of glutaraldehyde, but was bathed in 10% glutaraldehyde for 60 minutes. At removal, only 43% of stiff grafts were patent compared with 86% of compliant grafts. Although these results demonstrate increased patency with more compliant grafts, no effect on intimal hyperplasia was demonstrated.

In summary, operative manipulation and hemodynamic factors may both contribute to the development of intimal hyperplasia. Clearly, however, these factors are only part of the puzzle and numerous other contributing elements are probably necessary for the development of the full hyperplastic response.

Alterations in Lipid Metabolism

One feature that is immediately apparent when examining hyperplastic intimal lesions histologically is an architecture strikingly similar to that seen in specimens of atherosclerosis. Proliferating SMCs, as well as abundant lipid and connective tissue elements, are consistently identified in both lesions. This simple observation has led some investigators to speculate that both intimal hyperplasia and atherosclerosis may in fact share a common pathophysiologic pathway.

In this theory, atherosclerosis and intimal hyperplasia both represent lesions within the spectrum of atherogenesis and differ only in the kinetics of the lesion formation. Atherosclerosis forms over decades and appears to be connected to the slow accumulation of lipids. By contrast, endothelial damage following vascular reconstruction leads to a hyperplastic intimal response within days, and fully formed lesions often become clinically significant within months. Normally, the vascular SMCs regulate the accumulation of lipid and cholesterol at the level of a surface membrane high affinity low-density lipoprotein (LDL) receptor. These receptors bind LDL and internalize the bound compounds by endocytosis. The incorporated lipids and cholesterol are transported to liposomes where they are degraded and processed for use by the cell. In atherosclerosis, increased storage of intracellular cholesterol esters, due to many years of oversaturation with high concentrations of plasma LDL, leads to the development of foam cells. With time, necrosis of these cells, the release of their contents, and finally calcification, lead to the necrotic, lipid-rich extracellular debris seen in mature atherosclerosis. Intimal hyperplasia, however, is characterized by a higher proportion of SMC proliferation and less lipid-laden necrosis. This difference may be the result of a sudden loss of endothelial integrity immediately exposing the underlying SMCs to large amounts of plasma bound LDL. The SMCs respond by both initiating cellular replication as well as up-regulating the production of LDL receptors. LDL is a potent SMC mitogen. Therefore, if this theory is correct, both intimal hyperplasia and atherogenesis can be considered alterations in lipid metabolism. The rapid kinetics of intimal hyperplasia formation, however, lead to a predominantly cellular lesion with moderate amounts of extracellular matrix, whereas atherosclerosis develops slowly over many decades leading to necrotic, lipid-laden lesions with a relatively sparse cellular component.

Platelets

Platelets have long been known to play a central role in the reaction of a vessel wall to injury. To date, most research in this area has focused on the activation of platelets by the injured endothelium as the major factor in the development of intimal hyperplasia. Denudation of the arterial wall exposes the subendothelial matrix, which leads to adherence of platelets. This adherence requires the interaction of subendothelial collagen, a platelet membrane glycoprotein receptor GPIb, plasma von Willebrand factor, and fibronectin. Following adherence, platelets undergo a morphologic change, stretch to cover the exposed surface, and release a variety of stored granule products. Classically, these secreted products have been categorized according to the three types of granules in which they are stored: lysosomes, alpha granules, and dense granules. Lysosomes contain a large variety of hydrolases and other enzymes. Alpha granules contain the adhesive glycoprotein molecules, coagulation factors, and important cellular mitogens such as platelet factor 4 and platelet-derived growth factor (PDGF). Dense granules are primarily composed of ATP, ADP, serotonin, and calcium. Alternatively, when describing platelet interaction with an injured vessel wall, it can be helpful to distinguish those activated platelet products that act to promote platelet aggregation from those that are primarily involved in SMC activation.

Activated platelets subsequently release ADP and activate the arachidonic acid pathway to release thromboxane (TxA_2). Both of these factors lead to platelet aggregation. Recruitment of platelets requires the rapid expression of the platelet membrane receptor complex GPIIb and GPIIIa, both of which promote platelet aggregation through the binding of circulating fibrinogen. Platelet adhesion and granule release also lead to a parallel acceleration of the coagulation cascades. This activation of clotting pathways, combined with high local concentrations of fibrinogen mediated by binding to the glycoprotein IIb/IIIa complex, results in a fibrin protein network that further stabilizes the aggregated platelet plug. Once platelet aggregation is initiated by the pathways previously mentioned, its further formation is actively inhibited by an intact endothelium. Thus, a damaged endothelium not only initiates platelet activation but also impairs its inhibition.

With activation of platelets there is secretion of PDGF along with other granule constituents including platelet factor 4, thromboglobulin, and thrombospondin. PDGF is a cationic protein with a molecular weight of 28,000 to 31,000. It is comprised of two subunits (A and B). Physiologically, PDGF functions as both a chemo-attractant as well as a mitogen for SMCs and fibroblasts. Because it has been shown to bind with high affinity to SMCs, it has been suggested that PDGF may attract the SMCs from the media into the intima, bind to them, and stimulate their proliferation. Interestingly, recent evidence has shown that the platelet may not be the only source of this protein. PDGF (A and B subunits) is produced by human umbilical vein and saphenous vein endothelial cells. In fact, a large increase in PDGF production can be measured in injured endothelial cells. Also, both A- and B-subunit messenger ribonucleic acid (mRNA) have been noted in fresh endarterectomy specimens obtained during carotid surgery.[11] Lastly, SMCs themselves produce PDGF-like activity in response to arterial injury, and it has been shown that SMCs from human atheroma contain mRNA for the PDGF A-subunit.[12] Taken together, these findings may explain how intimal proliferation continues after re-endothelialization occurs. PDGF may be released by both platelets and endothelial cells causing activation migration of SMCs, which then secrete additional PDGF leading to proliferation.

Inflammatory Cell Pathways

For many years it has been suspected that the biologic pathways of inflammation and cellular proliferation are closely related. Frequently, these processes occur together during normal physiologic responses to injury. Evidence connecting these pathways is particulary strong in the case of vascular injury. At any time, a significant portion of the intravascular pool of polymorphonuclear leukocytes (PMNs) are adherent to the vascular endothelium. Furthermore, PMN adhesion and infiltration is a common finding following arterial wall injury. Electron microscopic studies, after a balloon catheter intimal injury, have shown that leukocytes attach to the de-endothelialized surface of an arterial lumen.[13] Both monocytes and lymphocytes also adhere to damaged endothelium and, in some instances, even penetrate it. Finally, in addition to being present at the site of vessel wall injury, white blood cells have been demonstrated to secrete substances capable of stimulating the growth of intimal lesions.[14]

The association between inflammation and intimal proliferation was recently demonstrated in an impressive *in vivo* model of vasculitis.[15] In this study, endotoxin-soaked thread was placed on one-half of a rat femoral artery to produce an inflammatory response. This technique consistently caused in a significant leukocyte infiltration that occurred only on the treated side of the vessel. Histologic examination 14 days later revealed nonuniform intimal lesions in which proliferating SMCs were located exclusively on the side of the lumen adjacent to the treated half of the arterial wall. Clearly, these findings again suggest an association between inflammatory and proliferative biologic pathways. The mechanisms controlling this relationship are an obvious target for therapeutic intervention and have therefore become an area of intense investigation.

Neutrophil adhesion to the surface of endothelial cells is controlled by several complex glycoproteins located on the surface of both endothelial and white blood cells. Together, these binding molecules constitute a sophisticated communications system.

To date, two endothelial cell adhesion molecules involved in neutrophil binding have been well characterized: the endothelial-leukocyte adhesion molecule-1 (ELAM-1) and the intercellular adhesion molecule-1 (ICAM-1). ELAM-1 is either unexpressed or simply remains intracellular in the nonactive endothelial cell. After activation by a variety of different cytokines, however, this adhesion complex is rapidly induced and can be seen on the membrane surface of the stimulated endothelial cell. Both the physiologic function of this molecule and the specific leukocyte receptor to which it binds remain unknown. ICAM-1 is located, in small amounts, on the surface of nonactive endothelial cells. Following activation by either injury or a variety of stimulating agonists, the expression of this binding complex is significantly increased. ICAM-1 is the binding ligand for the CD11a/CD18 receptor on the leukocyte membrane.

Histochemically, the adhesion molecules located in the surface membranes of white blood cells, which are responsible for leukocyte binding to endothelial cells, can be separated into three related heterodimers. Each of these heterodimer protein complexes are composed of an α and a β subunit. The α subunit differs between the three glycoprotein complexes (either CD11a, CD11b, or CD11c) whereas the β subunit remains constant (CD18). The CD11a/CD18 complex is found on the surface of all white blood cells and is thought to mediate the attachment of unstimulated neutrophils to stimulated endothelial cells. This binding is probably through an interaction with the ICAM-1 receptor, which, as mentioned, is expressed on the lumenal surface of activated or injured endothelial cells. The binding of the CD11a/CD18 complex to the ICAM-1 receptor has also been suggested as playing a role in cytokine induced transendothelial migration of neutrophils. The CD11b/CD18 adhesion complex is also referred to as either MAC-1 or the C3b complement receptor. This glycoprotein has been implicated in the adhesion of chemotactically stimulated neutrophils and controls several cellular functions such as aggregation and cytotoxicity. Finally, the third heterodimer complex CD11c/CD18 has been shown to exist both on PMNs and monocytes but its role in binding to endothelial cells remains undetermined.

During inflammatory states, the attachment of neutrophils to the involved endothelium is greatly increased due primarily to the up-regulation, and enhanced expression, of the binding glycoproteins. A variety of substances is known to be capable of stimulating this enhanced neutrophil adherence and together are thought to be the primary mediators of the inflammatory response to tissue injury. Interleukin-1, tumor necrosis factor-α, lymphotoxin, and bacterial endotoxins (lipopolysaccharides, LPS) all increase the production of both ELAM-1 and ICAM-1 on the surface of affected endothelial cells. In addition, PMN activation can be stimulated by several substances that are released after inflammation. Examples include the complement factors C5a and C3b, which stimulate PMN chemotaxis and phagocytosis, respectively. Likewise PMN adhesion and chemotaxis can also be stimulated by interleukin-1, xanthine oxidase, PDGF, as well as the lipid mediators leukotriene B and platelet activating factor. Finally, tumor necrosis factor is an important mediator of PMN phagocytosis and can lead to increased lysosomal enzyme release.

Following activation and adhesion to the damaged vessel lumen, white blood cells have been demonstrated to migrate into the arterial wall. In one study, 42 days after a denuding injury, leukocytes were shown to penetrate the arterial media and were seen deep within the hyperplastic lesions.[16] The mechanisms triggering this leukocyte migration remain unknown. One possibility is that this process is mediated by the exposure of medial SMCs that follows an endothelial injury. Serum containing media that has been conditioned with SMCs has been demonstrated to stimulate leukocyte migration. More important, others have shown that SMCs and macrophages elaborate potent chemotactic factors for leukocytes, suggesting that these cells could sustain continued white blood cell recruitment.[17] Other chemotactic agents for leukocytes include PDGF and, in some reports, factors released by fibroblasts. Finally, it is interesting that SMCs removed from atherosclerotic plaques express ICAM-1, indicating a possible connection between these medial cells and leukocyte recruitment and activation.

After penetrating the injured arterial wall, the mechanism by which leukocytes may initiate the formation of intimal hyperplasia also remains unknown. Again, several pathways have been suggested. After a denuding endothelial injury and the deposition of inflammatory cells, a variety of inflammatory products may be elaborated. These include chemotactic factors, growth factors, complement components, and enzymes. One of the most studied substances is monocyte and macrophage derived growth factor (MDGF). MDGF is a well-known stimulator of SMC and fibroblast proliferation. This growth factor is similar and may be identical to PDGF. Thus, the stimulation of SMC proliferation may be one mechanism by which inflammatory cells may contribute to the formation of intimal hyperplasia. A second possibility involves the production of lysosomal degradation enzymes. Activated leukocytes secrete several potent proteases capable of degrading collagen, basement membranes, and other important extracellular structural proteins. One example of a PMN derived enzyme, which has been implicated in peri-inflammatory extracellular damage, is myeloperoxidase. Liberation of these destructive enzymes into the wall of an injured vessel may weaken the extracellular matrix. This loosening of the vessel wall may facilitate the migration of SMCs from the medial layer toward the lumen. Lastly, leukocytes may also act directly at sites of vessel injury to worsen the degree of endothelial injury. PMNs can produce oxygen free radicals through the action of the NADPH oxidase system, which is present on their membranes. The toxic substances elaborated by these activated PMNs, including superoxide anion, hydrogen peroxide, and hydroxyl radicals, can damage endothelial cells and alter capillary permeability. With neutrophil activation, therefore, marginally injured endothelial cells bordering a lesion may be destroyed, increasing the magnitude of the damage to the vessel wall. This further exposure of the subendothelial layer allows for more platelet cell adherence, aggregation, and activation, as well as the recruitment of more leukocyte mediators and therefore the stimulation of a continued cycle of inflammatory injury.

The Renin-Angiotensin System

The classic physiologic role given to the renin-angiotensin system is primarily that of a feedback-controlled endocrine system designed for the homeostatic regulation of hemodynamic and electrolytic balance. The function of this system may be summarized as follows. Renin is released by renal tissue in response to decreased perfusion pressures and circulates in the plasma where it converts angiotensinogen, generated by the liver, into angiotensin I. Angiotensin I is cleaved into active angiotensin II by angiotensin-converting enzyme (ACE) found primarily in the lungs. Angiotensin II then binds to specific angiotensin II receptors located in peripheral vascular arterial beds, and thereby exerts its homeostatic hemodynamic effects. The blood pressure and electrolyte changes, mediated by the components of the renin-angiotensin system, are numerous. In addition to vasoconstriction, potent actions of angiotensin II include modulation of prostaglandin release, expression of angiotensin II receptors, stimulation of angiogenesis, as well as complex adrenal, renal, and central nervous system effects.

Recent work suggests that this classic view of the circulating renin-angiotensin requires revision. Briefly, given the accepted amounts of angiotensin II produced and cleared from the peripheral tissues, the quantity of both angiotensin I and angiotensin

II, which can be measured in venous blood, is higher than can be explained by their generation in blood alone. It has been hypothesized, therefore, that a second source of production for these circulating angiotensins may be the peripheral tissues. According to this theory, the primary role of the renin-angiotensin pathway is the delivery of renin and angiotensinogen to the peripheral tissues, not the systemic production of angiotensin II. The endothelial-based ACE in the tissues then acts on the plasma-derived renin and angiotensinogen to produce most angiotensin II. This explains the high plasma levels of angiotensin II measured in venous blood, which is the result of "spill over" from tissue production sites. More important, if a large fraction of angiotensin II is produced locally, it is possible that this production may be controlled by tissue-specific mechanisms of regulation. From these theories, the concept of an integrated but distinct tissue renin-angiotensin system has recently evolved.

The idea that angiotensin II in the vascular wall is produced locally, and not delivered by the systemic circulation, was originally suggested by Swales and Thurston.[18] Subsequent evidence, suggesting the existence of a locally active vascular renin-angiotensin system, operating independently of the classical systemic circuit, is convincing. First, angiotensinogen mRNA, the only known precursor of the angiotensin peptides, has been detected in extrahepatic tissues including the aorta. Also, using monoclonal antirenin antibodies, immunohistochemical studies have stained positively for the presence of renin in vascular cells. Subsequent tissue culture studies have shown that, both vascular smooth muscle and endothelial cells can produce renin *in vitro.* Also, mRNA coding for renin has been identified in human vascular SMCs. Finally, it is widely accepted that ACE is present in large quantities on the luminal surface of endothelial cells. Thus, the normally functioning vascular wall possesses all the components necessary for the independent local production of angiotensin II.

The biologic role of locally produced angiotensin II is unknown. Several possibilities have been postulated. One interesting theory regarding the physiologic function of a locally active renin-angiotensin system involves the autocrine balance of vascular wall metabolic activity and tone. As mentioned, angiotensin II receptors have been identified on vascular endothelial cells, SMCs, and circulating platelets. Stimulation of endothelial cell bound angiotensin II receptors leads to the secretion of prostacyclin (PGI_2) and possibly endothelial-derived relaxant factor (EDRF). Both of these substances are known to cause medial SMC relaxation. However, activation of SMC angiotensin receptors causes the opposite effect. Stimulation of SMC angiotensin II receptors causes increased protein production and proliferation *in vitro.*[19] Also, this stimulation is abolished by saralazin, an angiotensin II receptor antagonist. Thus, regulation of the tissue production and action of angiotensin II in the vessel wall may play a role in modulating vascular tone and angiogenesis.

The existence of a tissue renin-angiotensin system, complete with its own locally specific control mechanisms, has led some investigators to study the role angiotensin II may have on the subsequent development of intimal hyperplasia. One general theory holds that endothelial damage, which invariably accompanies vascular injuries, may alter the balance of the local renin-angiotensin system. This may allow the stimulatory effects of angiotensin II, on the medial SMCs, to proceed uncontrolled. Another possible mechanism for the promotion of hyperplastic intimal growth by the local production of angiotensin II involves the activation of platelet metabolic pathways. As mentioned, platelets specifically bind angiotensin II, and it is thought that platelet stimulation and release of PDGF may contribute to the formation of intimal hyperplasia. In a recent study by Swartz and Moore,[20] it was shown that angiotensin II increased both collagen-induced platelet aggregation and secretion of TxA_2. Finally, expression of PDGF by activated SMCs has been demonstrated to be enhanced by the presence of angiotensin II.[21]

Coagulation Pathways and the Locally Active Fibrinolytic System

The establishment of a mature intimal lesion following an arterial insult requires the combination of several biologic pathways. The components and pathways that make up the body's coagulation system are extremely complex. It is likely that the products of these pathways participate in important and diverse ways in the development of intimal hyperplasia. As mentioned, the formation of a fibrin matrix in an area of endothelial damage helps stablize the aggregating platelet plug. Furthermore, many other substances, released by the adjacent organizing thrombus, may affect nearby medial SMCs independently. One important and intensely studied of these coagulation products is plasmin.

Plasmin is a proteolytic enzyme and is the active end-product of the tissue plasminogen-plasmin system. Other important components of this system include the precursor plasminogen and its main endogenous activators, urokinase-type plasminogen activator (uPA) and tissue-type plasminogen activator (tPA). The catalytic action of these proteases are inhibited *in vivo* by the plasmin inhibitors α_2-antiplasmin, α_2-macroglobulin, as well as a group of related plasminogen activator inhibitory proteins. In recent years, much has been learned about the interactions of these components at the cellular level and their role in the formation of hyperplastic intimal lesions. The steps leading to intimal lesions include SMC activation within the media, migration of these cells across the internal elastic lamina, and, finally, replication within the neointima. Although the regulation and stimulation of SMC activity have been studied extensively, the mechanisms involved in SMC migration have not been studied as thoroughly, and exactly how these cells traverse the thick medial collagenous extracellular matrix remains an interesting and unresolved issue. One idea proposed to explain this phenomenon involves the proteolytic products of the tissue plasminogen-plasmin system.

The hypothesis that plasmin is involved in SMC migration has been derived from several related observations. While an intact endothelium impedes the penetration of circulating plasminogen (which is a large protein), a damaged endothelium, however, allows this protein to readily diffuse into the medial cell layer. Plasmin, produced by the extracellular conversion of this plasminogen, can matabolize several matrix proteins as well as activate several other potent collagenases. Conversion of accumulated plasminogen, of course, is dependent on the presence of specific plasminogen activators. In an *in vivo* model of arterial repair, Clowes and associates[22] have shown that vascular SMCs express large amounts of both uPA and tPA. These experimental observations have led to the following hypothesis. Endothelial damage may permit the local penetration of circulating plasminogen and other chemotactic substances (elaborated from activated platelets and leukocytes) into the arterial wall. Subsequent production of specific plasminogen activators by medial SMCs leads to the formation of plasmin. High levels of extracellular plasmin then cause the destruction of important structural matrix proteins. This process can be enhanced by the presence of leukocyte derived enzymes. Lastly, growth and chemotatic factors initiate activation of SMCs and stimulate migration of these cells across the weakened arterial wall. Also, because the gradient of plasminogen and mitogenic activity is greatest adjacent to the endothelial defect, the direction of migration is determined automatically. Precise characterization of the role of local plasminogen-plasmin pathways in the development of intimal hyperplasia requires further research.

Cellular Growth Factors

The stimulation of vascular SMC growth is the final common pathway of all postulated mechanisms leading to the development of intimal hyperplasia. Viewing the vascular wall as a complex integrated organ, complete with its own endogenous local autocrine system, is an emerging concept that is gaining support. In this theory, intimal hyperplasia is postulated to result from an imbalance of these local hormonal systems. This could be due to either an excess of stimulatory molecules or from the absence or reduction of inhibitory hormones.

PDGF, MDGF, and angiotensin II are all examples of cellular growth factors believed to be involved in the formation of hyperplastic intimal lesions; each has been reviewed in detail. In addition to these mitogens, basic fibroblast growth factor (bFGF) is another promotor of SMC growth deserving comment. bFGF is a potent stimulator of angiogenesis. Researchers studying intimal hyperplasia have become interested in this protein for several reasons. It has been suggested that direct SMC damage may be an important stimulus for subsequent SMC activation. These data come from research that shows that the response of an arterial wall to injury varies depending on the method of injury. Balloon catheterization, which damages both the medial SMCs as well as the endothelium, causes a large proliferative response.[23] However, wire denudation, which significantly damages the endothelium but does not injure the medial cells, results in much less SMC activation.[24] Furthermore, recent reports have shown that intimal lesions, following a balloon catheter injury, occur even in the absence of platelets.[25] This work implies that elaboration of PDGF, in this setting, may not be required for the subsequent stimulation of SMC replication. Thus, damaged SMCs may stimulate replication of adjacent undamaged medial cells by the release of an endogenous intracellular growth factor. Because bFGF is synthesized by SMCs, and the expression of bFGF mRNA in these cells is increased following injury, it has been postulated that bFGF is this endogenous growth factor.

Several studies have been undertaken to investigate the role of bFGF in the development of hyperplastic intimal lesions. In one such study by Lindner and associates,[26] arteries were exposed to bFGF following an injury with a balloon catheter. In this experiment, SMC replication increased from 11.5% to 54.8% after exposure to bFGF. Also, an equivalent increase was seen in vessels denuded by the wire loop technique, suggesting that bFGF is able to up-regulate undamaged medial cells. It is notable that when bFGF was administered to normal nondenuded arteries, no effect on SMC growth was observed. Lastly, prolonged exposure of the growth factor was found to result in a twofold increase in intimal thickness compared to control vessels. In a related study, Cuevas et al.[27] demonstrated that the direct local infusion of bFGF, into either normal adventitia or injured media, results in proliferation of both vasa vasorum and vascular SMCs.

The cellular growth factors discussed so far are all peptide cellular mitogens. Recently, nonpeptide molecules have also been shown to be important modulators of SMC growth. Nitric oxide (NO), previously identified as EDRF, is normally secreted by endothelium, and its levels are decreased following endothelial damage. Although the exact pathways are still being determined, NO has been shown to inhibit vascular SMC proliferation and DNA synthesis *in vitro*.[28] The manipulation of NO production at sites of arterial injury may be an important new tool in the pharmacologic control of intimal hyperplastic lesions.

In summary, it appears probable that the balance of locally produced cellular growth factors, such as bFGF and NO, play an important role in the regulation of SMC activity and the subsequent development of intimal hyperplasia. Clearly, research into ways to influence this balance will have meaningful implications for the pharmacologic management of these lesions.

PHARMACOLOGIC MANAGEMENT

The ability of various pharmacologic agents to inhibit the development of intimal hyperplasia has been well documented. The large variety of medications that has been effective in limiting this response is both striking and confusing. Many different classes of drugs, including antihypertensive agents, antilipid metabolites, antiplatelet agents, anti-inflammatory agents, and anticoagulants, have been shown to be at least partially effective. In addition, many other substances that interfere with normal cellular growth have also shown promise. Unfortunately, because of the nonuniformity of both the doses and duration of the agents studied and the models of intimal hyperplasia used, comparison of the results of these trials is difficult. As a result, clinical effectiveness of pharmacologic therapy, in this setting, remains undetermined. Clearly, this attests to the complexity of the biologic pathways involved in the development of this lesion and suggests that no one agent will likely be totally effective in its prevention. Combination treatments, local drug delivery systems, and other new methods to improve the specificity and local concentrations of therapeutic agents have shown some promise. To date, however, no treatment has achieved complete effectiveness. In this section we review several approaches to the pharmacologic control of intimal hyperplasia. For clarity, we have divided our discussion into sections determined by the biologic modulator being manipulated.

Modulation of Lipid Metabolism

The connection between atherogenesis and increased levels of plasma LDL has long been appreciated. Studies quantifying the plasma concentration of LDL among Eskimos have demonstrated much lower levels in this population group compared to age matched Danes.[29] This difference could play a role in the strikingly low incidence of atherosclerotic heart disease seen in the Eskimo population. Additional characterization of plasma lipid compositions has revealed that Eskimos possess extremely low levels of circulating arachidonic acid as well as unusually high concentrations of eicosapentanoic acid (EPA).[30] EPA is an omega-3 polyunsaturated fatty acid. It is present in large amounts in fish but humans cannot synthesize EPA *de novo*. Following ingestion, EPA competes directly with arachidonic acid in prostaglandin synthesis pathways. Whereas arachidonic acid metabolism leads to the formation of TxA_2, a potent stimulator of platelet aggregation, EPA is converted into TxA_3, which has no effect on platelet function.

Many studies have tested the theory that increased levels of EPA, present at the time of an endothelial injury, may alter the production of intimal hyperplasia. The ability of small doses of marine oils to inhibit intimal thickening has been reported in vein graft models by both Cahill et al.[31] and Landymore et al.[32] More recently, O-hara et al.[33] have demonstrated a marked reduction of intimal hyperplasia in a rabbit polytetrafluoroethylene (PTFE) graft model, following administration of EPA.

Additional studies will be required in order to establish both the specific pathways by which EPA alters intimal hyperplasia as well as the optimal dose and duration of exposure of this and related agents.

Modulation of Platelet Function

Attempts to inhibit intimal hyperplasia by interfering with platelet activation pathways have yielded disappointing results. One of the early studies, which suggested a role for platelets in these lesions, was reported by Friedman et al.[34] This group found that following an aortic balloon catheter injury, thrombocytopenic rabbits formed less intimal hyperplasia. Prevention of intimal hyperplasia was then attempted using a number of different antiplatelet drugs. Antiplatelet drugs block the synthesis of prostaglandins by inhibiting arachidonic acid metabolic pathways. Aspirin irreversibly inhibits platelet cell function by acetylating cyclooxygenase. Dipyridamole increases cytoplasmic cyclic AMP and blocks the precursors thromboxane A_1 and B_2. Therefore, because both aspirin and dipyridamole interfere with platelet adherence and aggregation by inhibiting the production of prostaglandin metabolites, it seemed logical to propose that these agents could be useful in preventing intimal hyperplasia. Unfortunately, attempts to inhibit this response using antiplatelet agents (aspirin, dipyridamole, and ibuprofen) have so far failed to yield encouraging results.

In experimental models and clinical trials, exposure to aspirin has resulted in decreased platelet adherence to prosthetic vascular grafts.[35] Whether or not the addition of dipyridamole enhances this effect remains inconclusive. Importantly, although antiplatelet agents decrease platelet aggregation and thrombus formation, data from other laboratories have demonstrated that they have no effect on initial platelet deposition.[36] The consequence of these agents on graft patency and hyperplasia formation has also been inconsistent. In one study using rhesus monkeys, iliac arteries were ligated bilaterally and autologous vein bypass grafts were constructed.[37] Beginning 3 weeks before the surgical procedure, the experimental animals were administered aspirin (165 mg, administered twice daily) and dipyridamole (25 mg, administered twice daily). At sacrifice, 16 weeks after the procedure, the intimal thickening was examined and found to be markedly reduced in the experimental group. In a follow-up study using a balloon catheter injury in rabbits, however, no difference between the two groups was observed with respect to tritiated thymidine incorporation, nuclear proliferation, or progression of intimal hyperplasia.[38] In a similar study, also performed in rabbits, aspirin greatly improved the patency of an end-to-side iliac anastomosis but had no effect on the formation of intimal hyperplasia.[39]

Thromboxane (TxA_2) is synthesized and stored in platelets. It is formed by the action of the enzyme TxA_2 synthetase on cyclic endoperoxide precursors from the arachidonic acid pathways and is a powerful mediator of both platelet aggregation and vascular constriction. Thromboxane synthetase inhibitors block this conversion of intermediate endoperoxide precursors into TxA_2. Furthermore, while doing so, the prostaglandin metabolic pathways are shifted toward the production of PGI_2. Thus, theoretically, TxA_2 synthetase inhibitors actually enhance the production of endothelial cell derived PGI_2 while blocking platelet derived TxA_2. It has therefore been postulated that these agents might be more specific inhibitors of platelet function than aspirin compounds. In a recent report the ability of TxA_2 synthetase inhibition to prevent distal anastomotic intimal hyperplasia was studied and compared to aspirin.[40] Two different types of grafts were evaluated in a bilateral aortoiliac bypass graft model: thin-walled PTFE and PTFE seeded with autologous endothelial cells. Treatment groups consisted of antiplatelet therapy with either the TxA_2 synthetase inhibitor U-63,577A or aspirin. Surprisingly, aspirin was significantly more effective in maintaining patency and preventing hyperplasia in both types of grafts. Considering the TxA_2 synthetase inhibitor group alone, however, the drug was more effective in seeded than nonseeded bypass grafts. Furthermore, patency of both seeded and nonseeded grafts was improved when compared to no therapy at all. It appears that, in combination with other antiplatelet drugs, these agents could prove to be important inhibitors of platelet function and may have a role in reducing the hyperplastic reaction of a vessel wall following an endothelial injury. No substantiated clinical trials, however, are as of yet available.

To summarize the available data at the present time, antiplatelet drugs would seem to improve the patency of vein and prosthetic bypass grafts, but do not appear to significantly inhibit the formation of intimal hyperplasia. New approaches and agents, however, are continually being studied. Platelet aggregation in response to collagen and ADP has been reduced by blocking GPIIb and GPIIIa with a murine monoclonal antibody (LJ-CP8).[41] Unfortunately, in an arteriovenous shunt model, this antibody failed to decrease deposition of platelets on Dacron or PTFE grafts.[42] Clearly, additional studies will be required in order to determine the clinical potential of these newer agents.

Modulation of Inflammatory Pathways

Several investigators have postulated that leukocyte pathways may play a role in the development of intimal hyperplasia. This theory is supported by the fact that leukocyte infiltration is observed in hyperplastic intimal lesions. Also, it has been demonstrated that these accumulated white blood cells possess sufficient enzymatic and mitogenic activity to stimulate medial SMCs. Although many approaches designed to modulate the inflammatory contribution to the formation of intimal hyperplasia have been described, most work in this area has focused on the immunosuppressive glucocorticoids and cyclosporin.

In 1979, Hoepp et al.[43] did not find any significant differences, in patency or intimal response, between steroid-treated and control groups in a canine femoropopliteal Dacron bypass graft model. However, the animals in this experiment were given a relatively low dose of a short acting steroid (methyl-prednisolone), and the agent was administered only after the procedure and preoperatively. In 1988, a report by Gordon and associates[44] was among the earliest to suggest that glucocorticoids could inhibit SMC proliferation after an endothelial injury. These investigators found that the administration of the endogenous steroid dehydroepiandrosterone led to a decrease in the production of atherosclerotic plaques in hypercholesterolemic rabbits. More recently, clinical trials have been attempted. The M-HEART project, a large, randomized, double-blind clinical study, investigated whether or not steroids could decrease the rate of restenosis following balloon angioplasty.[45] In this study, a single large dose of methylprednisolone (1 g) was given intravenously prior to the procedure. The results did not find any significant difference between steroid and placebo treated groups. It may be significant that it has been shown that the period of maximal intimal proliferation following an arterial injury is between 2 to 4 weeks.[23] Furthermore, the results of many studies have demonstrated that beginning steroid treatment prior to the arterial injury may be important. This may explain the negative results found in the M-HEART project study in which a relatively short-acting steroid was given as a single one-time dose. With these principles in mind, our laboratory recently investigated the use of steroids in a balloon catheter injury model performed in rabbits. Dexamethasone (0.10 mg/kg given intramuscularly) was administered 2 days before the endothelial injury and was continued for a period of 8 weeks. This treatment was found to result in a dramatic reduction of intimal growth.[46] Furthermore, in a follow-up study, this response to dexamethasone therapy was found to be dose dependent.[47]

How glucocorticoids prevent or suppress the development of intimal hyperplasia remains unclear. One theory involves the well-known actions these agents have on fibroblast growth and wound healing. Studies have shown that glucocorticoids can slow the growth of cultured fibroblast cell lines.[48] Also, *in vitro* studies clearly demonstrate decreased leukocyte aggregation to several chemotactic factors in the presence of steroids.[49] In addition, steroids have been observed to decrease adhesion between leukocytes and endothelial cells.[50] Although the mechanism of this inhibition remains unknown, in some neoplastic cell lines, dexamethasone has been related to ICAM-1 inhibition.[51] Lastly, steroids have been shown to alter white blood cell cytotoxic function. In this setting, steroids decrease the production of superoxide anions and inhibit the release of zymogen granules.[52] In addition to this experimental data, *in vivo* studies have also suggested a mechanism by which steroids may prevent intimal hyperplasia. In one such study, high dose methyl-prednisolone was found to prevent endothelial sloughing in vein grafts.[53] This effect on endothelial sloughing may decrease one of the main stimuli leading to SMC activation: an absent endothelium. Finally, studies have shown that dexamethasone has an inhibitory effect on tPA activity.[54] Therefore, inhibition of medial SMC migration may represent another mechanism by which steroids prevent the formation of intimal lesions.

The effect of cyclosporin treatment on the subsequent development of intimal hyperplasia was recently studied in a rat common iliac artery injury model.[55] Before the arterial injury, animals were given parenteral cyclosporin at a dose of 5 mg/kg/day. The drug was continued for 2 and 6 weeks. Results demonstrated that arteries treated with cyclosporin formed significantly less medial thickening at each time interval. Like steroids, the mechanism of cyclosporin's efficacy in this model has not been characterized. As mentioned, atherosclerotic plaques contain activated lymphocytes and SMCs, and these cells do express class II major histocompatibility antigens. Interaction of these antigens and immune cells may propagate an immune response that results in release of other inflammatory mediators and cytokines. The exact role of the immune system in the evolution of intimal hyperplasia, and whether modulation of these pathways will lead to a clinically useful strategy for preventing these lesions, will require further investigation.

Modulation of Components of the Renin-Angiotensin System

Powell and associates[56] were the first to report the ability of an ACE inhibitor to prevent intimal proliferation after a vascular injury. In this preliminary study, rats were given 10 mg/kg of cilazapril, mixed with their normal food, beginning 6 days before an endothelial injury. The drug was administered daily and continued for 14 days. The results demonstrated that the experimental group experienced a significant reduction in the amount of subsequent intimal thickening. In addition, this reduction was independent of any changes in several measured hemodynamic variables. Also, the same authors demonstrated the reversal of this effect following the intravenous infusion of angiotensin III.[57] Recently, using a vein graft model of intimal hyperplasia, O'Donohoe and associates[58] reported encouraging results following the long-term administration of an ACE inhibitor. In this study, experimental animals received daily enteral captopril doses of 10 mg/kg. The agent was begun 1 week prior to the procedure and continued 28 days until each animal was sacrificed. Impressively, histologic evaluation of the experimental grafts revealed a 40% reduction in intimal thickness when compared to controls. Finally, using a hyperlipidemic rabbit model, one recent study reported a statistically significant reduction in aortic atherosclerosis following the administration of captopril.[59]

In our laboratory we have studied the effect of chronic ACE inhibition with enalaprilat on the development of intimal hyperplasia following an arterial injury.[60] Enalaprilat was chosen because it is available in injectable form. One disturbing problem, common to all of these *in vivo* animal studies previously described, is that the models used rely on oral consumption of the pharmacologic agent. This route of drug administration in animal studies has frequently been criticized for making the interpretation of observed results difficult and perhaps unreliable. Also, enalaprilat is much longer-acting than the injectable form of captopril. It is therefore better suited for animal studies in which once-a-day dosing is better tolerated and more practical. In our study, a standardized carotid artery endothelial injury was produced in adult New Zealand white rabbits.[60] Control animals received injections of isotonic saline. Experimental animals were given enalaprilat at a dose of 0.07 mg/kg. All injections were begun 1 day before the arterial injury and continued daily, five times a week, for 8 weeks. After the arterial segments were removed, the degree of hyperplastic intimal change was calculated. The results demonstrated that experimental animals treated with enalaprilat developed significantly less intimal hyperplasia than control animals.

The biology of the renin-angiotensin system and its role in the pathophysiology of several disorders is currently undergoing intense research. Likewise, elucidation of the precise mechanisms by which ACE inhibitors prevent or suppress intimal hyperplasia are under investigation. Early studies suggest that this response is probably due to the interruption of the locally active renin-angiotensin system with the subsequent reduction of angiotensin II, a potent medial SMC mitogen. The possibility that these drugs possess a direct inhibitory effect on SMCs is another potential mechanism. In their study, however, Powell et al.[56] failed to demonstrate any effect on human SMC proliferation *in vitro* by ACE inhibitors or their metabolites. Clearly, a complete understanding of these pathways may lead to the development of clinically useful treatment protocols as well as more specific pharmacologic agents to control this response. At least one clinical trial designed to analyze the ability of ACE inhibitors to prevent restenosis following angioplasty procedures is already underway.

Modulation of Coagulation Pathways

As discussed, circulating coagulation cascades and their end products may be important components of the complex biologic system that leads to the development of intimal hyperplasia. Since heparin is a well characterized and available inhibitor of the plasma-bound clotting cascades, it was a logical starting point for studies investigating pharmacologic methods of inhibiting these pathways. It has been long accepted that heparin given perioperatively can prevent early thrombosis in peripheral bypass grafts. It has always been assumed that this action is due to the drug's effect on the thrombotic coagulation cascades. Recently, however, *in vitro* and *in vivo* studies have demonstrated that heparin can inhibit both SMC migration and proliferation.[61,62] The precise mechanism of this effect has not yet been established. Inhibition of bFGF, which is released by injured medial SMCs, is one hypothesis. Alternatively, Clowes and associates[57] have suggested that heparin reduces SMC migration by blocking degradation of the surrounding extracellular matrix. Supporting this view is evidence demonstrating that, in the arterial media, heparin decreases the expression of both tPA and collagenase.[57]

Low molecular weight (LMW) heparin is a preparation of short chain heparin polymers with much lower anticoagulant activity than standard heparin mixtures. Interestingly, new data seem to indicate that SMC antiproliferative activity is present in both anticoagulant and nonanticoagulant heparin fractions.[62] Excitement about these new LMW heparin molecules stems from their potential for controlling intimal hyperplasia without creating a systemic anticoagulated state. Evidence that LMW heparin may be effective in this regard has been published recently by at least one investigator.[62]

Modulation of Cellular Growth Factors

It has been suggested that medial SMC activation and the subsequent hyperplastic intimal lesions may be thought of as resulting from an imbalance in local vascular autocrine systems following an endothelial injury. Attempts to modulate this response through inhibition of important cellular growth factors has become a promising new area of investigation. One agent recently studied in this setting is somatostatin. Somatostatin is a widely occurring peptide hormone that acts as a modulator of a diverse class of endogenous growth promoters. Unfortunately, because of a very short half-life and instability in storage, it is difficult to use in *in vivo* models. Angiopeptin is a stable octapeptide somatostatin analog that has been shown to be an effective long-acting somatostatin receptor agonist. In animal models, this analog has been successful in suppressing the formation of intimal hyperplasia.[63] For example, Foegh et al.[64] reported that angiopeptin significantly reduced the amount of post-transplant coronary artery intimal hyperplasia in rabbits. This study was weakened, however, by the fact that these rabbits were also given cyclosporin. As discussed, cyclosporin has also been implicated as a potential inhibitor of hyperplastic intimal lesions. Whether or not angiopeptin is actually antagonizing the trophic effects of growth promoters in these studies is not clear. Direct SMC inhibition by angiopeptin has also been demonstrated in *in vitro* work, suggesting that the action of angiopeptin may not be related to activation of the somatostatin receptor. This view is further supported by the observation that some somatostatin analogs seem unable to inhibit intimal hyperplasia. Regardless, the concept of the vascular tree functioning as a complex local hormonal system, which can be controlled with pharmacologic therapy, remains an exciting area of investigation.

The use of conjugated toxins is another approach to inhibiting cellular growth factors that has recently been suggested. In this method, cellular growth mitogens are converted into "mitotoxins" by binding to specific cytotoxins. The new toxin is then delivered to the mitogenic receptor and prevents cellular growth by competitive inhibition. Recently, an example of one such cellular growth inhibitor has been constructed that competes for the bFGF receptor. This cytotoxin is made by conjugating the protein saporin to bFGF. Saporin is a potent inhibitor of cellular growth that works by inactivating cytoplasmic ribosomes. In one *in vivo* model of endothelial injury, administration of the bFGF-saporin compound resulted in significantly decreased numbers of replicating SMCs located in the arterial wall.[26] Further investigation is needed to determine if this, or other conjugated "mitotoxins," will be effective in controlling the development of intimal hyperplasia following an arterial injury.

Lastly, mention should be made of recent attempts to inhibit cellular growth by interfering with cellular proliferative pathways at the cytoplasmic level. It is well known that certain polyamines are critical substances involved in the regulation of cell growth and differentiation. Polyamines are synthesized from ornithine by the action of ornithine decarboxylase (ODC). Furthermore, this enzymatic reaction is the rate-limiting step that determines the amount of polyamine production. For this reason, ODC inhibition has been suggested as a possible way of preventing cellular proliferation. Evidence supporting this concept includes the fact that ODC activity has been shown to increase in tissues undergoing active cell division. To date, at least one animal model has been used to study the ability of ODC inhibition to prevent intimal hyperplasia.[65] Experimental animals were treated with α-difluoromethylornithine, an ODC inhibitor, and subsequently developed significantly less intimal hyperplasia than untreated controls.

FUTURE DIRECTIONS

Modulation of the Inflammatory Response

With increased information regarding the biologic pathways controlling leukocyte activation, it will probably be possible soon to specifically block receptors responsible for stimulating the development of intimal hyperplasia without inhibiting the systemic inflammatory response. MoAb 60.3 is a murine IgG monoclonal antibody that binds the CD18 epitope on the surface of leukocytes. Studies have shown that this antibody reduces neutrophil mediated tissue injury in a variety of physiologic settings. Administration of MoAb 60.3 to rabbits has reduced PMN adherence and prevented PMN tissue migration.[66] Of concern, however, is that patients exposed to this antibody could develop a symptom complex similar to that found in leukocyte adhesion molecule deficiency. In this disorder, the CD18 subunit is lacking and affected individuals suffer from severe recurrent bacterial infections and abnormal wound healing. Monoclonal antibody therapy directed at the leukocyte binding adhesion molecules that are expressed on the surface of vascular endothelial cells constitutes another, perhaps more promising, approach. This more specific therapy may reduce the severity of any adverse systemic effects of neutrophil inhibition. Several antibodies, which recognize both the ELAM-1 and ICAM-1 complexes, have already been developed and are potential candidates for this type of anti-intimal hyperplasia therapy. Despite the fact that these alternative approaches have not been specifically tested, they remain an exciting area of potential future research.

In Vivo Gene Transfer

The emergence of the necessary technology to isolate and transfer genetic material into human vascular cells has suggested new possibilities for the treatment of several disorders. Gene transfer methods are providing important information about the biology of vascular cells, and treatment strategies for problems such as thrombosis, atherosclerosis, vasculitis, and restenosis are already being evaluated.

The common denominator of most gene transfer techniques involves the introduction of new genetic information into the genome of specific vascular cells. These genetically altered cells subsequently express individual proteins or traits for which they have been engineered. The result is that the local biology of the vessel wall is altered in a specific and predetermined way. Most investigators have considered endothelial cells the ideal recipient for human gene therapy. This is because their location makes them easily accessible to recombinant vectors and allows for any produced products to be secreted directly into the bloodstream. Furthermore, endothelial seeding of vascular grafts and stents is an area of research that has already reached relatively advanced stages of development.

In vitro experiments have already been performed that have documented the ability to transfer specific genes into cultured endothelial cells.[67] Genes coding for neomycin resistance, β-galactosidase, growth hormone, prostacyclin, and tPA, have all been successfully transferred. In addition, transduced endothelial cells have been observed to survive and proliferate on both vascular prostheses and stainless steel stents. More recently, expression of recombinant gene products, by transduced endothelial cells, has also been achieved *in vivo*. In one series of experiments, genes responsible for β-galactosidase production were transferred into the iliofemoral arterial segments of pigs.[68] Following this gene transfer, detectable levels of the transduced gene were observed for as long as 5 months.[68] Likewise, the ability of a prosthetic vascular graft, lined with genetically modified endothelial cells, to express prolonged activity of a transduced gene has also been reported recently.[69]

The potential of genetically engineered vascular cells to modify the vessel wall and interfere with the development of intimal hyperplasia is obvious, and research into this possibility is developing rapidly. One workable avenue of research might be the establishment of a line of endothelial cells that are missing the DNA responsible for encoding the leukocyte adhesion molecules ELAM-1 and ICAM-1. When transduced into an endarterectomized or anastomosed vessel, these cells would then fail to initiate an inflammatory response and might thereby limit the development of intimal lesions. Clearly, the potential exists for this technology to someday play an important role in altering the complex pathways leading to the development of intimal hyperplasia.

Photodynamic Therapy

Proliferating intimal SMCs can be viewed as undifferentiated medial myofibroblasts whose growth fails to be inhibited by normal cellular controls. Seen in this way, intimal hyperplasia can be considered to be a benign neoplastic process. Because photodynamic therapy has been demonstrated to be safe and effective in the treatment of several rapidly growing benign neoplasms, it has recently been suggested as a possible means for controlling hyperplastic intimal lesions. Photodynamic therapy works by administering a chemosensitizing agent to living tissue. The agent is selectively concentrated in rapidly dividing cells, such as activated medial SMCs. Photoactivation of the chemosensitized tissue causes cell death and is achieved by exposing the tissue to light at a specific wavelength.

One of the first attempts to use this new method was reported by Neave et al.[70] in 1988. These investigators reported the destruction of fibrocellular atheroma in the aorta of rabbits treated with dihematoporphyrin ether porphyrin-II. Also, Mackie et al.[71] and Spear et al.[72] have shown that atherosclerotic plaque preferentially absorbs hematoporphyrin-II (photofrin) and that photodynamic therapy leads to a significant reduction in the fibrous portion of this atherosclerotic lesion. Unfortunately, due to the remaining calcified noncellular material, the atherosclerotic plaque could not be completely destroyed in these experiments. Nevertheless, since intimal hyperplasia is primarily fibrous and contains little if any calcified material, these early studies clearly show the potential of photodynamic therapy for the treatment of these lesions. Work in this area was also encouraged by Dartsch et al.[73] who found that human derived hyperplastic SMCs absorbed photofrin-II preferentially. Furthermore, this group demonstrated that subsequent exposure of these photofrin-II bound SMCs to light significantly inhibited their growth. Eton and associates[74] performed an *in vivo* study in which a photofrin compound was administered to rabbits following a carotid artery endothelial injury. Experimental animals were exposed to a standardized laser light energy source and the subsequent intimal thickening was compared to similarly injured controls. The results suggested that photodynamic therapy is able to diminish the amount of intimal hyperplasia following an arterial injury. Other investigators have demonstrated similar results recently.[75] This approach remains an intriguing area of study, and we and other researchers are pursuing ways to improve and control the results.

REFERENCES

1. Imparato AM, Bracco A, Kim GE, et al. Intimal and neointimal fibrous proliferation causing failure of arterial reconstructions. *Surgery*. 1972;72:1107–1117.

2. Colburn MD, Moore WS. Surgery or endovascular surgery for chronic lower extremity ischemia: what selection criteria should we use? In: Swedenborg J, Blohmé L, eds. *Risk Benefit Aspects of Vascular Surgery*. Stockholm: Scandinavian Surgical Society; 1994:249–276.
3. Carrel A, Guthrie CC. Anastomosis of blood vessels by the patching method and transplantation of the kidney. *JAMA*. 1906;47:1648–1651.
4. Imparato AM, Baumann FG, Pearson J, et al. Electron microscopic studies of experimentally produced fibromuscular arterial lesions. *Surg Gynecol Obstet*. 1974;139:497–504.
5. Berguer R, Higgins RF, Reddy DJ. Intimal hyperplasia: an experimental study. *Arch Surg*. 1980;115:332–335.
6. Zarins CK, Zatina MA, Giddens DP, et al. Shear stress regulation of artery lumen diameter in experimental atherogenesis. *J Vasc Surg*. 1987;5:413–420.
7. LoGerfo FW, Nowak MD, Quist WC, et al. Flow studies in a model carotid bifurcation. *Atherosclerosis*. 1981;1:235–241.
8. Phillips DJ, Greene FM, Langlois Y, et al. Flow velocity patterns in the carotid bifurcations of young, presumed normal subjects. *Ultrasound Med Biol*. 1983;9:39–49.
9. Lye CR, Sumner DS, Strandness DE. The transcutaneous measurement of the elastic properties of the human saphenous vein femoropopliteal bypass graft. *Surg Gynecol Obstet*. 1975; 141:891–895.
10. Abbott WM, Megerman J, Hasson JE, et al. Effect of compliance mismatch on vascular graft patency. *J Vasc Surg*. 1987;5:376–382.
11. Barrett T, Benditt E. Platelet-derived growth factor gene expression in human atherosclerotic plaques and in normal artery wall. *Proc Natl Acad Sci USA*. 1988;85:2810–2814.
12. Libby P, Warner S, Salomon R, et al. Production of platelet-derived growth factor-like mitogen by smooth muscle cells from human atheroma. *N Eng J Med*. 1988;318:1493–1498.
13. Cole C, Lucas J, Mikat E, et al. Adherence of polymorphonuclear leukocytes to injured rabbit aorta. *Surg Forum*. 1984;35:440–442.
14. Shimokado K, Raines E, Madtes D, et al. A significant part of macrophage-derived growth factor consists of at least two forms of PDGF. *Cell*. 1988;43:277–286.
15. Prescott MF, McBride CK, Venturini CM, et al. Leukocyte stimulation of intimal lesion formation is inhibited by treatment with diclofenac sodium and dexamethasone. *J Cardiovasc Pharmacol*. 1989;14:VI76–VI81.
16. Lucas J, Makhoul R, Cole C, et al. Mononuclear cells adhere to sites of vascular balloon catheter injury. *Curr Surg*. 1986;43:112–115.
17. Mazzone T, Jensen M, Chait A. Human arterial wall cells secrete factors that are chemotactic for monocytes. *Proc Natl Acad Sci USA*. 1983;80:5094–5097.
18. Swales JD, Thurston H. Generation of angiotensin II of peripheral vascular level: studies using angiotensin II antisera. *Clin Sci Mol Med*. 1973;45:691–700.
19. Campbell-Boswell M, Robertson AL. Effects of angiotensin II and vasopressin on human smooth muscle cells in vitro. *Exp Mol Path*. 1981;35:265.
20. Swartz S, Moore T. Effect of angiotensin II on collagen-induced platelet activation in normotensive subjects. *Thromb Haemo*. 1990;63:87–90.
21. Naftilan AJ, Pratt RE, Dzau VJ. Induction of platelet-derived growth factor A-chain and c-myc gene expressions by angiotensin II in cultured rat vascular smooth muscle cells. *J Clin Invest*. 1989;83:1419–1424.
22. Clowes AW, Clowes MM, Au YPT, et al. Smooth muscle cells express urokinase during mitogenesis and tissue-type plasminogen activator during migration in injured rat carotid artery. *Circ Res*. 1990;67:61–67.
23. Clowes AW, Reidy MA, Clowes MM. Kinetics of cellular proliferation after arterial injury. I. Smooth muscle growth in the absence of endothelium. *Lab Invest*. 1983;49:327–333.
24. Fingerle J, Au YPT, Clowes AW, et al. Intimal lesion formation in the rat carotid arteries after endothelial denudation in the absence of medial injury. *Arteriosclerosis*. 1990;10:1082–1087.
25. Fingerle J, Johnson R, Clowes AW, et al. Role of platelets in smooth muscle proliferation and migration after vascular injury in rat carotid artery. *Proc Natl Acad Sci USA*. 1989;86:8412–8416.
26. Lindner V, Lappi DA, Baird A, et al. Role of basic fibroblast growth factor in vascular lesion formation. *Circ Res*. 1991;68:106–113.

27. Cuevas P, Gonzalez AM, Carceller F, et al. Vascular response to basic fibroblast growth factor when infused onto the normal adventitia or into the injured media of the rat carotid artery. *Circ Res.* 1991;69:360–369.
28. Garg UC, Hassid A. Nitric oxide-generating vasodilators and 8-bromo-cyclicguanosine monophosphate inhibit mitogenesis and proliferation of cultured rat vascular smooth muscle cells. *J Clin Invest.* 1989;83:1774–1777.
29. Bang HO, Dyerberg J, Nielsen A. Plasma lipid and lipoprotein pattern in Greenlandic west-coast Eskimos. *Lancet.* 1971;1:1143–1145.
30. Dyerberg J, Bang HO, Stoffersen E, et al. Eicosapentanoic acid and prevention of thrombosis and atherosclerosis. *Lancet.* 1978;2:117–119.
31. Cahill PD, Sarris GE, Cooper AD, et al. Inhibition of vein graft intimal thickening by eicosapentanoic acid: reduced thromboxane production without change in lipoprotein levels or low-density lipoprotein receptor density. *J Vasc Surg.* 1988;7:108–117.
32. Landymore RW, Manku MS, Tan M, et al. Effects of low-dose marine oils on intimal hyperplasia in autologous vein grafts. *J Thor Cardiovasc Surg.* 1989;98:788–791.
33. O-hara M, Esato K, Harada M, et al. Eicosapentanoic acid suppresses intimal hyperplasia after expanded polytetrafluoroethylene grafting in rabbits fed a high cholesterol diet. *J Vasc Surg.* 1991;13:480–486.
34. Friedman RJ, Stemerman MB, Wenz B, et al. The effect of thrombocytopenia on experimental arteriosclerotic lesion formation in rabbits: smooth muscle cell proliferation and re-endothelialization. *J Clin Invest.* 1977;60:1191–1201.
35. McCollum C, Crow M, Rajah S, et al. Anti-thrombotic therapy for vascular prosthesis: an experimental model testing platelet inhibitory drugs. *Surgery.* 1980;87:668–676.
36. Plate G, Stanson A, Hollier L, et al. Drug effects on platelet deposition after endothelial injury of the rabbit aorta. *J Surg Res.* 1985;39:258–266.
37. McCann R, Hagen P-O, Fuchs J. Aspirin and dipyridamole decrease intimal hyperplasia in experimental vein grafts. *Ann Surg.* 1980;191:238–243.
38. Radic ZS, O'Malley MK, Mikat EM, et al. The role of aspirin and dipyridamole on vascular DNA synthesis and intimal hyperplasia following deendothelialization. *J Surg Res.* 1986;41:84–91.
39. Quiñones-Baldrich W, Ziomek S, Henderson T, et al. Patency and intimal hyperplasia: the effect of aspirin on small arterial anastomosis. *Ann Vasc Surg.* 1988;2:50–56.
40. Graham LM, Brothers TE, Darvishian D, et al. Effects of thromboxane synthetase inhibition on patency and anastomotic hyperplasia of vascular grafts. *J Surg Res.* 1989;46:611–615.
41. Hanson S, Pareti F, Ruggeri Z, et al. Antibody-induced platelet inhibition reduces thrombus formation in vivo. *Clin Res.* 1986;34:658.
42. Torem S, Schneide P, Hanson S. Monoclonal antibody-induced inhibition of platelet function: effects on hemostasis and vascular graft thrombosis in baboons. *J Vasc Surg.* 1988;7:172–180.
43. Hoepp LM, Elbadawi A, Cohn M, et al. Steroids and immunosuppression: effect on anastomotic intimal hyperplasia in femoral arterial Dacron bypass grafts. *Arch Surg.* 1979;114: 273–276.
44. Gordon GB, Bush DE, Weisman HF. Reduction of atherosclerosis by administration of dehydroepiandrosterone. *J Clin Invest.* 1988;82:712–720.
45. Pepine C, Hirshfeld JW, MacDonald RG, et al. A controlled trial of corticosteroids to prevent restenosis after coronary angioplasty. *Circulation.* 1990;81:1753–1761.
46. Chervu A, Moore WS, Quiñones-Baldrich WJ, et al. Efficacy of corticosteroids in suppression of intimal hyperplasia. *J Vasc Surg.* 1989;10:129–134.
47. Colburn MD, Moore WS, Gelabert HA, et al. Dose responsive suppression of myointimal hyperplasia by dexamethasone. *J Vasc Surg.* 1992;15:510–518.
48. Ruhmann AG, Berliner DL. Effect of steroids on growth of mouse fibroblasts in vitro. *Endocrinology.* 1965;76:916–927.
49. Majeski JA, Alexander JW. The steroid effect on the in vitro human neutrophil chemotactic response. *J Surg Res.* 1976;21:265–271.
50. Mishler J. The effects of corticosteroids on mobilization and function of neutrophils. *Exp Hematol.* 1977;5:15–32.

51. Hess AD, Esa AH, Colombanic PM, et al. Mechanisms of action of cyclosporin: effect on cells of the immune system and on subcellular events in T-cell activation. *Transplant Proc.* 1988;20:II29.
52. Goldstein I, Roos D, Weissmann G, et al. Influence of corticosteroids on human polymorphonuclear leukocyte function in vitro enzyme release and superoxide production. *Inflammation.* 1976;1:305–315.
53. Pearce J, Dujovny M, Ho K, et al. Acute inflammation and endothelial injury in vein grafts. *Neurosurgery.* 1985;17:626–634.
54. Cwikel BJ, Barouski-Miller PA, Coleman PL, et al. Dexamethasone induction of an inhibitor of plasminogen activator in HTC hepatoma cells. *J Biol Chem.* 1984;259:6847–6851.
55. Wengrovitz M, Selassie LG, Gifford RRM, et al. Cyclosporine inhibits the development of medial thickening after experimental arterial injury. *J Vasc Surg.* 1990;12:1–7.
56. Powell JS, Clozel JP, Müller RK, et al. Inhibitors of angiotensin-converting enzyme prevent myointimal proliferation after vascular injury. *Science.* 1989;245:186–188.
57. Clowes AW, Reidy MA. Prevention of stenosis after vascular reconstruction: pharmacologic control of intimal hyperplasia—a review. *J Vasc Surg.* 1991;13:885–891.
58. O'Donohoe MK, Schwartz LB, Radic ZS, et al. Chronic ACE inhibition reduces intimal hyperplasia in experimental vein grafts. *Ann Surg.* 1991;214:727–732.
59. Chobanian AV, Haudenschild CC, Nickerson C, et al. Antiatherogenic effect of captopril in the watanabe heritable hyperlipidemic rabbit. *Hypertension.* 1990;15:327–331.
60. Law MM, Colburn MD, Hajjar GE, et al. Suppression of intimal hyperplasia in a rabbit model of arterial balloon injury by enalaprilat but not dimethyl sulfoxide. *Ann Vasc Surg.* 1994;8:158–165.
61. Clowes AW, Clowes MM. Kinetics of cellular proliferation after arterial injury. II. Inhibition of smooth muscle growth by heparin. *Lab Invest.* 1985;52:611–616.
62. Dryjski M, Mikat E, Bjornsson TD. Inhibition of intimal hyperplasia after arterial injury by heparins and heparinoid. *J Vasc Surg.* 1988;8:623–633.
63. Calcagno D, Conte JV, Howell MH, et al. Peptide inhibition of neointimal hyperplasia in vein grafts. *J Vasc Surg.* 1991;13:475–479.
64. Foegh ML, Khirabadi BS, Chambers E, et al. Inhibition of coronary artery transplant atherosclerosis in rabbits with angiopeptin, an octapeptide. *Atherosclerosis.* 1989;78:229–236.
65. Endean ED, Kispert JF, Martin KW, et al. Intimal hyperplasia is reduced by ornithine decarboxylase inhibition. *J Surg Res.* 1991;50:634–637.
66. Arfors KE, Lundberg C, Lindbom L, et al. A monoclonal antibody to the membrane glycoprotein complex CD18 inhibits polymorphonuclear accumulation and plasma leakage in vivo. *Blood.* 1987;69:338.
67. Zwiebel JA, Freeman SM, Kantoff PW, et al. High-level recombinant gene expression in rabbit endothelial cells transduced by retroviral vectors. *Science.* 1989;243:220–222.
68. Nabel EG, Plautz G, Nabel GJ. Site-specific gene expression in vivo by direct gene transfer into the arterial wall. *Science.* 1990;249:1285–1288.
69. Wilson JM, Birinyi LK, Salomon RN, et al. Implantation of vascular grafts lined with genetically modified endothelial cells. *Science.* 1989;244:1344–1346.
70. Neave V, Giannotta S, Hyman S, et al. Hematoporphyrin uptake in atherosclerotic plaques: therapeutic potentials. *Neurosurgery.* 1988;23:307–312.
71. Mackie RW, Vincent GM, Fox J, et al. In vivo canine coronary artery laser irradiation: photodynamic therapy using dihematoporphyrin ether and 632nm laser. A safety and dose-response relationship study. *Lasers Surg Med.* 1991;11:535–544.
72. Spears JR, Serur J, Shopshire D, et al. Fluorescence of experimental atheromatous plaques with hematoporphyrin derivative. *J Clin Invest.* 1983;71:395–399.
73. Dartsch PC, Betz E, Ischinger T. Effect of dihematoporphyrin derivatives on cultivated human smooth muscle cells from normal and atherosclerotic vascular segments. Overview of results and implications for photodynamic therapy. *Z Kardiol.* 1991;80:6–14.
74. Eton D, Colburn MD, Shim V, et al. Inhibition of intimal hyperplasia by photodynamic therapy using photofrin. *J Surg Res.* 1992;53:558–562.
75. LaMuraglia GM, ChandraSekar NR, Flotte TJ, et al. Photodynamic therapy inhibition of experimental intimal hyperplasia: acute and chronic effects. *J Vasc Surg.* 1994;19:321–331.

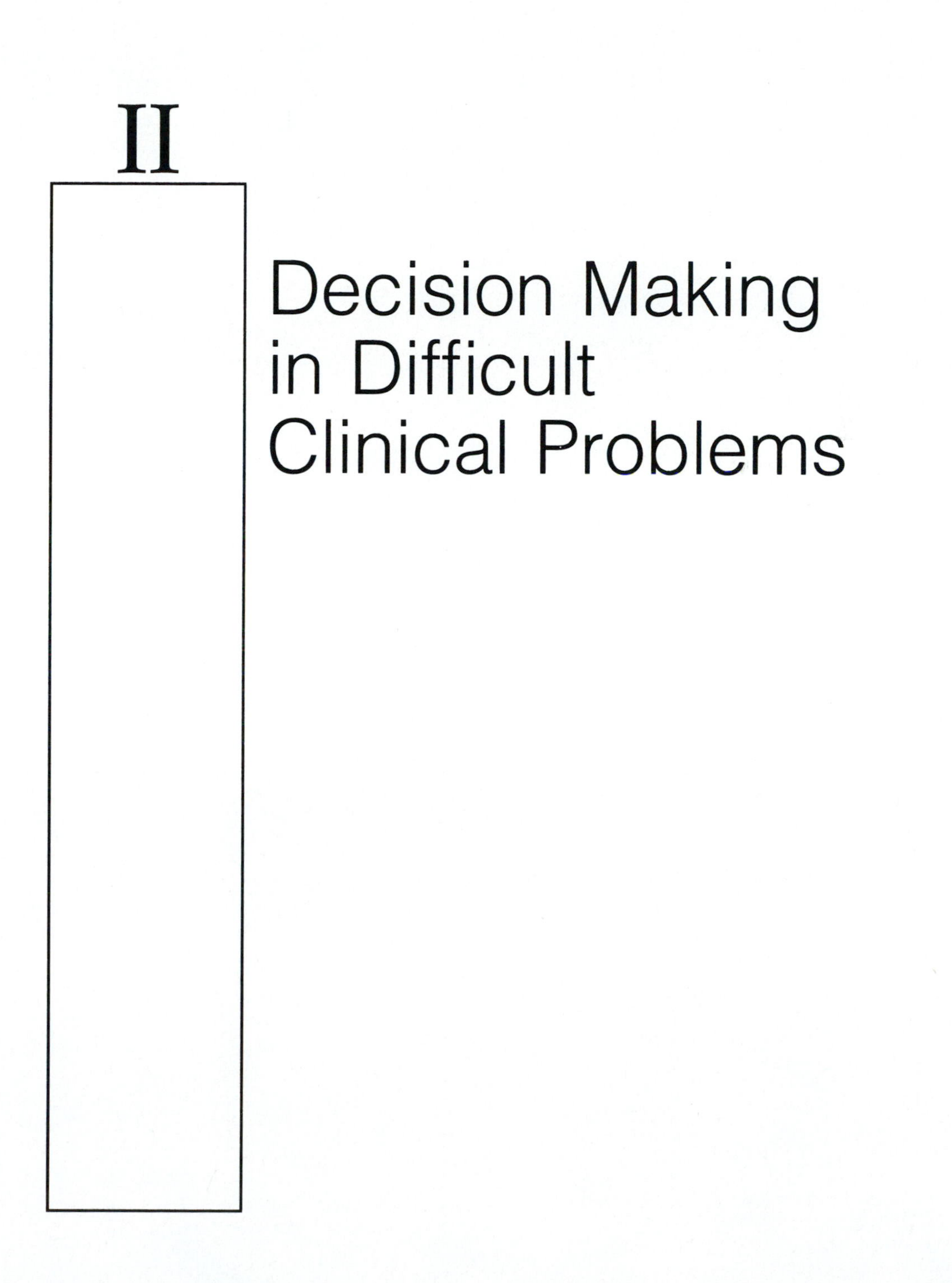

II

Decision Making in Difficult Clinical Problems

3

Diagnostic and Therapeutic Plan for Immediate and Late Reoperation After Carotid Endarterectomy

Thomas S. Riles, MD, Patrick J. Lamparello, MD, and Mark A. Adelman, MD

It is the hope of every surgeon and patient that once the decision has been made to undertake a carotid endarterectomy, the operation will be successful, free of complications, and that the reconstruction will restore normal blood flow to the brain and remove the risk of stroke for the remainder of the patient's life. Remarkably, this is true for the vast majority of carotid endarterectomies that are performed. As many as 5% of these operations, however, will be associated with problems that may require further evaluation and possible reoperation. In this chapter we explore some of the issues related to reoperation after carotid endarterectomy. Since the indications for surgery, preoperative evaluation, and surgical goals for early and late reoperation have few similarities, it is useful to divide this chapter into two sections.

EARLY REOPERATION

For the purposes of this chapter, *early reoperation* is defined as any reoperation of a carotid artery within 30 days of the original carotid endarterectomy. Early reoperations are usually performed for bleeding, a new neurologic deficit, or, in some cases, thrombosis or residual stenosis of the carotid artery. In the case of perioperative stroke, because of the emergent nature in most of these early operations, time is an important factor in the decision-making process. Often a choice must be made between diagnostic testing and therapy. Judgment and experience are often critical in deciding what information is essential before returning to the operating room. For this reason, the first step in any algorithm for a housestaff officer is to notify the responsible surgeon and to provide him or her with an accurate appraisal of the situation.

Postoperative Neurologic Symptoms

Perhaps no call causes more anxiety for a vascular surgeon than that which bears the message, "The postoperative carotid patient has a new neurologic deficit." Along with a mix of frustration, anger, and guilt, there is generally confusion regarding the cause and appropriate action. Well-meaning but inexperienced assistants, housestaff officers, and nurses may add to the confusion by initiating action not beneficial to the patient. The fact that perioperative stroke is a rare event in most hospitals (occurring in 1% to 5% of carotid endarterectomies)[1,2] adds to the uncertainty. In anticipation that some day every surgeon who performs carotid surgery will receive this call, it is worthwhile to prepare a plan of action with clear objectives and alternatives.

The first step in formulating a therapeutic plan is to have a clear understanding of the probable cause of perioperative stroke. In a recent review of our own experience with perioperative strokes over a 27-year period, we identified more than 20 mechanisms that led to neurologic injury.[1] Excluding those strokes that were unrelated to the carotid surgery, most perioperative strokes could be grouped into several broad categories: (1) strokes due to embolization or inadequate cerebral perfusion during the carotid endarterectomy, (2) strokes due to embolization of fresh thrombus or thrombotic occlusion after restoration of flow in the carotid artery, and (3) strokes due to intracerebral hemorrhage resulting from a reperfusion injury to the brain. These three mechanisms accounted for 51 : 66 (77%) strokes. Postendarterectomy thrombosis accounted for one-half of these events (26/51). In recent years, this mechanism has become the major cause of perioperative stroke since with improved cerebral monitoring and more frequent use of shunts, strokes due to ischemia during carotid clamping have become rare.

Embolization of plaque material during dissection of the carotid bulb, or at the moment of releasing the clamps, is often cited as a cause of perioperative stroke.[3,4] In our series, however, we found these events to be rare (2/66).[1] Unless there is clear evidence that the stroke did in fact occur during the dissection or at the moment of restoration of blood flow, one should not assume this to be the cause of the stroke. If one readily concludes this to be the mechanism of the stroke, there is a tendency to not consider other possibilities that may require emergency reoperation or other therapies. Although embolization to the cerebral circulation usually occurs with strokes due to technical problems at the site of the endarterectomy, the difference between this and embolization during the procedure is that with the former, the process may continue until the technical problem is repaired. Assuming that the problem was not related to clamp ischemia (a shunt was used or the patient was properly monitored during the clamping of the carotid), the two most likely causes for the postoperative stroke are thrombus formation at the site of the endarterectomy or reperfusion injury. Because the therapeutic goals are quite different, it is extremely important to differentiate between these two circumstances as quickly as possible. If the stroke is due to thrombus formation within the carotid artery, the surgical goal is to return to the operating room and remove the thrombus as quickly as possible and at the same time to repair the underlying defect that led to the thrombosis. If the patient has hemorrhaged into the brain, it may be important to consider evacuation of the hemorrhage or placement of an intraventricular shunt to prevent hydrocephalus.

We have occasionally noted some subtle differences between patients who had postoperative ischemic strokes and those who had hemorrhagic strokes. The patients with intracranial hemorrhage often are hypertensive and the stroke may be heralded by a seizure, particularly if it is a cortical bleed. This observation, however, is not sufficiently reliable to make a diagnosis. The definitive tests to diagnose carotid thrombosis and intracranial hemorrhage are an angiogram and a CT scan or an MRI. These tests, however, often require considerable time to arrange and perform. If the patient's carotid artery is thrombosing or embolizing from thrombus at the site of the endarterectomy, the ultimate outcome may be determined by the length of time it takes to correct the underlying problem.

If the patient is in the recovery room when the stroke occurs, our first response is to make plans for immediate return to the operating room. Generally this requires a few minutes of setup. While these arrangements are being made, we can often obtain an emergency Duplex scan. The Duplex scan has been extremely helpful in determining whether the artery has intraluminal thrombus or is open without obstruction. If the artery is found to be widely patent, and we have clinical suspicion that the patient is having an intracranial bleed, we may postpone the return to the operating room and obtain a CT scan. If, however, there is evidence of a flow defect, the patient is returned to the operating room as soon as possible. If a Duplex scanner is unavailable, the patient is taken to the operating room for reexploration of the artery. Although the patient may be suffering a bleed, we believe it is most important to be certain that the surgical repair is not the cause of the neurologic deficit, since the diagnosis and correction of a technical problem is the best chance of recovery for the patient. In the operating room an angiogram can be performed. More commonly the artery is simply opened and examined for intraluminal thrombus technical defects.

If thrombus is found, it is helpful to "read the clot" to determine the cause of the thrombus formation. Usually the point where platelets are aggregated is the site of technical defect. Common causes of platelet aggregation and thrombosis are retained plaque, ledges where the plaque was transected, kinking and/or narrowing of the internal carotid artery, a rough endarterectomy surface, and clamp injuries. These must be repaired; and if a patch was not used, it certainly should be used for the secondary closure.

If the artery is completely thrombosed, we usually try to restore flow by simply extracting the clot or using a Fogarty catheter on some occasions. It is important that the Fogarty not be passed more than 8 to 10 cm, the length of the extracranial carotid. A Fogarty passed into the siphon portion of the carotid may lead to a carotid cavernous fistula. If there is any doubt about complete removal of the clot, an intraoperative angiogram using 2 to 3 mL of contrast is necessary to delineate the distal internal carotid artery. This angiogram should be performed before restoration of flow through a rubber catheter approximately the same size as the internal carotid. It is important that the catheter is not securely fixed to the internal carotid. If there is distal obstruction, intraluminal pressure may not result from injection of the contrast dye. If the catheter is not secured, it will simply disengage. If it is occluded distally, one does not wish to push the thrombus into the intracranial circulation, nor does one wish to rupture the artery due to excessive pressure. If the artery is open, a few mL of dye will easily flow into the vessel and outline the distal carotid.

Occasionally the question is asked whether it is better to leave an artery thrombosed or to do the thrombectomy in a patient with a fresh stroke. We generally follow the principle that it is better to restore flow, except for the rare occasion when the patient has dense coma. Although no studies address this question, experience with patients with carotid trauma and neurologic deficits suggests that the individual is most likely to recover from the stroke with restoration of flow than not.[5] The risk of converting a bland stroke into a hemorrhagic stroke in the early minutes or hours after a complete occlusion seems to be minimal.

It is impossible to know if the reoperation will lead to improvement in the patient's stroke or change the clinical outcome. Since the decisions usually are made within the first hour after the onset of the neurologic symptoms, it is always possible that the patient would have recovered anyway—having experienced what would otherwise have been a transient ischemic attack (TIA). Even if a rapid reoperation is performed and the artery is successfully repaired, the patient may be left with a neurologic deficit from embolization of the thrombus. In spite of the lack of data to prove that reoperation is the best treatment, we continue to treat early neurologic deficits due to thrombosis in this manner for several reasons. First, we believe it is important to prevent any further embolization. Second, we hope recovery will be better with an open carotid artery than an occluded one. Third, we think it is important to examine the area of occlusion with the hope that the information gained will lead to better surgery in the future.

If a new neurologic deficit occurs 1 to 2 days after the carotid surgery, the diagnostic and therapeutic options may be quite different. It may be in the middle of the night, and the patient may be in an unmonitored room—or, in some cases, already at home. Thrombosis of the carotid artery may still be the cause, but the longer the interval between the surgery and the new stroke, the more likely it is that the stroke is due to intracerebral hemorrhage. Because of this, and also because the operating room is not immediately available, the Duplex and CT scan are used to guide treatment. If an intraluminal thrombus is found, plans are made for reexploration. With these delayed neurologic deficits, the surgeon must determine which resources are available and which will most expeditiously lead to the correct diagnosis and therapy.

Although postoperative intracranial hemorrhage is an extremely rare complication, it is one of the most devastating for carotid surgery. It generally occurs in patients with severe stenosis and a preoperative neurologic deficit.[1] Paradoxically, the indications for carotid surgery are rarely in dispute for these individuals. The operation itself is often uncomplicated and void of technical errors. Although these patients are often noted to be hypertensive at the onset of the neurologic event, it is never clear whether the hypertension contributed to the bleed or if it is the result of the bleed. Early evaluation of the carotid artery by Duplex scan, arteriogram, or reexploration will show unobstructed flow. CT scan of the head will confirm the diagnosis.

For patients with small intracranial hemorrhages, there is little to offer in the way of therapy other than careful control of the blood pressure and general supportive measures. For major bleeds, critical decisions must be made. It is advisable to enlist the aid of a neurosurgeon early since cranial surgery may be necessary. For patients with massive bleeds into the parenchyma of the brain, it may be necessary to evacuate the hematoma as a life-saving measure. In some cases, the hemorrhage may mainly involve the ventricle. Since bleeding into the ventricles may lead to obstruction, increased intraventricular pressure, and worsening of the neurologic deficit, a temporary intraventricular shunt may prove critical to the recovery of the patient.

Asymptomatic Residual Stenosis and Occlusion

What if a patient has successfully undergone a carotid endarterectomy and, in the course of a routine postoperative follow-up study, is found to have a critical stenosis (>80%) or total occlusion of the internal carotid artery? Should the patient be reoperated on, even though there are no neurologic symptoms? Some have argued that, unlike the atherosclerotic plaques that cause stenosis and possess the potential for embolization, asymptomatic postoperative early stenoses are unlikely to cause stroke and therefore do not require reoperation. It is important to note that most opinions are based on the observation of early restenoses (myointimal hyperplasia) and do not necessarily pertain to the residual lesions that are almost always technical problems. Following the principles that stenoses within the carotid circulation have the potential for causing intraluminal thrombus formation, embolization, and stroke, and that the surgery was performed to remove such a risk from the patient, we believe that any residual stenosis should be reoperated and surgically corrected as soon as possible. If a patch was not used in the first operation, it should be used for the secondary procedure.

More difficult is the question regarding the asymptomatic occlusion. The problem is that unless the occlusion is detected within the first 24 hours of the surgery, it is difficult to know how long the thrombus has been present. If the thrombosis is very recent, an attempt should be made to remove the clot. As outlined in the section on reoperation for neurologic symptoms, we would generally perform an intraoperative arteriogram before restoration of flow and would not hesitate to ligate the carotid artery if the thrombectomy were incomplete. The later in the course of the recovery the thrombosis is detected, the less likely the thrombectomy will be successful. For this reason, we would be less inclined to reexplore a thrombosis that may be more than a few days old.

LATE REOPERATION

Carotid reoperation more than 30 days after the initial carotid endarterectomy is usually for recurrent stenosis. Some lesions described as recurrent stenoses are in fact residual lesions that have gone undetected since the original operation. True recurrent lesions may develop within a few months or may not appear until years after carotid surgery. The actual incidence of recurrent stenosis varies from 1.2% to 36%,[6–17] depending on the type of surveillance, the definition of recurrent stenosis, the interval of follow-up, and the surgical technique used for the primary operation.

In general, lesions that occur in the first few years after carotid surgery are due to myointimal hyperplasia, whereas those that occur later are atherosclerotic plaques, which are similar in appearance to the primary disease.[6,8,10,18] Another lesion that is responsible for late recurrent stenosis is aneurysmal dilatation with intraluminal thrombus formation.[18–20] With the latter, the stenosis is due to the thrombus rather than a growth of tissue from the arterial wall. Also, these lesions are more commonly seen in patients who had vein patch closures at the time of the original carotid endarterectomy.

Some authors have recommended against surgery for asymptomatic recurrent stenosis, particularly if the lesion is early and therefore more likely to be due to myointimal hyperplasia.[14,18,21] We, however, have had patients develop neurologic symptoms with early myointimal hyperplasia, and therefore have become more aggressive in the treatment of early asymptomatic recurrent stenosis. For those patients with recurrent neurologic symptoms and recurrent stenosis involving the carotid artery ipsilateral to the affected hemisphere, few would argue against reoperation.

In preparing for reoperation for recurrent stenosis, we generally will obtain a digital subtraction angiogram (DSA) with selected views of the carotid artery. Whereas the magnetic resonance angiogram (MRA) is often adequate for primary surgery, the resolution is often insufficient for secondary carotid surgery. Specifically, we wish to know the relationship of the stenosis to the bony landmarks and the previous field of operation.

Consistent with our anesthetic preference for primary carotid surgery, we favor cervical block anesthetic for reoperation.[18] Whether it is better to use EEG, stump pressure, or monitor awake patient's neurologic status to determine if a patient requires a shunt is beyond the scope of this chapter. It is helpful to have the option not to shunt, since the scarring in the region of the internal carotid artery may be severe and dissection may be difficult. In some cases, we have begun the operation under regional anesthesia and, once we have determined the patient is tolerant of clamping, we have converted to general anesthesia that offers more relaxation and head rotation and therefore better exposure.

The dissection is usually begun low in the neck, exposing a virginal segment of the common carotid artery. When the scarring is severe, we prefer to develop a plane between the carotid and the jugular vein and follow this until past the stenosis on the internal carotid artery. An even more posterior plane along the vagus nerve may sometimes be necessary to reach the distal internal carotid artery. Once the distal artery is dissected, an attempt is made to locate the hypoglossal nerve and dissect it free from the carotid artery.

Although we formerly favored redo endarterectomy and patch angioplasty for recurrent stenosis, a follow up of our patients so treated revealed that up to 20% developed tertiary lesions, a tenfold increase over recurrence after primary endarterectomy. These results have led us to change our approach and to use a variety of reconstructive techniques for recurrent lesions.

For those patients with patch dilatation or aneurysmal formation, with or without intraluminal thrombus, the replacement of the entire segment with a vein or synthetic graft is the treatment of choice. For patients with myointimal hyperplasia, simple repair with a patch may sometimes be all that is needed. For more advanced lesions, we now favor reconstruction with an interposition graft—either vein, Dacron, or polytetrafluoroethylene (PTFE). Although it is not absolutely necessary, we will make an effort to preserve the external carotid artery either by using the proximal end of the graft or a long onlay patch to allow for safe removal of the shunt. Whether these techniques will improve the results with secondary carotid surgery remains to be seen.

Although some authors have stated that the higher operative risk for reoperation is a reason for a more conservative approach to recurrent stenosis, we have found the complication rates for secondary surgery to be no greater than for primary surgery. In a consecutive series of 47 reoperations on 42 patients, there were no strokes or deaths.[19] There is, however, a greater potential for cranial nerve injuries, and patients should be forewarned. Without question, these operations require more time and patience than primary carotid surgery. For this reason, it is advisable not to undertake a difficult reoperation when one is fatigued. Good assistance, good lighting, and good instruments are important to reduce the frustration that may develop due to difficulty identifying the anatomic landmarks, which are obscured by dense scar tissue.

CONCLUSION

Reoperative carotid surgery differs in many ways from primary carotid endarterectomy. The pathology is quite varied and the indications for surgery less well established. The dissection is always more difficult. The choices of reconstructions are multiple and must be tailored to the pathology. When the patient is threatened with stroke and corrective surgery is the best alternative for prevention, the surgeon must be prepared to meet the challenge. Understanding the issues that are in many ways unique to reoperative carotid surgery is essential to planning a successful operation. Because few vascular surgeons develop extensive experience with reoperative surgery, it is often worthwhile to discuss the case in advance with colleagues and seek outside advice in difficult cases. The surgeon should be prepared with several plans for reconstruction, depending on the pathology that is encountered. With good planning, patience, and diligence, the outcome is usually excellent and the effort professionally rewarding.

The most important lesson from reoperative carotid surgery is prevention. Early reoperations for recurrent neurologic symptoms, residual stenosis, thrombosis, and bleeding are almost always due to a technical failure. Many experienced surgeons have developed routines to minimize the chance of a technical mishap. A surgeon with more than a 1% to 3% early reoperation rate should seek further training from a center with a good record with carotid surgery and analyze their technique. Late reoperations may also be traced back to flaws in surgical technique. Unfortunately, we do not yet know which techniques offer the best long-term results. For example, failure to use a patch may cause more recurrent stenosis, but the use of a patch may lead to more aneurysm of the carotid artery.

As our experience with carotid surgery grows, it may become more obvious which techniques provide the best long-term results.

REFERENCES

1. Riles TS, Imparato AM, Jacobowitz GR, et al. The cause of perioperative stroke after carotid endarterectomy. *J Vasc Surg*. 1994;19:206–216.
2. North American Symptomatic Carotid Endarterectomy Trial Collaborators. Beneficial effect of carotid endarterectomy in symptomatic patients with high-grade stenosis. *N Engl J Med*. 1991;325:445–453.
3. Hertzer NR, Beven EG, Greenstreet RL, et al. Internal carotid artery back pressure, intraoperative shunting, ulcerated atheromata, and the incidence of stroke during carotid endarterectomy. *Surgery*. 1978;83:306–312.
4. Perdue GL. Management of postendarterectomy neurologic deficits. *Arch Surg*. 1982;117: 1079–1081.
5. Liekweg WG, Greenfield LJ. Management of penetrating carotid arterial injury. *Ann Surg*. 1978;188:587–592.
6. Stoney RJ, String ST. Recurrent carotid stenosis. *Surgery*. 1976;80:705–710.
7. Gagne PJ, Riles TS, Imparato AM, et al. Redo endarterectomy for recurrent carotid artery stenosis. *Eur J Vasc Surg*. 1991;5:135–140.
8. Cantelmo NL, Cutler BS, Wheeler HB, et al. Noninvasive detection of carotid stenosis following endarterectomy. *Arch Surg*. 1981;116:1005–1008.
9. Mattos MA, Hodgson KJ, Londrey GL, et al. Carotid endarterectomy: operative risks, recurrent stenosis, and long-term stroke rates in a modern series. *J Cardiovasc Surg*. 1992;33:387–400.
10. Das MB, Hertzer NR, Ratliff NB, et al. Recurrent carotid stenosis: a five-year series of sixty-five reoperations. *Ann Surg*. 1985;202:28–35.
11. Turnipseed WD, Berkoff HA, Crummy A. Postoperative occlusion after carotid endarterectomy. *Arch Surg*. 1980;115:573–574.
12. Shumway SJ, Edwards WH, Jenkins JM, et al. Recurrent carotid stenosis: incidence and management. *Ann Surg*. 1987;53:61–65.
13. Eikelboom BC, Ackerstaff RGA, Hoenveld H, et al. Benefits of carotid patching: a randomized study. *J Vasc Surg*. 1988;7:240–247.
14. Healy DA, Zierler RE, Nicholls SC, et al. Long-term follow-up and clinical outcome of carotid restenosis. *J Vasc Surg*. 1989;10:662–669.
15. DeGroote RD, Lynch TG, Jamil Z, et al. Carotid restenosis: long-term noninvasive follow-up after carotid endarterectomy. *Stroke*. 1987;18:1031–1036.
16. Norrving B, Nilsson B, Olsson JE. Progression of carotid disease after endarterectomy: a Doppler ultrasound study. *Ann Neurol*. 1982;12:548–552.
17. Hertzer NR, Beven BG, O'Hara PJ, et al. A prospective study of vein patch angioplasty during carotid endarterectomy: three-year results for 801 patients and 917 operations. *Ann Surg*. 1987;206:628–635.

18. Nitzberg RS, Mackay WE, Predniville E, et al. Long-term follow-up of patients operated on for recurrent carotid stenosis. *J Vasc Surg.* 1991;13:121–126.
19. Gagne PJ, Riles TS, Jacobowitz GR, et al. Long-term follow-up of patients undergoing reoperation for recurrent carotid artery disease. *J Vasc Surg.* 1993;18:991–1001.
20. Piepgras DG, Sundt TM, March WR, et al. Recurrent carotid stenosis: results and complications of fifty-seven operations. *Ann Surg.* 1986;203:205–213.
21. Ricotta JJ, O'Brien MS, DeWeese JA. Natural history of recurrent and residual stenosis after carotid endarterectomy: implications for postoperative surveillance and surgical management. *Surgery.* 1992;4:656–663.

4

Staged or Combined Procedures in Patients with Coexisting Aortoiliac and Femoropopliteal Occlusive Disease

R. Eugene Zierler, MD

Although atherosclerotic occlusive disease is a widespread process, it tends to be localized in specific segments of the lower extremity arterial circulation. From both the clinical and diagnostic points of view, it is useful to divide the lower extremity arteries into three regions or segments: aortoiliac, femoropopliteal, and tibioperoneal. Although occlusive lesions may be confined to a single segment, involvement of more than one segment is common.[1-3] The terms *multilevel disease, multisegment disease,* and *combined segment disease* have all been used to describe the combination of aortoiliac (inflow) disease with femoropopliteal or tibioperoneal (outflow) disease. Patients with both inflow and outflow lesions present the vascular surgeon with a complex diagnostic and therapeutic challenge.

Basic hemodynamic principles dictate that femoropopliteal or femorotibial bypass grafts performed distal to significant inflow disease are likely to fail.[4] Similarly, aortoiliac or aortofemoral reconstructions in limbs with significant outflow lesions may not improve distal blood flow and relieve ischemic symptoms. Thus, optimal therapeutic decision making in patients with suspected multilevel disease should be based on accurate methods for identifying hemodynamically significant inflow or outflow disease and predicting whether an inflow procedure alone will be clinically beneficial.

Reports published since the mid-1970s show that up to 57% of patients with multilevel disease do not heal ischemic ulcers or experience relief of claudication or rest pain with inflow reconstruction alone.[5-12] Clearly, more objective guidelines are needed for managing patients with multilevel disease. This chapter reviews the clinical features of multilevel lower extremity arterial occlusive disease, the various diagnostic approaches to this problem, and the options for treatment.

LOWER EXTREMITY ARTERIAL DISEASE

Clinical Presentation

While occlusive disease involving a single lower extremity arterial segment may be associated with intermittent claudication, ischemic rest pain and tissue loss typically require the presence of lesions at multiple levels. Thus, patients with inflow disease and evidence of ischemia at rest almost always have additional outflow lesions.[13] There are rare situations, however, in which single level disease can result in limb-threatening ischemia. For example, when the origin of the profunda femoris artery is occluded in combination with occlusion of the common femoral or superficial femoral arteries, the usual profunda-geniculate collateral pathways may be inadequate even at rest. Occlusive lesions in the foot at the junction of the plantar and digital arteries can also result in rest pain and ulceration due to a lack of collateral circulation.[14]

The ankle:brachial index, or ABI (ankle systolic pressure divided by brachial systolic pressure), reflects the hemodynamic effect of all lower extremity arterial lesions and correlates with the clinical presentation.[15,16] In the absence of arterial occlusive disease, the ABI has a mean value of 1.11; limbs with intermittent claudication have a mean ABI of 0.59; while the mean ABI is 0.26 in limbs with ischemic rest pain and 0.05 in limbs with impending gangrene.[17] Although the ABI does not discriminate among occlusions at various anatomic levels, it tends to be considerably lower in limbs with multilevel disease. In general, limbs with a single level of occlusion have ABI values greater than 0.5 and limbs with lesions at multiple levels have ABI values less than 0.5.[16]

Patients with multilevel arterial disease are more likely to require intervention for limb-threatening ischemia than patients with single level disease. Multilevel disease patients often have a history of intermittent claudication prior to developing ischemic rest pain or ulceration, suggesting progression from single level to multilevel involvement. As would be expected, these patients also tend to be older than those with more localized lower extremity arterial disease, and there is a higher prevalence of diabetes and hypertension as well as concomitant extracranial carotid and coronary artery disease.[1,12,18–20] Consequently, patients with ischemia at rest and multilevel disease carry a higher risk for perioperative complications than patients with claudication alone.

Distribution of Lesions

The lower extremity arterial segment most commonly affected by atherosclerotic lesions is the superficial femoral artery at the level of the adductor canal.[21,22] In a group of nondiabetic patients requiring amputation for lower extremity atherosclerosis, the distribution of lesions included the aortoiliac segment in 68%, the femoropopliteal segment in 89%, and the tibioperoneal segment in 57%.[22] For a similar group of patients with diabetes, atherosclerotic lesions involved the aortoiliac segment in 27%, the femoropopliteal segment in 80%, and the tibioperoneal segment in 80%.[22] Thus, although femoropopliteal occlusive disease is relatively common in both nondiabetic and diabetic patients, aortoiliac disease is less common and tibioperoneal disease is more common in patients with diabetes. Atherosclerotic lesions of the profunda femoris artery, particularly beyond the origin, are also more common in diabetic patients. While the reported incidence of combined aortoiliac and femoropopliteal occlusive disease varies widely, it is typically in excess of 50% in patients undergoing arteriography and who are being considered for surgical and radiologic intervention.[1,12,18,19,23,24]

Progression of lower extremity atherosclerosis is more common with multilevel disease than with lesions limited to a single segment. In a series of patients undergoing surgical procedures for aortoiliac disease, those with isolated aortoiliac lesions had only a 14% incidence of disease progression, while 38% of the patients with combined aortoiliac and more distal occlusive disease showed new areas of involvement.[11] Most of the disease progression was observed in the femoropopliteal segment. Progression of disease proximal to femoropopliteal reconstructions has also been described as a cause of infrainguinal bypass graft occlusion.[25]

EVALUATION OF MULTILEVEL ARTERIAL DISEASE

The clinical history and physical examination are important initial steps in identifying the patient with lower extremity arterial disease; however, further diagnostic studies are needed to define the anatomic location and severity of the lesions. For example, in a series of patients with significant aortoiliac disease proven by direct pressure measurements, thigh claudication was present in 76% and calf claudication alone was present in 24%; in a corresponding group of patients with isolated femoropopliteal disease, 23% had thigh claudication and 77% had claudication in the calf only.[26] Experience has also shown that femoral pulse palpation can be misleading. Palpable femoral pulses are classified as abnormally reduced in up to 30% of limbs with normal aortoiliac segments, while a similar proportion of limbs with hemodynamically significant inflow disease are considered to have normal femoral pulses.[26-28] Finally, bruits over the iliac or femoral arteries are absent in 42% of patients with hemodynamically significant aortoiliac disease and present in 51% of patients with normal aortoiliac segments.[26]

Although arteriography is relatively accurate for identifying hemodynamically significant disease in the femoropopliteal and tibioperoneal segments, arteriographic assessment of the aortoiliac segment is considerably less reliable. Asymmetric plaques and variability in arteriogram interpretation often make it difficult to estimate the hemodynamic effects of aortoiliac lesions, particularly when only a single-plane anteroposterior projection is available.[29-33] The use of lateral or oblique projections can improve the results of arteriography, but the determination of hemodynamic significance remains a problem.[28,31] Incorrect assessments of the aortoiliac segment are responsible for many of the unsatisfactory results reported after surgical treatment of multilevel disease.[33] The most common error appears to be the underestimation of the degree of aortoiliac involvement.

Based on the previous discussion, the key questions in patients with suspected combined aortoiliac and femoropopliteal occlusive disease are whether the inflow lesions are hemodynamically significant and whether correction of the aortoiliac disease alone will result in clinical improvement. Efforts to address these questions using both noninvasive and invasive approaches have generated an extensive body of literature. Noninvasive tests have been applied to the primary evaluation of arterial disease at various levels in the lower extremity and the prediction of the hemodynamic results of inflow procedures.

Noninvasive Methods

Indirect Testing

Table 4–1 lists the most widely used indirect and direct noninvasive methods for evaluating the aortoiliac segment. The techniques for performing these tests have been described in detail elsewhere.[34-36] Unfortunately, the hemodynamic significance of lesions in the aortoiliac segment has been difficult to determine by noninvasive testing, especially the indirect noninvasive methods.

TABLE 4–1. NONINVASIVE TESTS FOR AORTOILIAC DISEASE

Indirect Tests
- Segmental Leg Pressures
- Pulse Volume Recorder (PVR)
- Femoral Artery Waveform Analysis
  - Qualitative Interpretation
  - Pulsatility Index
  - LaPlace Transform

Direct Tests
- Duplex Scanning
  - B-mode Imaging
  - Pulsed Doppler Flow Detection
  - Spectral Waveform Analysis
  - Color-flow Imaging

While the ABI is a reliable guide to the overall severity of lower extremity arterial occlusive disease, it does not indicate the specific levels of involvement. Measurement of segmental leg pressures is based on the same general principles as the ABI and is an indirect approach to localizing occlusive lesions within the lower extremity. In theory, the pressure obtained with a pneumatic cuff on the proximal thigh should reflect the status of the aortoiliac segment. When the proximal thigh pressure is measured with a relatively narrow cuff, the thigh systolic pressure normally exceeds the brachial systolic pressure by a "cuff artifact" of 30 to 40 mm Hg, and the ratio of the thigh pressure to the brachial pressure (thigh pressure index) is 1.2 or greater.[37] Patients with decreased thigh pressure indices should have significant aortoiliac disease and benefit more from an inflow procedure than those with normal thigh pressure indices. Similarly, patients with large pressure gradients between the proximal thigh and ankle would be expected to have poor results from an inflow procedure since the segmental pressure gradients suggest significant occlusive lesions distal to the aortoiliac segment. However, the accuracy of segmental leg pressures for predicting the results of inflow procedures has been inconsistent.[9,38–42]

The main problem with indirect segmental pressure measurement is not with the theory, but with the practical difficulty in measuring the proximal thigh pressure accurately. Cuff artifacts, which depend on the relationship between cuff width and limb circumferance, can be quite variable. In addition, the presence of superficial femoral artery disease can result in a decreased thigh pressure, even when the aortoiliac segment is hemodynamically normal.

An alternative to indirect segmental pressure measurement is the pulse volume recorder (PVR). This instrument is a calibrated air plethysmograph with a series of segmental cuffs that are used to detect changes in the volume of the leg at various levels.[35,38,40,43] Interpretation is based on the amplitude and shape of volume tracings from the thigh, calf, and ankle. The PVR tracings are less likely to be affected by arterial wall calcification and incompressibility than segmental pressure measurements because air plethysmography does not require arterial occlusion. However, thigh tracings taken with the PVR are prone to the same errors as proximal thigh pressure measurements in the presence of superficial femoral artery lesions.

The difficulties encountered with segmental pressure measurement and plethysmography prompted interest in the use of Doppler-derived femoral artery velocity waveforms as an alternative method for assessing aortoiliac disease. Qualitative interpretation is the simplest approach and is based on visual inspection of the femoral artery velocity waveform.[42] Changes in the contour of the waveform from the normal triphasic configuration to a damped monophasic pattern with loss of the normal reverse flow phase signify the presence of disease in the proximal aortoiliac segment.[30,44] The reported results of this qualitative approach, however, are highly variable, and the false positive and negative rates appear to be high enough to make this method unsatisfactory for routine clinical use.[44,45]

Quantitative methods for analysis of femoral artery velocity waveforms include the pulsatility index (PI) and the LaPlace transform.[45,46] The most widely used of these approaches is the PI, which is defined as the ratio of the peak-to-peak range and the mean amplitude of the waveform. A femoral artery PI of 4 or greater is highly predictive of a hemodynamically normal aortoiliac segment; however, an abnormally low PI does not discriminate reliably between aortoiliac and superficial femoral artery disease.[46] The LaPlace transform is a complex computerized method for analysis of femoral velocity waveforms that appears to be less affected by superficial femoral artery disease.[35,45] While these quantitative methods are an improvement over simple qualitative waveform interpretation, they are cumbersome to use and still have significant limitations. As is discussed later, duplex scanning and direct measurement of arterial pressures across the aortoiliac segment overcome the major limitations of the indirect diagnostic methods.

Direct Testing

Duplex ultrasound, which uses a scanner that combines anatomic and physiologic tests in a single instrument, has been the most successful noninvasive technique for evaluating the aortoiliac segment.[36,47–49] As indicated in Table 4–1, the components of a duplex scanner include a B-mode imaging system, a pulsed Doppler flowmeter, and the capability to process Doppler signals by spectral waveform analysis and color-flow imaging. The vessels of interest are directly visualized on the B-mode image, and the pulsed Doppler sample volume is then used to assess the flow patterns within them. Certain features of the pulsed Doppler spectral waveforms allow the severity of disease at specific arterial sites to be classified according to criteria such as those given in Table 4–2.[36,48]

Duplex scanning offers several distinct advantages over the indirect noninvasive tests for lower extremity arterial disease: lesions can be detected at multiple levels in the same limb and accurately localized, stenoses can be classified according to their degree of severity, and severe stenoses can be distinguished from total occlusions. In a validation study of 383 lower extremity arterial segments evaluated by duplex scanning and arteriography, duplex scanning had a sensitivity of 82%, a specificity of 92%, a positive predictive value of 80%, and a negative predictive value of 93% for identifying hemodynamically significant stenoses (>50% diameter reduction).[48] A similar study reported sensitivities for detecting hemodynamically significant arterial stenoses that ranged from 89% in the iliac segment to 67% in the popliteal segment, and stenosis was correctly distinguished from occlusion in 98% of cases.[49]

The duplex scan findings often suggest whether a particular lower extremity arterial lesion is most suitable for an endovascular procedure or direct arterial surgery. For example, focal stenoses or short occlusions in the iliac arteries are usually amenable to balloon angioplasty, while arterial segments with long irregular stenotic lesions or extensive occlusions are better treated by direct arterial reconstruction. The anatomic features that are particularly important in making this determination are the site, severity, and length of the lesion. In addition, it is essential to assess the status of the

TABLE 4–2. CRITERIA FOR CLASSIFICATION OF LOWER EXTREMITY ARTERIAL OCCLUSIVE DISEASE BY DUPLEX SCANNING WITH SPECTRAL WAVEFORM ANALYSIS

Normal	Triphasic waveform, no spectral broadening
1%–19% diameter reduction	Triphasic waveform with minimal spectral broadening only; peak systolic velocities increased <30% relative to the adjacent proximal segment; proximal and distal waveforms remain normal
20%–49% diameter reduction	Triphasic waveform usually maintained, although reverse flow component may be diminished; spectral broadening is prominent with filling-in of the clear area under the systolic peak; peak systolic velocity is increased from 30%–100% relative to the adjacent proximal segment; proximal and distal waveforms remain normal
50%–99% diameter reduction	Monophasic waveform with loss of the reverse flow component and forward flow throughout the cardiac cycle; extensive spectral broadening; peak systolic velocity is increased >100% relative to the adjacent proximal segment; distal waveform is monophasic with reduced systolic velocity
Occlusion	No flow detected within the imaged arterial segment; pre-occlusive "thump" may be heard just proximal to the site of occlusion; distal waveforms are monophasic with reduced systolic velocities

inflow to the diseased arterial segment and the quality of the distal runoff. Duplex scanning provides a reliable method for obtaining this information without resorting to arteriography. In a series of 110 patients having lower extremity duplex scanning prior to arteriography, 50 lesions were considered suitable for balloon angioplasty on the basis of the duplex scan findings, and the procedure was actually performed in 47 (94%).[50] In the remaining three cases, lesions were present as predicted by the duplex scan, but angioplasty was not done for various technical reasons.

Predicting Results of Inflow Procedures

Numerous studies have investigated the role of noninvasive tests in predicting the hemodynamic results of proximal reconstructions and the need for combined inflow and outflow procedures in patients with multilevel disease.[9,11,23,38,51,52] However, no single test has emerged as completely reliable for this purpose. For example, the changes observed in the ABI immediately following completion of an inflow procedure are extremely variable and are not predictive of the eventual clinical outcome. An increase in the ABI of 0.10 or more is generally a favorable prognostic sign, but no change or even a decrease does not always predict a poor result.[5,6,8,53] Although maximal ABI values are attained within several weeks in most patients undergoing inflow procedures for multilevel disease, the ABI may continue to increase for many months postoperatively.[9]

In addition to identifying hemodynamically significant inflow disease, noninvasive tests have been used to assess the capacity of the collateral circulation in patients with occlusive lesions in the femoropopliteal and tibioperoneal segments. These techniques evaluate the profunda-geniculate system, which is the critical collateral route in the lower extremity.[19,54] Such methods are typically based on either segmental pressure measurements or PVR tracings and include the pressure decrease across the knee expressed as the profunda-popliteal collateral index (PPCI),[55] the difference in thigh and ankle PVR amplitudes (FPΩ),[38] and an index of runoff resistance (IRR) calculated by dividing the difference between the thigh and ankle pressures by the brachial pressure.[9] While these approaches may be of theoretic and historic interest, they have not proven particularly useful in the clinical setting.[23] The major problem with these techniques is that they rely on indirect methods of assessing the aortoiliac segment that, as discussed previously, are relatively inaccurate.

Direct Arterial Pressure Measurement

The direct measurement of arterial pressure avoids the cuff artifacts and other potential errors associated with indirect noninvasive pressure measurements. Specific approaches to the assessment of inflow disease include pull-through aortoiliac artery pressures during arteriography, percutaneous measurement of common femoral artery pressures, and intraoperative pressure measurements during arterial reconstructions.[28,55,56] Direct pressure measurements can be made both at rest and following some form of hemodynamic stress that increases flow rates above resting levels. Increased flow rates tend to augment pressure gradients that are not apparent in the resting state.[4] Pedal ergometer exercise has been used with percutaneous common femoral artery pressure measurements; however, many patients are unable to perform this test, and it has not been widely applied.[33,57] Intra-arterial injection of papaverine to produce peripheral vasodilatation is a simpler technique for increasing arterial flow rates and does not require patient cooperation or specialized equipment.

Percutaneous Pressure Measurement

Since the femoral puncture site is most commonly used for arteriographic procedures, direct measurements of arterial pressure during arteriography generally include the aortic, iliac, and femoral segments. Such pull-through pressures taken with the arteriogram catheter indicate the hemodynamic significance of any aortoiliac lesions. The intra-arterial injection of papaverine can serve as a pharmacologic stress test to assess the pressure gradients at higher flow rates. Studies of patients without inflow disease have shown that a hemodynamically significant lesion in the aortoiliac segment is present when the systolic pressure gradient is more than 10 mm Hg at rest or 20 mm Hg following injection of papaverine (30 mg) into the arteriogram catheter.[46]

Direct femoral artery pressure measurements are performed by percutaneous puncture of the common femoral artery with a needle that is connected by fluid-filled tubing to a calibrated pressure transducer. The femoral artery systolic pressure is divided by the brachial artery systolic pressure to obtain the femoral:brachial index (FBI).[56] A resting FBI of greater than or equal to 0.9 is considered normal, while values less than 0.9 indicate the presence of a hemodynamically significant lesion proximal to the common femoral artery.[58] If the resting FBI is normal, the injection of papaverine can be used to detect less severe aortoiliac lesions, as described previously for pressure measurements during arteriography. This is accomplished by injecting 30 mg of papaverine directly through the needle in the common femoral artery and monitoring both the common femoral and brachial artery pressures. A decrease in the FBI of 15% or more following papaverine injection is indicative of a hemodynamically significant lesion.[58]

Intraoperative Pressure Measurement

The basic techniques for intraoperative pressure measurement are similar to those of the percutaneous approach. Common femoral artery pressures, both before and after papaverine injection, can be used to assess the aortoiliac segment when it is not practical to obtain these measurements before surgery.

TREATMENT APPROACHES

Selection of the most appropriate surgical procedure for patients with multilevel disease is based on a combination of clinical factors, noninvasive test results, direct arterial pressure measurements, and arteriographic findings. The first priority is identification of hemodynamically significant inflow disease. As discussed previously, direct noninvasive testing with duplex scanning can be helpful, but some type of direct arterial pressure measurement is clearly the standard method for assessing the aortoiliac segment. The severity of outflow disease and the adequacy of the lower extremity collateral circulation are readily evaluated by a combination of indirect or direct noninvasive tests and arteriography.

Experience has shown that the clinical indication for lower extremity revascularization is also important in selecting the optimal treatment for multilevel disease. A technically successful procedure for hemodynamically significant inflow disease will frequently improve claudication, relieve ischemic rest pain, or promote healing of small superficial foot ulcers. However, the management of extensive distal tissue loss and infection, particularly in diabetic patients, generally requires simultaneous correction of both inflow and outflow lesions.[52,59] Thus, combined procedures are indicated in most patients with ischemic ulceration, especially when concomitant toe or foot amputations may be necessary for limb salvage. Even patients without tissue loss may benefit from combined inflow and outflow revascularization. Although patients with claudication are usually improved by inflow procedures, only about one-third will be asymptomatic.[7,9,11,23,60–62] In addition, patients who are relieved of rest pain by an inflow procedure may be left with disabling claudication.

Historically, the use of combined inflow and outflow procedures has been discouraged, except for extreme cases of ischemic necrosis and infection. This attitude was based on the belief that morbidity and mortality were higher for more complex and prolonged operations.[63] Furthermore, the results of isolated inflow procedures were often favorable, and it was difficult to predict which patients would subsequently require an outflow procedure. This led to the practice of performing a staged distal reconstruction in selected patients.[9] In one series of patients undergoing aortofemoral bypass grafting, a distal bypass was eventually performed in 21%, including 10% of the patients with intermittent claudication and 29% of those with limb-threatening ischemia.[23]

Improvements in vascular surgical techniques and perioperative care are now prompting the more frequent use of combined procedures.[52,64–66] Contemporary reports indicate that combined inflow and outflow procedures can be performed with virtually the same perioperative complication rates as inflow procedures and with improved clinical outcomes compared to inflow procedures alone.[52]

The ultimate choice between an inflow, outflow, combined, or staged arterial reconstruction depends on the clinical presentation, disease distribution, and general medical condition of the individual patient (Fig. 4–1). While the technical details of specific procedures are beyond the scope of this chapter, the following comments on the various management options pertain to the issue of staged or combined operations in patients with multilevel disease.

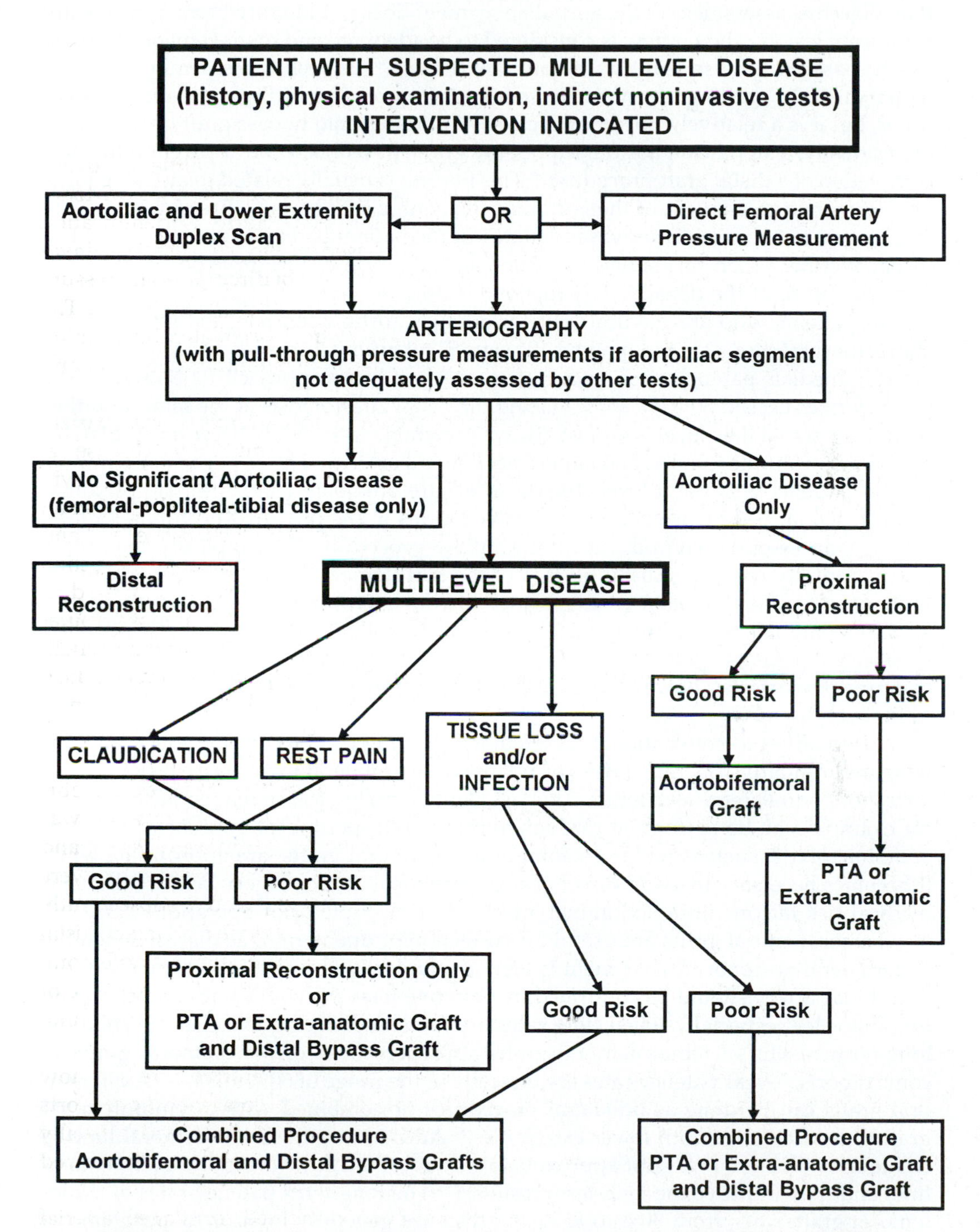

Figure 4–1. Algorithm for management of patients with suspected multilevel lower extremity arterial occlusive disease.

Single Level Reconstruction

If an objective assessment of the aortoiliac segment does not identify hemodynamically significant lesions, then inflow is considered to be adequate and management decisions can be based on the severity of the outflow disease.[67] In such cases, femoropopliteal or femorotibial grafting are typically required. Progression of proximal disease may occur, but it is a relatively uncommon cause of infrainguinal bypass graft occlusion.[25,68] Occasionally, a significant aortoiliac pressure gradient will become apparent only after completion of a distal graft procedure.[69] This finding is usually related to an inadequate hemodynamic assessment of the aortoiliac segment, either because pressure measurements were not obtained after vasodilatation or the patient had an insufficient response to papaverine. When this situation occurs, an inflow procedure may be necessary to prevent failure of the distal reconstruction.

In patients who are medically fit for a major aortic operation, the procedure of choice for correction of hemodynamically significant inflow disease in an aortobifemoral graft. Immediate patency rates for aortofemoral graft limbs approach 100%, and 5-year patency rates exceed 80%.[7,11,19,24,70,71] Placing the distal anastomosis at the femoral rather than the external iliac level is almost always preferable to provide direct revascularization of the profunda femoris and superficial femoral arteries. This is particularly important in patients with multilevel disease to ensure adequate runoff for the proximal reconstruction.[19,54,71,72] Correction of occlusive lesions in the proximal profunda femoris artery is an essential component of any inflow procedure. This typically requires a profundaplasty using the distal portion of the aortofemoral graft limb, either with or without an endarterectomy. A satisfactory proximal profunda femoris artery should accommodate at least a 4-mm diameter probe.[19,23] Aortoiliac endarterectomy is indicated in selected patients with occlusive lesions that are limited to the distal aorta and common iliac arteries; however, this lesion distribution is rarely found in patients with multilevel disease.[20]

Alternatives to conventional aortofemoral grafting can be considered for patients who are prohibitive operative risks or require only unilateral lower extremity revascularization. A unilateral aortofemoral bypass, iliofemoral bypass, or iliac endarterectomy, for example, can be performed through a limited retroperitoneal approach.[73–75] Extra-anatomic grafts, such as femorofemoral or axillofemoral grafts, are appropriate when it becomes necessary to avoid direct or retroperitoneal aortic surgery because of major medical risk factors, intra-abdominal infection, or multiple prior operations.[76–80]

Femorofemoral grafts are useful for correction of unilateral iliac disease when the contralateral or donor iliac segment is hemodynamically normal. The adequacy of the donor iliac artery should be confirmed by objective tests to avoid creating a steal from the donor leg, especially when flow rates are increased during exercise.[4,76] While the long-term results of femorofemoral grafts approach those of aortofemoral grafts in some reports, 5-year patency rates are typically in the range of 60% to 80%.[81] Axillofemoral grafts can be done as unilateral procedures or combined with a femorofemoral graft to revascularize both lower extremities.[82] Addition of the femorofemoral limb to create an axillobifemoral graft approximately doubles the flow rate in the axillofemoral limb and may improve the long-term results.[79,83] The long-term patency rates of axillofemoral grafts vary from 30% to 85%, but they are generally inferior to aortofemoral bypass.[78–84] This variability is probably due to differences in patient selection, since many series include cases done for nonocclusive disease along with patients treated for claudication and limb salvage.[81] In some reports, long-term patency of axillofemoral and femorofemoral grafts has been adversely affected by superficial femoral artery occlusion.[85] Therefore, whenever an extra-anatomic inflow procedure is used for multilevel disease, addition of an outflow procedure should be considered to improve runoff for the proximal graft.

Percutaneous transluminal angioplasty (PTA) is an alternative to direct arterial reconstruction for localized occlusive lesions.[50,86,87] The best results with PTA have been achieved with focal stenoses of the common iliac arteries in patients with good distal runoff.[86] Femoropopliteal and tibioperoneal lesions tend to include multiple stenotic areas and long segmental occlusions which are much less suitable for PTA, although some satisfactory results have been reported.[88]

Combined Inflow and Outflow Procedures

As previously mentioned, patients with multilevel lower extremity arterial occlusive disease can undergo complete revascularization in a single operation with acceptable morbidity and mortality rates.[52,65,66,89] The rationale for combined inflow and outflow procedures is based on the superior hemodynamic results compared to single level reconstructions and the avoidance of the technical difficulties associated with reoperative vascular procedures in the groins. In addition, performing a staged outflow procedure only after an inflow operation has failed to relieve ischemic symptoms may reduce the chances for limb salvage.[89] The potential for reducing health care costs by performing combined rather than staged procedures should also be considered.

Any of the inflow procedures previously described can be combined with an outflow procedure; however, patients who are considered to be medically unsuitable for direct aortic reconstruction should have an extra-anatomic inflow procedure combined with an expeditious distal reconstruction.[52,66,89] Combined procedures are easier when two surgical teams are used to minimize operating time. Using this approach, a variety of simultaneous inflow and outflow procedures were carried out on 62 patients with an operative mortality of 1.8%.[52] The operating time and perioperative complication rate were not significantly different from a group of patients at the same institution who had isolated inflow operations. Primary patency was 93% at 24 months for inflow procedures and 95% at 24 months for outflow procedures. Cumulative limb salvage was 91% at 36 months, and all patients with claudication were completely relieved of their symptoms.

A treatment option to consider in patients with multilevel disease that includes focal iliac artery lesions is a proximal PTA combined with an outflow procedure. This approach is particularly appropriate for patients with major medical risk factors who require intervention for limb salvage.[90–92] The PTA can be performed either as a separate procedure several days prior to surgery or intraoperatively. In a series of 79 patients undergoing staged iliac artery PTA and distal revascularization, the 5-year primary patency rate of the distal procedure was 76%, and the secondary patency rate was increased to 88% at 5 years by various repeated interventions.[90] Iliac stenosis at a new or previously dilated site was considered to be responsible for failure of the distal procedure in 5% of the patients. Among the patients with ischemic rest pain, 91% were relieved of symptoms, while limb salvage was achieved in 86% of those with ischemic tissue loss.

Finally, although lumbar sympathectomy has been recommended as an adjunct to lower extremity revascularization, there is no conclusive evidence that it improves graft patency rates or decreases the requirement for staged outflow procedures after proximal revascularizations.[93,94] However, since the predominant effect of sympathectomy appears to be on skin blood flow, the use of sympathectomy for cutaneous ischemia has a physiologic rationale.[95] Some favorable results have been reported in patients with mild rest pain and very superficial ischemic ulcers, but patients with severe rest pain and extensive tissue loss are unlikely to benefit.[96]

CONCLUSIONS

Multilevel occlusive disease is relatively common in patients with lower extremity atherosclerosis, particularly those with severe claudication, ischemic rest pain, and tissue loss. Therapeutic decision making for these patients requires determining the relative hemodynamic significance of the arterial lesions at various levels. While the indirect noninvasive tests are useful for evaluating the overall severity of lower extremity occlusive disease, they are less reliable for anatomic localization and hemodynamic assessment of specific lesions. In spite of its complexity, duplex scanning has become the standard noninvasive method for direct evaluation of the lower extremity arteries. When the necessary hemodynamic information is not provided by duplex scanning, some type of intra-arterial pressure measurement is indicated. It is usually most practical and convenient to obtain pull-through pressure measurements during arteriography.

The algorithm in Figure 4–1 outlines the management of patients with suspected multilevel lower extremity arterial disease. As for all treatment algorithms, it is intended to provide general guidelines, and management decisions must be tailored to the circumstances of each patient. The first consideration is whether the patient has hemodynamically significant inflow disease and whether correction of this disease alone will be sufficient. Patients having isolated proximal reconstructions require close follow-up to identify those who will need a staged outflow procedure.

Contemporary clinical experience suggests that combined inflow and outflow procedures should be used more often to provide maximal benefit to patients with multilevel disease. Combined procedures for multilevel disease may be indicated in the following situations: (1) when the aortoiliac lesions are relatively minor compared to the distal disease; (2) when the superficial femoral artery is occluded and the profunda femoris artery is diffusely diseased beyond its origin; (3) when the outflow disease involves both the femoropopliteal and tibioperoneal segments; and (4) when there is extensive ischemic necrosis and infection of the distal lower extremity.

Whether a single level or combined inflow and outflow procedure is selected, the operative approach must suit the medical risk profile of the individual patient. This requires the use of extra-anatomic bypass procedures and consideration of percutaneous transluminal angioplasty for proximal revascularization in a large proportion of patients with multilevel disease.

REFERENCES

1. Darling RC, Brewster DC, Hallet JW, et al. Aortoiliac reconstruction. *Surg Clin North Am.* 1979;59:565–579.
2. DeBakey ME, Lawrie GM, Glaeser DH. Patterns of atherosclerosis and their surgical significance. *Ann Surg.* 1985;201:115–131.
3. Veith FJ, Gupta SK, Wengerter KR, et al. Changing arteriosclerotic disease patterns and management strategies in lower-limb-threatening ischemia. *Ann Surg.* 1990;212:402–414.

4. Zierler RE, Strandness DE Jr. Hemodynamics for the vascular surgeon. In: Moore WS, ed. *Vascular Surgery—A Comprehensive Review.* 4th ed. Philadelphia: WB Saunders; 1993:179–204.
5. Garrett WV, Slaymaker EE, Heintz SE, et al. Intraoperative prediction of symptomatic result of aortofemoral bypass from changes in ankle pressure index. *Surgery* 1977;82:504–509.
6. Kozloff L, Collins CJ Jr, Rich NM, et al. Fallibility of postoperative Doppler ankle pressures in determining the adequacy of proximal arterial revascularization. *Am J Surg.* 1980;138:326–329.
7. Rutherford RB, Jones DN, Martin MS, et al. Serial hemodynamic assessment of aortofemoral bypass. *J Vasc Surg.* 1986;4:428–435.
8. Satiani B, Hayes JP, Evans WE. Prediction of distal reconstruction following aortofemoral bypass for limb salvage. *Surg Gynecol Obstet.* 1980;151:500–502.
9. Sumner DS, Strandness DE Jr. Aortoiliac reconstruction in patients with combined iliac and superficial femoral arterial occlusion. *Surgery.* 1978;84:348–355.
10. Edwards WH, Wright RS. A technique for combined aorto-femoral-popliteal arterial reconstruction. *Ann Surg.* 1974;179:572–579.
11. Mozersky DJ, Sumner DS, Strandness DE Jr. Long-term results of reconstructive aortoiliac surgery. *Am J Surg.* 1972;123:503–509.
12. Royster TS, Lynn R, Mulcare RJ. Combined aorto-iliac and femoro-popliteal occlusive disease. *Surg Gynecol Obstet.* 1976;143:949–952.
13. Mavor GE. The pattern of occlusion in atheroma of the lower limb arteries: the correlation of clinical and arteriographic findings. *Br J Surg.* 1956;43:352–364.
14. Strandness DE Jr. Chronic arterial occlusion. In: Strandness DE Jr, ed. *Collateral Circulation in Clinical Surgery.* Philadelphia: WB Saunders; 1969:368–404.
15. Yao JST, Hobbs JT, Irvine WT. Ankle systolic pressure measurements in arterial diseases affecting the lower extremities. *Br J Surg.* 1969;56:676–679.
16. Carter SA. Clinical measurement of systolic pressures in limbs with arterial occlusive disease. *JAMA.* 1969;207:1869–1874.
17. Yao JST. Hemodynamic studies in peripheral arterial disease. *Br. J Surg.* 1970;57:761–766.
18. Samson RH, Scher LA, Veith FJ. Combined segment arterial disease. *Surgery.* 1985;97:385–396.
19. Brewster DC, Darling RC. Optimal methods of aortoiliac reconstruction. *Surgery.* 1978; 84:739–748.
20. Brewster DC. Clinical and anatomical considerations for surgery in aortoiliac disease and results of surgical treatment. *Circulation.* 1991;83(suppl 2):I42–I52.
21. Lindbom A. Arteriosclerosis and arterial thrombosis in the lower limb: a roentgenological study. *Acta Radiol.* 1950;80(suppl):1–80.
22. Strandness DE Jr, Priest RE, Gibbons GE. Combined clinical and pathologic study of diabetic and nondiabetic peripheral arterial disease. *Diabetes.* 1964;13:366–372.
23. Brewster DC, Perler BA, Robison JG, et al. Aortofemoral graft for multilevel occlusive disease: predictors of success and need for distal bypass. *Arch Surg.* 1982;117:1593–1600.
24. Szilagyi DE, Elliot JP, Smith RF, et al. A thirty-year survey of the reconstructive surgical treatment of aortoiliac occlusive disease. *J Vasc Surg.* 1986;3:421–436.
25. Mozersky DJ, Sumner DS, Strandness DE Jr. Disease progression after femoropopliteal surgical procedures. *Surg Gynecol Obstet.* 1972;135:700–704.
26. Johnston KW, Demorais D, Colapinto RF. Difficulty in assessing the severity of aortoiliac disease by clinical and arteriographic methods. *Angiology.* 1981;32:609–614.
27. Sobinsky KR, Borozan PG, Gray B, et al. Is femoral pulse palpation accurate in assessing the hemodynamic significance of aortoiliac occlusive disease? *Am J Surg.* 1984;148:214–216.
28. Brewster DC, Waltman AC, O'Hara PJ, et al. Femoral artery pressure measurements during aortography. *Circulation.* 1979;60:120–124.
29. Bruns-Slot H, Strjbosch L, Greep JM. Interobserver variability in single plane aorto-arteriography. *Surgery.* 1981;90:497–503.
30. Breslau PJ, Jorning PJG, Greep JM. Assessment of aorto-iliac disease using hemodynamic measures. *Arch Surg.* 1985;120:1050–1052.
31. Sethi GK, Scott SM, Takaro T. Multiple plane angiography for more precise evaluation of aortoiliac disease. *Surgery.* 1975;78:154–159.
32. Udoff EJ, Barth KH, Harrington DP, et al. Hemodynamic significance of iliac artery stenosis: pressure measurements during angiography. *Radiology.* 1979;132:289–293.

33. Moore WS, Hall AD. Unrecognized aortoiliac stenosis: a physiologic approach to the diagnosis. *Arch Surg.* 1971;103:633–638.
34. Zierler RE, Strandness DE Jr. Nonimaging physiologic tests for assessment of extremity arterial disease. In: Zwiebel WJ, ed. *Introduction to Vascular Ultrasonography.* 3rd ed. Philadelphia: WB Saunders; 1992:201–221.
35. Baker JD. Hemodynamic assessment of the aortoiliac segment. *Surg Clin North Am.* 1990;70:31–40.
36. Zierler RE, Zierler BK. Duplex sonography of lower extremity arteries. In: Zwiebel WJ, eds. *Introduction to Vascular Ultrasonography.* 3rd ed. Philadelphia: WB Saunders; 1992:237–251.
37. Cutajar CL, Marston A, Newcombe JF. Value of cuff occlusion pressures in assessment of peripheral vascular disease. *Br J Med.* 1973;2:392–395.
38. O'Donnell TF, Lahey SJ, Kelly JJ, et al. A prospective study of Doppler pressures and segmental plethysmography before and following aortofemoral bypass. *Surgery.* 1979;86:120–128.
39. Bone GE, Hayes AC, Slaymaker EE, et al. Value of segmental limb blood pressures in predicting results of aortofemoral bypass. *Am J Surg.* 1976;132:733–738.
40. Rutherford RB, Lowenstein DH, Klein MF. Combining segmental systolic pressures and plethysmography to diagnose arterial occlusive disease of the legs. *Am J Surg.* 1979;138:211–218.
41. Heintz SE, Bone GE, Slaymaker EE, et al. Value of arterial pressure measurements in the proximal and distal part of the thigh in arterial occlusive disease. *Surg Gynecol Obstet.* 1978;146:337–343.
42. Faris IB, Jameson CW. The diagnosis of aortoiliac stenosis: a comparison of thigh pressure measurements and femoral artery flow velocity profile. *J Cardiovasc Surg.* 1975;16:597–602.
43. Kempczinski RF. Segmental volume plethysmography in the diagnosis of lower extremity arterial occlusive disease. *J Cardiovasc Surg.* 1982;23:125–129.
44. Persson AV, Gibbons G, Griffey S. Noninvasive evaluation of the aortoiliac segment. *J Cardiovasc Surg.* 1981;22:539–542.
45. Baker JD, Machleder HI, Skidmore R. Analysis of femoral artery Doppler signals by LaPlace transform damping method. *J Vasc Surg.* 1984;1:520–524.
46. Thiele BL, Bandyk DF, Zierler RE, et al. A systematic approach to the assessment of aortoiliac disease. *Arch Surg.* 1983;118:477–481.
47. Jager KA, Phillips DJ, Martin RRL, et al. Noninvasive mapping of lower limb arterial lesions. *Ultrasound Med Biol.* 1985;11:515–521.
48. Kohler TR, Nance DR, Cramer MM, et al. Duplex scanning for diagnosis of aortoiliac and femoropopliteal disease: a prospective study. *Circulation.* 1987;76:1074–1080.
49. Moneta GL, Yeager RA, Antonovic R, et al. Accuracy of lower extremity arterial duplex mapping. *J Vasc Surg.* 1992;15:275–284.
50. Edwards JM, Coldwell DM, Goldman ML, et al. The role of duplex scanning in the selection of patients for transluminal angioplasty. *J Vasc Surg.* 1991;13:69–74.
51. Williams LR, Flanigan DP, Schuler JJ, et al. Prediction of improvement in ankle blood pressure following arterial bypass. *J Surg Res.* 1984;37:175–179.
52. Dalman RL, Taylor LM, Moneta GL, et al. Simultaneous operative repair of multilevel lower extremity occlusive disease. *J Vasc Surg.* 1991;13:211–221.
53. O'Donnell TF, Cossman D, Callow AD. Noninvasive intraoperative monitoring: a prospective study comparing Doppler systolic occlusion pressure and segmental plethysmography. *Am J Surg.* 1978;135:539–546.
54. Strandness DE Jr. Functional results after revascularization of the profunda femoris artery. *Am J Surg.* 1970;119:240–245.
55. Boren CH, Towne JB, Bernhard VM, et al. Profunda-popliteal collateral index: a guide to successful profundaplasty. *Arch Surg.* 1980;115:1366–1372.
56. Flanigan DP, Ryan TJ, Williams LR, et al. Aortofemoral or femoropopliteal revascularization? A prospective evaluation of the papaverine test. *J Vasc Surg.* 1984;1:215–223.
57. Sobinsky KR, Williams LR, Gray B, et al. Supine exercise testing in the selection of suprainguinal versus infrainguinal bypass in patients with multisegmental arterial occlusive disease. *Am J Surg.* 1986;152:185–189.

58. Flanigan DP, Williams LR, Schwartz JA, et al. Hemodynamic evaluation of the aortoiliac system based on pharmacologic vasodilatation. *Surgery*. 1983;93:709–714.
59. Imparato AM, Sanoudos G, Epstein HY, et al. Results in 96 aortoiliac reconstructive procedures: preoperative angiographic and functional classifications used as prognostic guides. *Surgery*. 1970;68:610–616.
60. Martinez BD, Hertzer NR, Beven EG. Influence of distal arterial occlusive disease on prognosis following aortobifemoral bypass. *Surgery*. 1980;88:795–805.
61. Hill DA, McGrath MA, Lord RSA, et al. The effect of superficial femoral artery occlusion on the outcome of aortofemoral bypass for intermittent claudication. *Surgery*. 1980;87:133–136.
62. Galland RB, Hill DA, Gustave R, et al. The functional results of aortoiliac reconstruction. *Br J Surg*. 1980;67:344–346.
63. Benson JR, Whelen TJ, Cohen A, et al. Combined aortoiliac and femoropopliteal occlusive disease: limitations of total aortofemoropopliteal bypass. *Ann Surg*. 1966;163:121–130.
64. Harris PL, Cave Bigley DJ, McSweeney L. Aortofemoral bypass and the role of concomitant femorodistal reconstruction. *Br J Surg*. 1985;72:317–320.
65. Eidt J, Charlesworth D. Combined aortobifemoral and femoropopliteal bypass in the management of patients with extensive atherosclerosis. *Ann Vasc Surg*. 1986;1:453–459.
66. Harward TR, Ingegno MD, Carlton L, et al. Limb-threatening ischemia due to multilevel arterial occlusive disease: simultaneous or staged inflow/outflow revascularization. *Ann Surg*. 1995;221:498–506.
67. Kikta MJ, Flanigan DP, Bishara RA, et al. Long-term follow-up of patients having infrainguinal bypass performed below stenotic but hemodynamically normal aortoiliac vessels. *J Vasc Surg*. 1987;5:319–328.
68. Brewster DC, LaSalle AJ, Robison JG, et al. Femoropopliteal graft failures: clinical consequences and success of secondary reconstructions. *Arch Surg*. 1983;118:1043–1047.
69. Gupta SK, Veith FJ, Kram HB, et al. Significance and management of inflow gradients unexpectedly generated after femorofemoral, femoropopliteal, and femoroinfrapopliteal bypass grafting. *J Vasc Surg*. 1990;12:278–283.
70. Jones AF, Kempczinski RF. Aortofemoral bypass grafting: a reappraisal. *Arch Surg*. 1981;116:301–305.
71. Malone JM, Goldstone J. The natural history of bilateral aortofemoral bypass grafts for ischemia of the lower extremities. *Arch Surg*. 1975;110:1300–1306.
72. Baird RJ, Feldman P, Miles JT, et al. Subsequent downstream repair after aortoiliac and aortofemoral bypass operations. *Surgery*. 1977;82:785–792.
73. Kram HB, Gupta SK, Veith FJ, et al. Unilateral aortofemoral bypass: a safe and effective option for the treatment of unilateral limb-threatening ischemia. *Am J Surg*. 1991;162:155–158.
74. Kalman PG, Hosang M, Johnston KW, et al. Unilateral iliac disease: the role of iliofemoral bypass. *J Vasc Surg*. 1987;6:139–143.
75. Taylor LM Jr, Freimanis IE, Edwards JM, et al. Extraperitoneal iliac endarterectomy in the treatment of multilevel lower extremity arterial occlusive disease. *Am J Surg*. 1986;152:34–39.
76. Sumner DS, Strandness DE Jr. The hemodynamics of the femorofemoral shunt. *Surg Gynecol Obstet*. 1972;134:629–636.
77. Lamarton AJ, Nicolaides AN, Eastcott HHG. The femorofemoral graft: hemodynamic improvement and patency rate. *Arch Surg*. 1985;120:1274–1278.
78. Savrin RA, Record GT, McDowell DE. Axillofemoral bypass. *Arch Surg*. 1986;121:1016–1020.
79. Johnson WC, LoGerfo FW, Vollman RW, et al. Is axillo-bilateral femoral graft an effective substitute for aorto-bilateral iliac/femoral graft? An analysis of ten years' experience. *Ann Surg*. 1977;186:123–129.
80. Harris EJ, Taylor LM Jr, McConnell DB, et al. Clinical results of axillobifemoral bypass using externally supported polytetrafluoroethylene. *J Vasc Surg*. 1990;12:416–421.
81. Whittemore AD, Donaldson MC, Mannick JA. Aortoiliac occlusive disease. In: Moore WS, ed. *Vascular Surgery—A Comprehensive Review*. 4th ed. Philadelphia: WB Saunders; 1993:451–464.
82. Ascer E, Veith FJ, Gupta SK, et al. Comparison of axillounifemoral and axillobifemoral bypass operations. *Surgery*. 1985;97:169–175.
83. Moore WS, Hall AD, Blaisdell FW. Late results of axillary-femoral bypass grafting. *Am J Surg*. 1971;122:148–154.

84. O'Donnell TF, McBride KA, Callow AD, et al. Management of combined segment disease. *Am J Surg.* 1981;141:452–459.
85. Rutherford RB, Patt A, Pearce WH. Extra-anatomic bypass: a closer view. *J Vasc Surg.* 1987;6:437–446.
86. Johnston KW, Rae M, Hogg-Johnston SA, et al. Five-year results of a prospective study of percutaneous transluminal angioplasty. *Ann Surg.* 1987;206:403–413.
87. Wilson SE, Wolf GL, Cross AP. Percutaneous transluminal angioplasty versus operation for peripheral atherosclerosis: report of a prospective randomized trial in a selected group of patients. *J Vasc Surg.* 1989;9:1–9.
88. Rush DS, Gewertz BL, Lu CT, et al. Limb salvage in poor risk patients using transluminal angioplasty. *Arch Surg.* 1983;118:1209–1212.
89. Nypaver TJ, Ellenby MI, Mendoza O, et al. A comparison of operative approaches and parameters predictive of success in multilevel arterial occlusive disease. *J Am Coll Surg.* 1994;179:449–456.
90. Brewster DC, Cambria RP, Darling RC, et al. Long-term results of combined iliac balloon angioplasty and distal surgical revascularization. *Ann Surg.* 1989;210:324–331.
91. Peterkin GA, Belkin M, Cantelmo NL, et al. Combined transluminal angioplasty and infrainguinal reconstruction in multilevel atherosclerotic disease. *Am J Surg.* 1990;160:277–279.
92. Katz SG, Kohl RD, Yellin A. Iliac angioplasty as a prelude to distal arterial bypass. *J Am Coll Surg.* 1994;179:577–582.
93. Barnes RW, Baker WH, Shanik G. Value of concomitant sympathectomy in aortoiliac reconstruction: results of a prospective randomized study. *Arch Surg.* 1977;112:1325–1330.
94. Satiani B, Liapis CD, Hayes JP, et al. Prospective randomized study of concomitant lumbar sympathectomy with aortoiliac reconstruction. *Am J Surg.* 1982;143:755–760.
95. Moore WS, Hall AD. Effects of lumbar sympathectomy on skin capillary blood flow in arterial occlusive disease. *J Surg Res.* 1973;14:151–157.
96. Strandness DE Jr. Role of sympathectomy in the treatment of arteriosclerosis obliterans and thromboangiitis obliterans. In: Strandness DE Jr, ed. *Collateral Circulation in Clinical Surgery.* Philadelphia: WB Saunders; 1969:450–459.

5

Timing of Carotid Endarterectomy in Patients with Acute Ischemic Attacks, Crescendo Transient Ischemic Attacks, or Coexisting Coronary Artery Disease

James A. DeWeese, MD

The onset of neurologic deficit secondary to acute ischemia of the brain with involvement of the internal carotid artery is almost always sudden. The severity of the symptoms immediately after the onset, however, bears little relationship to the eventual neurologic status. The episode may be merely a transient ischemic attack (TIA), which will disappear within a short time, or a reversible ischemic neurologic deficit (RIND), which will require more than 24 hours to completely resolve. More serious situations include a continued worsening of neurologic symptoms resulting in death (progressive stroke) and persistent deficits, which suggest an infarction has occurred (completed stroke). Other patients will experience repeated TIAs that occur with greater duration, increased severity, or both (crescendo TIAs). The management of all these situations should be influenced by the patients' associated risk factors, particularly coronary artery disease. We discuss the timing of carotid endarterectomy in patients with acute strokes of more than 24 hours duration, crescendo TIAs, or a coexisting coronary artery disease.

ACUTE STROKES

The severity of the neurologic deficit must be considered when determining the timing of an operation. Patients with severe deficits are those with hemiplegia, aphasia, possible blindness, or an altered level of consciousness. The results of the Joint Study of Extracranial Arterial Occlusion,[1] published in 1969, discouraged almost all surgeons from performing early operations or operations at all on this group of patients. Of 50 patients with profound strokes who had carotid endarterectomies within 13 days, only 34% were improved and 42% died. Of 18 patients on whom operations were performed after 14 days, there was an improvement rate of 72% but a mortality rate of 17%. This was compared to similar results in 187 patients on whom no operation was performed, of which 53% were improved and 20% died. It was believed that at least part of the reason for the increased morbidity among the patients operated on early was the restoration of blood flow to an area of ischemic brain; it was thought that this produced a hemorrhagic infarct and eventually a massive hemorrhage into the area of infarction. This speculation was supported by reports of such occurrences by Caplan et al.,[2] Gonzalez, and Lewis[3] and Wylie et al.[4] It thus became an accepted policy to delay surgery for 4 to 6 weeks in patients diagnosed with acute stroke, regardless of the severity. This conservative approach was supported by Giordano et al.'s report in 1985.[5] They reported experiences with 49 endarterectomies performed on patients with a neurologic deficit lasting more than 24 hours. Twenty-seven endarterectomies were performed less than 5 weeks after the initial stroke, and 22 operations were performed 5 to 20 weeks after the stroke. Postoperative strokes occurred in 18.5% (5:27) of the patients operated on within 5 weeks. None of the patients operated on after 5 weeks had worsening of their preoperative neurologic status.

More recent reports, however, suggest that early operation should be considered in some patients with mild to moderately severe acute strokes (Table 5–1). Whittemore et al.[6] described 28 patients with "small fixed neurologic deficits" and a carotid artery stenosis of greater than 75%. The neurologic deficits included isolated speech deficits in 6 patients, monoparesis of the upper extremity in 10, hemiparesis in 6, and a combination of speech deficit and hemiparesis in 6. Endarterectomies were performed 2 to 30 days after onset. Fifteen of the 28 operations were performed within 7 days of onset of the stroke. There were no new in-hospital strokes nor any extensions of previous deficits; 1 patient died of a pulmonary embolus. Rosenthal et al.[7] operated on 29 post-stroke patients who had "limited stable strokes" 9 to 21 days after onset. These patients had internal carotid artery stenosis of greater than 75% or had complex macroulcerated plaques. There was one postoperative stroke and 3 patients sustained focal minor TIAs. Similar results were obtained with patients who had RINDs. Piotrowski et al.[8] admitted 82 patients to the hospital with acute strokes with the intent to perform endarterectomy when "neurologic

TABLE 5–1. EARLY OPERATIONS FOR ACUTE STROKES

Source	Symptoms	Stenosis	No.	Timing (Days)	Postoperative Strokes	Death
Whittemore et al.[6]	Small fixed neurologic deficit	75%–99%	15	0–7	0	0
			13	8–30	0	1 (pul. emb.)
Rosenthal et al.[7]	Limited stable strokes	75%–99%	29	9–21	1	0
Piotrowski et al.[8]	Neurologic deficit plateaued		31	0–14	1	1 (stroke)
			31	15–28	0	0
			20	19–42	0	0
Gasecki et al.[9]	Minor nondisabling stroke	70%–99%	42	3–30	2	0
		Total	181		4 (2.2%)	2 (1.1%)

recovery had plateaued." Eight patients recovered completely. There were 25 patients with mild deficits on admission and 56 with mild deficits after observation. There were 47 patients with moderate deficits on admission and only 16 following observation. There were 10 patients with severe deficits on admission and only 2 following observation. Progressive strokes were not included as acute strokes in this study. Thirty-one patients were operated on within 2 weeks of onset and 1 of these patients who was operated on 3 days after onset had fluctuating blood pressure and suffered a hemorrhagic infarction 2 days postoperatively and died. Thirty-one patients were operated on 2 to 4 weeks after acute onset and 20 were operated on 4 to 6 weeks after onset without postoperative complications. Gasecki et al.[9] reported on 100 patients who were a subgroup of patients enrolled in the North American Symptomatic Carotid Endarterectomy Trials (NASCET) who were admitted with "minor nondisabling strokes." A nondisabling stroke was defined as persistence of symptoms or signs of hemispheric ischemia greater than 24 hours that they determined would have resulted in no significant impairments restricting activities of daily living. The patients all had internal carotid artery stenosis of 70% to 99%. Strokes occurred in 4.8% (2:42) patients operated on from 3 to 30 days after their stroke.

The major reason for delaying operations for acute strokes has been the fear of hemorrhage into the infarct. In the past, the severity of the stroke was thought to be related to the size of the infarct. With the development of the CT scan, however, it became possible to objectify the presence and extent of the infarct. Some reports supported the position that endarterectomies on patients with positive CT scans increased the risk of postoperative strokes. For example, Ricotta et al.[10] performed endarterectomies on 27 patients with unstable neurologic symptoms within 10 days of onset. Of the 17 patients with normal CT scans, only 1 patient suffered a postoperative stroke. Of the 10 patients with positive CT scans, 4 patients had neurologic deterioration.

Some authors did not choose to challenge the standard thinking and withheld urgent operations from patients with positive CT scans. Whittemore[11] did not operate on patients with acute "large infarcts." Dosick et al.[12] performed CT scans 1 and 5 days after onset of acute strokes with mild to moderate deficits on 245 patients. Patients with normal CT scans were operated on within 14 days. Patients with positive scans were followed for 4 to 6 weeks before angiograms and appropriate operations were performed.

Some studies found a postoperative stroke rate that was the same or higher in those who had normal preoperative scans. Gasecki et al.[9] reported two postoperative strokes in 25 patients operated on in less than 30 days who had normal preoperative CT scans and none in 17 patients who had abnormal CT scans. The strokes were secondary to carotid occlusion. Piotrowski et al.[8] performed endarterectomy on 82 patients less than 6 weeks after onset of strokes who had CT scans. Separate analysis of patients with cortical infarcts on CT scans did not reveal any increase in the stroke or death rate compared to the group as a whole or to those patients with lacunar infarcts or normal CT scan findings. Giordano et al.[5] reported four postoperative strokes in patients operated on in less than 5 weeks. Only 1 patient had a positive preoperative scan. One of the three who had a negative scan had a hemorrhagic infarct.

There are other anecdotal examples of the uselessness of CT scanning in determining the timing of endarterectomy. For example, in Ricotta et al.'s[10] series of one death in the early operation group was due to a hemorrhagic infarct in a patient who had had a normal preoperative scan. Martin et al.[13] reported 3 patients with abnormal CT scans who underwent endarterectomy less than 6 weeks after acute onset of their stroke without morbidity. In their overall use of CT scans in the preoperative evaluation of

469 patients considered for carotid endarterectomy, no correlation was found between the presence of an infarct on the preoperative CT scan and postoperative neurologic morbidity. They conceded, however, that CT scans were of "potential" use in determining timing in patients with acute strokes, but for other patients CT scanning is unnecessary before carotid endarterectomy and is not cost effective.

Pomposelli et al.[14] believed that factors other than timing alone might be responsible for intracranial hemorrhage following carotid endarterectomy. They reviewed the records of 11 such patients of a total of 1,500 patients who had endarterectomy at their institution. The only recognizable significant predisposing factor was relief of stenosis greater than 90%, as has been recognized by others. Only 1 of 5 patients had positive preoperative CT scans. Although none of the patients were extraordinarily hypertensive (systolic pressure 120–160) preoperatively, postoperative systolic blood pressures were 200 to 240 mm Hg in 6 of 11 patients. The possible danger of uncontrolled hypertension has been recognized by Caplan and others.[2]

The timing of a carotid endarterectomy for an acute stroke is a multifactorial decision, and each case must be judged on its own merit. The following may be of some help in evaluating patients with strokes for timing of operation.

1. Patients with acute completed strokes or RINDs with minor to moderate severity have been successfully operated on within a few days of the onset of stroke with low postoperative stroke and death rates.

However, there are no similar extensive experiences of good results of carotid endarterectomy reported for patients with acute, severe, or profound strokes, particularly in patients with altered levels of consciousness.

2. The reports of successful results have been when operations were performed on patients with 70% to 99% stenosis of their carotid arteries. The severity of the lesion can be determined initially with a duplex scan. Angiography is performed for confirmation of the stenosis and the demonstration of ulceration.

In addition, duplex scan evidence of a thrombus or extremely severe stenosis may prompt an earlier performance of an angiogram to demonstrate a floating thrombus that might dictate an earlier operation.

Confirmation of the value of carotid endarterectomy for symptomatic carotid diameter stenosis of less than 70% requires an extension of the NASCET.[15]

Since then, the Asymptomatic Carotid Arteriosclerosis Study (ACAS) concluded that carotid endarterectomy is indicated for an asymptomatic carotid diameter stenoses of greater than 60%.[16]

3. CT scanning is required for the evaluation of an acute stroke to rule out hemorrhage as the cause of the stroke.

The preoperative presence or absence of an infarct demonstrated on a CT scan has not correlated with postendarterectomy infarcts.[13] It is doubtful, however, that a "large infarct" seen on preoperative CT scan has ever been submitted to the test of a carotid endarterectomy.[11]

4. Since postoperative systolic blood pressures of 200 to 240 mg have been correlated with hemorrhagic infarcts it is prudent to gain control of significantly elevated pressures prior to submitting a patient to a carotid endarterectomy.[2]

5. The possibility that a patient might have a stroke while awaiting operation has been used as a justification for earlier operations. Dosick et al.[12] report the occurrence of strokes in waiting patients with strokes to be 21% (4:19). With increased experience, however, he found it to occur in 9.5% (7:74) of patients. Rosenthal et al.[7] observed recurrence of stroke to be only 4% (4:99) within 1 year of an acute stroke.

CRESCENDO TRANSIENT ISCHEMIC ATTACKS

Crescendo TIAs are transient ischemic neurologic deficits that occur with increasing frequency, greater duration, or greater severity, and may eventually occur several times a day. There are no residual deficits between attacks.

In 1976 Goldstone and Moore[17] described 3 patients with transient episodes of arm and leg hypesthesia in one, hemiparesis in another, and monoparesis and amaurosis fugax in the third, which were increasing in frequency and, in 2 of the 3, were occurring several times per day. All 3 had carotid artery stenoses of greater than 90%. All underwent carotid endarterectomy with uneventful recovery. All patients were operated on immediately after the diagnosis was established. Carson et al.[18] later performed carotid endarterectomy emergently on 24 patients with crescendo TIAs. There were no postoperative neurologic deficits. Wilson et al.[19] reported the experience of the Trialists in the Department of Veterans Affairs (VA) Cooperative Study Program Number 309. Twelve of the 98 patients with TIAs assigned to medical treatment developed a "crescendo" pattern of symptoms. All underwent successful operation with uncomplicated courses. All operations were performed within 12 to 24 hours of admission.

There are no extensive natural history studies of patients with untreated crescendo TIAs. Mentzer et al.[20] offer some useful information. Twelve patients with crescendo TIAs and high grade carotid stenosis were evaluated. Five were not operated on, of which one recovered, three were moderately to severely impaired at discharge, and one died of complications of cerebral infarction. The seven patients who underwent carotid endarterectomy recovered completely.

McIntyre and Goldstone [21] have reported their experience with an additional 24 patients. All had uncomplicated courses except for 1 who did not have a preoperative arteriogram and operation resulted in a fixed deficit later attributed to a lacunar infarction.

Rothrock et al.'s[22] experience with 47 patients with symptoms of crescendo TIAs emphasizes the need for complete evaluation of these patients prior to endarterectomy including arteriograms and CT scans. Only 55% of their patients had arteriographic evidence of significant carotid artery disease as defined by a luminal stenosis of greater than 75%, ulceration of greater than 2 mm in depth, or both. Twelve of the 47 angiograms were completely normal. Negative arteriograms were most frequently found in patients with only "numbness/weakness" or "typical lacunar" pure sensory or pure motor symptoms.

COEXISTING CORONARY HEART DISEASE

Strokes occur in less than 5% of patients undergoing coronary bypass, not all of which are secondary to carotid artery disease. If stroke does occur, it is a devastating problem for the patients and their families.[23] Carotid artery disease is sometimes suspected on the basis of bruits or symptoms in approximately 10% of patients being evaluated for myocardial revascularization. Symptomatic or high-grade (>70% diameter) carotid lesions were identified on 275 (2.8%) of 9,714 patients scheduled for coronary artery bypass grafting (CABG) at Cleveland Clinic.[24] Two recent randomized trials have resulted in the establishment of recommendations for indications for carotid endarerectomy. The NASCET determined that in patients with symptomatic carotid territory TIAs or nondisabling strokes, and carotid diameter stenoses of 70% to 99%, that the cumulative risk of ipsilateral stroke 2 years after carotid endarterectomy was 9% as compared to 26% ($p<.001$) for those who did not have an operation.[15] The perioperative stroke or death rate was 5.8%. The ACAS concluded that patients who were asymptomatic but had carotid diameter stenoses of greater than 60% and had carotid endarterectomies had a 5-year aggregate risk rate of stroke or death of 4.8% as compared to 10.6% for those not assigned to surgery, ($p = 0.0006$).[16] The operative stroke or death rate was 2.3%. It would seem logical therefore that symptomatic patients with stenoses greater than 60% should also be considered as candidates for carotid endarterectomy.

Also of importance, coronary artery disease is commonly found in patients being evaluated for carotid endarterectomies. On the basis of EKG alone 24% of patients in our institution had coronary artery disease.[25] O'Donnell et al.[26] found that 66% of patients undergoing carotid surgery had clinical evidence of coronary artery disease. Hertzer et al.[27] identified 37% of 506 carotid patients with coronary artery disease severe enough to warrant a CABG. Coronary artery disease is also the most common cause of late death following carotid endarterectomy. It was responsible for 24% of deaths occurring within 5 years following carotid endarterectomy in our institution.[25]

The indications for carotid endarterectomy alone and coronary artery bypass alone are becoming more standardized. When patients are found to have both coronary artery and carotid artery disease, the timing of and sequence of each operation becomes important. It is necessary to decide if the carotid operation should be performed before, at the same time as, or after the CABG. The decision is based on consideration of the operative risk of stroke and death for each individual patient.

Carotid Endarterectomy Prior to Coronary Bypass

Performance of carotid endarterectomy before CABG may be appropriate in some patients. Hertzer performed staged carotid endarterectomies prior to CABG in patients with "frequent TIAs and severe carotid stenosis" who also had asymptomatic or stable coronary atherosclerosis and were candidates for CABG.[28] Permanent postoperative strokes occurred following only 1.5% (1:65) of carotid operations followed later by CABG. There were no deaths. Hertzer et al.[24] reported on 24 patients with unilateral carotid diameter stenosis of greater than 70% of whom 10 were asymptomatic, 4 had TIAs, and 6 had completed strokes with good functional recovery. One patient (4.2%) suffered a stroke and died. Cosgrove quotes a review of five reported surgical series in which the stroke rate following the staged procedure was 3.2% with a mortality rate of 7.5%, with most deaths secondary to fatal myocardial infarctions during the staging interval.[23]

Combined Carotid Endarterectomy and Coronary Bypass

Combined operations are appropriate for many patients. Patients with TIAs, prior strokes, or severe bilateral carotid lesions as well as unstable angina, left main disease, triple vessel disease, or poor ventricular function have been typical candidates for combined procedures.[23,24] Hertzer et al.[24] described 170 patients who underwent combined operations with a stroke rate of 5.3% and a mortality rate of 5.3%. The postoperative stroke rate was 1% and the mortality rate was 1% for the isolated CABGs at the same institution.[24] Rizzo et al.[29] reported combined operations on 127 patients of which one-third had asymptomatic carotid stenosis and all had severe coronary artery disease. There were eight (6.3%) strokes. Six of the eight strokes were ipsilateral to the carotid endarterectomy. There were seven (5.5%) heart-related deaths. Other centers have also observed increased stroke and mortality rates for combined operations as compared to isolated CABGs.[30-32] Other institutions have reported no increased stroke rates for combined operations as compared to CABGs alone.[33-35] Differences in results can be at least partially attributed to the selection of the patients. Gardner et al.[36] observed stroke rates following CABG of 6.3% in patients older than 70 years of age as compared to 3% for those 61 to 70, and 1.3% for those 51 to 60. The stroke rate may also be influenced by the preoperative symptoms and extent of the carotid lesions. Hertzer et al.[24] observed stroke rates of 6.7% for combined operations on patients with bilateral carotid stenosis who had had preoperative TIAs or strokes, with an additional stroke rate for 10% for the subsequent endarterectomy for the contralateral stenosis, as compared to a stroke rate for only 2.8% for patients with unilateral stenosis who were asymptomatic preoperatively and had a combined operation. Rizzo et al.[29] observed a stroke rate of 10.1% (8:84) in symptomatic carotid patients as compared to a 0% (0:42) frequency rate of stroke in patients without carotid symptoms. Hertzer et al.[24] found that patients with severe bilateral carotid stenosis who required a combined operation before their contralateral endarterectomy had total stroke rates for the two procedures of 16.7% (5:30), as compared to 0% stroke rates for 9 patients with stable enough coronary heart disease that they could have their carotid operation before their combined operation.

Coronary Bypass Followed by Carotid Endarterectomy

Patients with severe coronary artery disease and stable carotid artery disease have undergone CABGs prior to their carotid endarterectomy. Hertzer et al.[24] reported an 8.7% stroke rate with no deaths in 23 such patients who required urgent CABGs before their delayed carotid endarterectomy. Hertzer et al.[24] performed a randomized study of 129 patients with severe coronary disease and with asymptomatic unilateral greater than 70% diameter carotid stenosis. There were 71 patients who had combined operations and 58 who had CABG followed by carotid endarterectomy. The 14.4% (6.9% + 7.5%) stroke rate and 5.3% mortality rate for the two procedures required in the 58 patients who were staged was significantly greater than the 2.8% stroke rate and 4.2% mortality rate in the 71 patients who had combined procedures. Stroke rates were improved in patients who had their carotid operations delayed. The stroke rate was 11% in 61 patients operated on less than 2 weeks after their CABG, but only 2.2% in 46 patients operated on more than 2 weeks after their CABG.

The timing of carotid endarterectomies for a patient with associated coronary artery disease must be judged on its own merit. The following may be of some help in evaluating each patient:

1. Carotid endarterectomies can be performed prior to a CABG with a low risk of stroke and death and increased longevity of the patient.

The patient should have a carotid diameter stenosis greater than 60%, as well as asymptomatic and stable coronary artery disease for which CABG is indicated to increase longevity.

The coronary operation should not be unduly delayed after the carotid operation.

2. Combined carotid endarterectomy and CABG operations are most suited to patients without neurologic symptoms but with severe (60% diameter) carotid stenoses. They typically also have unstable angina, left main disease, triple vessel disease, or poor ventricular function.

Stroke and mortality rates following such patients approach those for CABG alone.

Although patients with TIAs or strokes may have increased longevity, perioperative stroke rates may be 5% to 10% and mortality rates in the 5% range.

Older patients, particularly those older than 70 years of age, are four times more likely to have strokes than those less than 60.

Patients who have severe bilateral carotid stenosis and stable enough coronary artery disease to allow performance of the endarterectomy before a combined procedure for the contralateral carotid lesion have much lower stroke rates than those who require their combined operation prior to contralateral endarterectomy.

3. CABGs have on occasion been performed on patients with unstable coronary artery disease urgently before carotid endarterectomy is even considered. This may be because of the severity of the coronary artery disease or the lack of recognition of the carotid disease.

The stroke rates have been significantly increased in such patients. The randomized study of Hertzer et al.[24] suggest that even patients with an asymptomatic carotid diameter stenosis of greater than 70% should rarely have CABG performed first. Those patients had total stroke rates for their two operations of 14.4% and mortality rate of 5.3%, compared to only 2.8% and 4.2% rates if a combined operation was performed.

If the carotid endarterectomy is delayed until after the CABG, it should be performed no sooner than 2 weeks after the CABG.

REFERENCES

1. Blaisdell WF, Clauss RH, Galbraith JG, et al. Joint study of extracranial arterial occlusion. *JAMA.* 1969;209:1889–1895.
2. Caplan LR, Skillman J, Ojemann R, et al. Intracerebral hemorrhage following carotid endarterectomy: a hypertensive complication? *Stroke.* 1978;9:457–463.
3. Gonzalez LL, Lewis CM. Cerebral hemorrhage following successful endarterectomy of the internal carotid artery. *Surg Gynecol Obstet.* 1962;122:73–76.
4. Wylie EJ, Hein MF, Adams JE. Intracranial hemorrhage following surgical revascularization for treatment of acute strokes. *J Neurosurg.* 1964;21:212–216.
5. Giordano JM, Trout HH III, Kozloff L, et al. Timing of carotid endarterectomy after stroke. *J Vasc Surg.* 1985;2:250–254.
6. Whittemore AD, Ruby ST, Couch NP, et al. Early carotid endarterectomy in patients with small, fixed neurologic deficits. *J Vasc Surg.* 1984;1:795–799.
7. Rosenthal D, Borrero E, Clark MD, et al. Carotid endarterectomy after reversible ischemic neurologic deficit or stroke: is it of value? *J Vasc Surg.* 1988;4:527–534.
8. Piotrowski JJ, Bernhard VM, Rubin JR, et al. Timing of carotid endarterectomy after acute stroke. *J Vasc Surg.* 1990;11:45–52.
9. Gasecki AP, Ferguson GG, Eliasziw M, et al. Early endarterectomy for severe carotid artery stenosis after a nondisabling stroke: results from the North American Symptomatic Carotid Endarterectomy Trial. *J Vasc Surg.* 1994;20:288–295.
10. Ricotta JJ, Ouriel K, Green RM, et al. Use of computerized cerebral tomography in selection of patients for elective and urgent carotid endarterectomy. *Ann Vasc Surg.* 1985;202:783–787.
11. Whittemore AD. Discussion of paper by Piotrowski JJ, Bernhard VM, Rubin JR, et al. Timing of carotid endarterectomy after acute stroke. *J Vasc Surg.* 1990;11:45–52.
12. Dosick SM, Whalen RC, Gale SS, et al. Carotid endarterectomy in the stroke patient: computerized axial tomography to determine timing. *J Vasc Surg.* 1985;2:214–219.
13. Martin JD, Valentine RJ, Myers SI, et al. Is routine scanning necessary in the preoperative evaluation of patients undergoing carotid endarterectomy? *J Vasc Surg.* 1991;13:267–270.
14. Pomposelli FB, Lamparello PJ, Riles TS, et al. Intracranial hemorrhage after carotid endarterectomy. *J Vasc Surg.* 1988;7:248–255.
15. North American Symptomatic Carotid Endarterectomy Trial (NASCET) collaborators. Beneficial effect of carotid endarterectomy in symptomatic patients with high-grade carotid stenosis. *N Engl J Med.* 1991;325:445–463.
16. Clinical advisory: carotid endarterectomy for patients with asymptomatic internal carotid artery stenosis. *Stroke.* 1994;25:2523–2524.

17. Goldstone J, Moore WS. Emergency carotid artery surgery in neurologically unstable patients. *Arch Surg*. 1976;111:84–91.
18. Carson SN, Demling RH, Ewquivel CO. Aspirin failure in symptomatic atherosclerotic carotid artery disease. *Surgery*. 1981;90:1084–1092.
19. Wilson SE, Mayberg MR, Yatsu F, et al. Crescendo transient ischemic attacks: a surgical imperative. *J Vasc Surg*. 1993;17:249–256.
20. Mentzer RM Jr, Finkelmeier BA, Crosby IK, et al. Emergency carotid endarterectomy for fluctuating neurologic deficits. *Surgery*. 1981;89:60–66.
21. McIntyre KE Jr, Goldstone J. Carotid surgery for crescendo TIA and stroke in evolution. In: Bergan JJ, Yao JST, eds. *Cerebrovascular Insufficiency*. New York: Grune & Stratton; 1983;220–226.
22. Rothrock JF, Lyden PD, Yee J, et al. 'Crescendo' transient ischemic attacks: clinical and angiographic correlations. *Neurology*. 1988;38:198–201.
23. Cosgrove DM, Hertzer NR, Loop FD. Surgical management of synchronous carotid and coronary artery disease. *J Vasc Surg*. 1986;3:690–694.
24. Hertzer NR, Loop FD, Beven EG, et al. Surgical staging for simultaneous coronary and carotid disease: a study including prospective randomization. *J Vasc Surg*. 1989;9:455–463.
25. DeWeese JA, Rob CG, Satran R, et al. Results of carotid endarterectomies for transient ischemic attacks—five years later. *Ann Surg*. 1973;178:258–264.
26. O'Donnell TF Jr, Gallow AD, Willet C, et al. The impact of coronary artery disease on carotid endarterectomy. *Ann Surg*. 1983;198:705–712.
27. Hertzer NR, Young JR, Beven EG, et al. Coronary angiography in 506 patients with extracranial cerebrovascular disease. *Arch Intern Med*. 1985;145:849–852.
28. Hertzer NR, Loop FD, Taylor PC, et al. Staged and combined surgical approach to simultaneous carotid and coronary vascular disease. *Surgery*. 1978;84:803–811.
29. Rizzo RJ, Whittemore AD, Couper GS, et al. Combined carotid and coronary revascularization: the preferred approach to the severe vasculopath. *Ann Thorac Surg*. 1992;54:1099–1109.
30. Brener BJ, Brief DK, Alpert J, et al. The risk of stroke in patients with asymptomatic carotid stenosis undergoing cardiac surgery: a follow-up study. *J Vasc Surg*. 1987;5:269–277.
31. Lord RSA, Graham AR, Shanahan MX, et al. Rationale for simultaneous carotid endarterectomy and aortocoronary bypass. *Ann Vasc Surg*. 1986;1:201–206.
32. Mehigan JT, Buch WS, Pipkin RD, et al. A planned approach to coexistent cerebrovascular disease in coronary artery bypass candidates. *Arch Surg*. 1977;112:1403–1409.
33. Perler BA, Burdick JF, Willian GM. The safety of carotid endarterectomy at the time of coronary artery bypass surgery: analysis of results in a high-risk patient population. *J Vasc Surg*. 1984;2:558–562.
34. Emery RW, Cohn LH, Whittemore AD, et al. Coexistent carotid and coronary artery disease: surgical management. *Arch Surg*. 1983;118:1035–1038.
35. Craver JM, Murphy DA, Jones EL, et al. Concomitant carotid and coronary artery reconstruction. *Ann Surg* 1982;195:712–720.
36. Gardner TJ, Homeffer PJ, Manolio TA, et al. Major stroke after coronary artery bypass surgery: changing magnitude of the preferred approach to severe vasculopath. *Ann Thorac Surg*. 1992;54:1099–1109.

6

Management of the Infected Aortic Graft

Staged or Single Surgical Procedures

William D. Turnipseed, MD

Infection of an abdominal aortic prosthetic graft is one of the most serious postoperative complications that can occur in vascular surgery, challenging the skill and judgment of even the most experienced surgeon. Historically, the management of infected aortic prosthetics has been associated with poor clinical outcome, as manifested by high perioperative mortality rates, frequent amputation, and poor long-term survival.[1–3] Although the incidence of aortic graft infections is relatively low (2%), the aging of our population and the increased number of graft placements over time almost guarantee that surgeons performing vascular procedures will eventually have to deal with this problem. The best clinical outcomes will undoubtedly belong to those surgeons who develop treatment strategies based on good judgment and the experience of their predecessors.

Although improved surgical techniques, better suture and graft materials, and the use of more effective antibiotic prophylaxis have helped reduce the incidence of infection, the complication continues to occur, posing a serious threat to life and limb. Clinical experience suggests that vascular graft infections are often related to breaks in intraoperative technique, postoperative wound complications, and episodes of sepsis that cause direct or hematogenous contamination of prosthetic graft material. The idea that careful preoperative preparation and surgical technique are important cannot be overemphasized since proper handling of tissues is probably more important than antibiotics in preventing the environment that promotes vascular graft infection. Once the diagnosis of a prosthetic graft infection has been made, priorities of management should include systemic control of the infection based on the use of culture-specific antibiotics, the removal of all infected prosthetic graft material, and the prevention of limb-threatening ischemia. Although the use of broad spectrum antibiotics is universally agreed upon, surgeons commonly disagree about the indications for graft removal and often are at odds as to the most appropriate timing and reconstruction technique for reducing postoperative mortality and preserving limb function.

Although antibiotics can suppress some of the systemic consequences of graft infection, they cannot prevent suture line breakdown or pseudoaneurysm formation—nor can they sterilize *in situ* prosthetic graft material. Therefore, it is essential that all contaminated elements of an infected prosthesis be removed in order to achieve long-term control of sepsis. Most surgeons accept the caveat that complete removal of an infected prosthetic is the most effective way to prevent persistent or recurrent sepsis.[4,5] Despite this fact, many seem willing to test this thesis by performing only limited or partial resection of an infected graft because of the magnitude of surgery required to reconstruct and preserve blood flow to the lower extremities while removing offending graft material.[6,7] Basically, it is impossible to be absolutely sure that residual graft material does not harbor bacteria that can cause recurrent infections in the future. Although preoperative arteriography, CT scanning, indium-labeled white cell scans, and contrast scintigraphy can provide the surgeon with important information regarding the patency, anastomotic integrity, and the extent of infection, the decision of whether or not to completely remove a prostheses can only be made at the time of surgery.[8]

The traditional (gold standard) operation for treatment of infected aortic grafts, including graft enteric fistulae, mandated complete excision of the intra-abdominal graft followed by the remote placement of an extracavitary subcutaneous prosthetic bypass graft from the axillary artery to femoral or more distal run-off vessels in the lower extremity. This sequence of infected graft excision followed by remote bypass to the lower extremities was time-consuming, tedious, bloody, and created prolonged periods of pelvic and lower extremity ischemia. These procedures often had perioperative mortality rates ranging from 25% to 75% and amputation rates in excess of 30%. As a result of lower extremity wound healing problems and graft failure, recurrent infection was common (40%). Consequently, surgeons began looking for ways to reduce morbidity and mortality by altering risks of operative treatment.[9,10] Since the early 1980s, clinical experience documented in the surgical literature suggests that the malignant effects of prolonged pelvic and lower extremity ischemia can be favorably altered by reversing the operative sequence of the traditional gold standard operation so that lower extremity revascularization *precedes* removal of the infected graft and/or repair of the graft enteric fistula.[10,11] This sequence change allowed the surgeon to perform a clean bypass operation using uninfected tissue planes remote from the abdominal cavity, prevented prolonged lower extremity ischemia (and all of its adverse metabolic consequences), and reduced the likelihood of direct contamination or recurrent infection caused by breaks in sterile technique. Selective review of clinical studies utilizing this "reverse sequence" operative technique demonstrate a favorable trend toward reduced perioperative mortality.[12] This reverse sequence operation is most appropriate for patients who are not systematically septic, who are hemodynamically stable, and who are not bleeding from enteric fistula or disrupted suture lines. The reverse sequence operation can be performed under the same anesthesia when extracavitary bypass can be done in a straightforward and timely fashion. This approach is most feasible for treating chronically infected aortic tube grafts or iliac bifurcation grafts that do not compromise access to the common femoral vessels. Although many authors believe that the risk for new graft infection is inordinately high with this approach and that competitive flow will result in graft occlusions, there is no objective data to confirm these opinions.[10] It would appear that new graft infection rates are significantly reduced for the reverse sequence procedures (18% to 27%) when compared to the traditional gold standard operation (25% to 40%). New graft infection rates do not change significantly when a "staged" interval between extracavitary bypass and complete graft excision is employed (18% to 24%).[11,12] New graft infections, when they do occur, may not be as threatening to the patient's life, but often result in a much higher likelihood of lower extremity amputation (40%) because access to distal runoff vessels is usually compromised. Although reverse sequence arterial reconstruction may reduce the likelihood of new graft infections, its major advantage is prevention of prolonged pelvic and lower extremity ischemia. This has significantly reduced the incidence of perioperative amputation when compared to the traditional procedure (15% vs. 46%).

A conceptual extension of the reverse sequence operation led to the idea that vascular reconstruction could be performed several days prior to elective removal of the infected graft. This "staged" technique was first proposed by Elliott et al. in 1974 and championed by Reilly and colleagues in 1987.[3,10] By interposing a time delay between extracavitary bypass and excision of the infected abdominal prosthesis, operative stress was reduced for patient and surgeon alike. Operative times were shorter and anesthesia requirements less demanding. Lower extremity ischemia was prevented and breaks in sterile technique were less likely to occur. Despite the fact that there is no significant difference between the staged and reverse sequence procedures with respect to perioperative mortality (26% vs. 24%), amputation rate (16% vs. 11%), or reinfection (16% vs. 18%), the staged operative approach is preferred because it affords a better opportunity for soft tissue debridement, surgical drainage of local infections, and drug control of sepsis before graft excision.[11,12]

A variation of the staged reverse sequence surgery algorithm has been used at our institution for more than 15 years.[13] We originally felt that complete excision of an infected graft was mandatory. Upon completion of graft removal, we discovered that it was possible to patch arteriotomy sites with autogenous vein or endarterectomized segments of occluded superficial femoral artery in nearly 40% of our patients. By doing this we were able to preserve collateral perfusion beds to the lower extremity and to reduce the need for acute limb salvage bypass surgery. This staged delay between infected graft excision and secondary vascular reconstruction, which ranged from 8 hours to 9 months (average = 2 weeks), makes it possible to control sepsis and to prevent reinfection of newly placed grafts.

When staged delay in secondary vascular reconstruction was used instead of the synchronous (gold standard) procedure, operative mortality dropped from 57% to 23%. Although amputation rates were identical for the two procedures (15%), reinfection of remotely placed vascular bypass dropped from 43% to 10%. This drop in recurrent graft infection was due to better control of local and systemic sepsis, made possible by aggressive debridement of all infected perigraft soft tissue in the groin and retroperitoneum, complete excision of the infected prosthesis, control of any enteric fistula, and use of culture-specific antimicrobial coverage. Staged delay in vascular reconstruction should be considered whenever complete removal of an infected intra-abdominal graft is deemed necessary because the body or proximal anastomosis of the graft is involved; the aortic graft or one of its limbs is obstructed; a graft enteric fistula is present; suture line breakdown with hemorrhage or pseudoaneurysm occur; or infection develops early after surgery with no host fixation to the graft. Staged delay in vascular repair may be most appropriate in select circumstances where autogenous patching can maintain collateral blood flow to the lower extremity. Since ligation of the iliac and femoral vessels destroys vascular continuity to the lower limb, ligation should be avoided whenever possible. Debridement of the artery wall at anastomotic sites may be necessary in order to prevent recurrent infection. The possibility of recurrent infection at patch sites may be further reduced by using omental flaps to cover aortic and iliac artery repairs. Myocutaneous rotational flaps can be used to assure healthy soft tissue coverage for femoral patch sites and to obliterate large soft tissue defects in the groin resulting from primary surgical debridement.[14]

The timing and method of delayed arterial reconstruction is critical for limb salvage and rehabilitation of the patient. Although there is no precise way to determine who really needs immediate reconstruction after removal of an infected graft, we have found that the presence of a good Doppler signal in the groin, an ankle pressure of 44 mg/Hg, or an index of 0.3 or more correlates with successful delayed reconstruction. Although limb function may be significantly impaired, viability can be maintained provided collateral pathways to the leg are preserved. When initial surgery can be limited to removal of the infected graft and repair of injured bowel, operating time and transfusion requirements may be significantly reduced. This makes it easier to stabilize the patient, eliminate the source of infection, and plan a clean secondary vascular reconstruction when necessary. Clinical circumstances favoring the staged delay of vascular reconstruction include: the presence of systemic sepsis and bacteremia; infected aortoiliac and aortofemoral bypass grafts with proximal end-to-side anastomoses; occluded aortoiliac or aortofemoral grafts; infected iliofemoral reconstructions; and infected femoral crossover conduits. Delayed secondary vascular reconstruction requires very careful monitoring in the intensive care unit and should be reserved for treatment of limb-threatening ischemia that develops after graft excision in the acutely ill or septic patient. By linking secondary vascular reconstruction to clinical development of limb-threatening ischemic symptoms, limb salvage rates and patient survival improve. As long as a digital motor function and positional sensation are preserved, limbs are considered to be viable. Loss of sensation and motor function mandates surgical intervention. If secondary revascularization is necessary within the first week of graft excision, it is best to use autogenous material for reconstruction. Several techniques have been proposed including extensive host vessel endarterectomy,[15] graft bypasses using superficial femoral vein,[16] and cadaver aortic allografts.[17]

Synchronous graft excision and vascular reconstruction may be necessary when acute shock results from suture line bleeding or enteric fistula hemorrhage and when lower extremity ischemia is complicated by the presence of uncontrolled sepsis. Surgical emergencies of this nature do not allow for safe use of reversed sequence or staged delay procedures because of the coexistent need to control hemorrhage and infection, as well as to maintain lower extremity perfusion. These patients are seriously ill and at high risk for death and morbid complications. Infection in these individuals is most commonly caused by *Staphylococcus aureus, Staphylococcus epidermidis, Escherichia coli, Pseudomonas,* or a mixture of gram-positive and gram-negative organisms (Table 6–1). Gram-positive bacteria often produce a glycocalyx mucin that protects them from the host immune system and that promotes adherence to prosthetic material such as Dacron. Gram-negative organisms tend to be more virulent, with more aggressive tissue inva-

TABLE 6–1. MOST COMMON ORGANISMS ASSOCIATED WITH AORTIC GRAFT INFECTIONS SINCE 1980

Organism	Prevalence (%)
Staphylococcus aureus	24
Staphylococcus epidermidis	17
Escherichia coli	10
Pseudomonas	8
Streptococcus	7
Other	34

sion and a higher incidence of vessel wall necrosis and suture line disruption. The most virulent organism is *Pseudomonas aeruginosa.* Gram-negative and gram-positive organisms are also capable of producing proteases that will break down elastin, collagen, and fibrin and often produce lysins, which are hemolytic and result in cell necrosis and white cell destruction. The malignant consequences of soft tissue invasion and impaired host response mandate aggressive debridement of perigraft soft tissues and complete graft excision. Reinfection rates can be very high even when prosthetic materials such as PTFE are used for vascular reconstruction (>20%) under these circumstances. For this reason, autogenous materials are preferred.[18] Ehrenfeld et al.[15] advocated the use of extended aortoiliac endarterectomy in patients with occlusive disease requiring graft excision. This surgery was long, technically difficult, and bloody, and was associated with a high mortality rate (>35%). Amputations were common (25%). The major advantage of the synchronous *in situ* reconstruction using endarterectomy was a significant reduction in the incidence of new graft infection among patients that survived the initial operative procedure. Clagett and others[16] have recently described the use of superficial femoral vein as an autograft to reconstruct the aortoiliac system. In contrast to greater saphenous veins, which are prone to failure because they develop focal stenoses and intimal hyperplasia, the superficial femoral veins have an excellent size match with the iliac and femoral arteries, seem more resistent to fibrointimal hyperplasia and recurrent infection, and maintain durable patency. This neoaortoiliac system (NAIS) repair has most commonly been employed as a means of preserving lower extremity circulation when more conservative local procedures such as extracavitary bypass, muscle flap coverage, and *in situ* limb replacement have failed. The NAIS procedure should be considered as an alternative to extended aortoiliac endarterectomy when extracavitary prosthetic bypass is not feasible and when inline arterial reconstruction appears necessary. An alternative to use of autogenous superficial femoral vein has been proposed by Kieffer and associates[17] who have utilized cadaveric allografts as a means of *in situ* graft replacement. These biologic conduits appear to be resistant to recurrent infection. The inline allograft repair makes vascular reconstruction simpler and has the potential of reducing early perioperative death and morbidity. Unfortunately, these grafts are not routinely available and they are susceptible to late structural degeneration that causes occlusion and pseudoaneurysm.

When autogenous or allograft conduits are not available, *in situ* prosthetic graft replacement may be the only means of preserving flow to the lower extremity. Because the risk of subsequent reinfection is significant, *in situ* prosthetic reconstructions should be avoided whenever possible. Contraindications to *in situ* prosthetic vascular repair include systemic sepsis, grossly purulent drainage from graft bed, and extensive perigraft tissue necrosis. Clinical experience suggests that *in situ* replacement may succeed when there is localized graft infection without purulence and when complete excision of that involved segment and adequate debridement of perigraft soft tissues can be achieved. In select circumstances, both gram-positive and gram-negative infections can be managed by combined *in situ arterial* reconstruction, aggressive debridement, and antibiotic administration. Exceptions include *Pseudomonas aeruginosa* infections as well as yeast and fungal infections in immunocompromised patients.[18,19]

Leather and colleagues[20] have recently described a synchronous inline retroperitoneal prosthetic bypass using a PTFE bifurcation graft. This procedure requires an adequate length of uninfected aorta between the renals and the graft to allow for a clean division of the aorta and a new anastomosis. This operation is performed through a retroperitoneal incision and requires a clean left retroperitoneal gutter through which to tunnel the graft limbs into the groin once the proximal anastomosis has been completed. The infected graft is removed through a separate transabdominal incision. Initial experience with this technique has been encouraging because of low recurrent infection rates and minimal perioperative morbidity.

The decision to remove less than the entire graft, attempt graft preservation, or perform limited graft replacement should only be considered when isolated graft infection is identified; limb patency is angiographically confirmed; the anastomoses remain structurally intact; the patient is not systemically septic; and virulent organisms such as *Pseudomonas* are absent. Fungal and yeast infections in immunocompromised patients require complete graft excision. Any attempt at primary salvage of a functional, intact, but infected iliofemoral graft limb requires aggressive soft tissue debridement and excision of all contaminated perigraft soft tissues including the pseudocapsule that surrounds the prosthetic. Graft limb salvage procedures of this nature require a staged surgical approach. The first objective is to eradicate perigraft infection by aggressive surgical debridement. Sterilization of the exposed graft and groin wound may be achieved by irrigating or packing the soft tissue defect with Povidone–iodine-soaked sponges or by using Sulfamylon cream for 4 to 5 days prior to attempted wound closure. Quantitative cultures should confirm less than 10^5 organisms in soft tissues surrounding the graft before any attempt at graft replacement or wound coverage is made. Rotational myocutaneous flaps constructed from the rectus femoris or rectus abdominis muscles can be used to fill in the soft tissue defects in the groin and to circumferentially wrap the sterilized graft or its *in situ* replacement. *In situ* graft replacement with delayed myocutaneous flap coverage has been very effective in obliterating local perigraft infection, preventing recurrent graft sepsis, and in preserving functional lower extremity perfusion.[14]

CONCLUSION

There is no correct answer to the question, "Should staged or single surgical procedures be done for prosthetic aortic graft infections?" Synchronous operations are necessary when treating unstable septic patients with GI hemorrhage, bleeding suture lines, coexistent lower extremity ischemia, gross perigraft purulence, or extensive soft tissue necrosis. Complete graft removal is essential, and protection of lower extremity circulation may require regional use of autogenous or allograft conduits or remote replacement with extracavitary prosthetic bypass grafts. Postoperative mortality and the risk for new graft infection will be high. The need for perioperative amputation can be greatly reduced when secondary bypass reconstruction can safely precede infected graft removal. Staged operations are most appropriate for treatment of patients with clinically stable and oftentimes localized perigraft infections. As expected, perioperative mortality will be lower for staged procedures when compared to single operations. This usually relates to patient selection. Staged procedures afford a better opportunity to control infection, to protect lower extremity circulation, and to prevent new graft infections. When isolated perigraft infection involves a patent bypass with intact anastomoses, the first operation should be used to drain and debride infected tissues. Lower extremity perfusion can be maintained through the contaminated graft and delayed vascular repair performed after clearance of the infection. When complete graft excision is anticipated, the surgeon must determine whether it is possible to preserve reasonable collateral perfusion to the lower extremity by using autogenous patching at the anastomotic sites or whether bypass reconstruction is necessary. The likelihood of new graft infection will be much lower if autogenous patching and graft excision can be per-

TABLE 6–2. SURGICAL TREATMENT VERSUS OUTCOME

	Death (%)	Amputation (%)	New Graft Infection (%)
Synchronous Surgery			
Graft excision + A. fem. bypass (Gold Standard)	26–43	45–57	23–43
Reverse sequence ax. fem. bypass then graft excision	21–24	11	10
Graft excision and aorto iliac endarterectomy	35	25	0
Graft excision + NAIS*	10	10	0
Graft excision + cadaver allograft	14	0	7
Graft excision + prosthetic *in situ* bypass	32	11	11
Staged Surgery			
Graft excision + patch + delayed graft replacement	20	15	0
Remote bypass + delayed graft excision	26	16	16
Perigraft debridement + graft preservation + myocutaneous coverage	0	0	8
Perigraft debridement + partial graft removal and repair	11	13	10

* NAIS, neoaortoiliac system.

formed. Most surgeons, however, favor remote placement of a prosthetic graft through clean tissue planes several days prior to excision of the infected graft, even though there is a higher likelihood of encountering new graft infection (Table 6–2).

REFERENCES

1. Fry WJ, Lindenauer SM. Infections complicating use of plastic arterial implants. *Arch Surg.* 1967;94:600–609.
2. Bunt JF. Synthetic vascular graft infections, I: graft infection. *Surgery.* 1983;93:733–746.
3. Elliott JP, Smith RF, Szilagyi DE. Aortoenteric and paraprosthetic enteric fistulas: problems of diagnosis and management. *Arch Surg.* 1974;108:479–490.
4. Yeager RA, Moneta GL, Taylor LM, et al. Can prosthetic graft infection be avoided? If not, how do we treat it? *Acta Chir Scand.* 1990;555(suppl):155–163.
5. Ricotta JJ, Faggioli GL, Stella A, et al. Total excision and extra-anatomic bypass for aortic graft infection. *Am J Surg.* 1991;162:145–149.
6. Kwaan JHM, Connolly JE. Successful management of prosthetic graft infection with continuous povidone-iodine irrigation. *Arch Surg.* 1981;116:716–720.
7. Popovsky J, Singer S. Infected prosthetic grafts: local therapy with graft preservations. *Arch Surg.* 1980;115:203–205.
8. Szilagyi DE, Smith RF, Elliot JP, et al. Infection in arterial reconstruction with synthetic grafts. *Ann Surg.* 1972;176:321–333.
9. Vieth J, Gupta SK, Sampson RH. Progress in limb salvage by reconstructive arterial surgery combined with new or improved adjunctive procedures. *Ann Surg.* 1981;194:386–401.
10. Reilly LM, Stoney RJ, Goldstone J, et al. Improved management of aortic graft infection: the influence of operation sequence and staging. *J Vasc Surg.* 1987;5:421–431.

11. O'Hara PJ, Hertzer NR, Beven EG, et al. Surgical management of infected abdominal aortic grafts: review of a 25-year experience. *J Vasc Surg.* 1986;3:725–731.
12. Yeager RA, Porter JM. Arterial and prosthetic graft infection. *Ann Vasc Surg.* 1992;6:485–491.
13. Turnipseed WD, Berkoff HA, Detmer DE, et al. Arterial graft infections: delayed vs. immediate vascular reconstruction. *Arch Surg.* 1983;118:410–414.
14. Mixter RC, Turnipseed WD, Smith DJ, et al. Rotational muscle flaps: a new technique for covering infected vascular grafts. *J Vasc Surg.* 1989;9:472–478.
15. Ehrenfeld WK, Wilbur BG, Oceott CN IV, et al. Autogenous tissue reconstruction in management of infected prosthetic grafts. *Surgery.* 1979;85:82–92.
16. Clagett GP, Bowers BC, Lopez-Viego MA, et al. Creations of a neo-aortoiliac system from lower extremity deep and superficial veins. *Arch Surg.* 1993;218:239–249.
17. Kieffer E, Bahnini AM, Koskas F, et al. *In situ* allograft replacement of infected infrarenal aortic prosthetic grafts: results in forty-three patients. *J Vasc Surg.* 1992;17:349–355.
18. Bandyk DF, Esses GE. Prosthetic graft infection. *Surg Clin North Am.* 1994;74:571–590.
19. Gelabert HA, Moore WS. The role of *in situ* graft replacement in abdominal aortic infections. In: Calligaro KD, Fjeds V. *Management of Infected Arterial Grafts.* St. Louis: Quality Medical Publishing; 1994:142–159.
20. Leather RP, Darling C, Chang BB, et al. Retroperitoneal in-line aortic bypass for treatment of infected infrarenal aortic grafts. *Surg Gyn Obstet.* 1992;175:491–494.

III

Cerebrovascular Revascularization Procedures

7

High Cervical Internal Carotid Artery Exposure

Richard W. Chitwood, MD, and Calvin B. Ernst, MD

Over the last few years, the superiority of the surgical treatment of symptomatic and asymptomatic internal carotid artery (ICA) stenosis has been confirmed.[1,2] Carotid artery bifurcation endarterectomy (CEA) reduces both the risk of subsequent stroke and stroke-related death when compared to medical management alone in randomized clinical trials.[1,2] As a result of these trials, CEA for hemodynamically significant carotid arterial stenoses has achieved widespread acceptance. Consequently, the number of atherosclerotic carotid artery lesions requiring surgical repair will probably increase.

The ICA cephalad to a line between the angle of the mandible and the tip of the mastoid is considered inaccessible using standard operative techniques.[3,4] Some atherosclerotic lesions are complex and extend into the mid- to distal segments of the ICA (Fig. 7–1). Because of anatomic constraints posed by the mandible, the base of the skull, the cervical musculature, and the proximity of nerves, various technical maneuvers may be required to provide adequate ICA exposure to assure precise and complete removal of the offending plaque. Fortunately, atherosclerotic lesions extending into the distal ICA represent only a small proportion (less than 1%) of all carotid artery atherosclerotic lesions.[5] With an anticipated increase in carotid operations, a proportional increase in the number of lesions with distal ICA extension may be expected. In addition, owing to the growing violence in American society, an increase in distal ICA traumatic lesions requiring repair can be expected. For these reasons, knowledge of safe and reliable techniques for exposure of the distal ICA is necessary.

INDICATIONS FOR HIGH CERVICAL CAROTID ARTERY EXPOSURE

While distal extension of carotid atherosclerosis and carotid artery traumatic lesions are among the most common indications for high ICA exposure, several other abnormalities may require distal ICA exposure as well (Table 7–1).[5] In two reports involving 38 patients and describing temporomandibular subluxation (TMS) techniques, indications

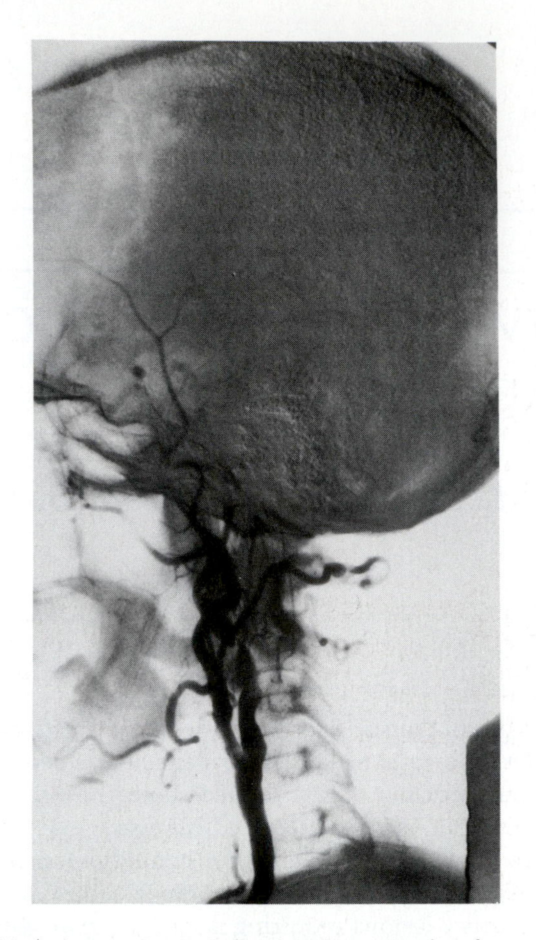

Figure 7–1. Carotid arteriogram demonstrating 4- to 5-cm extension of a preocclusive atherosclerotic plaque into the distal internal carotid artery. (*Reprinted with permission from Ernst CB. Surgical exposure of the distal internal carotid artery. In: Schmidek HH, Sweet WH, eds. Operative Neurosurgical Techniques. 3rd ed. Philadelphia: WB Saunders; 1995:891–895.*)

for such exposure included requirement for extended CEA in 22 (57.9%), resection of carotid body tumor in 6 (15.8%), repair of carotid injury in 4 (10.5%), repair of post-CEA pseudoaneurysm in 2 (5.3%), dilation of fibromuscular dysplasia in 2 (5.3%), repair of an aneurysm in 1 (2.6%), and ligation of an external carotid arteriovenous fistula in 1 (2.6%).[6,7]

TABLE 7–1. INDICATIONS FOR HIGH CERVICAL CAROTID ARTERY EXPOSURE

Distal extension of carotid atherosclerotic plaque
Trauma
Carotid body tumor or other neoplasm
Fibromuscular dysplasia
Congenital abnormalities (kinking or coiling)
Irradiation arteritis
Post endarterectomy pseudoaneurysm
Mycotic aneurysm

Preoperative identification of a patient who may require distal exposure of the ICA is essential since some of the maneuvers, such as TMS, must be performed before making the incision. The consequences of not recognizing the need for distal ICA exposure may complicate the operation and result in a cerebral ischemic event or technical mishap.

TECHNIQUES FOR DISTAL CERVICAL CAROTID EXPOSURE

Exposure of the distal cervical ICA can be obtained through lateral, anterolateral, and posterolateral approaches (Table 7–2).[6] The options for exposure vary in amount of time required, complexity, and potential complications. In general, time-consuming, complex exposures at the base of the skull are indicated only for elective ICA reconstruction and are impractical or even dangerous when urgent or emergent operation is required.

Lateral Approach

When using the lateral approach to the high cervical ICA, no bony resections, osteotomies, or extensive muscular sectioning are required. This approach has emerged as the easiest and least debilitating method for providing high ICA exposure. In an anatomic study of 12 human cadaver specimens, Mock and his colleagues[8] documented that division of the posterior belly of the digastric muscle improved distal ICA exposure by 1 cm, and TMS provided an additional 1 cm of exposure to that obtained by digastric division. They further noted that lateral mandible osteotomy did not significantly improve exposure beyond that obtained by TMS and styloidectomy. Division of the styloid group of muscles (styloglossus, stylopharyngeus, and stylohyoid) and resection of the styloid process can extend exposure by another 5 mm.

First reported in a series of trauma patients, bilateral mandibular subluxation with the use of fixation arch bars facilitates exposure of the distal ICA.[9] Enthusiasm for this subluxation technique led to development of a unilateral subluxation method stabilized by circum-mandibular and transnasal wiring.[7] Unilateral mandibular condylar subluxation provides 10 to 15 mm of anterior displacement of the vertical ramus of the mandible and converts the narrow triangular operative field into a larger rectangular one (Figs. 7–2 and 7–3).

Anterolateral Approach

Anterolateral access to the high ICA is limited by the vertical ramus of the mandible. Techniques designed to permit such exposure require mandibular osteotomies. Several types of osteotomies have been described, including transverse and vertical ramus osteotomies, osteotomy through the angle of the mandible, and osteotomy through the anterior body of the mandible.[10–12] Vertical subperiosteal mandibular osteotomy is performed from the angle of the mandible to the mandibular notch after dissection and retraction of the facial nerve and division of the masseter muscle. The vertical ramus can then be rotated outward to expose the ICA near the base of the skull.[10,12] Alternatively, a subperiosteal osteotomy can be performed through the anterolateral aspect of the mandible near the mental foramen. Outward rotation of the posterior mandibular segment provides similar exposure to vertical osteotomy.[11] Both vertical and anterolateral mandibular osteotomies can be performed through the operative incision; however, they are time-consuming procedures that may require postoperative maxillomandibular fixation and may result in mandibular nonunion. These techniques

TABLE 7–2. TECHNIQUES FOR EXPOSURE OF THE HIGH CERVICAL CAROTID ARTERY

Approach	Primary Investigators (Ref)	No. of Patients	Advantages	Disadvantages
Posterolateral				
Division of sternocleidomastoid	Shaha (13)	2	Simple	Potential neck deformity External carotid division may be required
Partial mastoidectomy	Purdue (14) Pellegrini (15)	1 1	Exposure of carotid at base of skull	Time consuming Possible cranial nerve VII dysfunction
Radical mastoidectomy	Fisch (16)	5	Exposure within carotid canal	Time consuming Possible cranial nerve VII dysfunction Hearing loss
Anterolateral				
Vertical osteotomy	Welsh (12)	7 2	Access from operative field	Time consuming Possible mandibular nonunion Possible postoperative maxillomandibular fixation
Anterolateral osteotomy	Dichtel (11)	1	Access from operative field	Time consuming Possible mandibular nonunion Postoperative maxillomandibular fixation Possible oral flora wound contamination
Lateral-Temporomandibular Subluxation				
Arch bars	Fry (9)	8	Nondeforming Minimal morbidity	Time consuming Must be performed before incision Not applicable to edentulous patients Unnecessary contralateral subluxation
Circum-mandibular/ transnasal wiring	Fisher (7)	12	Fast Nondeforming Applicable in edentulous patients	Must be performed before incision Bleeding in some patients
Diagonal wiring	Ernst (5)	26	Fast Nondeforming Applicable in edentulous patients	Must be performed before incision

Adapted from Dossa C, Shepard AD, Wolford DE, et al. Distal internal carotid exposure: a simplified technique for temporary mandibular subluxation. *J Vasc Surg.* 1990;12:319.

provide approximately 2 cm of additional high cervical ICA exposure over standard techniques.

Posterolateral Approach

Posterolateral exposure of the distal cervical ICA can be obtained by division of the sternocleidomastoid muscle near its origin, the posterior belly of the digastric muscle,

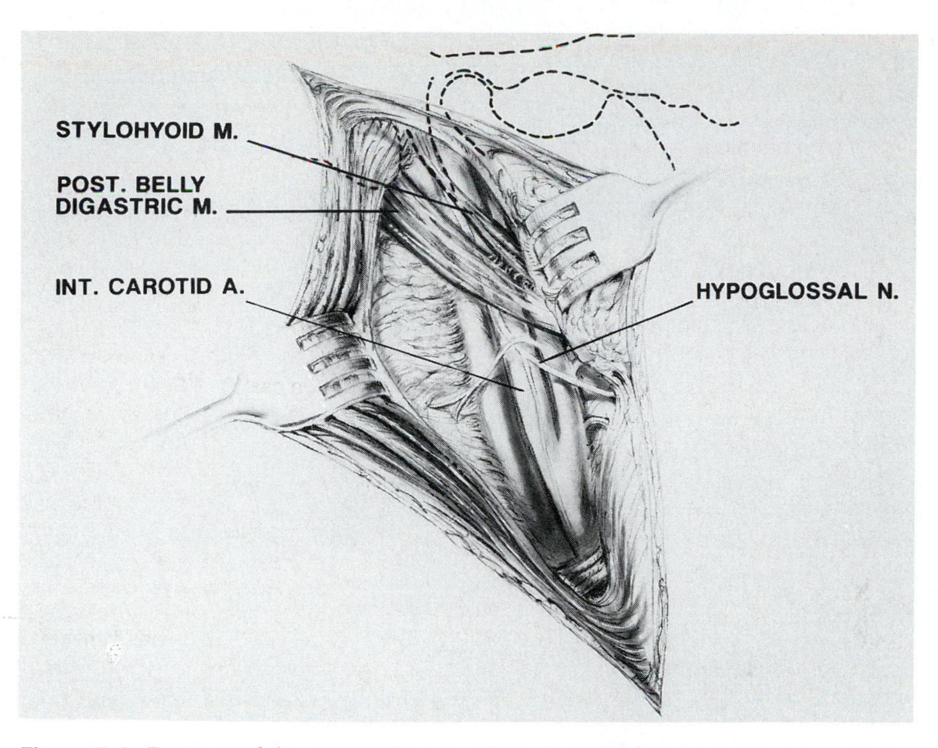

Figure 7–2. Exposure of the carotid bifurcation through a standard cervical incision with the temporomandibular joint in its anatomic position (*dotted line*). The distal one-third of the internal carotid artery is obscured by structures at the apex of the triangle. (*Reprinted with permission from Dossa C, Shepard AD, Wolford DG, et al. Distal internal carotid exposure: a simplified technique for temporary mandibular subluxation. J Vasc Surg. 1990;12:319–325.*)

and styloid group of muscles. This muscular dissection allows reasonable visualization of the high cervical carotid and can be performed rapidly; however, ligation of the external carotid artery, facial nerve dissection and retraction, and resection of the tail of the parotid gland may be necessary to obtain the desired exposure.[13] Some residual neck deformity may result from this procedure.

Partial resection of the mastoid process provides reasonable exposure of the ICA near the base of the skull. Such exposure is facilitated by division or resection of the posterior digastric muscle and styloid muscle group.[14,15]

More extensive resection of the mastoid and subtotal petrosectomy with permanent anterior displacement of the facial nerve and obliteration of the middle ear permits exposure of the ICA not only at the base of the skull but also in its bony canal into the cranial vault.[16] Mastoidectomies performed for carotid exposure are time consuming, risk injury to the facial nerve, and may result in hearing loss.[14–16]

APPROACH TO THE HIGH CERVICAL CAROTID ARTERY WITH UNILATERAL MANDIBULAR SUBLUXATION BY THE DIAGONAL WIRING TECHNIQUE

Since 1990 a simplified approach to unilateral TMS for exposure of the high ICA has been used at the Henry Ford Hospital.[6] Distal ICA exposure has been reliably obtained with minimal morbidity using this technique. Mandibular osteotomy techniques have

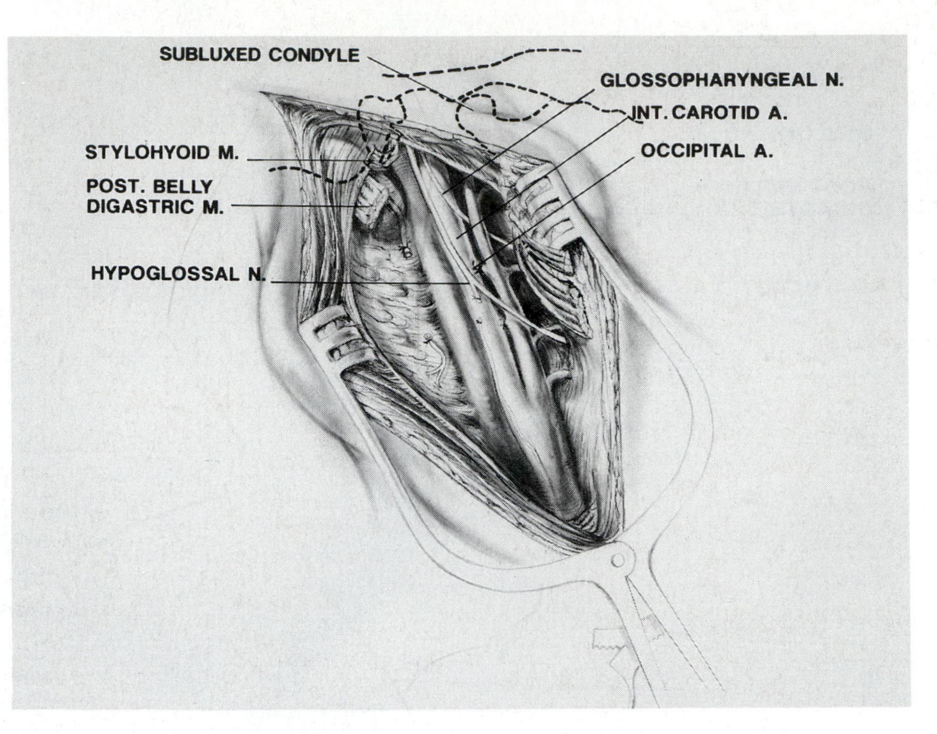

Figure 7–3. The temporomandibular joint appearance after subluxation (*dotted line*). The apex of the triangle is now rectangular in configuration, which provides an additional 1 to 2 cm of distal internal carotid exposure beyond that in Figure 7–2. *(Reprinted with permission from Dossa C, Shepard AD, Wolford DG, et al. Distal internal carotid exposure: a simplified technique for temporary mandibular subluxation. J Vasc Surg. 1990;12:319–325.)*

not been used. In addition, to the authors' knowledge, no symptomatic ICA lesion that would require mastoidectomy for exposure and repair has been identified at Henry Ford Hospital over the last 10 years.

Lesions located in the ICA at or above the level of the upper body of the second cervical vertebra are exposed using the unilateral TMS technique. Occasionally, division of the posterior belly of the digastric muscle along with the styloid muscle group and styloidectomy may provide distal ICA exposure, particularly when the need for high exposure was not recognized by preoperative arteriography and preparations were not made for TMS.

Preoperative Preparation and Anesthetic Management

Preoperative identification of patients who require exposure of the distal ICA is important because TMS requires satisfactory nasotracheal intubation anesthesia before the cervical incision. Such subluxation maneuvers are performed in cooperation with an oral surgeon. It is important to only sublux, and not dislocate, the ipsilateral mandible. Dislocation may damage the temporomandibular joint cartilage.

Mandibular Subluxation by Diagonal Wiring

Once satisfactory general nasotracheal anesthesia is obtained and before prepping and draping, unilateral mandibular subluxation is performed. In dentate patients, the subluxed position is held by Ivy loop interdental diagonal wiring of an ipsilateral mandibular cuspid or bicuspid tooth to a contralateral maxillary cuspid or bicuspid tooth using 25-gauge stainless steel wire. Gentle manual anterior mandibular subluxation is performed while the diagonal wires are tightened. In edentulous patients, TMS stabilization is maintained by intermaxillary-mandibular wiring around two 3/32 inch Steinmann pins drilled intraorally at the gingival margins into the ipsilateral mandible and the contralateral maxilla. The first Steinmann pin is placed by retracting the ipsilateral lower lip and drilling the pin through the oral mucosa into the mandible 2 cm from the midline, anterior to the mental foramen, and 1 to 2 cm from the alveolar crest, aiming at the contralateral mandibular angle. In a similar fashion, a second pin is drilled into the contralateral maxilla. This pin is placed 2 cm from midline and 1 to 2 cm above the alveolar crest. When the pins are adequately placed the tips can be palpated beneath the mucosa. Both pins are trimmed so that approximately 1 cm protrudes. Loops of 25-gauge stainless steel wire are attached to the pins and then tightened as the ipsilateral mandible is gently subluxed. Such subluxation maneuvers can be performed in 10 to 15 minutes.

Carotid Exposure

After preparation and draping, a skin incision along the anterior to the border of the sternocleidomastoid is made, with preauricular or postauricular extension, if necessary. If the parotid gland restricts exposure, it can be mobilized and anteriorly retracted or divided. The sternocleidomastoid muscle is mobilized and retracted posteriorly as the carotid sheath is exposed. The carotid bifurcation is gently dissected and the common, internal, and external carotid arteries encircled with polyethylene tubing (PE-90). The superior thyroid artery is ligated, if necessary, for exposure and mobilization of the bifurcation.

The vagus nerve, hypoglossal nerve, and carotid sinus branch of the glossopharyngeal nerve are identified. Subluxation may result in displacement of the hypoglossal nerve, which positions it cephalad from its normal anatomic position. The ansa cervicalis branch of the hypoglossal nerve is usually divided to improve exposure. As dissection proceeds cephalad, the posterior belly of the digastric muscle and the styloid group of muscles are divided (Fig. 7–3). The mastoid attachment of the sternocleidomastoid muscle may be divided and styloid process resected, if necessary. It must be kept in mind, however, that the spinal accessory nerve is vulnerable when the mastoid insertion of the sternocleidomastoid muscle is mobilized in order to excise the styloid process.

Dissection of the high ICA is facilitated by division of the occipital branch of the external carotid artery and the small muscular branches of the external carotid supplying the sternocleidomastoid muscle. Careful ligation and division of these vessels and the many delicate veins in the area will ensure a dry operative field in which nerves can be easily identified and protected.

Once the distal ICA is exposed, a balloon shunt may be placed if the criteria for shunting, determined by the operating surgeon, have been met. If a shunt is not required and it is difficult to clamp the distal ICA, a No. 3 balloon embolectomy catheter may be used to occlude the distal ICA.

Standard carotid endarterectomy is performed as previously described.[17] After carotid reconstruction is completed, the wound is closed with interrupted absorbable sutures in the platysma layer and staples in the skin. Drains are not usually used. The subluxation is reduced by removing the wires (and pins where required), and gently returning the mandible to its normal anatomic position.

Results

At the Henry Ford Hospital from 1986 to 1991, 26 patients underwent exposure of the high ICA using the TMS technique described.[5] This represented 5% of the carotid reconstructions performed during that 6-year period. Three patients suffered temporary temporomandibular joint pain related to the procedure, and 3 others suffered temporary cranial nerve deficits. One patient had a permanent cranial nerve deficit related to intentional enbloc excision of the hypoglossal and glossopharyngeal nerves for a malignant carotid body tumor. All patients except the 1 with intentional nerve excisions resumed oral diets on the first postoperative day. No early or late temporomandibular joint dysfunction has been recognized.

CONCLUSION

Unilateral TMS provides safe and reliable exposure of the distal ICA. The procedure is easily performed, requires little time, and results in minimal morbidity. The only drawback is the need for arteriography to identify patients who require subluxation prior to carotid reconstruction.

REFERENCES

1. North American Symptomatic Carotid Endarterectomy Trial (NASCET) Collaborators. Beneficial effect of carotid endarterectomy in symptomatic patients with high-grade carotid stenosis. *N Engl J Med*. 1991;325:445.
2. Endarterectomy for Asymptomatic Carotid Artery Stenosis Executive Committee for The Asymptomatic Carotid Atherosclerosis Study. *J Am Med Assn*. 1995;273:1421–1428.
3. Schwartz J, Turner D, Sheldon G, et al. Penetrating trauma of the internal carotid artery at the base of the skull. *J Cardiovasc Surg*. 1987;28:542.
4. Blaisdell W, Clauss R, Galbraith J, et al. Joint study of extracranial arterial occlusion. *JAMA*. 1969;209:1889.
5. Ernst CB. Surgical exposure of the distal internal carotid artery. In: Schmidek HH, Sweet WH, eds. *Operative Neurosurgical Techniques*, 3rd ed. Philadelphia: WB Saunders; 1995:891–895.
6. Dossa C, Shepard AD, Wolford DG, et al. Distal internal carotid exposure: a simplified technique for temporary mandibular subluxation. *J Vasc Surg*. 1990;12:319.
7. Fisher DF, Clagett GP, Parker JI, et al. Mandibular subluxation for high carotid exposure. *J Vasc Surg*. 1984;1:727.
8. Mock CN, Lilly MP, McRae RG, et al. Selection of the approach to the distal internal carotid artery from the second cervical vertebra to the base of the skull. *J Vasc Surg*. 1991;13:846.
9. Fry RE, Fry WJ. Extracranial carotid artery injuries. *Surgery*. 1980;88:581.
10. Larsen PE, Smead WL. Vertical ramus osteotomy for improved exposure of the distal internal carotid artery: a new technique. *J Vasc Surg*. 1992;15:226–231.
11. Dichtel WJ, Miller RH, Feliciano DV, et al. Lateral mandibulectomy: a technique of exposure for penetrating injuries of the internal carotid artery at the base of the skull. *Laryngoscope*. 1984;94:1140.
12. Welsh P, Pradier R, Repetto R. Fibromuscular dysplasia of the distal cervical internal carotid artery. *J Cardiovasc Surg*. 1981;22:321.
13. Shaha A, Phillips T, Scalea T, et al. Exposure of the internal carotid artery near the skull base: the posterolateral anatomic approach. *J Vasc Surg*. 1988;8:618.
14. Purdue GF, Pellegrini RV, Arena S. Aneurysms of the high internal carotid artery: a new approach. *Surgery* 1981;89:268.

15. Pellegrini RV, Manzetti GW, DiMarco RF, et al. The direct surgical management of lesions of the high internal carotid artery. *J Cardiovasc Surg*. 1984;25:29.
16. Fisch UP, Oldring DS, Senning A. Surgical therapy of internal carotid artery lesions at the skull base and temporal bone. *Otolaryngol Head Neck Surg*. 1980;88:548.
17. Ernst CB: Technical aspects of carotid endarterectomy for atherosclerotic disease. In: Ernst CB, Stanley JC, eds. *Current Therapy in Vascular Surgery*. 3rd ed. St. Louis: Mosby–Year Book; 1995:40–43.

8

Revascularization for Extensive Extracranial Occlusions

Ramon Berguer, MD, PhD

This chapter reviews the techniques used and the results obtained in the repair of extensive extracranial arterial occlusions using the cervical approach. Patients operated on were those in whom a transthoracic repair was considered risky because of advanced age, poor cardiopulmonary reserve, previous midsternotomy, or mediastinal radiation or infection. The thoracic approach to these complex lesions of the supra-aortic trunks is discussed in Chapter 12.

We define *patients with extensive extracranial arterial occlusions* as those presenting with severe disease or occlusion of two of the first-order branches of the aortic arch (innominate, common carotid, and subclavian artery) and, in addition, severe disease or occlusion of the second-order branch (internal carotid or dominant vertebral artery). Severe disease is qualified as a 75% or greater occluding stenosis. We limit this review to the years 1985 through 1994 because our protocols for revascularization have changed in the last decade. During this period, we gave preference to transposition over bypass operations and to the retropharyngeal rather than the pretracheal route to cross the neck, and we used routine intraoperative digital arteriography at the conclusion of every reconstruction.

MATERIAL AND METHOD

We searched the records of patients undergoing one or more operations in the extracranial arteries to reconstruct extensive disease as previously defined (Fig. 8–1). There were a total of 46 patients with severe disease or occlusion of two or more of the branches of the aortic arch associated with disease of the internal carotid artery (ICA) or dominant vertebral artery. A second-order branch, either an ICA or a single and dominant vertebral artery, was severely diseased or occluded in all 46 patients. Five of the 46 patients had bilateral ICA occlusion.

In these patients, we attempted to revascularize their brain combining a reconstruction of their common carotid arteries (CCA) with an internal carotid endarterec-

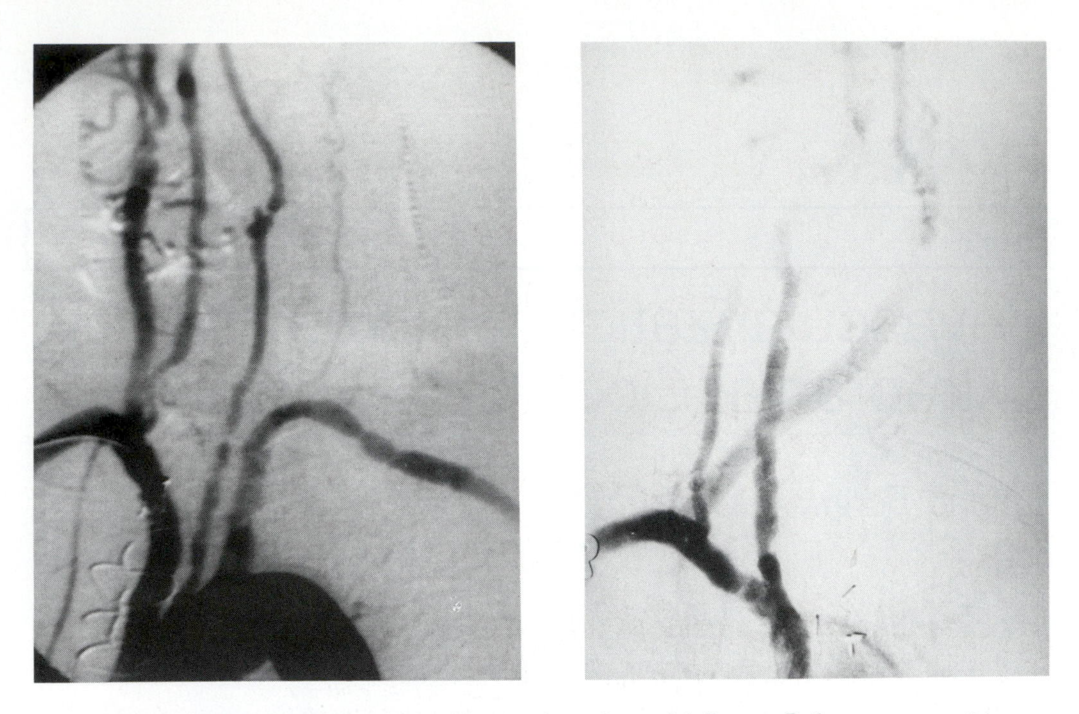

Figure 8–1. Arteriogram in patient with extensive extracranial disease. Both common carotid and the left subclavian arteries are diseased. There is severe stenosis of the left internal carotid artery, occlusion of the external carotid artery, and moderate disease of the first segment of the right single vertebral artery. (*Reprinted with permission from Berguer R, Gonzalez JA. Revascularization by the retropharyngeal route for extensive disease of the extracranial arteries. J Vasc Surg.* 1994;19:217–225.)

tomy. In those who had occlusion of the ICA, inflow to the brain was improved by bypassing occluded or severely diseased vertebral or external carotid arteries (Fig. 8–2).

The CCA lesion was revascularized preferentially from the ipsilateral subclavian artery (35 of 46 cases). This was accomplished by either a transposition or a bypass (Fig. 8–3). The second-order branch was revascularized by means of an internal carotid endarterectomy in 22 of 46 cases, an external carotid angioplasty or endarterectomy in 7 of 46 cases or a vertebral bypass or transposition in 4 of 46 cases. The diseased second-order branch was on the opposite side and not revascularized in 13 of 46 instances. The repair of the ICA was either part of the proximal reconstruction (as in the case of a bypass from the subclavian artery to the carotid bifurcation) or a concomitant procedure following a CCA to subclavian artery transposition.

In 7 of 46 cases, the ipsilateral ICA was chronically occluded and the bypass was anastomosed to the external carotid artery[1] (Fig. 8–3). These were patients in whom the external carotid artery was shown to contribute to the intracranial supply via the ophthalmic artery, or when the origin of the external carotid artery was occluded and one could demonstrate a distal vertebral to external carotid steal via the occipital artery. In four cases this was the dominant intracranial supply. This vertebral artery was used as the intracranial outflow for the proximal common carotid or subclavian reconstruction (Fig. 8–4).

In 11 cases the ipsilateral subclavian could not be used as a source artery because of severe disease or occlusion. In these patients, the bypass was originated in the

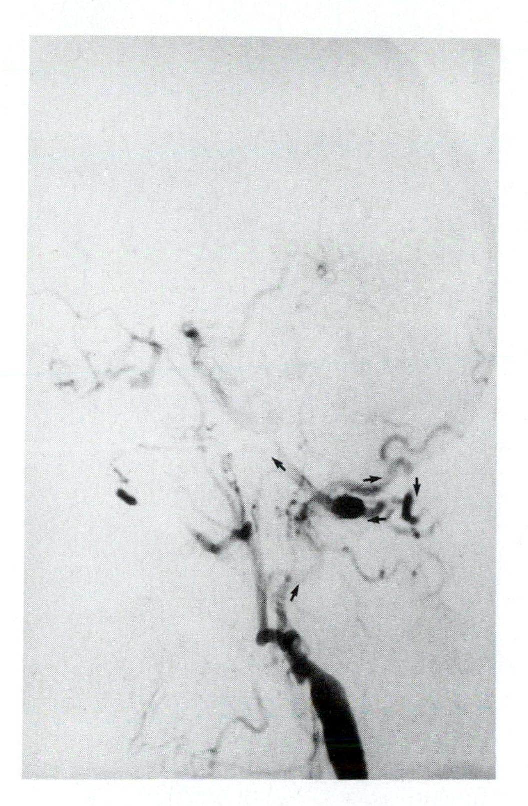

Figure 8–2. In this patient with the internal carotid artery occluded, a bypass to the external carotid artery provides inflow into the vertebrobasilar system via important collaterals from the occipital artery (the first and second segments of this single vertebral artery are occluded). The angular branch of the external carotid, via the ophthalmic artery, opacifies the supraclinoid internal carotid artery that is proximally occluded.

opposite side of the neck (CCA or, more commonly, subclavian artery) and was tunneled through the shorter retropharyngeal route[2] across the midline and into the receiver vessel.

TECHNICAL POINTS

On either side of the neck, the transposition of the CCA to the ipsilateral subclavian artery is a straightforward technique. If the CCA is severed low in the neck, there is sufficient length for its implantation in the second (retroscalene) or third segment of the subclavian artery. The site of implantation is determined by the anatomy and condition of the subclavian. We most often use the segment of subclavian artery between the scalenus anticus and the brachial plexus as a donor site. This precludes the division of the scalenus muscle and the dissection of (and potential injury to) the phrenic nerve.

If most of the length of the CCA is involved by disease, we place a prosthetic bypass in the subclavian artery and tunnel it under the internal jugular vein and up to the bifurcation of the CCA. Since an endarterectomy of the ICA is nearly always necessary (unless done before), we divide the distal CCA across below the bifurcation,

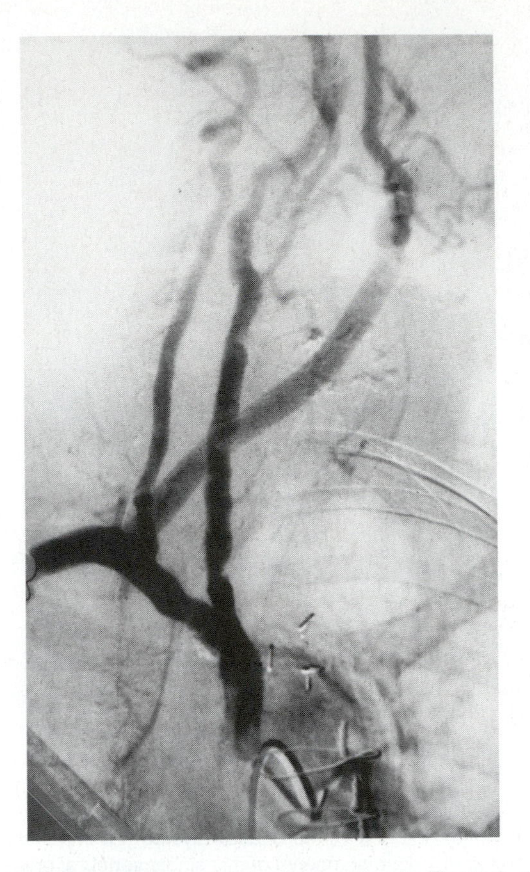

Figure 8–3. Postoperative arteriogram of the patient shown in Figure 8–1. There is a patent right subclavian to left carotid bifurcation bypass with endarterectomy of the branches of the latter.

do an eversion endarterectomy of both branches of the latter, and anastomose the bypass to the distal rim of CCA (Fig. 8–3). If the CCA was occluded, no shunt is used. In the rare instance when a shunt is advisable, its proximal end is inserted into the prosthesis and its distal end in the ICA.

This transposition is often coupled with an eversion endarterectomy of the proximal subclavian and/or vertebral arteries. On the left side a low (intrathoracic) origin of the vertebral artery may make it unadvisable to transpose the subclavian artery to the CCA. A subclavian to common carotid transposition is contraindicated in any patient who has had the corresponding internal mammary artery used for myocardial revascularization.

If the ipsilateral subclavian artery is occluded or diseased and cannot be used as an inflow source for a bypass, the contralateral subclavian artery (or CCA) may be a suitable source. Whenever we tend a bypass across the midline of the neck we use the retropharyngeal (prevertebral) tunnel (Fig. 8–5) as opposed to a pretracheal route. The retropharyngeal route is shorter (about half the length) and more direct than the conventional route in front of the trachea (Fig. 8–6). The endotracheal tube is placed in the midline (Fig. 8–7), and the neck is draped in such a manner that will permit exposure of each side alternately. Access to the retropharyngeal tunnel is achieved on both sides of the neck dissecting behind the CCA and over the sympathetic chain. The bodies of the cervical vertebrae are easily palpable and

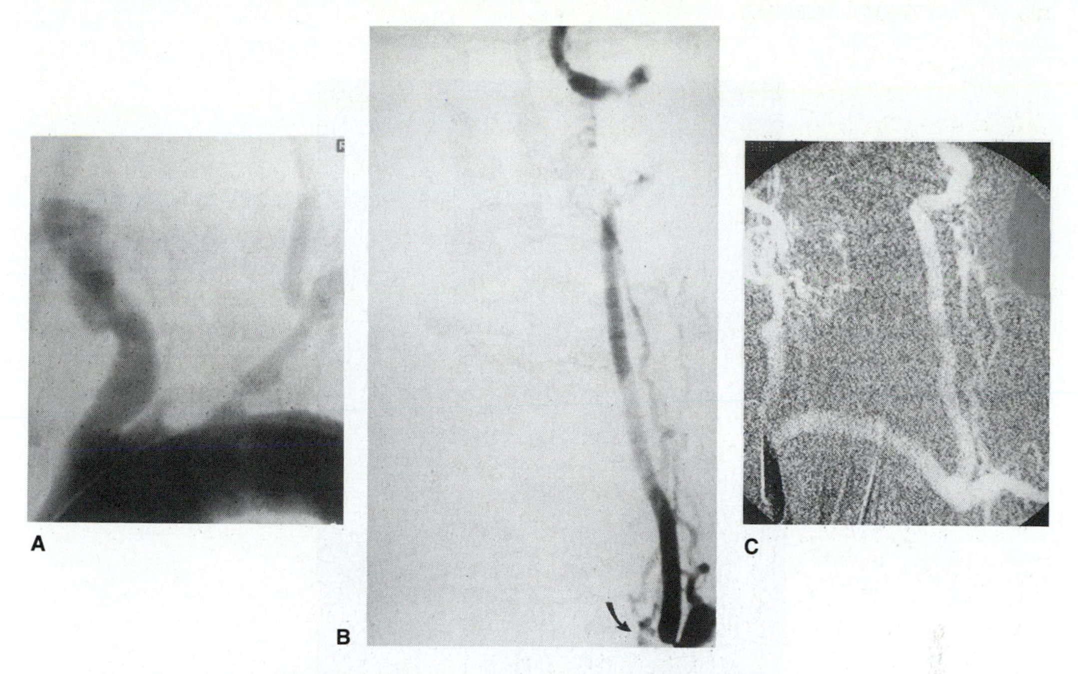

Figure 8–4. (A) Patient with bilateral internal carotid occlusion, left common carotid occlusion, and severe disease of the left subclavian artery and **(B)** left dominant vertebral artery. **(C)** A right subclavian to left proximal subclavian bypass and eversion endarterectomy of the vertebral artery origin provide the sole direct intracranial inflow in this patient.

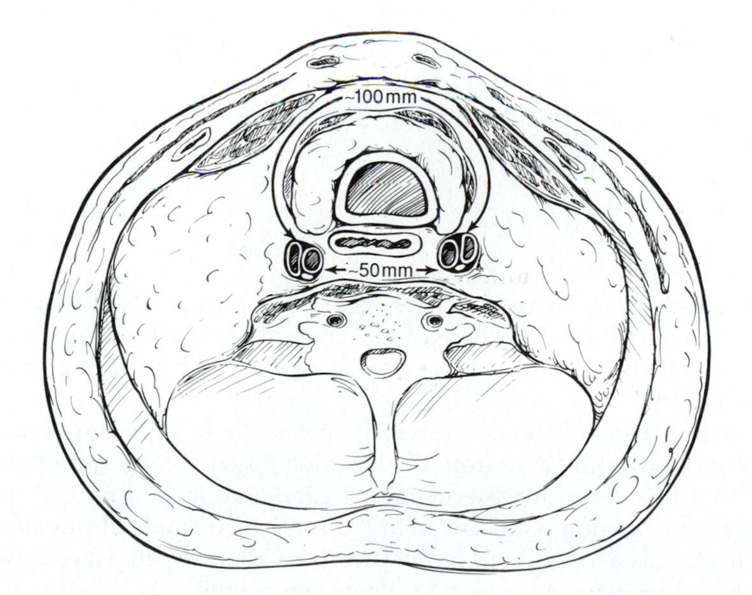

Figure 8–5. Diagram showing the shorter distance of the retropharyngeal tunnel compared with the conventional pretracheal route. (Reprinted with permission from Berguer R, Gonzalez JA. Revascularization by the retropharyngeal route for extensive disease of the extracranial arteries. *J Vasc Surg.* 1994;19:217–225.)

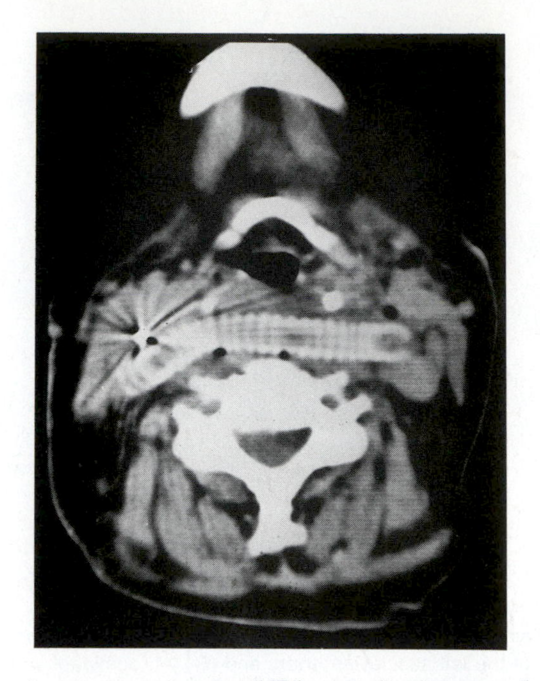

Figure 8–6. Magnetic resonance imaging (MRI) scan showing a prosthetic retropharyngeal bypass in place.

the tunnel is developed in this space with a finger. The anastomosis to the donor artery is done first and the bypass is drawn across the midline through the retropharyngeal tunnel to the carotid bifurcation. At this level the distal anastomosis is handled in the same manner as previously described for the ipsilateral subclavian-carotid bifurcation bypass.

RESULTS

The mean follow-up was 5.6 years. There were three strokes (6.5%) recorded within 30 days of the operation: 1 patient had a small cortical bleed with symptoms subsiding in 2 days, 1 patient had dysphasia for 3 days, and 1 had a mild hemiparesis that subsided in 1 month.

There was one death (2.1%) due to sepsis secondary to suppurative tenosynovitis occurring 2 weeks post discharge from the hospital. Patency rates were determined by duplex and, in a few cases, by arteriographic examination. Thrombosis was seen in two proximal reconstructions (subclavian to external carotid and subclavian to common carotid) and in one distal (vertebral) reconstruction. Clinically, 40 patients were asymptomatic and 6 had recurrent or new neurologic symptoms.

DISCUSSION

When confronted with symptomatic disease of the supra-aortic trunks, the surgeon is confronted with the choice of transthoracic versus cervical repair. While cervical repairs

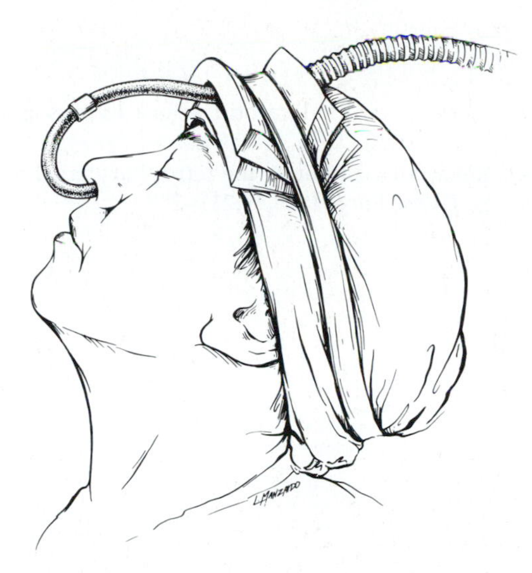

Figure 8–7. Taping the endotracheal tube in the midline permits rotating the neck to alternately expose each side.

are less morbid, they are also less durable. In our protocols for treatment of occlusive disease of the supra-aortic trunks, we favor a cervical approach for single lesions of the subclavian or CCAs and a thoracic approach for lesions of the innominate artery or for those involving more than one trunk on different sides of the neck. Patients with severe emphysema, history of congestive heart failure, angina pectoris, previous myocardial revascularization, or mediastinal infection or radiation are also candidates for a cervical approach.

The group of patients discussed here had extensive disease of their brain supply involving the first-order branches of the aortic arch (supra-aortic trunks) and the second-order branches (ICA and vertebral arteries). The cervical approach was chosen either because (1) one of the contraindications previously listed was present, or (2) the occluded or severely diseased branches of the arch were both on the left side (common carotid and subclavian) while the right-sided trunks (innominate, right common carotid, and right subclavian arteries) were either normal or moderately diseased. In these patients, a cross-over retropharyngeal bypass appeared to be a less risky operation than a transthoracic reconstruction.

The stroke rate was substantial (6.5%), probably reflecting the extensive involvement by atherosclerotic disease in these patients. Fortunately, none of the three observed strokes resulted in a permanent deficit.

CONCLUSION

In patients with extensive disease of the first- and second-order branches of the aortic arch, arterial reconstruction is possible by means of a cervical bypass based on any remaining branch of the aortic arch. These techniques are preferentially used in individuals that present a high risk for transthoracic repair. Their long term follow-up results show that, at 5 years, 86% are asymptomatic and 93% have patency proven by arteriography or duplex.

REFERENCES

1. Berguer R. Subclavian artery to external carotid artery bypass graft. *Arch Surg*. 1976;111: 893–896
2. Berguer R, Gonzalez JA. Revascularization by the retropharyngeal route for extensive disease of the extracranial arteries. *J Vasc Surg*. 1994;19:217–225.

9

Optimal Exposure and Technique for Vertebral Artery Operations

William H. Pearce, MD, and William D. McMillan, MD

Despite a relatively high incidence of atherosclerotic occlusive disease of the vertebral artery (VA), vertebral artery surgery is uncommon in most surgical practices. In a classic study by Hutchinson and Yates,[1] the incidence of VA occlusive disease in patients dying of cerebrovascular accidents was 39%. However, the collateral circulation is often sufficient to prevent symptoms; and, when present, vertebrobasilar insufficiency may be misdiagnosed due to the variable nature of the presenting symptoms. Transient ischemic attacks (TIAs) caused by carotid artery disease are readily recognized by most clinicians, but manifestations of vertebrobasilar TIAs are more variable and subtle. Symptoms of posterior circulation ischemia include dizziness, loss of balance, motor dysfunction consisting of paralysis and weakness, visual symptoms, and aphasia. Finally, direct VA surgery may be avoided by correcting critical stenosis of the internal carotid arteries (ICAs).[2] Humphries et al.[2] reported the improvement in vertebrobasilar symptoms in patients with stenotic lesions of both the carotid and vertebral arteries. By improving the perfusion pressure in the anterior circulation (ICA), blood flow is increased to the posterior circulation via the circle of Willis, thus avoiding the need for VA surgery.

When symptomatic lesions that cannot be corrected by carotid surgery are identified in the vertebral system, direct surgical repair of the vertebral artery then becomes unavoidable. If such lesions are untreated, the outcome of patients with infarctions in the posterior circulation is extremely poor. This chapter reviews the history of the most commonly recommended surgical procedures for VA stenosis and describes the operative technique.

HISTORICAL PERSPECTIVE

The history of vertebral surgery has been carefully reviewed by Carney.[3] Early surgery of the VA was primarily performed for trauma or its complications (aneurysms). Ligation of the VA, or packing, was recommended. Ligation of the VA was also recommended for the treatment of epilepsy in the 1880s but was soon abandoned.

Reconstructive surgery of the VA did not evolve until the second half of the twentieth century. During the 1950s, many new techniques were developed both for the radiographic visualization of the arterial system and for surgical repair. Throughout this era, Dr. Michael DeBakey was a pioneer, authoring or co-authoring more than 50 papers on VA surgery (of which 10 representative references are listed here).[4–13] These papers described techniques for cerebral and vertebral angiography, the brachial basilar syndrome, surgery of the innominate and subclavian vessels, carotid endarterectomy, and direct VA surgery. Based on his work, techniques of reimplantation, bypass, and angioplasty of the proximal VA were developed by later surgeons.

Surgery of the distal VA is less common and was first reported in 1881 for the ligation of a distal VA aneurysm. Contemporary surgery of the distal VA was later popularized by Carney[3,14] and Berguer.[15] Exposure of the distal VA is necessary when the proximal VA is occluded or the second portion of the VA is diseased, as occurs with osseous spurs.

PROXIMAL VERTEBRAL ARTERY

The vast majority of VA surgery is performed on the proximal segment. The VA has been divided anatomically into four segments, V-1 through V-4. The V-1 segment is that portion of the VA that extends from the subclavian artery to the bony canal. The VA on the left may take origin from the aortic arch or from a more proximal subclavian artery. In these instances, a direct surgical approach may not be feasible. In 95% of patients, the VA will enter the transverse process of C-6 to begin its intraosseous portion. Unfortunately, the VA may enter at other levels, including C-5 (4.5%), C-7 (1.2%), and C-4 (0.7%).[16] Therefore, in planning a surgical procedure on the first portion of the VA, it is important to know the location of both its origin from the subclavian and its entrance into the intraosseous canal. Short segments or very proximal origins may alter the planned surgical procedure.

The surgical approach to the proximal portion of the VA has not changed significantly since the description by Crawford, DeBakey, and Fields[4] in 1958 (Fig. 9–1).

> With the patient under local anesthesia an incision was made on the left 3 cm above and parallel to the clavicle. The clavicular head of the sternocleidomastoid muscle and the anterior scalenus were severed, exposing the subclavian artery and its branches. Due to the deep mediastinal origin of the vertebral artery in this case, additional exposure was obtained with the patient under general anesthesia when the mediastinum was opened through a combined cervical thoracic incision, splitting the sternum in the midline. . . . [B]ecause of the localized nature of the lesion to such a small segment of the artery the technique of endarterectomy was employed. Temporary occlusion clamps were placed on the subclavian artery both proximal and distal to the origin of the vertebral artery and temporary ligatures were placed around the thyro-cervical and internal mammary arteries. With the vertebral artery temporarily occluded with a soft bulldog clamp to prevent backbleeding a longitudinal incision was made in the subclavian artery opposite to the origin of the vertebral artery. The edges of the arterial incision were everted with temporary retraction sutures. From the intraluminal side of the subclavian artery the origin of the vertebral artery appeared as a dimple with an opening in the center of approximately 1 mm. A circumferential incision was made through the intima of the subclavian artery around the edge of the dimple and through the circumferential incision a cleavage plane was developed between the involved intima and the involved media layers of the vertebral artery. The occluding hypertrophied intima containing the atheromatous material was removed by retraction. . . .

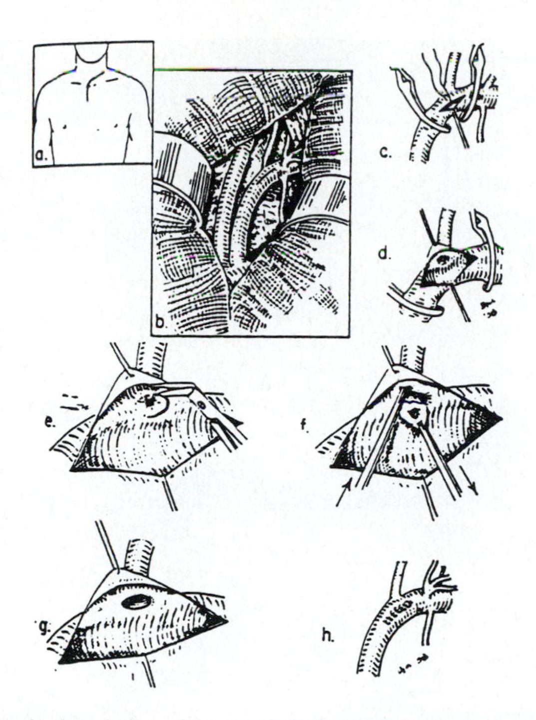

Figure 9–1. DeBakey's description of trans-subclavian vertebral artery endarterectomy. Diagrams showing technique of operation: **(a)** Cervicothoracic incision, splitting sternum, was made, exposing **(b)** great vessels originating on aortic arch, including subclavian artery in region of vertebral artery. **(c)** Longitudinal incision was made in subclavian artery opposite origin of vertebral artery; incision was retracted with fine silk sutures, exposing **(d)** origin of vertebral artery from lumen of subclavian artery. **(e)** Circular incision was made in intima of subclavian artery surrounding origin of vertebral artery and by development of proper plane of dissection. **(f)** Occluding tissues were removed, restoring **(g)** normal lumen to origin of vertebral artery. **(h)** Circulation was restored by repair of subclavian arterial wound with continuous fine silk suture and removal of clamps. *(Reprinted with permission from Crawford ES, DeBakey ME, Fields WS. Roentgenographic diagnosis and surgical treatment of basilar artery insufficiency. JAMA. 168(5):509–514, 1958. Copyright 1958, American Medical Association.)*

This description of direct VA endarterectomy was later popularized by Wylie and others.[17]

Several anatomic details warrant consideration in order to avoid potential complications during operative approach to the proximal VA (Figs. 9–2 and 9–3). First, it is important when identifying the scalene muscle to identify the phrenic nerve on the interior surface of this muscle. The phrenic nerve is small and passes from the lateral aspect of the scalene muscle to the medial side. As the scalene muscle is gradually divided, care must be taken to avoid injury to both the phrenic nerve and the subclavian artery. After the subclavian artery is identified in the region of the VA, several important landmarks should be noted. The inferior thyroid artery passes directly over the anterior surface of the VA. To gain exposure of the VA, this vessel must be ligated. Second, the vertebral vein is found in association with the VA. This vessel also needs to be ligated. Finally, the sympathetic chain is identified in close apposition to the VA. There are several ramifications of the sympathetic chain that pass around the VA to the stellate ganglion. The precise location of the stellate ganglion and the sympathetic chain is variable, but generally the sympathetic chain passes posterior to the VA. Care must be taken not to injure

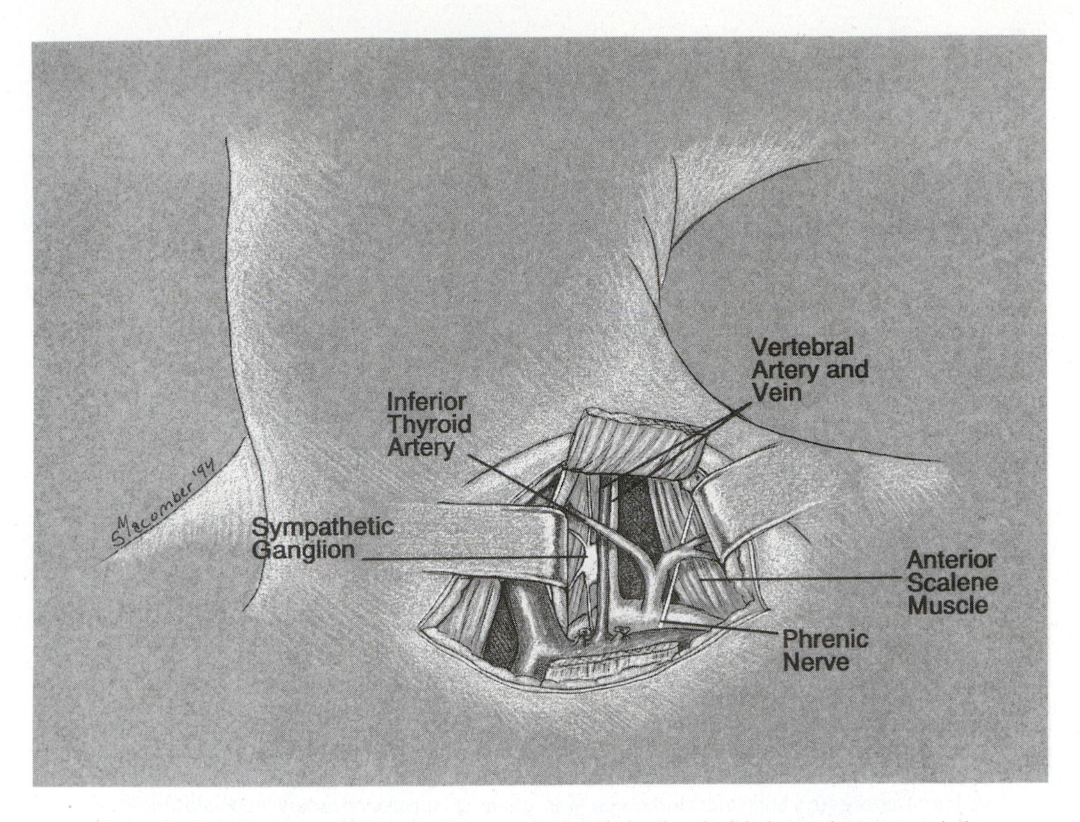

Figure 9–2. A transverse cervical incision made directly by the clavicle is used to approach the vertebral artery at the base of the neck. Following division of the anterior scalene muscle the subclavian artery is identified as well as its branches. By tracing the subclavian proximally, the vertebral artery is encountered. The vertebral artery lies adjacent to the vertebral vein, which must be transsected. The sympathetic ganglion lies in close apposition to the vertebral artery. Care must be taken to avoid damage to sympathetic outflow. The inferior thyroid artery also lies directly over the vertebral artery and must be transsected.

the stellate ganglion or the sympathetic outflow. If the sympathetic outflow is interrupted, the patient will suffer from Horner's syndrome. Therefore, patients should be cautioned about the possibility of Horner's syndrome preoperatively. If a more proximal exposure is required, a limited median stenotomy may be performed, although this is rarely necessary unless an endarterectomy is planned. This exposure provides a variety of surgical options for VA reconstruction. These include trans-subclavian endarterectomy, patch angioplasty, and modifications of the patch angioplasty as described by Imparato[18] (Fig. 9–4). Alternative techniques include vertebral artery reimplantation[19–21] on either the subclavian artery or the carotid artery, or bypasses from either the carotid or subclavian arteries (Fig. 9–5).[22–24]

DISTAL VERTEBRAL ARTERY

Exposure of the distal VA is uncommon. With proximal occlusion, the VA will thrombose to the next major collateral vessel. For this reason a small segment of the distal VA (V-3) is patent via collaterals from the external carotid artery. In some patients, a saphenous vein graft from the carotid artery to a patent V-3 segment of the VA may be performed. The incision for this operation is placed anterior to the sternocleidomastoid,

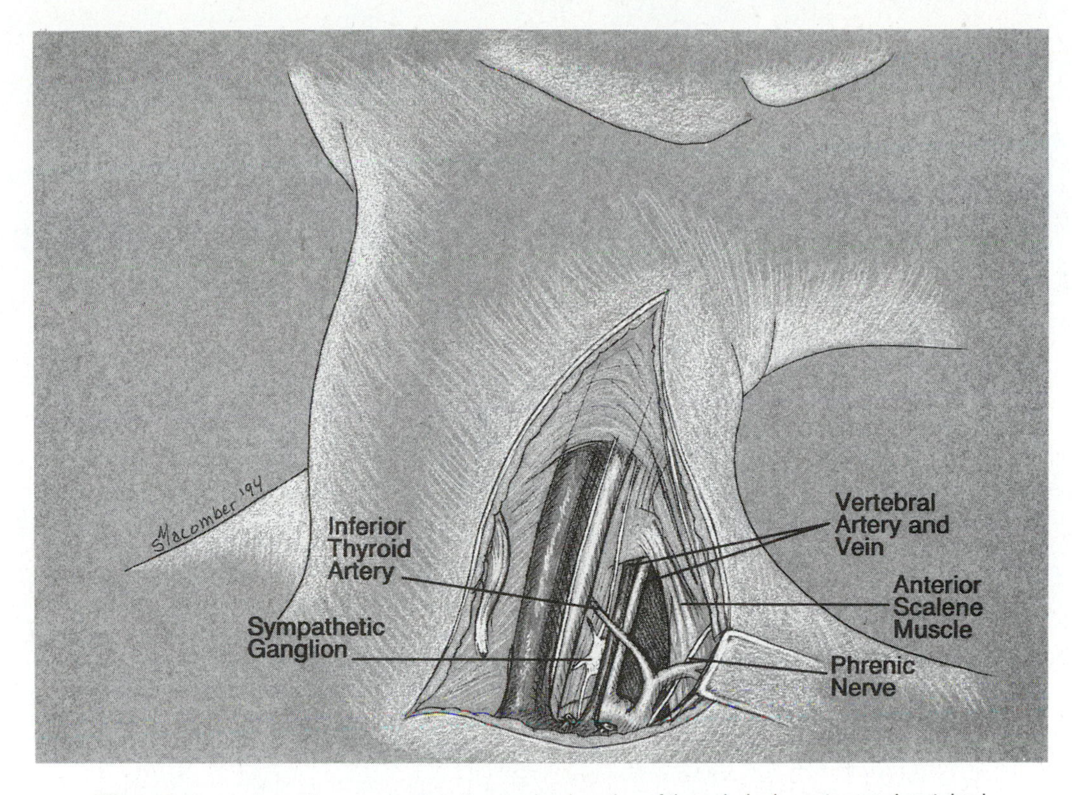

Figure 9–3. An alternative approach to the proximal portion of the subclavian artery and vertebral arteries is obtained through a vertical incision. Through this incision the carotid artery and jugular vein is identified and retracted medially. Just posterior to the structure lie the vertebral artery sympathetic chain and vertebral vein. This incision is particularly useful for carotid transpositions.

passing posterior to the earlobe near the mastoid process (Fig. 9–6). The carotid artery is exposed in a standard fashion. Important landmarks for this procedure include the spinal accessory nerve and the process of C-1. Once the carotid artery has been dissected, the operation is carried posteriorly to the internal jugular vein with identification of the spinal accessory nerve. This nerve is dissected free from the digastric muscle, across the internal jugular vein to the sternocleidomastoid muscle. With the nerve free, the transverse process of C-1 is identified. Next, the fascia of the underlying muscles is opened, allowing identification of the levator scapula. This muscle is recognized by the emergence of the anterior ramus of C-2 below the muscle belly. This muscle is carefully transected over a right angle or other instrument. During this procedure, the splenius cervicis muscle is also transected. Both muscles are excised to provide optimal exposure of the underlying VA. The ramus of C-2 is anterior to the VA, which also must be divided. At this point a small segment of the VA is seen with the adjacent vertebral veins. It is important to use optical magnification and extreme care in dissecting the VA, as many collaterals enter at this point. The distal artery is controlled using a microhemoclip, while the remaining vessels are clipped using standard surgical staples. Adequate distal control of the artery is mandatory since any slippage of the microhemoclip will result in uncontrolled hemorrhage. Saphenous vein graft is used for these bypasses. The artery is transected in such a fashion that it can be rotated in the field to be spatulated and prepared for the end-to-end anastomosis. Following completion of the distal anastomosis, the proximal anastamosis is performed to the common carotid artery (CCA) in a standard fashion.

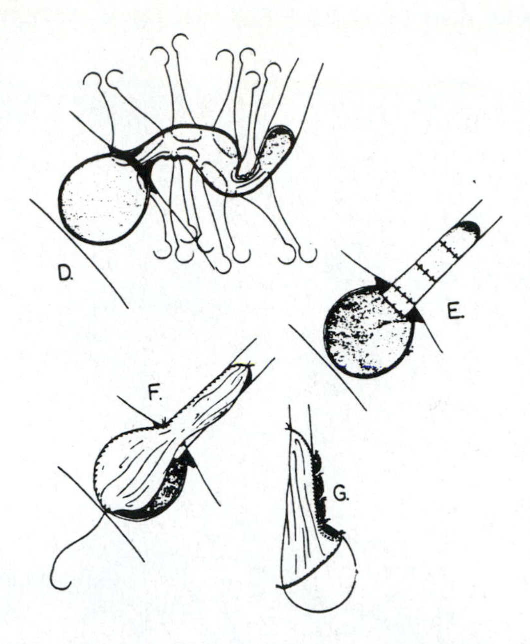

Figure 9–4. Reproduction of the vertebral artery plication procedure described by Imparato. In this procedure an endarterectomy is performed on the vertebral artery and a patch angioplasty performed. Due to lengthening of the artery, the plication is performed. *(Reprinted with permission from Imparato AM, Lin JPT. Vertebral arterial reconstruction: internal plication and vein patch angioplasty. Ann Surg. 1967; 166:213–221.)*

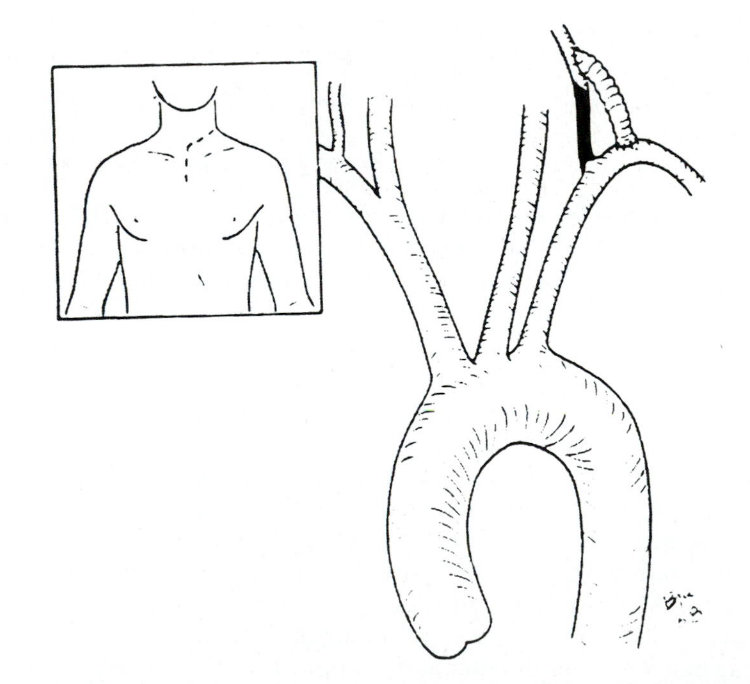

Figure 9–5. Original reproduction of the bypass procedure described by DeBakey and colleagues for proximal occlusion of the vertebral artery. Here dacron graft is interposed between the subclavian artery and vertebral artery. Diagrammatic drawing showing location of incision, extent of occlusion and bypass graft. *(Reprinted with permission from DeBakey ME et al. Surgical considerations of occlusive disease of innominate, carotid, subclavian, and vertebral arteries. Ann Surg. 1959; 149:703.)*

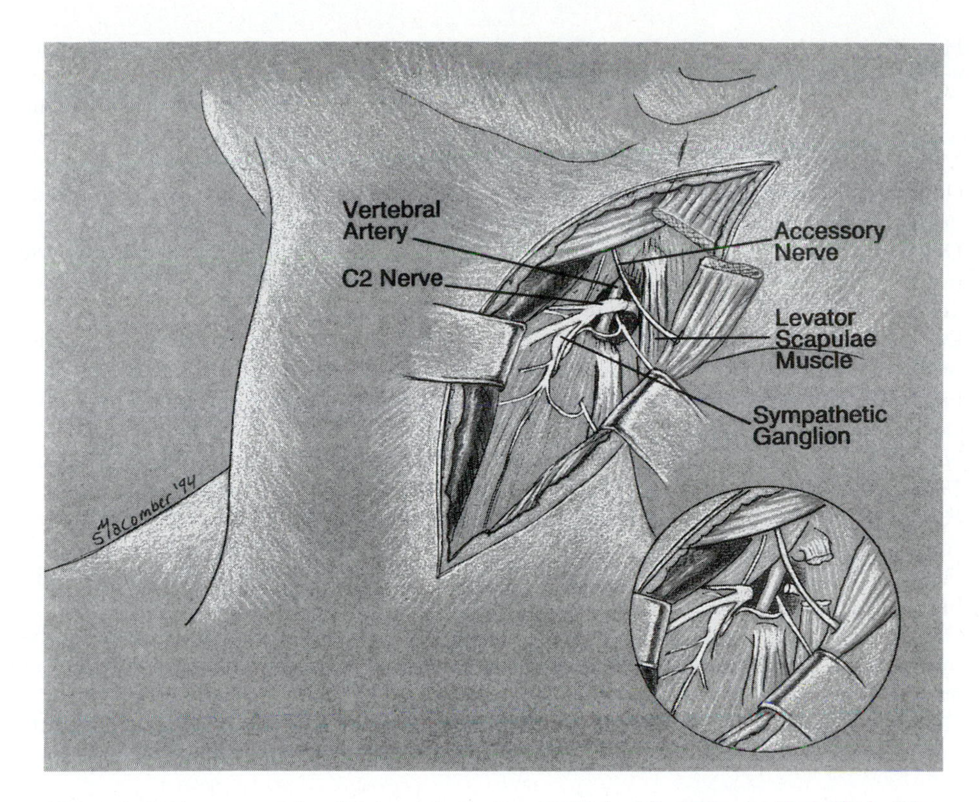

Figure 9–6. Exposure of the distal vertebral artery is obtained through a vertical skin incision that passes just posterior to the ear. Initially the carotid artery and internal jugular veins are identified. Posterior to these structures lies the spinal accessory nerve as well as the C-2 nerve root. Both of these important structures need to be identified during the dissection. Just posterior to the C-2 nerve root lies the vertebral artery. During the dissection of the levator the scapular muscle is transsected. Arterial collaterals are common in this area and care must be taken to avoid injury.

CONCLUSION

From the time of the earliest ligations of the VAs to modern reconstructive surgery, steady progress has occurred in the surgical management of patients with vertebral basilar insufficiency. New noninvasive diagnostic methods provide a more complete evaluation of the posterior circulation, while duplex ultrasound scans and magnetic resonance angiography provide a detailed anatomy and hemodynamic evaluation of the cerebral circulation. Using the meticulous techniques developed by Dr. Michael DeBakey and his colleagues at Baylor, we can now achieve excellent results. Furthermore, the surgical advances made by Carney and Berguer have allowed us to approach the third portion of the VA in some patients. In short, modern surgical management of patients with vertebral basilar insufficiency due to occlusion or stenosis of the VA has become reliable and safe.

REFERENCES

1. Hutchinson EC, Yates PO. Cervical portion of vertebral artery: clinico-pathological study. *Brain.* 1956;70:319–331.

2. Humphries AW, Young JR, Beven EG, et al. Relief of vertebrobasilar symptoms by carotid endarterectomy. *Surgery*. 1965;57:48–52.
3. Carney AL. Vertebral artery surgery: historical development, basic concepts of brain hemodynamics, and clinical experience of 102 cases. In: Carney AL, Anderson EM, eds. *Advances in Neurology*. New York: Raven Press; 1981;30:249–282.
4. Crawford ES, Debakey ME, Fields WS. Roentgenographic diagnosis and surgical treatment of basilar artery insufficiency *JAMA*. 1958;168:509–514.
5. DeBakey ME, Crawford ES, Fields WS. Surgical treatment of lesions producing arterial insufficiency of the internal, carotid, common carotid, vertebral, innominate and subclavian arteries. *Ann Intern Med*. 1959;51:436–448.
6. DeBakey ME, Crawford ES, Morris GC Jr, et al. Surgical considerations of occlusive disease of the innominate, carotid, subclavian, and vertebral arteries. *Ann Surg*. 1961;154:698–725.
7. Fields WS, Crawford ES, DeBakey ME. Surgical considerations in cerebral arterial insufficiency. *Neurology*. 1958;8:801–808.
8. North RR, Fields WS, DeBakey ME, et al. Brachial-basilar insufficiency syndrome. *Neurology*. 1962;12:810–820.
9. Henly WS, Morris JC Jr, Balas PE, et al. Vertebral arteriography by an infraclavicular route. *Am J Surg*. 1964;107:656–659.
10. DeBakey ME, Morris GC Jr, Jordan GL Jr, et al. Segmental thrombo-obliterative disease of branches of aortic arch: successful surgical treatment. *JAMA*. 1958;166:998–1003.
11. DeBakey ME, Crawford ES, Fields WS. Surgical treatment of lesions producing arterial insufficiency of the internal carotid, common carotid, vertebral, innominate and subclavian arteries. *Ann Intern Med*. 1959;51;436–448.
12. DeBakey ME, Crawford ES, Fields WS. Surgical treatment of patients with cerebral arterial insufficiency associated with extracranial arterial occlusive lesions. *Neurology*. 1961;11: 145–159.
13. DeBakey ME, Crawford ES, Morris GC Jr, et al. Arterial reconstructive operations for cerebrovascular insufficiency due to extracranial arterial occlusive disease. *J Cardiovasc Surg*. 1962; 3:12–25.
14. Carney AL, Anderson EM. Carotid distal vertebral artery bypass for carotid artery occlusion. *Clin Electroencephalogr*. 1978;9:105–109.
15. Berguer R. Selection of patients, choice of surgical technique, and results with vertebral artery reconstruction. In: Berguer R, Bauer RB, eds. *Vertebrobasilar Arterial Occlusive Disease: Medical and Surgical Managements*. New York: Raven Press; 1984:297–303.
16. Feldman AJ. Surgical approach to disease of the first portion of the vertebral artery. In: Berguer R, Bauer RB, eds. *Vertebrobasilar Arterial Occlusive Disease: Medical and Surgical Management*. New York: Raven Press; 1984:231–239.
17. Roon AJ, Ehrenfeld WK, Cooke PD. Vertebral artery reconstruction. *Am J Surg*. 1979;138:29–36.
18. Imparato AM, Lin JPT. Vertebral arterial reconstruction: internal plication and vein patch angioplasty. *Ann Surg*. 1967;166:213–221.
19. Edwards WH, Mulherin JL. The surgical approach to significant stenosis of vertebral and subclavian arteries. *Surgery*. 1980;87:20–28.
20. Edwards WH, Mulherin JL Jr. The management of brachiocephalic occlusive disease. *Am Surg*. 1983;9:465–471.
21. Edwards WH, Mulherin JL. The surgical reconstruction of the proximal subclavian and vertebral artery. In: Berguer R, Bauer RB, eds. *Vertebrobasilar Arterial Occlusive Disease: Medical and Surgical Management*. New York: Raven Press; 1984:241–256.
22. Cormier JM, Laurian C. Surgical management of vertebral-basilar insufficiency. *J Cardiovasc Surg*. 1976;17:205–223.
23. Kieffer E, Rancurel G, Richard T. Reconstruction of the distal cervical vertebral artery. In: Berguer R, Bauer RB, eds. *Vertebrobasilar Arterial Occlusive Disease: Medical and Surgical Management*. New York: Raven Press; 1984:265–290.
24. Piepgras DG, Sundt TM Jr. Bypass procedures for vertebrobasilar occlusive disease. In: Berguer R, Bauer RB, eds. *Vertebrobasilar Arterial Occlusive Disease: Medical and Surgical Management*. New York: Raven Press; 1984:321–330.

10

Vertebral Arteriovenous Fistulae

Eric J. Russell, MD

SOLITARY VERTEBRAL ARTERIOVENOUS FISTULAE

Solitary connections that develop between the vertebral artery (VA) or one of its muscular branches and the surrounding intraspinal (epidural) and paraspinal venous plexus result in redirection of blood flow away from the intracranial vertebrobasilar system toward adjacent venous channels. This may result in symptoms related to secondarily induced brainstem and cerebellar ischemia, or to compression of neural tissues by dilated arteries and veins.

Vertebral-venous fistulae (VVF) can occur spontaneously.[1–4] Spontaneous or congenital fistulae may present during childhood by the detection of an asymptomatic audible bruit during routine physical examination. Other persons present with symptoms later in life, when flow through the fistula increases for some reason—during pregnancy, for example, or in association with systemic hypertension.[5,6] A number of spontaneous cases are associated with vessel wall abnormalities related to collagen deficiencies and have been reported in patients with neurofibromatosis, Ehlers-Danlos syndrome, and fibromuscular dysplasia.[7,8]

The majority of VVFs result from blunt or penetrating neck injuries, iatrogenic trauma related to direct puncture vertebral arteriography (now outmoded), and internal jugular venipuncture, or inadvertent injury during surgery of the neck or cervical spine.[9–21] Sugar et al.[22] first suggested the possibility of iatrogenic VVF in their paper describing percutaneous vertebral angiography in 1949. The first report of postangiographic VVF was written by Sutton in 1963.[23] Local referral patterns may result in varying proportions of traumatic cases appearing for treatment at any one institution.[24]

Anatomy

The VA may be divided into three segments: the lowest segment from the subclavian artery to C-6, the middle segment in the foramen transversarium from C-6 to C-1, and the highest segment from C-1 to the foramen magnum. The artery is surrounded by the perivertebral venous plexus, which is quite dense around the artery in the middle segment. This venous plexus in turn communicates with the intraspinal anterior longitudinal venous plexus through connecting foraminal or uncinate veins, permitting fistulous flow to distend intraspinal veins that may potentially compress the spinal cord. The veins connect inferiorly to form the vertebral vein, which joins the jugular vein in the lower neck. Venous drainage from the fistula may course cephalad to produce intracranial venous hypertension. Since clinical findings are often related to the pattern of venous drainage, some authors have investigated this. In one large series of 45 patients,[11] venous drainage was directed outside the foramen transversarium in 41%, inside in 26%, and in both directions in 33%. Venous flow was toward the vertebral vein in 33%, toward the internal jugular vein in 30%, toward the epidural venous plexus in 26%, and toward the perimedullary veins in 2%.

Most traumatic VVFs involve the middle VA segment, while spontaneous fistulae tend to occur in the upper cervical region.[25–27] Intracranial fistulae may also occur.[28]

Clinical and Angiographic Findings

Solitary VVFs most commonly present with pulse synchronous tinnitus (50%), although 30% are asymptomatic at the time of discovery.[11] Fistulae are occasionally discovered by detection of a localized bruit during routine physical examination. Neurologic complaints such as ataxia, vertigo, diplopia, hearing loss, cranial neuropathy, and cervical radiculopathy are uncommon (<10%), but may occur due to ischemia related to a steal phenomenon or venous engorgement resulting in spinal cord or nerve root compression.[15,24,25,29,30] Radiculopathy may result from compression of the intraforaminal segment of the nerve root at the affected level by distension of foraminal veins connecting the perivertebral artery venous plexus with intraspinal veins.[15,30] High-flow fistulae may produce varices sufficiently large to compress the spinal cord[31] and the brainstem.[32] Rarely, subarachnoid hemorrhage may result when flow is directed toward the intracranial or perimedullary venous plexus or when vessels coursing through the subarachnoid space are directly injured by trauma. Pseudoaneurysms related to the initial trauma may be found in association with VVF in 15% of cases.[11]

The angiographic assessment of VVF should define all vascular supply (direct and collateral) toward the fistula. Injections should include the ipsilateral and contralateral VAs, the ipsilateral internal and external carotids, and the remaining branches of the ipsilateral subclavian artery (costocervical and thyrocervical trunks). When the fistulous VA has been surgically trapped, collateral flow from subclavian branches to the blind VA segment may continue to keep the fistula open. The constancy of such anastomotic connections is predicted by developmental considerations. The thyrocervical trunks and VAs develop as longitudinal anastomoses between the first six pairs of embryonic dorsal intersegmental arteries, which are paired branches from the primitive aortic arches,[33] and connections exist between them at many levels through muscular branches. Collateral flow to the vertebral artery may also arise from other sources, including the ascending pharyngeal arteries.[34]

Injection of collateral (indirect) routes to the fistula may better define the pathologic anatomy than direct injection of the VA, flow through collaterals is typically slower and the fistula will be less obscured at angiography by rapid filling of the draining veins. Very rapid filming sequences (cine or 5–7 frames/s, digital subtraction) should also be considered for anatomic definition of the fistula site.

There is a significant incidence of fistula closure following diagnostic angiography alone.[33–37] I have witnessed complete closure with full symptomatic relief immediately following angiography in two cases Fig. 10–1. This may be related to contrast viscosity or catheter and guide wire manipulation.

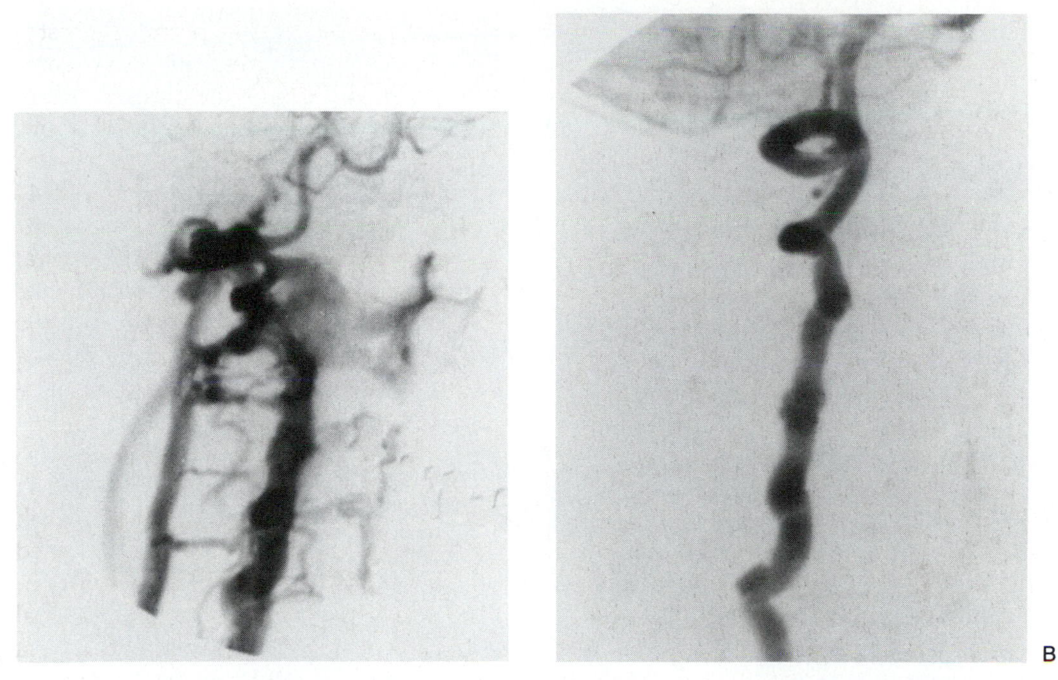

Figure 10–1. Spontaneous closure of right-sided VVF following diagnostic angiography, in a middle-age woman with pulsatile tinnitus and an audible cervical bruit. Conventional digital subtraction angiography with injections of the right vertebral artery performed on Day 1 **(A)** and Day 2 **(B)**. Note on the initial study (**A**), filling of the perivertebral venous plexus diagnostic of a vertebral-venous fistula (VVF). Follow-up study performed the next day **(B)** reveals an intact and patent vertebral artery, and complete closure of the fistula without treatment.

Surgical Treatment

Proximal surgical ligation, or proximal and distal VA trapping procedures, have been employed in the past for control of solitary VVFs.[12,38] Proximal ligation alone almost always fails because the fistula fills via retrograde from the opposite VA, across the vertebrobasilar junction. In fact, proximal ligation may induce or worsen neurologic signs and symptoms related to the steal phenomenon because of further flow reversal. Proximal ligation is also contraindicated because it obliterates direct endovascular access to the fistula.[30,39]

Surgical trapping of the VA should theoretically result in cure; there is, however, a significant failure rate.[40] Muscular collaterals arising from ascending and dorsal cervical branches of the thyrocervical and costocervical trunks of the subclavian arteries, and small collaterals from external carotid branches may continue to supply the blind vertebral segment, maintaining patency of the fistula[41] Fig. 10–2. As noted by Dutton,[42] it is "mandatory not to allow a segment of patent vessel to persist between ligatures with the fistula undiscovered." The goal of any therapy, therefore, should be local and permanent occlusion of the fistula.

Attempts to directly occlude the fistula operatively have met with limited success due to relative inaccessibility of the fistula site within the foramen transversarium or intervertebral foramen and the presence of large draining veins, which may totally obscure the fistula site.[43]

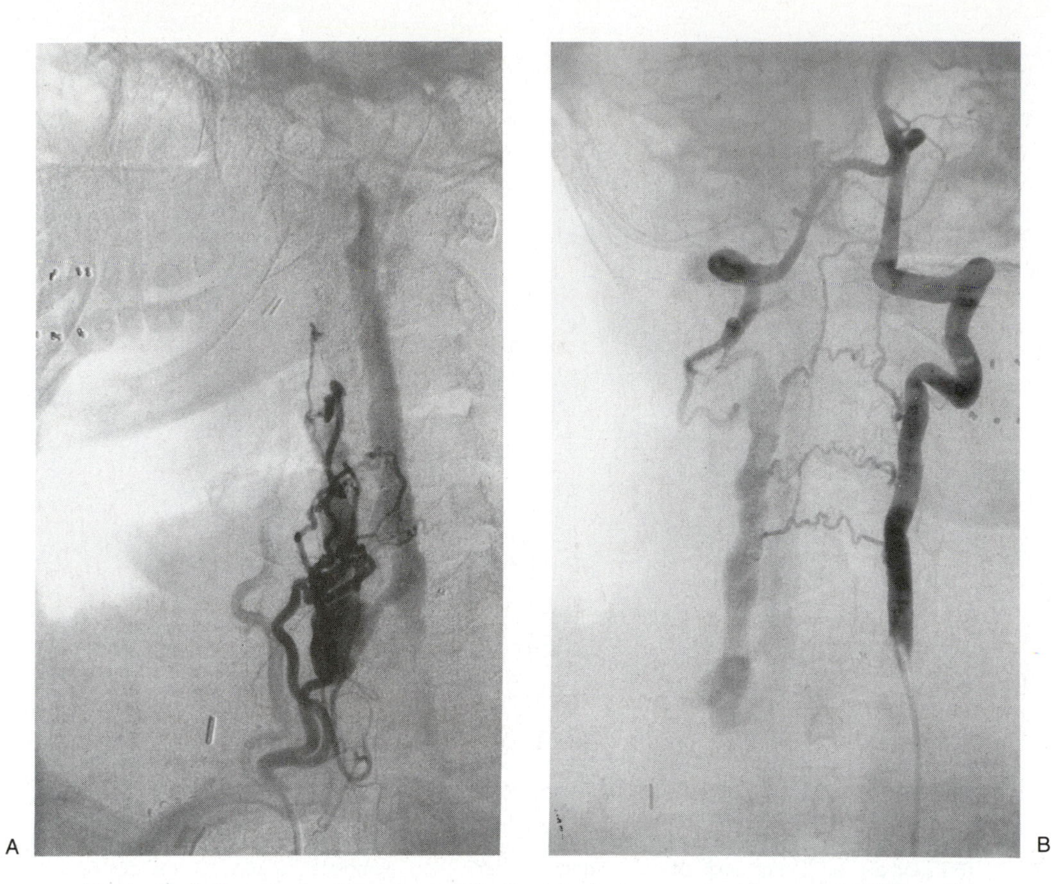

Figure 10–2. Percutaneous puncture of blind vertebral artery segment for cure of a VVF persistent following operative trapping procedures, in a 52-year-old woman presenting with right-sided tinnitus and recurrent neurologic symptoms. Twelve years before, the patient had transient right arm paresis and radiculopathy following a stab wound to the right lower neck. Four years before, a right neck bruit was discovered, and 2 years before, she developed dizziness and unsteady gait. The proximal and distal right vertebral artery were ligated in two procedures, without symptomatic relief.

(A) Initial injection of the thyrocervical branch of the right subclavian artery revealed enlarged collateral channels reconstituting the blind right vertebral artery segment, which then filled the longitudinal vertebral venous plexus by communication a single fistula. **(B)** Left vertebral arteriogram (frontal view with head turned to left) reveals trans-spinal vertebral–vertebral anastomotic channels filling the blind right vertebral artery segment. The longitudinal venous plexus then fills from the fistula hole via the foraminal vein at the C-6 level. Note also retrograde filling of the distal right vertebral artery down to the upper surgical clip. Right thyrocervical angiogram after fluoroscopically guided percutaneous deposition of steel coils into the blind vertebral sac at the fistula site, early **(C)** and delayed **(D)** phases. Note coils at fistula (**C**) and stagnant contrast within the blind vertebral segment (**D**). The fistula and spinal veins did not fill. *(Reprinted with permission from Russell EJ, Goldblatt D, Levy JM et al. Percutaneous obliteration of a postoperatively persistent vertebral arteriovenous fistula. Am J Neuroradiol. 1989;10:196–200.)*

Combined surgical and endovascular approaches have met with some success. Mullan described a combined operative and endovascular approach, using exposure of the C-7 level VA to introduce an occluding balloon catheter. Particulate agents have also been injected intraoperatively following surgical access to the fistula.[43a] Larger fistulae have been treated with the use of a venous bypass graft from the subclavian

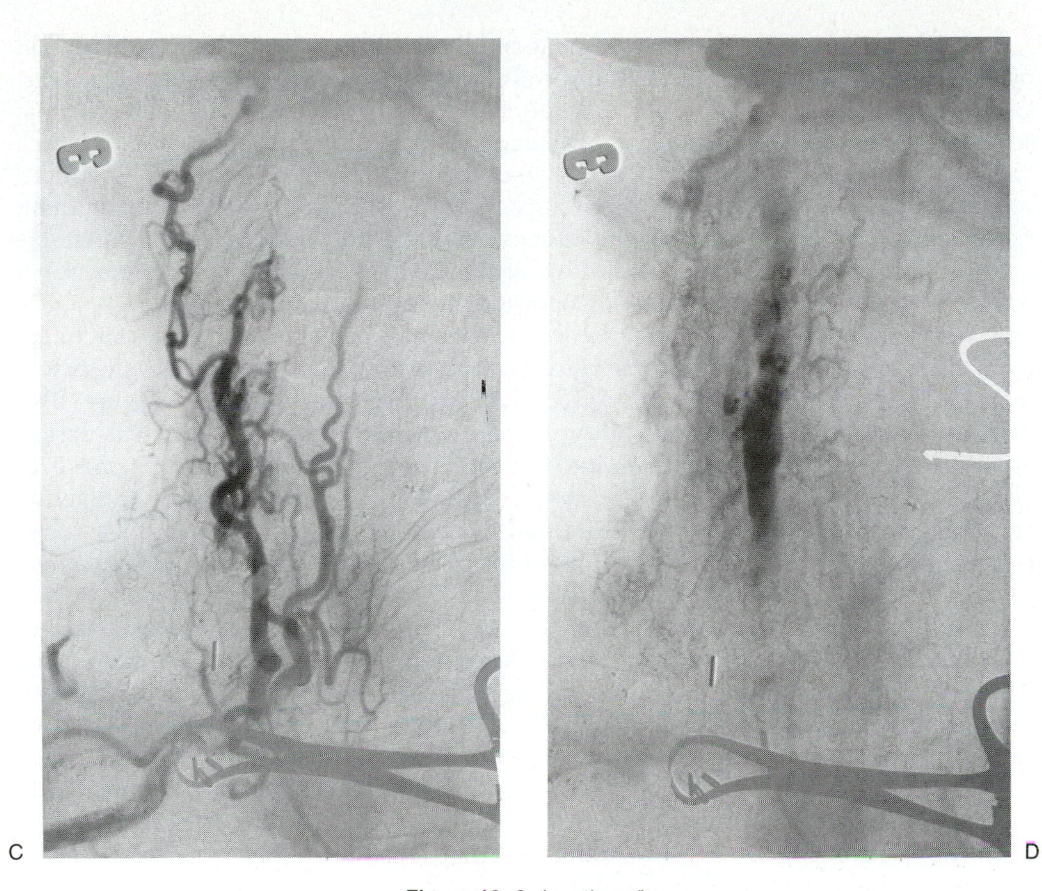

Figure 10–2. (*continued*)

artery to the VA beyond the fistula, combined with endovascular techniques to occlude the fistula.[43a]

Endovascular Treatment

The initial step in the process of performing any vascular interventional procedure is the development of a functional angiographic map of the lesion.[45] This is essential for determination of the contribution of individual vessels to the lesion, determining compartmentalization, and identification of potentially dangerous anastomoses between the vessels supplying the lesion and neurologically functional tissue. Identification of dangerous anastomoses is of utmost importance. During the embolization procedure, collateral arterial flow volume and direction can change rapidly, thus changing the destination of any embolic material injected. For example, collateral channels toward the VA territory are commonly encountered with lesions supplied by the ascending pharyngeal and occipital arteries. Meticulous angiographic technique with superselective catheterization is essential for safety.

VVFs must be carefully studied angiographically to determine the anatomy of the pathologic arteriovenous connection. Single-hole fistulae may be difficult to distinguish from complex arteriovenous malformations (AVMs) without selective angiographic injections of all regional arterial supply. It is imperative that treatment of these lesions be performed by occlusion at the site of the fistula, and the nagiographic map must be reviewed to select the safest and most effective route to reach the lesion.

Embolization of the fistulous segment is the goal. Large fistulas may be occluded by endovascular placement of platinum coils or detachable balloons at the fistula site. Occlusion proximal to the fistula site should be avoided at all cost, since, like proximal surgical ligation, it will result in persistence of the lesion by recruitment through collateral channels. Frequently (10% to 40% of the time[11,24]), the VA must be sacrificed by detachable balloon occlusion or coil deposition in order to close the fistula without risk of inadvertant distal embolization. When a complete steal is not present, a preferable goal is obliteration of the venous outflow at the fistula site, with preservation of VA patency. Endovascular treatment may occasionally require occlusion of the VA above and below the ends of a severed vessel.[24,25,46] When a direct ipsilateral approach to the fistula is not possible (due to prior surgical ligation or traumatic transection) the fistula may be catheterized and cured by a contralateral vertebral approach. Figure 10–3 illustrates a case demonstrating both principles, wherein a microcatheter was passed around the vertebrobasilar junction into the contralateral distal vertebral segment for obliteration of a fistula distal to a transected vessel.[47] When prior operative ligation and trapping has failed to cure a fistula, and there is no available endovascular route, cure may require percutaneous puncture of the blind VA segment (with direct deposition of embolic material directly at the fistula site[30]) (Fig. 10–2).

With some high-flow chronic fistulae, a chronic steal phenomenon may so impair local cerebral autoregulation that abrupt closure of the fistula will cause brain edema due to overperfusion. This "perfusion pressure breakthrough phenomenon" may lead to neurologic deficits related to swelling and hemorrhage. In such cases, functional testing of the artery may be performed with a nondetachable balloon, and a slow staged closure may be possible. An initial trial of temporary occlusion should be made with the patient awake to permit neurologic testing. Intermittent attempts at closure over a short period of time may allow autoregulation to return and permit final closure even when the first attempt is unsuccessful.[48–50]

Endovascular therapy has been reported to be curative in 91%, with minimal morbidity.[11] Clinical improvement is usually immediate following fistula closure, although deficits related to spinal cord and nerve root compression may incompletely resolve, or resolve in a delayed fashion.

Technical Considerations

First efforts to employ an endovascular technique to embolize solitary arteriovenous fistulae were made in casaes of carotid–cavernous fistulae, using muscle,[51] or a porridge of gelfoam, gauze, and saline.[52] Balloon-tipped nondetachable (Fogarty) catheters were employed later on. The catheters were placed via carotid puncture, inflated at the fistula site, and then left in place with the proximal portion buried subcutaneously.[53,54]

A tremendous advance in management of all carotid and vertebral fistulae resulted from the development of detachable balloon catheters.[55–57] The balloon attached to a flexible catheter can be guided through fistula and then inflated and detached in the venous compartment, preserving parent artery flow. Balloons may be filled with isosmotic contrast media, or solidified with polymerizing materials such as silicone and hydro xy-ethyl methacrylate (HEMA) to prevent premature deflation and pseudoaneurysm formation. Detachable balloons are effective devices for the treatment of VVFs.[58–60] If direct arterial access through the VA is not available, collateral channels may used to approach the site of the fistula, including the use of suboccipital collaterals from the occipital branch of the external carotid artery to the C-1 level vertebral.[61]

Thrombogenic coils have been used for the treatment of arteriovenous fistulae since 1973[62–65] and are quite effective for treating some VVFs as well,[66] (Figs. 10–2 and

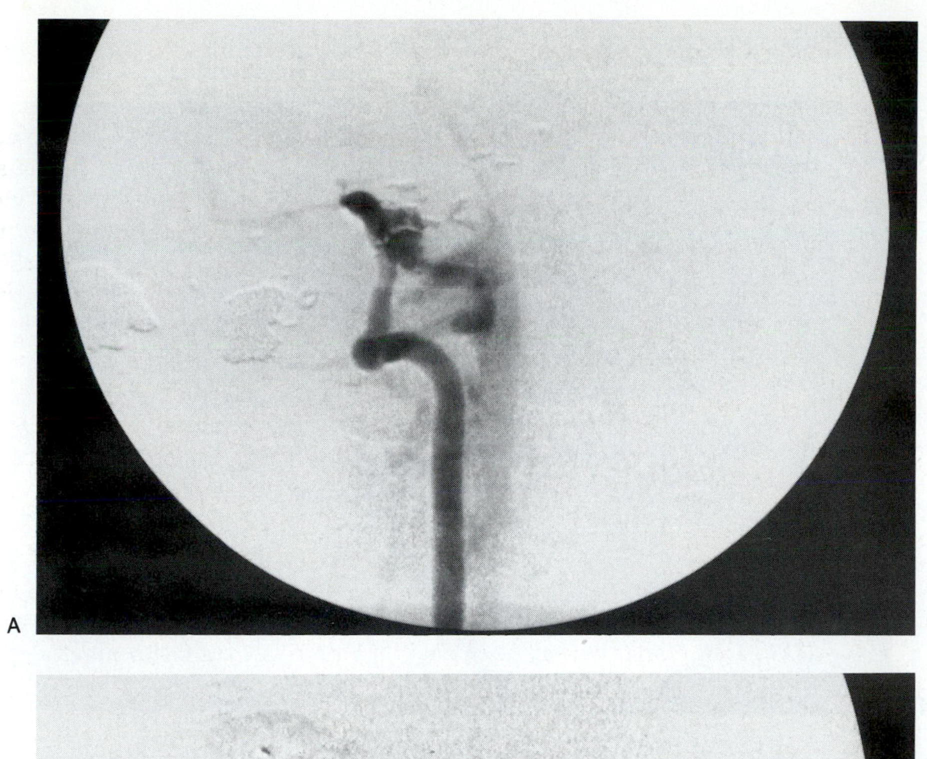
A

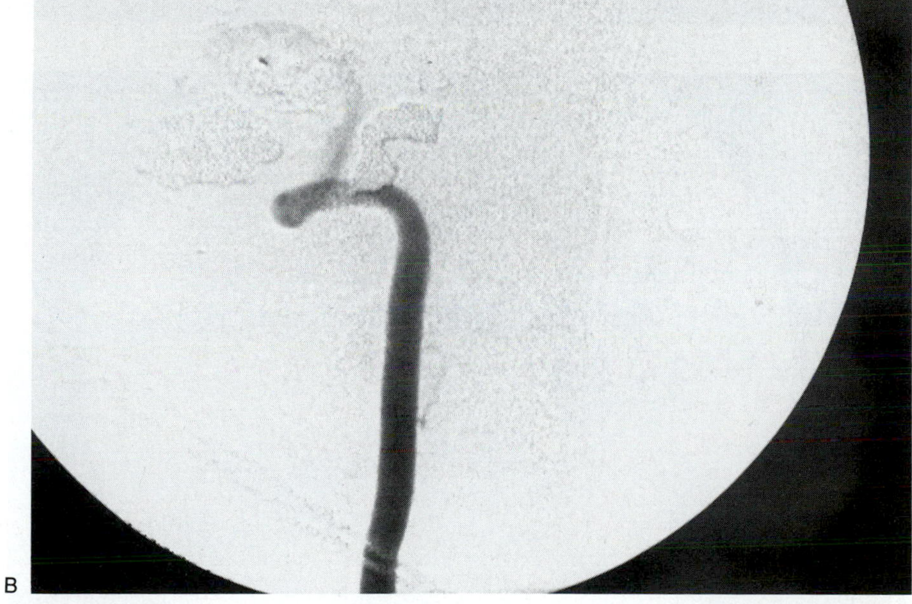
B

Figure 10–3. Traumatic VVF associated with arterial transection, in a 30-year-old man following a gunshot wound to the neck. The fistula was treated by separate ipsilateral and contralateral endovascular approaches to the proximal and distal segments of the injured vertebral artery. **(A)** Right vertebral angiogram demonstrates complete steal of flow from the proximal vertebral toward a fistula, which directly fills the right vertebral venous plexus. **(B)** Following closure of the proximal fistula with coils, there is sluggish flow within the right vertebral, with no filling of the fistula or the distal vertebrobasilar junction. **(C)** Left vertebral artery injection, performed after closure of proximal right vertebral fistula, demonstrates retrograde filling of the distal right vertebral artery, which then fills a second fistula to suboccipital venous channels. Note bullet fragments **(B)**. **(D)** Superselective angiogram of the distal right vertebral artery segment, midway through deposition of coils **(C)** at the second fistula site. Note the course of the variable stiffness catheter introduced through the contralateral left vertebral artery. The upper loop of the catheter traverses the vertebrobasilar junction (see Fig. 10–3C). Also note filling of the right posterior inferior cerebellar artery (PICA). **(E)** Post-embolization left vertebral angiogram demonstrates the distal right vertebral segment, which fills retrograde. All fistulas have been occluded. The patient did well, without any neurologic deficit.

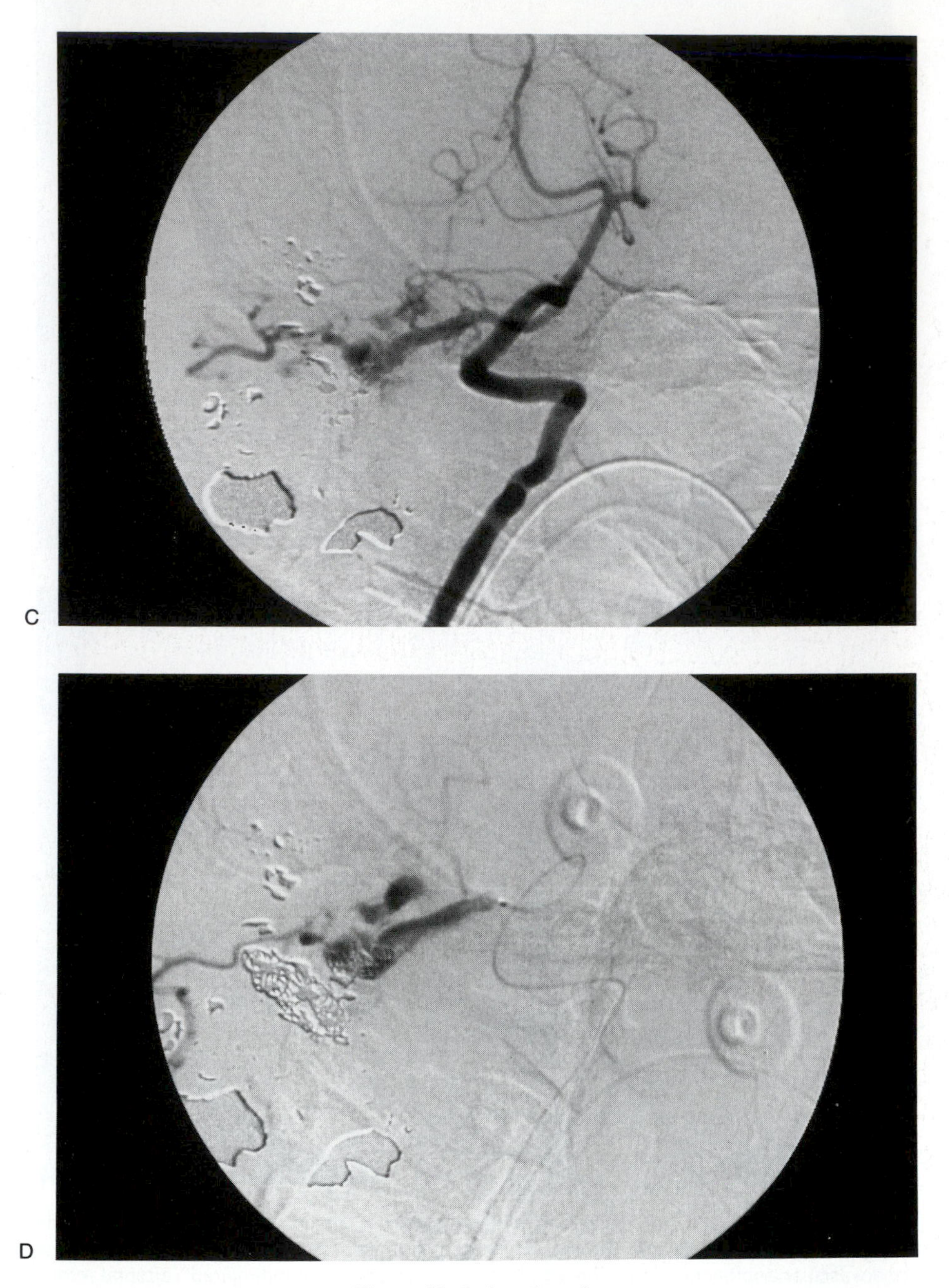

Figure 10–3. (*continued*)

10–3). Coils may also be deployed for treatment of fistulae affecting the intracranial brances of the vertebrobasilar system[67] (Fig. 10–4). A risk of releasable coil deployment is inadvertent migration of the coil in the parent artery, or through the fistula to the venous side and the lung. This risk may be lessened by the use of detachable coils, although these remain investigational. If coils become dislodged inadvertently, they may be manipulated back into place under some circumstances.[68]

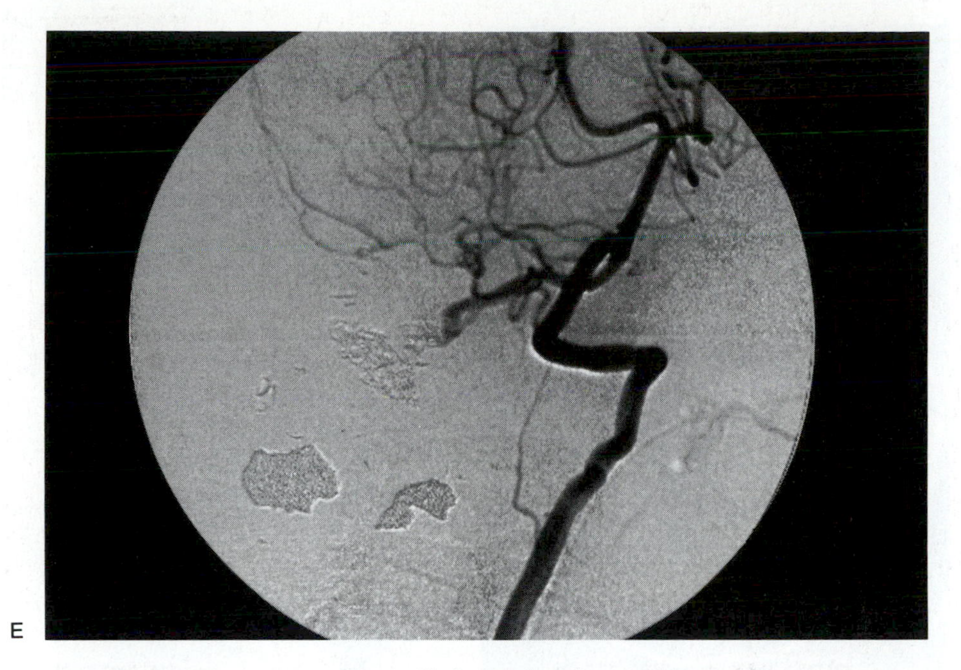

Figure 10–3. (*continued*)

If arterial navigation fails, a transvenous approach may be used, a technique pioneered in the carotid system.[69,70] This may be necessary when the parent VA is too small to accommodate a balloon catheter, and no suitable site can be found for coil placement. A transvenous approach is usually effective and safe for treatment of lower VA fistulae, when a balloon can be detached on the venous side, preserving parent artery patency.[71,72] If no endovascular access can be achieved, direct puncture of the artery may be feasible,[73] or surgical exposure of the fistula may be attempted with direct introduction of embolic material.[74,75]

Clinical follow-up after treatment may be supported by plain radiographs, which verify the position of the opacified balloon or radiopaque coils. Color doppler flow ultrasound or MR/MRA may be used to detect fistula recurrence if symptoms recur or persist.

DURAL ARTERIOVENOUS VERTEBRAL FISTULAE

Dural fistulae account for 10% to 15% of all intracranial AVMs, and one third of posterior fossa AVMs are purely dural. They are usually acquired lesions, which tend to develop at sites of venous thrombosis and recanalization.[76] A discreet nidus or core of arteriovenous communications may exist, although more diffuse lesions, containing many microfistulae, also occur. The nidus usually is located in the wall of a dural venous sinus, or along a dilated sinus tributary. Frequently, there is associated stenosis or occlusion of a portion of the sinus. These lesions are typically supplied by dural arteries arising from the external carotid, internal carotid, and vertebral meningeal arteries. Spinal dural arteriovenous fistulae in the cervical region also derive supply from the vertebral radiculomedullary branches.

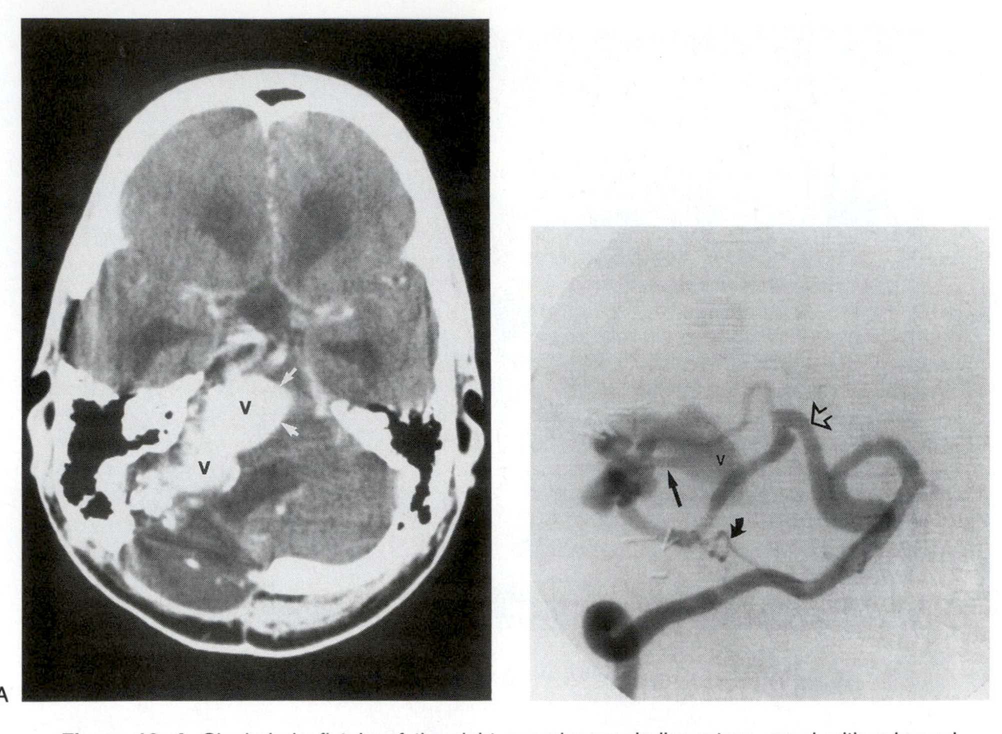

Figure 10–4. Single-hole fistula of the right superior cerebellar artery cured with released coil delivered by variable stiffness catheter, in a 46-year-old man with progressive neurologic deterioration. Embolization was undertaken in light of rapid progression of brainstem dysfunction and mental status changes, which had been slowly progressive until just prior to admission. Fistula closure resulted in immediate neurologic improvement with the patient still on the angiographic table.

(A) Post-contrast CT scan reveals post-operative changes of a suboccipital craniotomy approach to a presumed arteriovenous malformation 28 years earlier. There is a small pseudomeningocele (*arrows*). Large enhancing structures in the right cerebellopontine angle cistern, which compress the brainstem (*white arrows*), are varices draining a single-hole arteriovenous fistula supplied by the right superior cerebellar artery. **(B)** Right vertebral angiogram demonstrates markedly enlarged right superior cerebellar artery (*open arrow*), which bifurcates into two dilated distal vessels that course toward the prior operative site (marked by surgical clips). A jet of contrast through the single fistula hole (straight arrow) begins to fill the most proximal varix. An anterior inferior cerebellar artery branch (*curved arrow*) also supplies the fistula. **(C)** Right vertebral angiogram 7 months after embolization of the fistula hole and more proximal superior cerebellar artery feeder with platinum coils reveals undisturbed coil positions (*arrows*) and no filling of the fistula. Interval scans revealed thrombosis and shrinkage of the varices. The anterior inferior cerebellar artery also decreased in size (*curved arrow*). The patient returned to work with almost complete neurologic recovery. *(Reprinted with permission from Smith MD, Russell EJ, Levy R, et al. Transcatheter obliteration of a cerebellar arteriovenous fistula with platinum coils. Am J Neuroradiol. 1990;11:1199–1202.)*

Clinical Presentation

Dural vertebral arteriovenous fistulae (DAVF) present with a wide spectrum of signs and symptoms depending on location, size, and venous drainage pattern.[77] When flow is directed toward a patent dural venous sinus near the temporal bone, headache and pulsatile tinnitus usually result. Fistulae draining toward the cavernous sinus and ophthalmic venous system present with visual loss with raised intraocular pressure, diplopia, proptosis, and chemosis/conjunctival edema. Subarachnoid and intracerebral

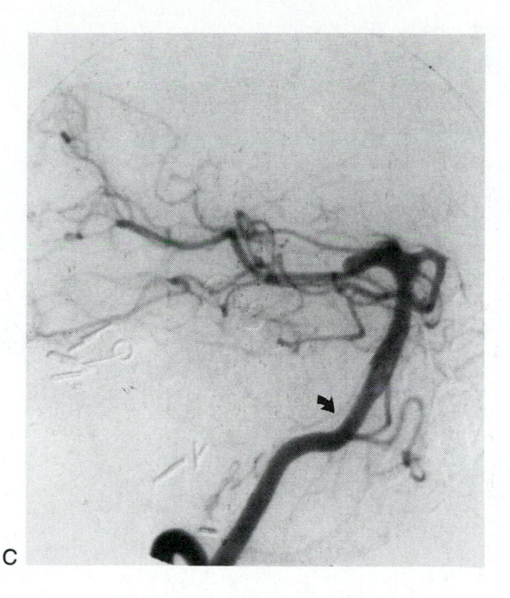

Figure 10–4. *(continued)*

hemorrhage and infarction may result when there is cortical venous drainage, typically in cases where there is partial or total occlusion of the adjacent dural venous sinus. Most at risk for bleeding are those fistulae located at the floor of the anterior cranial fossa (away from a large dural sinus) and along the tentorium cerebelli. Fistulae at the transverse/sigmoid and cavernous sinuses rarely hemorrhage.[78]

Headache may be related to intracranial venous hypertension. When severe, this may induce poor cerebrospinal fluid (CSF) resorption and communicating hydrocephalus. The venous hypertension may be reversible following fistula occlusion by endovascular or surgical techniques. Deficits such as hemiparesis and disorientation may promptly resolve after embolization.[79]

In the spine, the main clinical manifestation is ascending myelopathy, related to high-pressure flow from the fistula transmitted to the perimedullary venous plexus, resulting in venous hypertension, decreased arterial perfusion, and venous infarction. Clinical deterioration is usually progressive with a stepwise pattern related to episodes of ischemic tissue loss (Foix–Alajouanine syndrome). Hemorrhage may result from spinal DAVF, although it is uncommon.[80]

MR is the procedure of choice for the initial investigation of symptoms that may be related to dural arteriovenous fistulae. Identification of dilated cortical veins without an identifiable parenchymal nidus suggests the presence DAVF with cortical venous drainage. This may be facilitated by observing prominent flow voids (low signal in vessels related to high flow) on proton–density-weighted spin echo images, or linear high-signal intensity on flow-sensitive MR angiographic (MRA) images. However, when cortical venous drainage is not present, MR may be normal. In such cases, MRA is essential, since dilated meningeal vessels may be detected on reconstructions, which highlight increased vascularity near the fistula site.[81]

Angiography is required to define all feeders and categorize venous outflow. Multiple dural arterial feeders are usually demonstrated, often partly arising from cerebral vessels (meningohypophyseal trunk) and transosseous vessels (occipital artery).

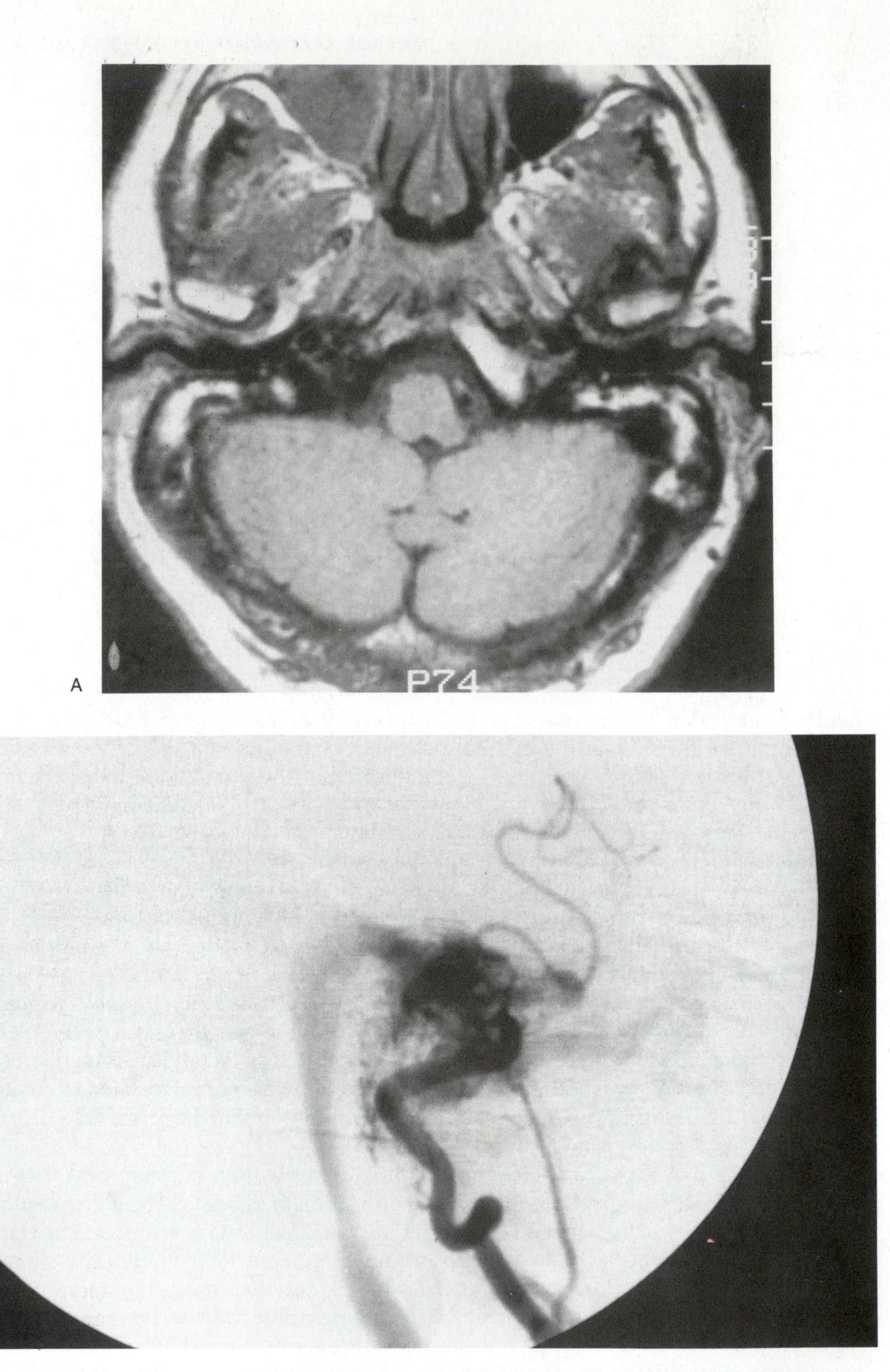

Figure 10–5. Dural arteriovenous fistula of the sigmoid sinus/jugular bulb, in a 58-year-old man with pulsatile tinnitus and intermittently severe headaches. **(A)** T1-weighted MRI showing low intensity within the lower right clivus and adjacent tissues, due to high-flow signal loss (flow void) related to the dural fistula. **(B)** Lateral view of digital subtraction right vertebral angiogram, showing a complete steal of flow from the vertebral artery, which fills a diffuse complex tangle of arterial feeders to the fistula along the surface of the distal sigmoid sinus (*arrows*). Note early filling of the jugular vein.

Fistulae involving the sigmoid and transverse dural sinuses frequently have some arterial supply from the dural or muscular branches of the VAs. These are typically acquired lesions related to venous thrombosis and subsequent recanalization.[76,82] Single or multiple microfistulae may exist (Fig. 10–5). Regional dural sinus thrombosis may occur due to turbulent flow. These patients usually present with pulsatile tinnitus.[83] There is a small incidence of spontaneous resolution.[36]

While techniques at surgical closure are well described,[84] endovascular techniques have recently added significantly to treatment planning.[85–87] Endovascular obliteration of the affected segment of the dural venous sinus is the procedure of choice if the venous compartment of the fistula is reachable and there are no functional cortical veins draining toward that segment of the nidus. Arterial embolization of all available feeders may also be successful, but failure is frequent since unembolizable feeders may arise from the VAs and ICAs, and it may not be possible to deposit embolic materials directly within the fistulous communications throughout the lesion.

REFERENCES

1. Goody W, Schechter MM. Spontaneous arterio-venous fistula of the vertebral artery. *Brit J Radiol.* 1960;33:709–711.
2. Jefferson G, Bailey RA, Kerr AS. Suboccipital arteriovenous aneurysms of the vertebral artery. *J Bone Joint Surg.* 1956;38B:114.
3. Tsuji HK, Redington JV, Kay JH. Vertebral arteriovenous fistula. *J Thor Cardiovasc Surg.* 1968;55:746–753.
4. Sutton D, Pratt AE. Vertebral arterio-venous fistula. *Clin Radiol.* 1971;22:289–295.
5. Ehrlich FE, Carey L, Kitrinos NP. Congenital arteriovenous fistula between the vertebral artery and vertebral vein. *J Neurosurg.* 1968;629–630.
6. Lawson TL, Newton TH. Congenital cervical arteriovenous malformations. *Radiology.* 1970;97:565–570.
7. Bahar S, Chiras J, Carpena JP, et al. Spontaneous vertebro-vertebral arterio-venous fistula associated with fibro-muscular dysplasia. *Neuroradiol.* 1984;26:45–49.
8. Hieshima GB, Cahan LD, Mehringer CM, et al. Spontaneous arteriovenous fistulas of cerebral vessels in association with fibromuscular dysplasia. *Neurosurgery.* 1986;18:454–458.
9. Morelli RJ. An angiographic complication of vertebral arteriovenous fistula. *J Neurol Neurosurg Psychiatry.* 1967;30:264–266.
10. Hayward R, Swanton H, Treasure T. Acquired arteriovenous communication: complication of cannulation of internal jugular vein. *Br Med J.* 1984;288:1195–1196.
11. Beaujeux RL, Reizine DC, Casasco A, et al. Endovascular treatment of vertebral arteriovenous fistula. *Radiology.* 1992;183:361–367.
12. Matas R. Traumatisms and traumatic aneurysms of the vertebral artery and their surgical treatment with the report of a cured case. *Ann Surg.* 1893;18:477–521.
13. Weinberg PE, Flom RA. Traumatic vertebral arteriovenous fistula. *Surg Neurol.* 1973; 1:162–167.
14. Cosgrove GR, Theron J. Vertebral arteriovenous fistula following anterior cervical spine surgery. Report of two cases. *J Neurosurg.* 1987;66:297–299.
15. Olson RW, Baker HL Jr, Svien HJ. Arteriovenous fistula: a complication of vertebral angiography. Report of a case. *J Neurosurg.* 1963;20:73–75.
16. Aronson NI. Traumatic arteriovenous fistula of the vertebral vessels. Angiographic demonstration and a rationale for treatment. *Neurology.* 1961;11:817–823.
17. Gokalp HZ, Egemen N, Ustun M, et al. Vertebral arteriovenous fistula caused by angiography catheter: case report. *Acta Neurochir.* 1993;124:153–155.
18. Jamieson KG. Vertebral arteriovenous fistula caused by angiography needle. *J Neurosurg.* 1965;23:620–621.

19. Sher MH, Meyer NI, Lenhardt HF, et al. Arteriovenous fistula involving the vertebral artery: report of three cases. *Ann Surg*. 1966;163:408–413.
20. van Tets WF, van Dullemen HM, Tjan GT, et al. Vertebral arteriovenous fistula caused by puncture of the internal jugular vein. *Eur J Surg*. 1992;158:627–628.
21. Waga S, Handa J, Jervara T. Traumatic vertebral arteriovenous fistula. *Surg Neurol*. 1974;2:279–281.
22. Sugar O, Holden LB, Powell CB. Vertebral angiography. *Am J Roentgenol*. 1949;61:166.
23. Sutton D. *Arteriography*. Edinburgh: E & S Livingstone Ltd; 1962:321.
24. Halbach VV, Higashida RT, Hieshima GB. Treatment of vertebral arteriovenous fistulas. *Am J Neuroradiol*. 1987;8:1121–1128.
25. Reizine D, Laouiti M, Guimaraens L, et al. Vertebral arteriovenous fistulas: clinical presentation, angiographic appearance, and endovascular treatment. A review of twenty-five cases. *Ann Radiol (Paris)*. 1985;28:425–438.
26. Deans WR, Bloch S, Leibrock L, et al. Arteriovenous fistula in patients with neurofibromatosis. *Radiology*. 1982;144:103–107.
27. Merland JJ, Reizine D, Riche MC, et al. Traitment endovasculaire des fistules arterio-veineuses vertebrales: a propos de vingt-deux cas. *Ann Chir Vasc*. 1986;1:73–78.
28. Halliday AL, Ogilvy CS, Crowell RM. Intracranial vertebral arteriovenous fistula. Case report. *J Neurosurg*. 1993;79:589–591.
29. Nagashima C, Iwasaki T, Kawanuma S, et al. Traumatic arteriovenous fistula of the vertebral artery with spinal cord symptoms. *J Neurosurg*. 1977;46:681–687.
30. Russell EJ, Goldblatt D, Levy JM, et al. Percutaneous obliteration of a postoperatively persistent vertebral arteriovenous fistula. *Am J Neuroradial*. 1989;10:196–200.
31. Johnson CE, Russell EJ, Huckman MS. Resolution of spinal epidural vascular pseudotumor following balloon occlusion of a postoperative vertebral arteriovenous fistula. *Neuroradiology* 1990;31:529–532.
32. Smith MD, Russell EJ, Levy R, et al. Transcatheter obliteration of a cerebellar arteriovenous fistula with platinum coils. *Am J Neuroradiol*. 1990;11:1199–1202.
33. Arey LB. *Developmental Anatomy: Textbook and Laboratory Manual of Embryology*. 7th ed. Philadelphia: WB Saunders; 1965.
34. Nierling DA, Wollschlaeger PB, Wollschlaeger G. Ascending pharyngeal-vertebral anastomosis. *Am J Roentgenol*. 1966;98:599–601.
35. Kubota M, Watanabe O, Takase M, et al. Spontaneous disappearance of arteriovenous fistula between the vertebral artery and deep cervical vein—case report. *Neurol. Med Chir (Tokyo)*. 1992;32:84–87.
36. Pritz MB, Pribram HFW. Spontaneous closure of a high-risk dural arteriovenous malformation of the transverse sinus. *Surg Neurol*. 1991;36:226–228.
37. Svetilas C, Dean DC. Intermittent vertebral arteriovenous fistula due to cervical stab wound. *N Y State J Med*. 1972;735–738.
38. Chou SN, Story JL, Seljeskog E, et al. Further experience with arteriovenous fistulas of the vertebral artery in the neck. *Surgery*. 1967;62:779–788.
39. Markham JW. Spontaneous arterio-venous fistula of the vertebral artery and vein. *J Neurosurg*. 1969;31:220–223.
40. Elkin DC, Harris MH. Arteriovenous aneurysm of the vertebral vessels. Report of ten cases. *Ann Surg*. 1946;124:934–951.
41. Doppman JL, Pevsner P. Embolization of arteriovenous malformations by direct percutaneous puncture. *Am J Roentgenol*. 1983;140:773–778.
42. Dutton J, Isherwood I. Iatrogenic vertebral arteriovenous fistulae. *Neurochirurgia (Stuttg)*. 1970;13:49–60.
43. George B, Laurian C. Techniques of vertebral artery surgery: arteriovenous malformations. In: George B, Laurian C, eds. *The Vertebral Artery: Pathology and Surgery*. Vienna: Springer–Verlag, 1987; pp 167–170.
43a. Mullen S, Duda EE, Pratronas NJ. Balloon techniques in neurosurgery. *J Neurosurg*. 1980;52:321–329.
44. Latchaw RE, Harris RD, Chou SN, et al. Combined embolization and operation in the treatment of cervical arteriovenous malformations. *Neurosurgery*. 1980;6:131–137.

45. Russell EJ. Functional angiography of the head and neck. *Am J Neuroradiol.* 1986;7:927–936.
46. Debrun G, Legre J, Kasbarian M, et al. Endovascular occlusion of vertebral fistulae by detachable balloons with conservation of the vertebral blood flow. *Radiology.* 1979; 130:141–147.
47. Freitag HJ, Grzyska U, Zeumer H. The use of the "cross over technique" in the management of a traumatic vertebro-vertebral fistula. *Neuroradiol.* 1989;31:174–176.
48. Kondoh T, Tamaki N, Taeda N, et al. Fatal intracranial hemorrhage after balloon occlusion of an extracranial vertebral arteriovenous fistula. *J Neurosurg.* 1988;69:945–948.
49. Halbach VV, Higashida RT, Hieshima GB, et al. Normal perfusion pressure breakthrough occurring during treatment of carotid and vertebral fistulas. *Am J Neuroradiol.* 1987;8:751–756.
50. Spetzler RF, Wilson CB, Weinstein P, et al. Normal perfusion pressure breakthrough theory. *Clin Neurosurg.* 1978;25:651–672.
51. Brooks B. Discussion of Noland and Taylor. *Trans South Surg Assoc.* 1931;43:176–177.
52. Speakman TJ. Internal occlusion of a carotid-cavernous fistula. *J Neurosurg.* 1964;21:303–305.
53. Prolo DJ, Hamberry JW. Intraluminal occlusion of a carotid cavernous sinus fistula with a balloon catheter. Technical note. *J Neurosurg.* 1971;35:237–242.
54. Picard L, Lepoire J, Montaut J, et al. Endarterial occlusion of carotid–cavernous sinus fistulas using a balloon tipped catheter. *Neuroradiology.* 1974;8:5–10.
55. Serbinenko FA. Balloon catheterization and occlusion of major cerebral vessels. *J Neurosurg.* 1974;41:125–145.
56. Debrun GM, Lacour P, Caron JP, et al. Experimental approach to treatment of carotid cavernous fistulas with an inflatable and isolated balloon. *Neuroradiology.* 1975;9:9–12.
57. Debrun GM, Lacour P, Vinuela F, et al. Treatment of 54 traumatic carotid cavernous fistulas. *J Neurosurg.* 1981;55:678–692.
58. Fox AJ, Vinuela F, Pelz DM, et al. Vertebral and external carotid fistulas. *Semin Interven Radiol.* 1987;4:249–260.
59. Higashida RT, Halbach VV, Tsai FY, et al. Interventional neurovascular treatment of traumatic carotid and vertebral artery lesions: results in 234 cases. *Am J Roentgenol.* 1989;153:577–582.
60. Scialfa G, Vaghi A, Valsecchi F, et al. Neuroradiological treatment of carotid and vertebral fistulas and intracavernous aneurysms. *Neuroradiol.* 1982;24:13–25.
61. Moret J, Lasjaunias P, Doyon D. Occipital approach for treatment of arteriovenous malformation of the verebral artery by balloon occlusion. *Neuroradiol.* 1979;17:269–273.
62. Bookstein JJ, Goldstein HM. Successful management of post-biopsy arteriovenous fistula with selective arterial embolization. *Radiology.* 1973;109:535–546.
63. Gianturco C, Anderson JH, Wallace S. Mechanical devices for arterial occlusion. *Am J Roentgenol.* 1975;124:428–435.
64. Anderson JH, Wallace S, Gianturco C, et al. "Mini" Gianturco stainless steel coils for transcatheter vascular occlusion. *Radiology.* 1979;132:301–303.
65. Clark RA, Gallant TE, Alexander ES. Angiographic management of traumatic arteriovenous fistulas: clinical results. *Radiology.* 1983;145:9–13.
66. Rossi P, Passariello R, Simonetti G. Control of a traumatic vertebral arteriovenous fistula by a modified Gianturco coil embolus system. *Am J Roentgenol.* 1978;131–333.
67. Smith MD, Russell EJ, Levy R, et al. Transcatheter obliteration of a cerebellar arteriovenous fistula with platinum coils. *Am J Neuroradiol.* 1990;11:1199–1202.
68. Teng MM, Chang T, Huang CI, et al. Percutaneous reposition of dislodged coils in the treatment of a vertebral arteriovenous fistula with CT follow-up. *Neuroradiol.* 1991;33:195–199.
69. Halbach VV, Higashida RT, Hieshima GB, et al. Transvenous embolization of direct carotid cavernous fistulas. *Am J Neuroradiol.* 1988;9:741–747.
70. Manelfe C, Berenstein A. Treatment of carotid cavernous fistulas by venous approach. *J Neuroradiol.* 1980;7:13–21.
71. Kendall B, Hoare R. Percutaneous transvenous balloon occlusion of arteriovenous fistula. *Neuroradiol.* 1980;20:203–205.
72. Kendall B. Results of treatment of arteriovenous fistulae with the Debrun technique. *Am J Neuroradiol.* 1983;4:405–408.
73. Halbach VV, Higashida RT, Hieshima GB, et al. Direct puncture of proximally occluded internal carotid artery for treatment of carotid cavernous fistulas. *Am J Neuroradiol.* 1989;10:151–154.

74. Batjer HH, Purdy PD, Neiman M, et al. Subtemporal transdural use of detachable balloons for traumatic CCF. *Neurosurgery*. 1988;22:290–297.
75. Goodman SJ, Hasso A, Kirkpatrick D. Treatment of vertebrojugular fistula by balloon occlusion. *J Neurosurg*. 1975;43;362–367.
76. Chaudhary MY, Sachdev VP, Cho SH, et al. Dural arteriovenous malformations of the major venous sinuses: an acquired lesion. *Am J Neuroradiol*. 1982;3:13–19.
77. Lasjaunias P, Chiu M, Terbrugge K, et al. Neurological manifestations of intracranial dural arteriovenous malformations. *J Neurosurg*. 1986;64:724–730.
78. King WA, Martin NA. Intracerebral hemorrhage due to dural arteriovenous malformations and fistulae. *Neurosurg Clin N Am*. 1992;3:577–590.
79. Hurst RW, Hackney DB, Goldberg HI, et al. Reversible arteriovenous malformation-induced venous hypertension as a cause of neurological deficits. *Neurosurgery*. 1992;30:422–425.
80. Morimoto T, Yoshida S, Basugi N. Dural arteriovenous malformation in the cervical spine presenting with subarachnoid hemorrhage: case report. *Neurosurgery*. 1992;31:118–120.
81. Chen JC, Tsuruda JS, Halbach VV. Suspected dural arteriovenous fistula: results with screening MR angiography in seven patients. *Radiology*. 1992;183:265–271.
82 Nishijima M, Takaku A, Endo S, et al. Etiological evaluation of dural arteriovenous malformations of the lateral and sigmoid sinuses based on histopathological examinations. *J Neurosurg*. 1992;76:600–606.
83. Arenberg IK, McCreary HS. Objective tinnitus aurium and dural arteriovenous malformations of the posterior fossa. *Ann Otol Rhinol Laryngol*. 1971;80:111–120.
84. Mullan S. Surgical therapy: indications and general principles. In: Awad IA, Barrow DL, eds. *Dural Arteriovenous Malformations*. Park Ridge, IL: American Association of Neurologic Surgeons Publishing; 1993:213–229.
85. Barnwell S. Endovascular therapy of dural arteriovenous malformations. In: Awad IA, Barrow DL, eds. *Dural Arteriovenous Malformations*. Park Ridge, IL: American Association of Neurologic Surgeons Publishing; 1993:193–211.
86. Halbach VV, Higashida RT, Hieshima GB, et al. Dural fistulas involving the transverse and sigmoid sinuses: results of treatment in 28 patients. *Radiology*. 1987;163:443–447.
87. Halbach VV, Higashida RT, Hieshima GB, et al. Transvenous embolization of dural fistulas involving the transverse and sigmoid sinuses. *Am J Neuroradiol*. 1989;10:385–392.

11

Management of Spontaneous Dissection and Fibromuscular Dysplasia of the Carotid Artery

Richard M. Green, MD

Dissection of the carotid artery is a significant nonatherosclerotic cause of stroke in middle-age patients. It is a rapidly evolving process that may occur spontaneously or in certain predisposing conditions, such as fibromuscular dysplasia (FMD) or carotid kinking or coiling, and in a variety of primary arteriopathies, such as Ehlers-Danlos syndrome, Marfan's syndrome, pseudoxanthoma elasticum, polycystic kidney disease, and α-one antitrypsin deficiency.[1,2] Strokes may be due to embolization or carotid thrombosis. The role of minimal trauma is unclear, although there are anecdoctal reports describing dissections after coughing, nose blowing, head turning, and neck flexion. The yearly incidence of extracranial cervical dissection in population-based studies is 2.6 per 100,000.[3] Most reports originate in Western Europe or from areas with large European populations. Unlike atherosclerotic occlusions, carotid artery dissections usually resolve spontaneously. Prompt diagnosis and antithrombotic treatment are essential in order to avoid the embolic and thrombotic complications associated with this disorder.

INITIAL CLINICAL PRESENTATION

Spontaneous dissection of the internal carotid artery (ICA) was first described in 1959 by Anderson and Schecter. Neurologic symptoms are often preceded by the rapid onset of head pain, Horner's syndrome, and tinnitus.[4] These so-called "local" symptoms are inaugural in almost two-thirds of the patients with this condition. The remaining patients present with neurologic symptoms. The majority of patients presenting with local symptoms develop neurologic symptoms anywhere from a few minutes to several months, with a median time of roughly 10 days. Cranial nerve palsies are a prominent although not a universal component of carotid dissection.

The incidence of local symptoms varies between 5% and 96% and is a function of the method of diagnosis of the dissection (Table 11–1). Early reports made the diagnosis using arteriography after neurologic symptoms occurred. The series reported by Ehren-

TABLE 11–1. THE INCIDENCE OF LOCAL SYMPTOMS IN CAROTID DISSECTION

Author	As the First Symptom	Interval to Neurologic Symptoms	As an Isolated Symptom (%)
Ehrenfeld & Wylie[5] (1976)	1:19 (5%)	—	5
Fisher (1982)	25:26 (96%)	1 hour–several weeks	16
Hart (1983)	22:140 (16%)	Several hours–days	—
Biousse et al.[4] (1995)	53:80 (66%)	Minutes–66 days	18

—, no data.

feld and Wylie in 1976 included 19 patients, and only 1 had local symptoms as the presenting complaint.[5] Later series, using a combination of Doppler ultrasound and magnetic resonance (MR) scans, often detected the dissection prior to the onset of neurologic symptoms. There are several important concepts about the incidence of local symptoms and the interval to the onset of neurologic symptoms. First, local symptoms are common but rarely isolated; second, the process is unstable, often with neurologic progression in minutes; and third, antithrombotic treatment should begin immediately after the diagnosis is made.

Head pain is inaugural in 60% of patients with dissection, and its recognition is important for early diagnosis and treatment. The pain is usually homolateral to the dissection and lasts from 1 hour to 1 month with a median duration of 5 days. In addition, patients may complain of tenderness over the carotid bulb. The local signs of cranial nerve palsy and Horner's syndrome are due to compression by the enlarging hematoma. The incidence of carotid dissection may be underestimated in the setting of isolated cranial nerve palsy if only arteriography is used for diagnosis. Palsies alone or in combination of nerves IX through XII have been reported. These lesions produce the syndrome of dysphonia, dysarthria, dysphagia, and numbness of the throat.

The mean age of patients with a cervical carotid dissection is 43 years. Men and women are probably affected equally, although some series show a small preponderance of men. Associated factors include a history of migraine headaches (34%), an exogenous estrogen and progesterone intake (48% of affected women), fibromuscular dysplasia and related conditions (21%), and redundant arteries due to kinks or coils. Redundancy was noted at the time of angiography in 65% of carotid dissections as compared to 12% of normals. Since the process of ICA and vertebral artery (VA) dissections are identical, the two should be considered as one entity.

The pathology of the dissected extracranial artery is fairly typical. Externally there is a sharp transition between the normal and the dissected vessel (Figs. 11–1 and 11–2). The dissected artery has a cylindrical dilatation with a dark blue discoloration. There is a vertically oriented intimal rent usually several centimeters from the bifurcation. The hematoma pulsates into the tunica media creating a subadventitial dissection plane. Reentry and significant atherosclerotic changes are rare. The pattern is slightly different in patients less than 30 years old where subintimal rather than medial dissection is the rule. This difference is probably related to the increasing vulnerability of the media with age.

DIAGNOSTIC EVALUATION

With the advent of newer imaging modalities, the diagnosis of carotid dissection has become more accurate, and the natural history of the process has been defined. This

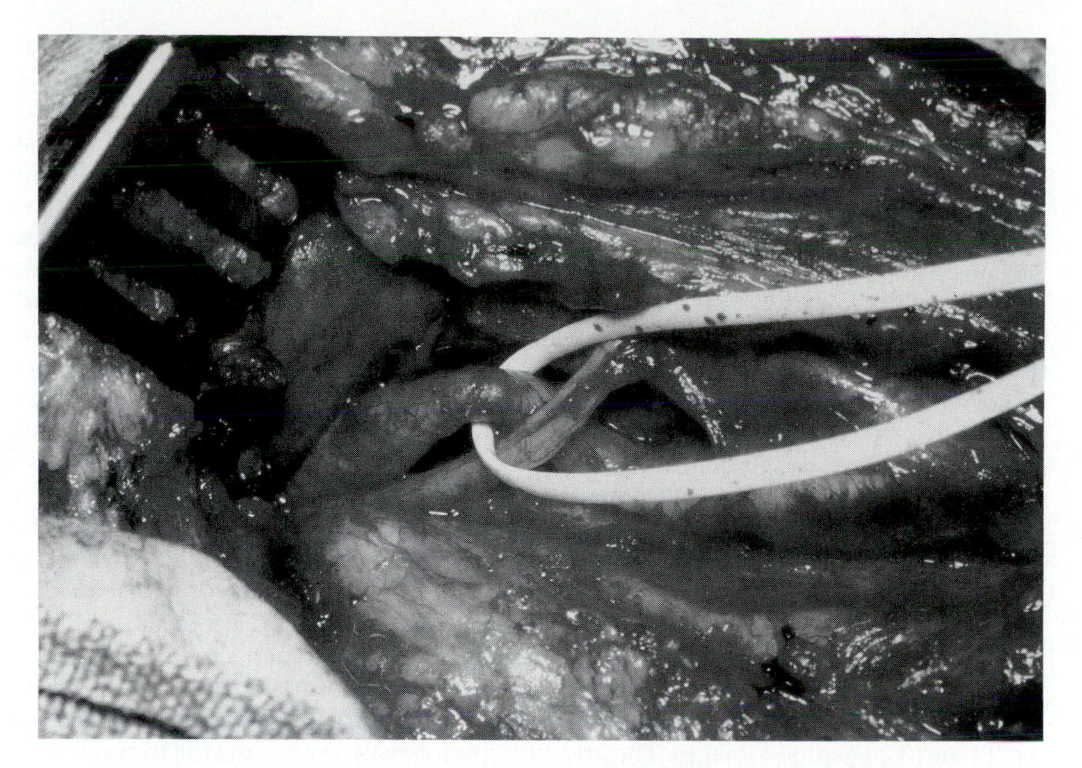

Figure 11–1. Operative photograph showing the external appearance of a dissection in the distal extracranial ICA. The hypoglossal nerve is seen crossing the ICA proximal to the dissection. There is a sharp transition between the normal and abnormal artery and a bulbous configuration at the site of the dissection just beyond the vessel loop. Note the redundancy in the ICA.

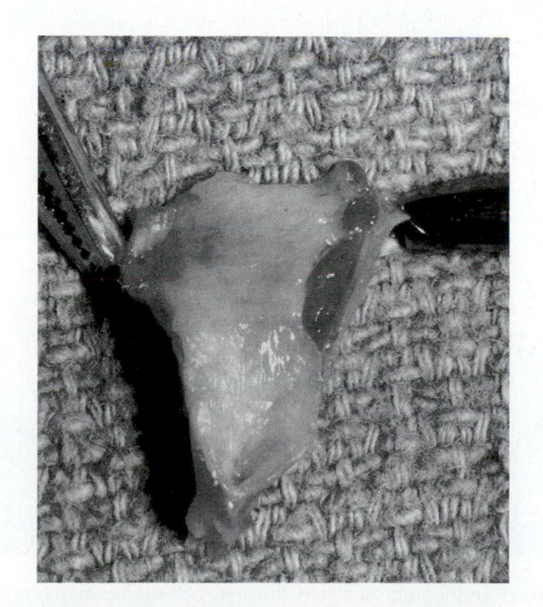

Figure 11–2. The artery has been opened and the dissected area resected. There is a vertical rent in the artery. The subadventitial hematoma is visible.

is a rapidly changing rather than a stable condition and serial studies are critical. Spontaneous carotid artery dissection may not be diagnosed on the basis of a single angiogram. Definitive diagnosis often requires serial ultrasonography, MRI, and/or angiography. The Doppler examination is abnormal in all of these patients. The most common abnormality is a high resistance, bidirectional flow pattern, which occurs in 90% of patients. B-mode analysis shows no morphologic abnormalities in 40% of patients, a tapering lumen of the ICA in 29%, a moving, thin echogenic intravascular structure in 15% (Fig. 11–3), and a wall hematoma in 4% of patients. The most important associated finding is the absence of significant atherosclerotic disease at the carotid bifurcation. The angiogram in Figure 11–4 illustrates the difficulty in distinguishing a pseudo-occlusion from dissection versus atherosclerotic plaque by angiography alone. Color analysis shows the complexity of the hemodynamics at the carotid bifurcation (Fig. 11–5). A zone of blue-coded flow reversal at the origin of the ICA occurs in all patients with reduced orthograde flow in the proximal common and distal ICAs. The duplex scan can trace the signal along the entire extracranial course of the ICA, which can distinguish between a dissection and an atherosclerotic process in many patients. This is important when the differential diagnosis is dissection versus an atherosclerotic occlusion, as is demonstrated in Figure 11–4.

The role of CT scanning and MRI is not completely defined. In most cases, the diagnosis can be made with either. Each method has the disadvantage of being costly and of providing no hemodynamic information. The MR pattern with dissection consists of a narrowed eccentric signal void surrounded by a semilunar signal hyperintensity on T1 and T2 weighted images. The area of hyperintensity represents the mural hematoma and is specific for cervical dissections. This pattern identifies 78% of carotid and

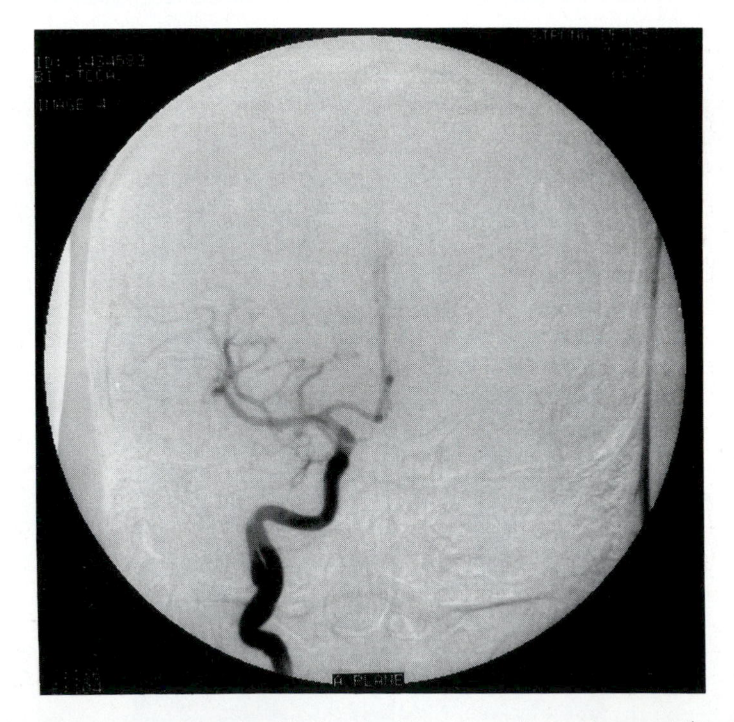

Figure 11–3. Carotid arteriogram showing the thin echogenic membrane at the site of the dissection and the bulbous configuration of the involved segment. This corresponds to the dilated area seen in the operative photograph in Figure 11–1.

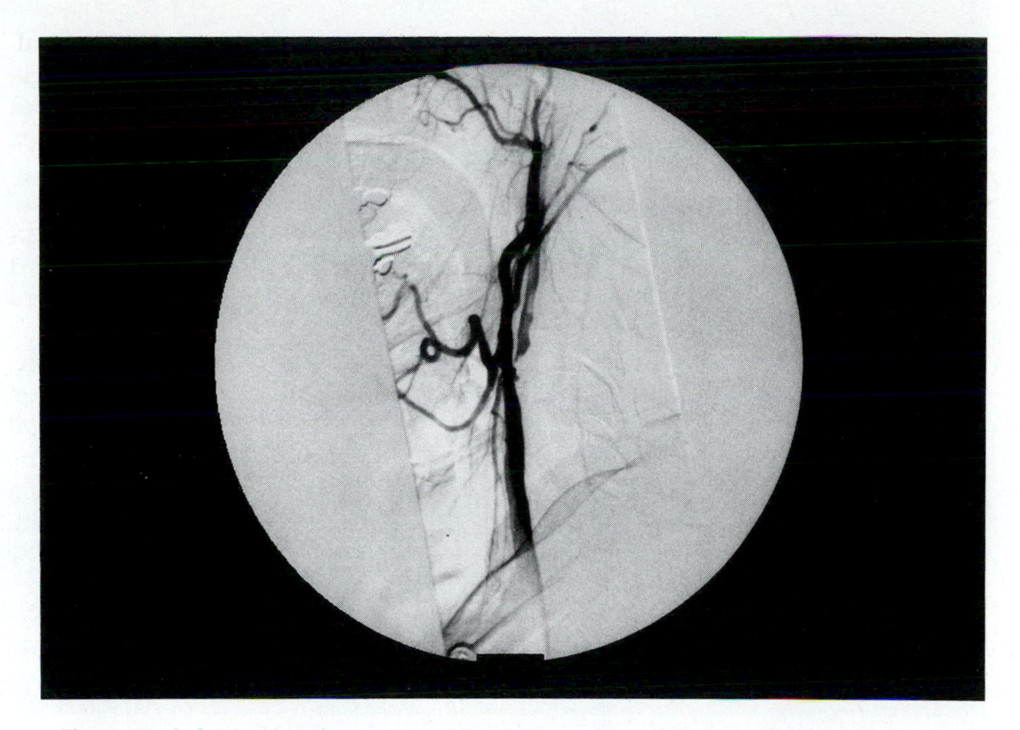

Figure 11–4. A carotid angiogram in a patient with a pseudo-occlusion and the appearance of a dissection. The duplex scan, however, identified a large bifurcation plaque. At operation the ICA was completely normal and a bifurcation endarterectomy was performed.

60% of VA dissections. The addition MR angiography identifies more carotid dissections, but conventional angiography is required to identify VA dissections. One clear role for the MR scan is the follow-up of hematomas at the base of the skull. Visualization of a hematoma adds to the reliability of the duplex scan.

Angiography may miss cervical dissections when the dissection does not encroach upon the arterial lumen. Four patterns are seen on conventional angiography: a "string-sign," a pseudo-occlusion, a pseudo-aneurysm, or an occlusion (Fig. 11–6). The intriguing aspect of carotid dissection is that these changes are not persistent. Resolution or recanalization is the norm rather than the exception. Repeat angiograms reveal that complete resolution occurs in 62% of cases and that the initial finding represents the stage of resolution rather than different types of dissection. The time course of the recanalization is described in Table 11–2. None of the pseudo-occlusions persist and only a small percentage of the other angiographic findings are present at follow-up. There are no correlations between the Doppler or the angiographic findings with the clinical presentation. Since there is in an increased incidence of intracranial aneurysms in patients with cervical dissection, angiograms are important for the evaluation of the intracranial vessels. Saccular aneurysms occur in 5.5% of patients with a cervical carotid dissection, compared to a 1% incidence in patients without a dissection.

CLINICAL COURSE

A completed stroke will occur in almost 50% of patients with carotid dissection, usually within the first week of symptoms. Age, sex, hypertension, a history of migraine, use

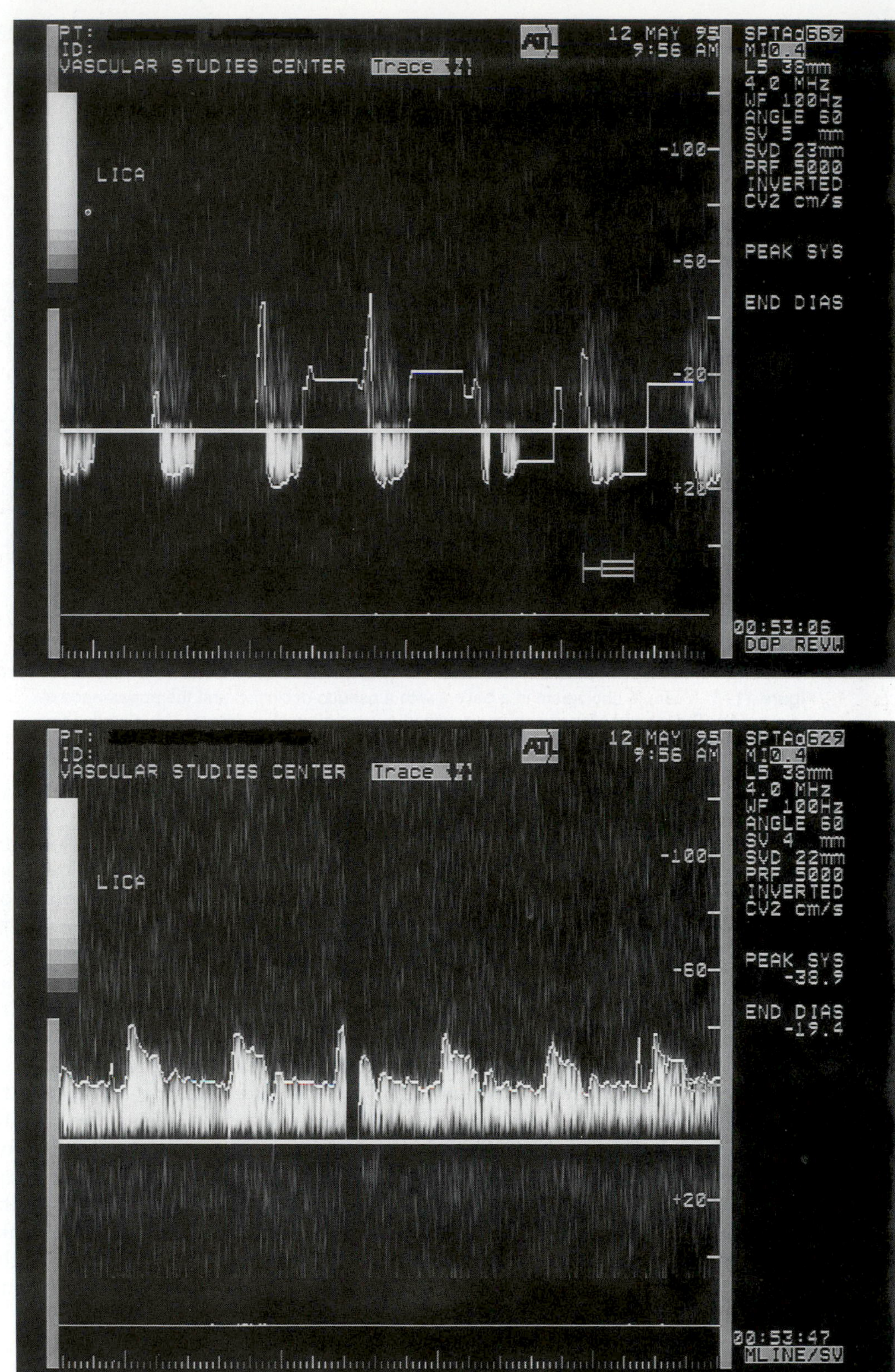

Figure 11–5. Duplex scans showing the complicated hemodynamics at the carotid bifurcation in a patient with a dissection. **(A)** Classical "to and fro" Doppler pattern at the bulb. Note that this is not the site of the dissection. **(B)** Color Doppler of carotid bulb reflecting the phenomena of "to and fro" flow. (See color plate following page 138.) **(C)** Doppler signal in distal ICA. The velocity is reduced, but in distinction to the occlusion of the ICA in atherosclerotic disease, there is demonstrable flow in the entire ICA.

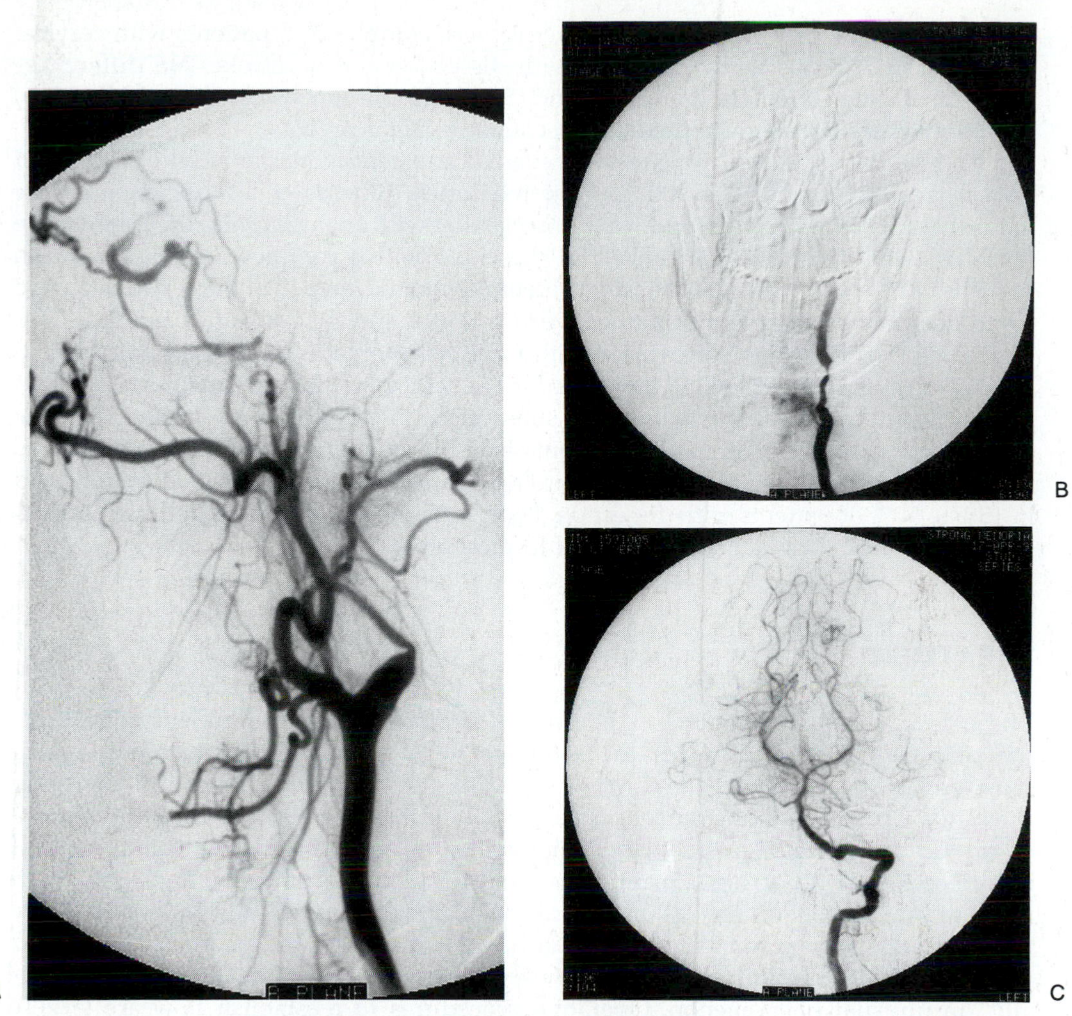

Figure 11–6. (A) The left ICA dissection has the typical appearance of a patient with FMD. There is a string sign beginning beyond the bifurcation and a "string of beads" appearance to the distal ICA. Doppler findings are shown in Figure 11–5. **(B)** Vertebral artery dissection with a critical distal stenosis. **(C)** This arteriogram shows a false aneurysm in an area of a VA dissection.

TABLE 11–2. ANGIOGRAPHIC FINDINGS IN CAROTID DISSECTION

Abnormality	Frequency (%)	Follow-up (%)	Interval
Pseudo-occlusion	28	0	—
Distal stenosis	20	5	42 days
Long dissection	36	11	12 days
Pseudo-aneurysm	10	11	35 weeks
Normal but irregular wall	4	62	30 days
Occlusion	2	11	80 weeks

—, no data.

of contraceptives, and angiographic patterns were compared in patients with cervical dissection and stroke and in patients with dissection but no stroke. No differences between the two populations were found. Similarly, the presence of local inaugural symptoms does not seem to predict subsequent ischemic events.

The overall incidence of neurologic events (transient ischemic attacks [TIAs] and CVAs) ranges from 50% to 95% in reported series. Biousse et al.[4] documented the natural history of carotid dissection and correlated it with angiographic and noninvasive findings. Nine of their 80 patients (11%) presented with a completed stroke. Eighteen patients (22%) presented with transient cerebral ischemia, and 10 of these patients went on to develop a completed stroke between 6 hours and 31 days after the first TIA. The remaining 53 patients presented with local symptoms; 14 (27%) did not develop neurologic symptoms; 23 (43%) developed a TIA, and 16 (30%) developed a completed stroke. Seven of the patients who had a subsequent TIA developed a stroke. The time interval between the inaugural symptoms and the development of a stroke ranged from a few minutes to 31 days. Severe neurologic deficits without resolution are reported in 15% to 50% of patients with dissection. Poor outcomes are common in those patients with embolic strokes and those who fail to recanalize.

TREATMENT

The delay in the development of neurologic symptoms and the known findings in the involved arteries provides the rationale for antithrombotic treatment, which must be begun as soon as the diagnosis of dissection is made. Heparin is currently the initial drug of choice. Anticoagulation is recommended because the maintenance of carotid patency and avoidance of a luminal thrombus is important while natural clot retraction is occurring. Current treatment protocols recommend anticoagulation until recanalization occurs, as measured by duplex scans. If the patient is ready for hospital discharge and recanalization has not occurred, the patient is converted to oral warfarin. Heparin should not be used when the dissection extends intracranially, an unusual phenomenon. Operative procedures to reestablish flow are largely unsuccessful and should be reserved to reconstruct arteries if spontaneous recanalization does not occur. Rarely, a delayed neurologic event occurs from a partially recanalized artery. Surgical options consist of local repair when possible or extracranial to intracranial bypass when low cerebral flow conditions exist as a result of ICA thrombosis.

THE ROLE OF FIBROMUSCULAR DYSPLASIA AND RELATED DISORDERS

Fibromuscular dysplasia (FMD) is often implicated in the pathogenesis of spontaneous carotid dissection. Arterial fibromuscular dysplasia was described in 1938 by Leadbetter and Burkland.[6] FMD of the carotid artery was described by Connett and Lansche in 1965 almost 30 years later.[7] FMD usually involves the renal arteries, followed by the internal carotid, iliac, subclavian, and vertebral arteries. The large review from the Mayo Clinic did not find any association between FMD of the carotid and renal arteries.[8]

FMD is a generalized nonatherosclerotic angiopathy that affects segments of long, medium-sized arteries with few branches. Its incidence in the carotid artery, based on angiographic studies, is 0.25% to 0.68%.[9] Angiographic changes of FMD are found in 10% to 20% of patients with cervical carotid dissection.[10] Despite this association, the pathologic significance of these angiographic changes is unknown. It is known that there is a high incidence of FMD in patients with collagen type III gene mutations, aortic coarctation, α-one antitrypsin deficiency, and other conditions associated with mesenchymal dysplasia.[11] The predisposition to arterial dissection in each of these conditions may be due to their shared high incidence of cystic medial necrosis.

Fibromuscular dysplasia is a cause of neurologic symptoms independent of arterial dissections. Strokes may occur in as many as 25% of patients, so it is not a benign entity. Despite this, the natural history of the asymptomatic lesion is unknown. The mean age upon diagnosis of FMD of the carotid arteries is 59 years, older than the population with involvement of the renal arteries and renovascular hypertension. Patients are predominantly women, and the majority have symptoms due to atheroembolization rather than flow reduction. Presenting symptoms in the large San Francisco[12] experience include TIA in 42% of the patients, nonhemispheric symptoms in 28%, stroke in 23%, a noise heard by the patient in 22%, amaurosis fugax in 22%, and a reversible neurologic deficit (RND) in 4%.

Angiographic findings in fibromuscular dysplasia of the carotid artery include a longer internal carotid with kinks and coils. The disease is usually located in the middle and distal third of the cervical ICA. The proximal ICA and the intracranial segment are largely spared. The most stenotic lesions are at the level of the first and second cervical vertebrae (Fig. 11–7). The findings are usually bilateral. There are three types of FMD: (1) the "string of beads," (2) tube-shaped stenoses with areas of stenosis or

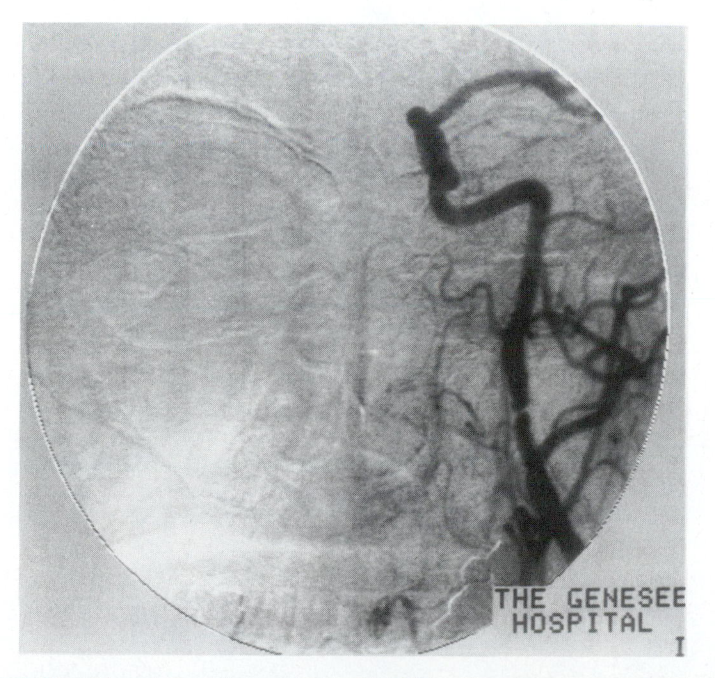

Figure 11–7. Carotid angiogram in a patient with FMD and a stenosis at the level of the first cervical vertebra. Graduated dilatation up to 3.5 mm was performed through an arteriotomy in the carotid bulb.

aneurysm (Fig. 11–8), or (3) localized stenoses. Pathologically, the medial fibroplastic variant is most often seen in the carotid artery. This particular form of FMD is associated with the angiographic pattern of the "string of beads." Microscopically, this consists of ridges of proliferative tissue which disrupt the normal smooth contour of the vessel. The areas of intervening dilatation are characterized by deficient smooth muscle and elastic lamellae.

There are two forms of operative management, graduated dilatation and direct excision with or without a bypass. Graduated dilatation was described in Houston by Morris et al.[13] in 1968 and remains the most commonly performed procedure for symptomatic FMD. The essential element in this procedure is a complete mobilization of the ICA so that it can be straightened during the dilatation (Fig. 11–9). This straightening is essential in order to avoid perforation. An arteriotomy is made at the carotid bulb and a 1.5-mm vascular dilator is inserted until resistance is felt. The resistance is broken with gentle pressure. This process is repeated until a 4-mm dilator can be easily inserted. The vessel is then repaired. If the ICA is

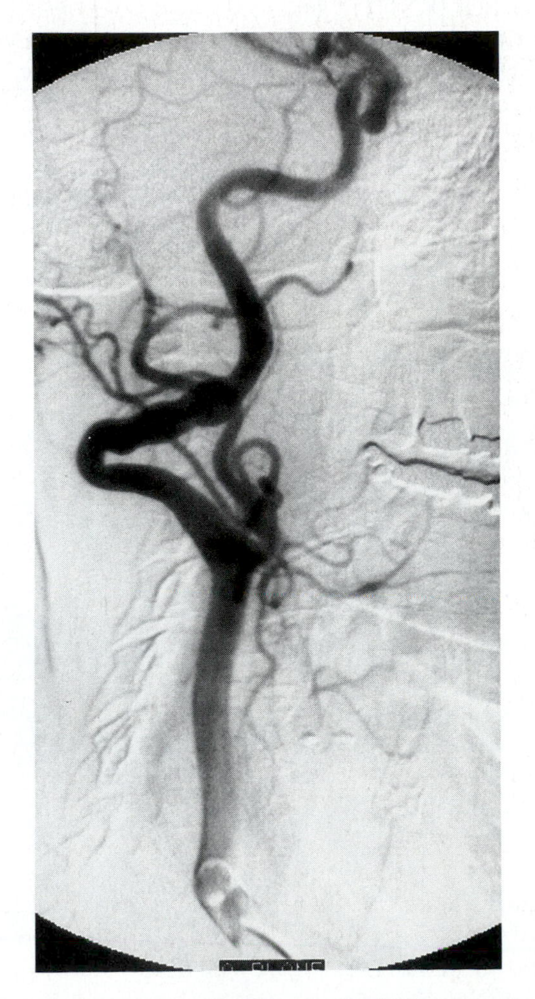

Figure 11–8. Arteriogram in a patient with FMD. The involved segment is ectatic with several areas of stenoses. This lesion was resected with a vein graft interposition. Note once again the redundancy in the artery. This patient also had a contralateral occlusion from a dissection.

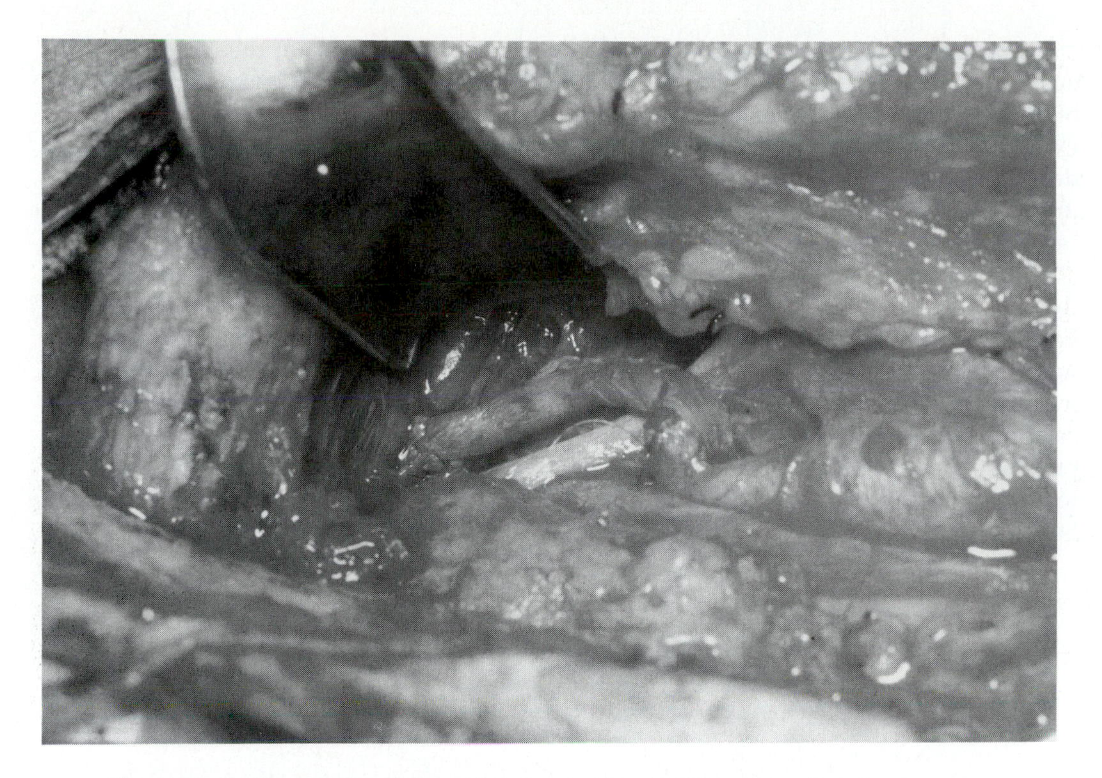

Figure 11–9. This operative photograph shows an ICA with FMD prior to dilatation. The vessel is elongated and complete mobilization is necessary in order to straighten out the artery during dilatation.

small, the dilatation can stop at 3.5 mm. Usually only the first and second probes are met with significant resistance. Angiographic confirmation of the dilatation is then performed prior to completion of the procedure. The results of dilatation are excellent. Patients have been followed for as long as 25 years. The incidence of recurrence requiring reoperation in the San Francisco series was 2%. Interestingly, there were no reported cases of dissection once the FMD was treated. Anecdotal cases of percutaneous angioplasty have been reported but the concern about embolization has prevented most interventionalists from attempting this procedure without distal control.[14] Resection and anastomosis are sometimes feasible for short segments of the middle third of the ICA. Long excised segments can be replaced with a saphenous vein interposition graft.

There are other generalized connective disorders other than FMD that are associated with carotid dissection. The Ehlers-Danlos syndrome type IV is the most life-threatening variant and was described in 1967.[15] There is a tendency toward spontaneous rupture or dissection of large and medium-sized arteries. It is inherited as an autosomal dominant trait. The skin is fragile and translucent. Easy bruising is common. The most common neurovascular event is the development of a carotid artery to cavernous sinus fistula. Carotid dissection also occurs.[16] The basic abnormality is a defect in type III collagen, which is a major component of the extracellular matrix. Diagnostic angiography and endovascular treatment of vascular abnormalities are very dangerous in this condition.[17]

Marfan's syndrome is another condition in which dissection of the carotid artery occurs. Usually the dissection is an extension of an aortic process but isolated dissections of the carotid artery have been reported. Pathologic changes are characterized by extensive cystic medial necrosis often with the loss of elastic fibers. The molecular defect is a deficiency in the microfibrillar protein fibrillin. Cystic medial necrosis is not unique to Marfan's, as it has been identified in patients with dissections of the cervical carotid artery and no stigmata of Marfan's syndrome.

These generalized disorders of connective tissue and others mentioned earlier that may predispose to a carotid artery dissection share a common denominator. Each has a distinct but a different defect in a single component of the extracellular matrix. The defect in FMD is unknown but the finding of cystic medial necrosis in patients without the stigmata of Marfan's suggests that there is a still undefined relationship between these arteriopathies. Since carotid dissection is such a significant problem due to the high incidence of unfavorable outcomes, careful consideration to treating asymptomatic FMD and elongated ICAs in appropriate patients should be given.

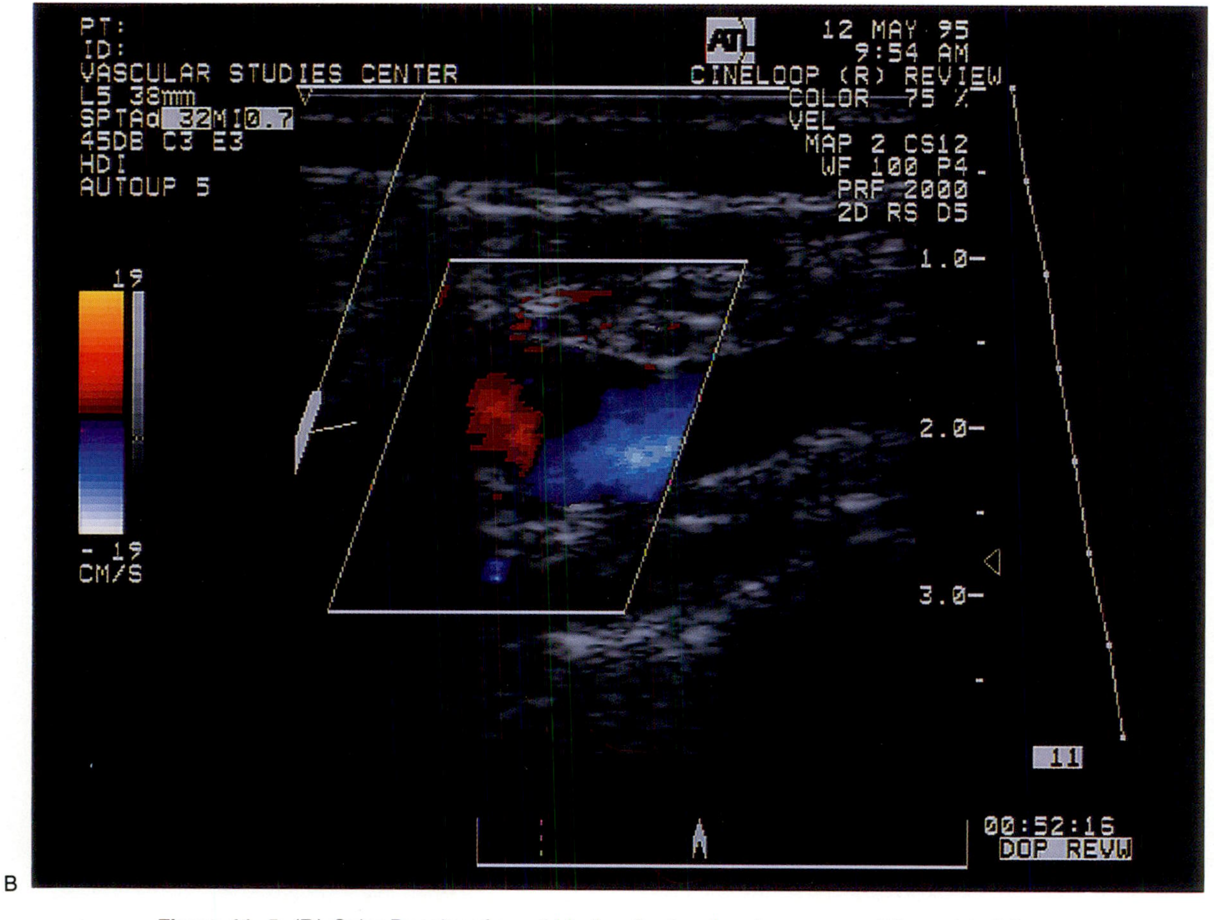

B

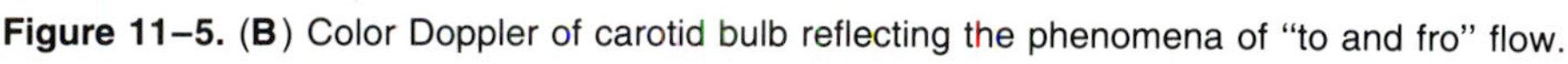

Figure 11–5. (**B**) Color Doppler of carotid bulb reflecting the phenomena of "to and fro" flow.

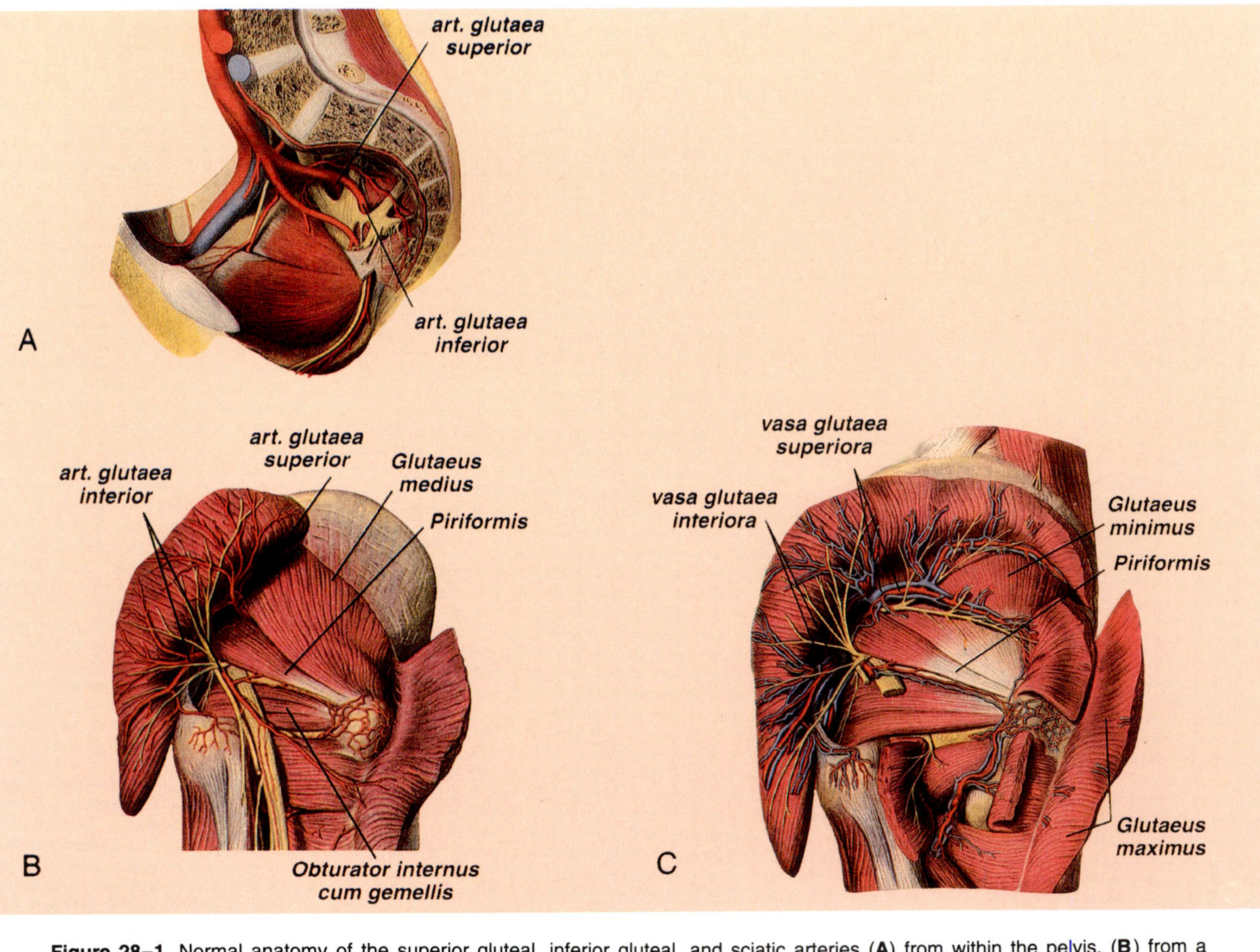

Figure 28–1. Normal anatomy of the superior gluteal, inferior gluteal, and sciatic arteries (**A**) from within the pelvis, (**B**) from a posterior approach, and (**C**) with detailed relationships to the sciatic nerve. (*Adapted from Sobotta J. Atlas der dekriptiven Anatomie des Menschen. Munich: JF Lehmanns Verlag; 1992.*)

REFERENCES

1. Schievink WI, Michels VV, Piepgras DG. Neurovascular manifestations of heritable connective tissue disorders: a review. *Stroke.* 1994;25:889–903.
2. Schievink WI, Prakash UBS, Piepgras DG, et al. Alpha-one antitrypsin deficiency in intracranial aneurysms and cervical carotid artery dissection. *Lancet.* 1994;343:452–453.
3. Gould DB, Cunningham K. Internal carotid artery dissection after remote surgery. Iatrogenic complications of anesthesia. *Stroke.* 1994;25:1276–1278.
4. Biousse V, D'Anglejan-Chatillon J, Touboul PJ, et al. Time course of symptoms in extracranial carotid dissection: a series of 80 patients. *Stroke.* 1995;26:235–239.
5. Ehrenfeld WK, Wylie EJ. Spontaneous dissection of the internal carotid artery. *Arch Surg.* 1976;111:1294–1301.
6. Leadbetter WF, Burkland CE. Hypertension in unilateral renal disease. *J Urol.* 1938;39:611.
7. Connett MC, Lansche JM. Fibromuscular hyperplasia of the internal carotid artery: report of a case. *Ann Surg.* 1965;162:59.
8. Kincaid OW, Davis GD, Hallermann FJ, et al. Fibromuscular dysplasia of the renal arteries: arteriographic features, classification, and observations on natural history of the disease. *Am J Roentgenol.* 104:271–282.
9. Osborn AG, Anderson RE. Angiographic spectrum of cervical and intracranial fibromuscular dysplasia. *Stroke.* 1977;8:617.
10. Schievink WI, Bjornsson J, Piepggras DG. Coexistence of fibromuscular dysplasia and cystic medial necrosis in a patient with Marfan's syndrome and bilateral carotid artery dissections. *Stroke.* 1994;15:2492–2496.
11. Luscher TF, Stanson AW, Houser OW, et al. Arterial fibromuscular dysplasia. *Mayo Clin Proc.* 1987;62:931–952.
12. Ehrenfeld WK, Wylie EJ. Fibromuscular dysplasia of the internal carotid artery: surgical management. *Arch Surg.* 1974;109:215.
13. Morris GC Jr, Lechter A, DeBakey ME. Surgical treatment of fibromuscular dysplasia of the carotid arteries. *Arch Surg.* 1968;96:636.
14. Jooma R, Bradshaw JR, Griffith HB. Intimal dissection following percutaneous transluminal carotid angioplasty for fibromuscular dysplasia. *Neuroradiology.* 1985;27:181.
15. Barabas AP. Heterogeneity of the Ehlers-Danlos syndrome: description of three clinical types and a hypothesis to explain the basic defects. *Br Med J.* 1968;3:612–613.
16. Krog, Almgren B, Eriksson I, et al. Vascular complications of the Ehlers-Danlos syndrome. *Acta Chir Scand.* 1983;149:279–282.
17. Cikrit DF, Miles JH, Silver D. Spontaneous arterial perforation: the Ehlers-Danlos spectre. *J Vasc Surg.* 1987;5:248–255.

12

Brachiocephalic Arterial Reconstruction

Edouard Kieffer, MD, Jean Sabatier, MD, Fabien Koskas, MD, Amine Bahnini, MD, and Carlo Ruotolo, MD

Although successful reconstruction of the innominate artery (IA) and subclavian arteries (SAs) was described in the 1950s,[1-3] and the Joint Study of Extracranial Arterial Occlusion reported a significant incidence of proximal arterial disease[4] in patients undergoing arteriography for cerebrovascular disease, brachiocephalic reconstruction is still rarely performed by most vascular surgeons. Indications, especially in patients with asymptomatic occlusive disease, and technical aspects, including the choice of surgical approach and type of reconstruction, have remained largely controversial. Only a limited number of large series of brachiocephalic arterial reconstruction has been reported.[5-16]

This chapter describes our current approach to brachiocephalic arterial reconstruction. Emphasis is placed on the wide pathologic spectrum of brachiocephalic lesions, the importance of versatility in surgical approaches and reconstructive techniques as well as the combined skills in thoracic and cerebrovascular surgery that are mandatory for the successful surgical management of these patients. Technical aspects of reoperative surgery are also described in some detail since complications may be expected to be seen more frequently with the future development of brachiocephalic reconstructive surgery.

ANATOMIC LESIONS

Although it remains the most common indication for brachiocephalic arterial reconstruction, pathology of the brachiocephalic arteries is far from being limited to atherosclerotic occlusive disease.[17-21] Nonatherosclerotic occlusive disease, aneurysms and congenital lesions account for almost 20% of our brachiocephalic arterial reconstructions.

Atherosclerotic Occlusive Disease

Atherosclerotic occlusive disease of the brachiocephalic vessels is usually detected in the fifth or sixth decade (i.e., significantly earlier than atherosclerotic carotid or vertebrobasilar arterial disease). Its predominance in males seems less apparent than in other localizations of atherosclerotic arterial disease. Lesions are commonly segmental in nature. They are usually located at the origin of the brachiocephalic arteries, often in continuity with a plaque of the upper aspect of the transverse aortic arch. Lesions of the left common carotid artery (CCA) are commonly located at its origin, while lesions of the IA and left SA may extend more distally, up to the bifurcation of the IA and origin of the left vertebral artery (VA), respectively. Lesions of the right SA and CCA are usually located at the origin of the vessels. Although some atherosclerotic lesions of the brachiocephalic arteries may be strictly isolated, they usually combine in various ways. Involvement of the origin of the three brachiocephalic vessels with an extensive plaque of the upper aspect of the transverse aortic arch has been described as the "aortic dome syndrome"[18] (Fig. 12–1).

Diffuse lesions of the brachiocephalic vessels extending to the distal SA and CCA are seen mostly in elderly, hypertensive, and/or diabetic patients. Carotid, vertebrobasilar, coronary, visceral, and peripheral atherosclerotic occlusive disease is often associated with atherosclerotic lesions of the brachiocephalic vessels. In many patients they have major prognostic as well as technical implications. They should be thoroughly evaluated in the preoperative work-up of atherosclerotic patients scheduled for brachiocephalic arterial reconstruction.

Takayasu's Arteritis

Takayasu's arteritis has been our second most common indication for brachiocephalic reconstruction.[19] This disease of unknown etiology may involve the entire aorta and all its major branches. It is more prevalent in Japan, India, South Africa, and Central

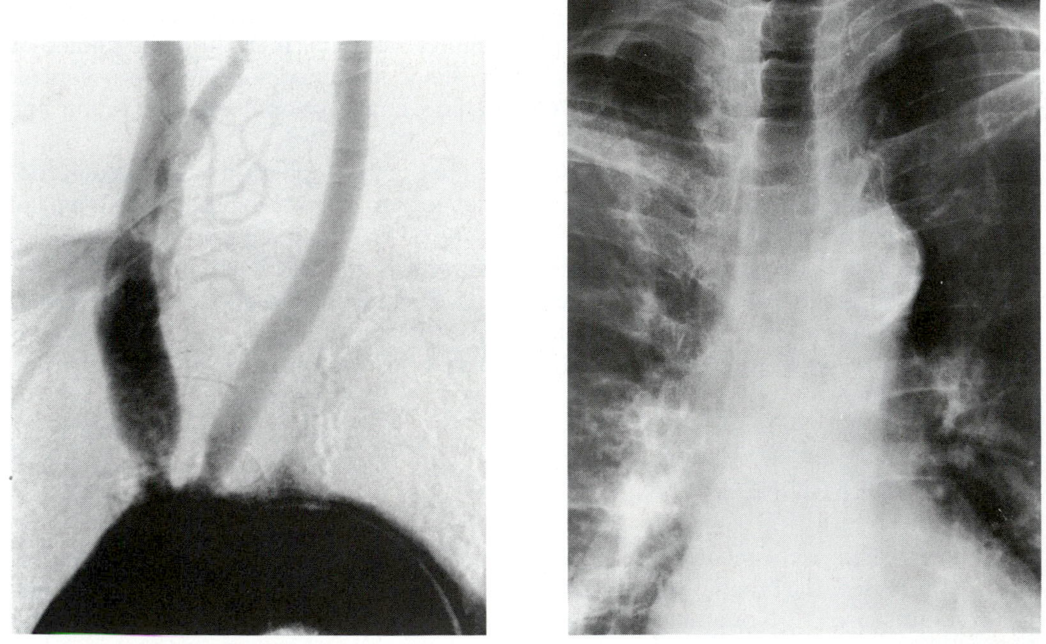

Figure 12–1. Aortic dome syndrome. **(A)** Arch aortography shows typical plaque of the transverse aortic arch with occlusive disease of the three brachiocephalic vessels. **(B)** Plain chest roentgenogram shows extensive calcification of the transverse aortic arch.

and South American than in Western countries. Most patients operated on in France originate from North Africa, the West Indies, Italy, or Spain. Lesions of the brachiocephalic vessels are frequent but not constant in Takayasu's arteritis. They may be located either at the origin of the vessel, in continuity with aortic lesions, or more distally. Lesions of the midportion of the CCA and distal SA extending to the axillary and brachial arteries are typical for Takayasu's arteritis and differ significantly from atherosclerotic lesions. The ICAs and VAs are usually patent in patients with Takayasu's arteritis, except in cases with extensive thrombosis complicating proximal arterial disease.

Radiation Arteritis

Radiation arteritis of the brachiocephalic vessels is increasingly frequent due to better long-term survival of patients with throat, neck, or breast malignancies or Hodgkin's disease. It usually takes 5 to 10 years before radiation-induced occlusive disease becomes clinically apparent. Although radiation-induced lesions basically consist of accelerated atherosclerosis, they differ from classical atherosclerotic lesions by their inflammatory or fibrous nature and their exclusive or predominant location to the irradiated arterial segment, usually the cervical portion of the CCA or distal portion of the SA. Associated lesions of the soft tissues and/or the presence of a tracheostomy may cause surgical problems. Radiation arteritis of the distal SA is often associated with brachial plexitis, causing significant pain and disability of the upper extremity.

Occlusive Disease of Miscellaneous Origin

Occlusive disease of the brachiocephalic vessels complicating kinking, embolism, fibromuscular dysplasia, temporal arteritis, neurofibromatosis, or mediastinal fibrosis has been described sporadically. Trauma to the brachiocephalic vessels may as well be responsible for late thromboembolic complications due to intimal lesions. Although proximal (Stanford type A) aortic dissections may extend to branches of the aortic arch in a significant number of patients, localized dissections of the brachiocephalic vessels are distinctly uncommon. They are usually associated with diffuse connective tissue disorders.

Aneurysmal Disease

Aneurysms of the proximal brachiocephalic vessels are uncommon. They are usually atherosclerotic or luetic in origin. Chronic aneurysms complicating Takayasu's arteritis or dissections are also seen occasionally. Most, if not all, of these proximal aneurysms are associated with thoracic aortic aneurysms calling for simultaneous surgical treatment. More distal, isolated, aneurysms may be caused by fibromuscular dysplasia, Marfan syndrome, trauma, radiation, or hematogenous infection. The major potential complication of aneurysms of the brachiocephalic vessels is rupture into the mediastinum, pleural cavity, trachea, esophagus, or pericardium. Less commonly, aneurysms of the brachiocephalic vessels may cause compression of the mediastinal structures or thromboembolism to the brain or upper extremity.

Congenital Disease

Aberrant SAs are not uncommon. Most are incidental and do not require treatment. Surgical repair of an aberrant SA is, however, indicated in four circumstances: the presence of dysphagia lusoria, occlusive disease, aneurysmal disease complicating

Kommerel's diverticulum, or associated thoracic aortic disease.[20] Isolation, atresia, or congenital stenosis of the IAs or SAs usually occur in patients with a right aortic arch. They have the same clinical consequences as acquired occlusive lesions.

PATIENT SELECTION

Patient with brachiocephalic arterial disease may present with symptoms of the carotid or vertebrobasilar distribution or both, and/or symptoms of upper limb ischemia. The mechanism for production of symptoms is either severe restriction of flow due to clinical lesions, usually at the origin of the brachiocephalic vessels, or embolization from irregular or ulcerated atherosclerotic plaques.

Our current indications for brachiocephalic arterial reconstruction are as follows[21]:

1. Symptomatic lesions causing ischemic symptoms of carotid, vertebrobasilar or upper limb distribution. Symptoms often involve the carotid and vertebrobasilar territories simultaneously and the upper extremities occasionally.
2. Asymptomatic patients with complex plaques in the IA or CCA and no evidence of carotid or intracranial arterial disease who present an ipsilateral silent hemispheric infarction on brain CT scan.
3. Asymptomatic but severe (>75% of diameter) lesions of the IA or CCA because we believe that these lesions have the same potential risks as those found in the carotid bifurcation.
4. Severe asymptomatic lesions of the SA (>75% of diameter) in patients who are candidates for coronary artery revascularization to ensure adequate internal mammary artery inflow. Asymptomatic occlusions of the SA are also revascularized to allow blood pressure measurement in patients with bilateral subclavian occlusion (especially in Takayasu's arteritis) and to provide inflow in those patients who require hemodialysis.
5. Revascularization of the SA is also indicated in patients who have had a previous myocardial revascularization using the internal mammary artery and have a recurrence of angina due to progression of disease in ipsilateral SA.
6. Finally, aneurysms of the brachiocephalic vessels should be operated on whenever they are large (>3–4 cm), expanding, and/or symptomatic.

PREOPERATIVE WORK-UP

Biplane arch aortography is routinely obtained in patients scheduled for brachiocephalic arterial reconstruction. In addition to the brachiocephalic vessels, it should display both carotid bifurcations, the cervical course of both VAs, and the intracranial arteries. Delineation of the distal vasculature, including the carotid bifurcations, may be difficult in patients with proximal arterial occlusions, despite late films and digital subtraction. Although patency of the ICA may be assessed by Duplex scanning, surgical exploration of the carotid bifurcation may be needed as the ultimate diagnostic procedure, especially in patients with extensive carotid occlusion in whom external carotid artery reconstruction is contemplated.

Brain CT scan is also performed routinely prior to brachiocephalic arterial reconstruction, even in clinically asymptomatic patients.[11] Silent hemispheric brain infarction may be present in up to 10% of patients with asymptomatic lesions of the IA or CCA. Because of an increased risk of reperfusion syndrome, operation should be delayed by at least 1 month in patients with recent stroke and/or contrast enhancement of brain infarction on CT scan. Patients with multiple occlusions of the brachiocephalic vessels should have their "hemodynamic cerebral reserve" assessed using regional cerebral blood flow studies. Loss of cerebral blood flow autoregulation entails a definite risk of reperfusion syndrome, even in asymptomatic patients and in the absence of hemispheric brain infarction. In our experience, this unexpected complication occurred mostly in patients with Takayasu's arteritis and extensive lesions, including bilateral carotid occlusion.[19]

Because of the frequent association of coronary artery disease, we advocate routine coronary arteriography for atherosclerotic patients in whom an intrathoracic brachiocephalic arterial reconstruction is planned.[11] Significant coronary artery disease should be corrected at the same operation[21–23] unless it is amenable to preoperative balloon angioplasty. This practice avoids the difficulty of having to do a later myocardial revascularization through a secondary trans-sternal approach with a crowded ascending aorta. In patients with isolated lesions of the SA or CCA, coronary arteriography is performed only on clinical grounds. In our experience, noninvasive testing using Thallium-dipyridamole scintigraphy has not proven useful in selecting asymptomatic patients for coronary arteriography.

A thoracic CT scan or MRI should be performed in patients with aneurysmal disease of the brachiocephalic vessels. It helps delineate the true diameter of the aneurysm and its relationships to the neighboring structures, including the sternum.

THORACIC PROCEDURES

Endarterectomy of the Innominate Artery

A median sternotomy extended slightly to the right along the anterior edge of the sternomastoid muscle provides easy access to the ascending aorta, the IA and its branches. The thymic remnants should be preserved and dissected as a flap since it will be used at the time of closure to isolate the arterial repair from the sternum. After exposing the ascending aorta, the origin of the IA lies behind the brachiocephalic vein and the exposure is extended over the origins of the right CCA and SA, avoiding injury to the right recurrent laryngeal nerve as it curves behind both branches of the IA.

Endarterectomy of limited lesions of the innominate artery bifurcation may be performed by clamping of the proximal IA. The usual extensive or proximal lesions of the IA call for partial exclusion clamping of the aortic arch.[11,21,24] The convexity of the aortic arch should therefore be widely dissected and the origin of the left CCA identified. Two anatomic criteria should be fulfilled in order to permit an IA endarterectomy: (1) there should be no extensive or calcific disease of the aortic arch around the origin of the IA, and (2) there should be enough space between the origins of the IA and left CCA to allow for exclusion clamping of the origin of the IA. If the endarterectomy appears feasible, systemic heparin is given (50 units/kg) and systolic arterial pressure is lowered to 100 mm Hg using pharmacologic agents. The distal vessels (i.e., right CCA and SA) are clamped first to avoid embolization. A Wylie clamp is then applied to the transverse aortic arch around the origin of the IA, taking care to preserve normal flow through the left CCA.

A longitudinal arteriotomy of the IA is then made and extended into the wall of the transverse aortic arch already excluded by the clamp. The endarterectomy is done in a plane more superficial than usually to avoid ending with a friable artery. Proximally, the IA plaque usually needs to be cut (Fig. 12–2) and the intima/media affixed to the aortic wall by tacking sutures. A thin IA wall with a jagged edge usually requires a prosthetic patch graft for closure. The suture is done with 5-0 monofilament. The sequence of the declamping is designed to avoid any embolization into the CCA. With the patient in the head-down position, the clamp on the right CCA is briefly released first and then reapplied. The clamp on the right SA is then released in order to flush the VA and SA. The clamp on the aortic arch is then released progressively in order to restore flow to the right SA. The clamp on the right CCA is released last, after gentle massage of the small proximal carotid cul-de-sac.

Especially difficult problems may result from the distal extension of the lesions. In these cases, the right SA is exposed medial to the jugular vein for separate clamping of the right VA and distal SA, with care taken not to injure the vagus nerve or its recurrent laryngeal branch. The arteriotomy of the IA is extended to the SA as far as needed to perform endarterectomy under direct vision. If the lesion is extended on the right CCA, a complete transsection of the CCA permits an eversion endarterectomy.[17] In presence of a common trunk bifurcating into an IA and a left CCA, endarterectomy remains possible using a Javid shunt from the ascending aorta to either CCA[21] (Fig. 12–3).

Bypass from the Ascending Aorta to Innominate Artery and/or Left Common Carotid Artery

The proximal portion of the ascending aorta is chosen because this segment is generally spared from the calcification and atheroma that may involve the dome of the transverse aortic arch. The proximal anastomosis is made easier if heparin is not used during this part of the procedure. The IA and origins of the right SA and CCA are dissected, avoiding injury to the right recurrent laryngeal nerve. If the left CCA is to be revascularized, it is exposed at the desired level through a separate presternomastoid incision.

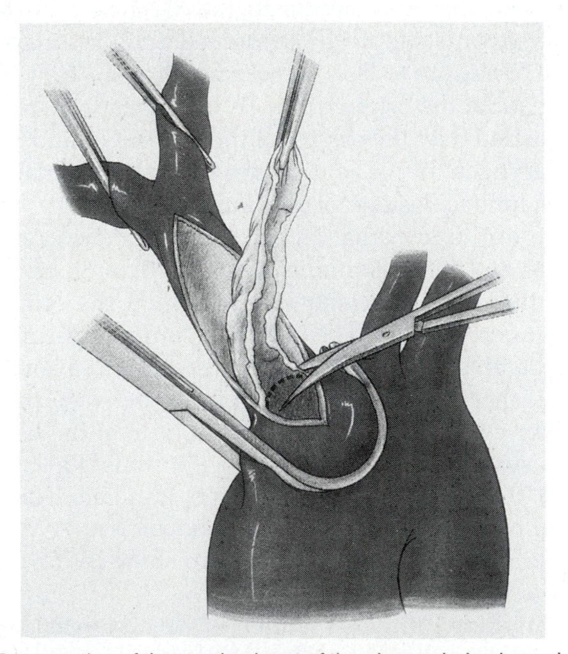

Figure 12–2. Transsection of the proximal part of the plaque during innominate artery endarterectomy.

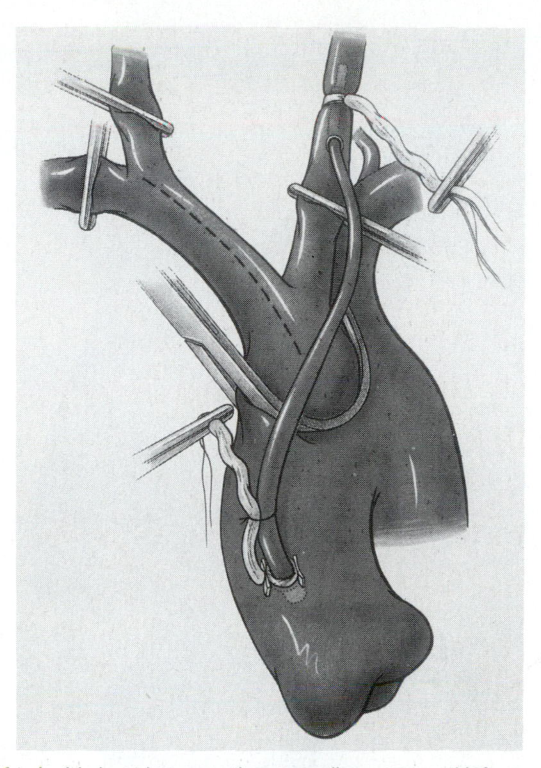

Figure 12–3. Use of a Javid shunt between the ascending aorta and left common carotid artery to allow safe clamping of a common trunk for the innominate and left common carotid arteries.

The aortic systolic pressure is lowered to about 100 mm Hg using pharmacologic agents. A Lemole–Strong clamp is placed on the right anterolateral portion of the aorta (Fig. 12–4A). It is most important not to use the more accessible anterior aspect of the ascending aorta since this may result in compression of the graft by the sternum or graft involvement should a sternal infection occur. Complete exclusion of the aorta is checked by verification that it remains empty after aspiration of blood through a fine needle. An 8- to 12-mm Dacron or polytetrafluoroethylene graft is anastomosed end to side to the ascending aorta using a continuous 3-0 monofilament suture and taking large bites on the aorta. If the aortic wall is friable or the sutures cut through, the anastomosis is made with a strip of Teflon felt applied outside.

Distal anastomosis to the brachiocephalic vessel should be performed end to end in order to avoid competitive flow and embolization from proximal lesions (Fig. 12–4B). In patients with associated lesions of the IA and left CCA the sequence of distal anastomoses is determined by the severity and location of the existing lesions. The most severely stenotic vessel is repaired first to take advantage of the collateral support provided by the less diseased vessel. The distal anastomosis is usually performed end to end to the distal IA. In patients with extension of the lesions to the proximal part of the right SA and/or CCA, the following techniques may be used: (1) eversion endarterectomy of a limited lesion of one or both vessels through the transected distal IA, (2) a longitudinal arteriotomy of the proximal part of one vessel allowing for a beveled anastomosis, or (3) complete transection of both vessels with the graft being anastomosed end to end to the largest vessel (usually the SA) and the remaining vessel being anastomosed end to side to the graft.[17,21]

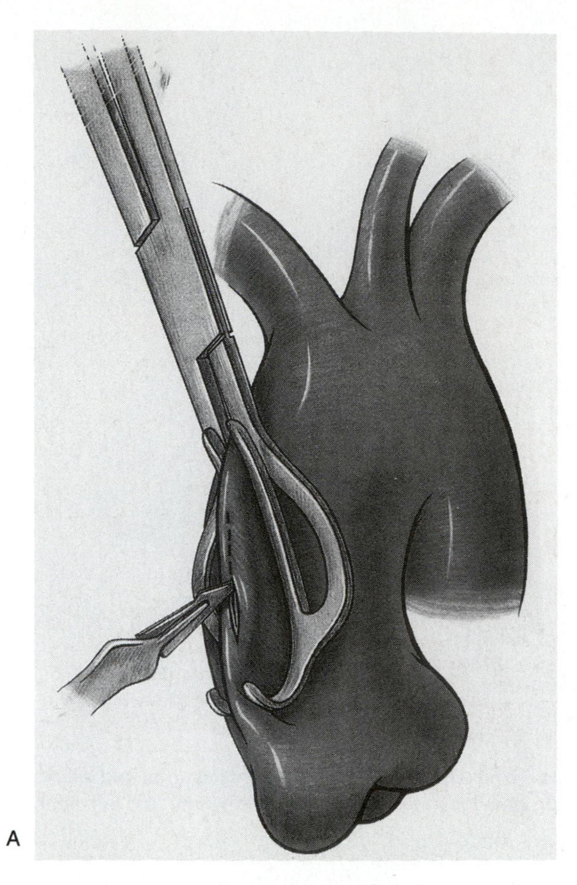

Figure 12–4. Aorto-inhominate artery bypass. **(A)** Partial exclusion-clamping and longitudinal incision of the lateral aspect of the ascending aorta for proximal implantation of a prosthetic bypass graft. **(B)** Various solutions for the distal end-to-end anastomosis of a bypass between the ascending aorta and the bifurcation of the innominate artery.

The surgical technique is the same for the reconstruction of the left CCA using a bypass from the ascending aorta. Either for left and right CCA, the distal anastomosis may be performed to the endarterectomized carotid bifurcation due to extensive carotid lesions (Fig. 12–5).

The stump of the IA and/or left CCA is closed with a double running suture, often using Teflon felt strips, depending on the quality of the arterial wall.

Thoracic Approach to the Left Subclavian Artery

The left SA may be approached through a median sternotomy incision with ligation of the left brachiocephalic vein. This approach is used to perform transposition of the left SA into the CCA in patients with a concomitant myocardial revascularization using the left internal mammary artery. The technique of SA to CCA transposition is described as follows.

The usual transthoracic approach to the left SA is through a left posterolateral incision in the fourth intercostal space. Care must be taken to avoid injury to the vagus, the phrenic, and the left recurrent laryngeal nerves. The SA is dissected from its origin up to the origin of the VA. The extent of the SA disease may be assessed by palpation.

The usual technique is a bypass graft originating from the descending aorta (Fig. 12–6). The lateral aspect of the proximal descending aorta is partially excluded using

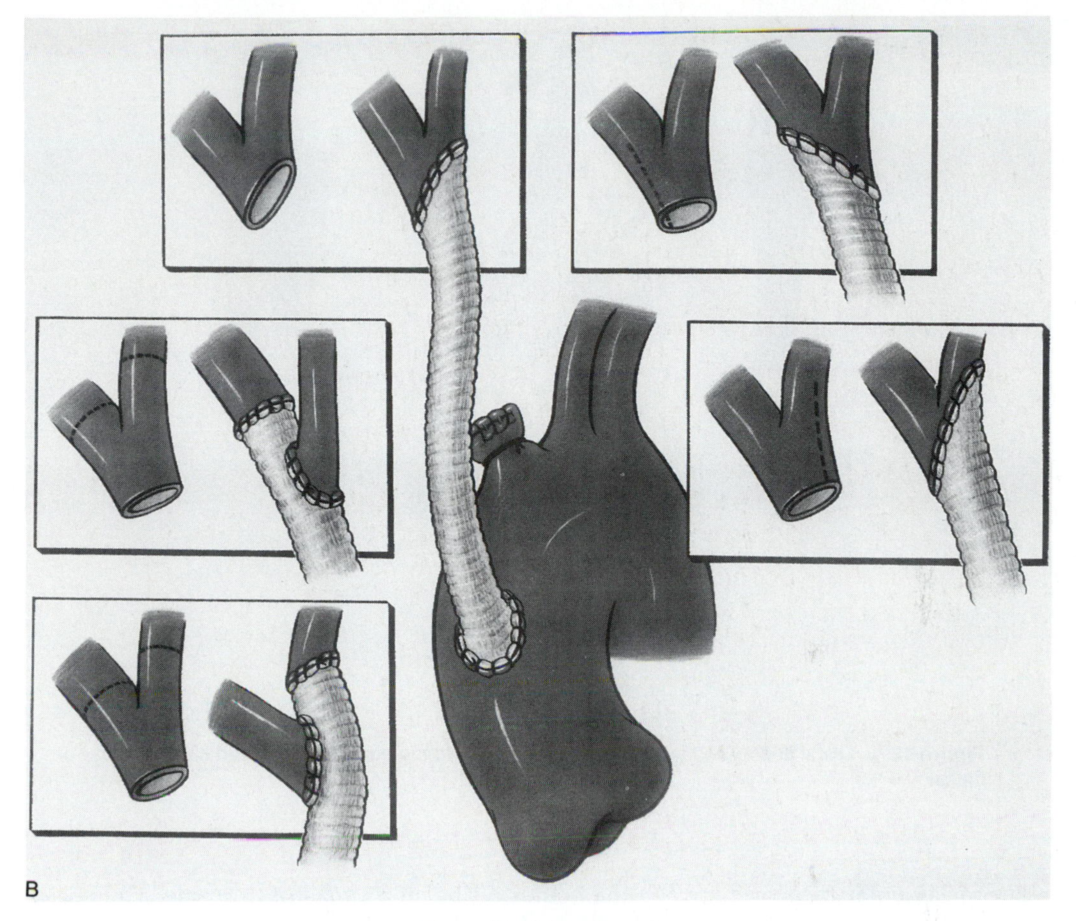

Figure 12–4. (*continued*)

a satinsky clamp. a 7- or 8-mm dacron (obtained from a limb of a bifurcation graft) or polytetrafluorethylene graft is anastomosed end to side to the aorta using 4-0 or 5-0 monofilament continuous suture. Then the graft is anastomosed end to end to the SA with 5-0 monofilament. Flow is reestablished first to the arm and then to the VA, which was clamped separately.

If the distal transverse aortic arch is free of disease, SA endarterectomy may be performed. The distal transverse aortic arch is excluded with a Wylie clamp around the origin of the SA taking care to preserve normal flow through the left CCA. The SA endarterectomy should not extend into the aortic arch. Tacking sutures may be needed to fix the aortic intima at the origin of the SA. The distal limit of the endarterectomy should be either proximal to or at the level of the VA, which can be endarterectomized using an eversion technique. The arteriotomy is closed with a continuous 5-0 monofilament suture, with or without prosthetic patch angioplasty, depending on the size of the SA and the quality of the arteriotomy edges.

CERVICAL PROCEDURES

Transpositions

Transposition of the SA into the CCA is our preferred technique for treating proximal occlusive disease of the SA[21,25] (Fig. 12–7). The SA and CCA are approached through

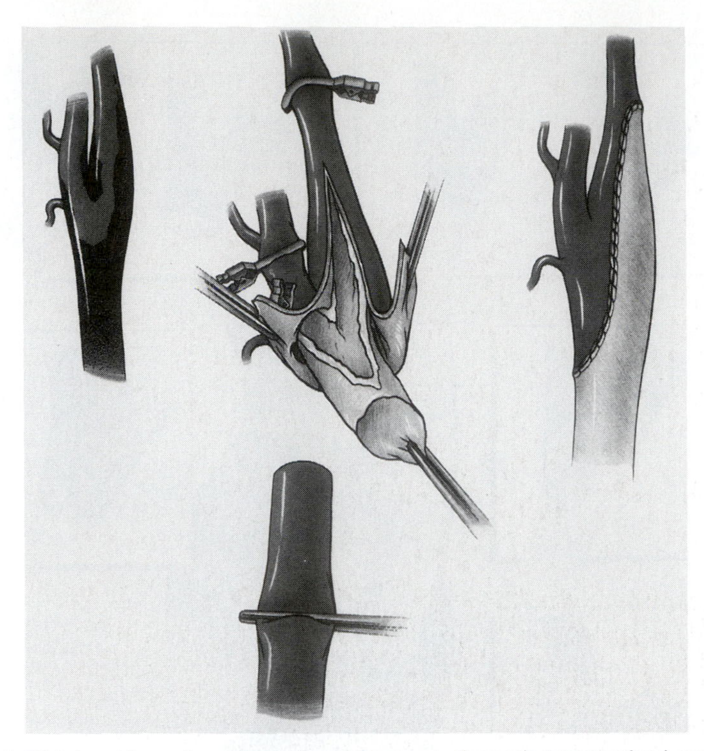

Figure 12–5. Distal end-to-end anastomosis of a bypass to the endarterectomized carotid bifurcation.

a supraclavicular incision between the bellies of the sternomastoid muscle. The entire dissection is performed medial to the internal jugular vein, vagus nerve, and prescalene fat pad. The CCA is bluntly dissected proximally along its intrathoracic course down to the transverse aortic arch. The proximal SA is also dissected toward its origin after the thoracic duct (on the left side) and the vertebral vein are divided. The VA is mobilized to the level at which it disappears into the cervical spine dividing the upper aspect of the stellate ganglion. Complete mobilization of the left SA to near the transverse aortic arch is most important. When mobilizing the right SA, the vagus nerve and its recurrent laryngeal branch must be identified and protected. After systemic heparinization the proximal SA is clamped using a small Satinsky or Castaneda pediatric clamp. It is then ligated with heavy silk and the stump is sutured with 5-0 monofilament. Following separate clamping of the VA and distal SA, the SA is transected obliquely about 1 cm proximal to the origin of the VA. If needed, an eversion endarterectomy of the VA may be done. The anticipated site of the anastomosis to the CCA is chosen, bearing in mind that the anastomosis should be low and result in an oblique takeoff of the SA from the CCA without kinking of the proximal VA. Then the CCA is cross-clamped and an arteriostomy made in the posterolateral wall of the CCA. The anastomosis is done in an open manner with 6-0 monofilament suture.

Transposition of the CCA into the SA for treatment of proximal lesions of the CCA is done less frequently. Transposition of a CCA into the opposite CCA is indicated in poor-risk patients who have stenosis of the left CCA and extensive disease of the left SA. In these circumstances this technique is preferable to crossover bypass or to a riskier aortocarotid bypass. However, it entails simultaneous clamping of both CCA and can be done only if the right VA has been shown to supply the hemispheres

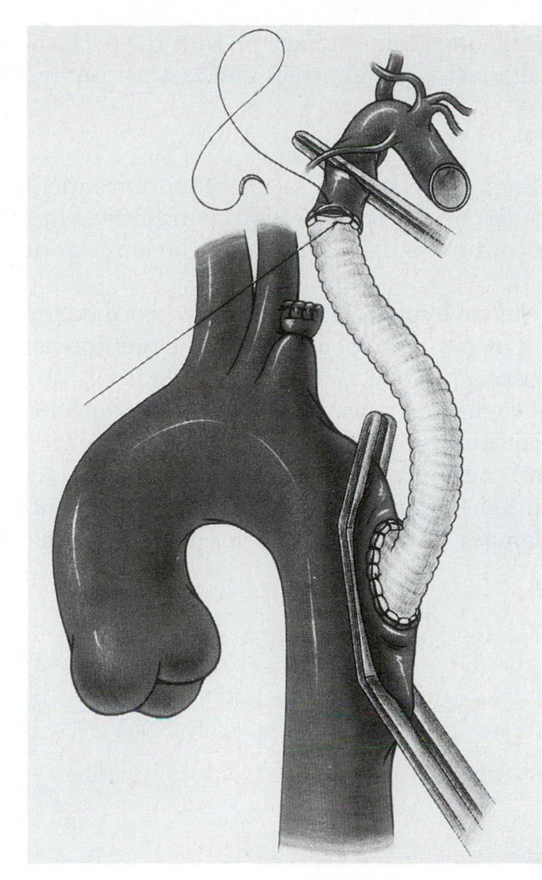

Figure 12–6. Aortosubclavian bypass through left thoracotomy incision.

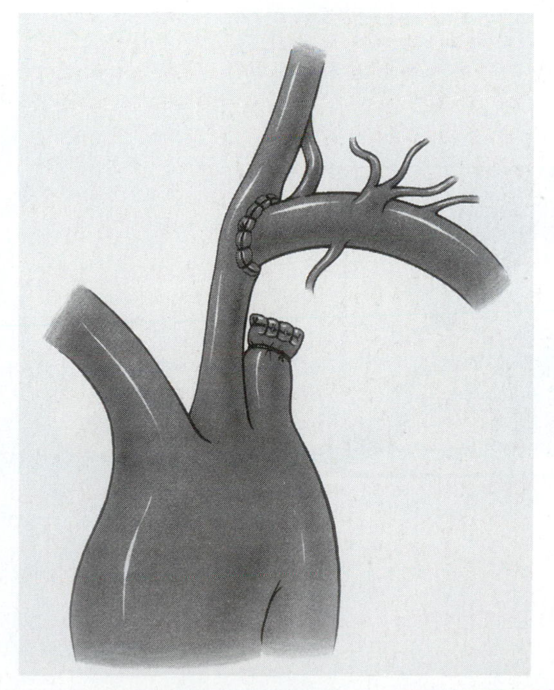

Figure 12–7. Transcervical left subclavian to carotid transposition: This procedure may be performed alternatively through a midsternotomy incision in unusual situations.

(through posterior communicating arteries) or with the protection of a shunt. A retropharyngeal route is shortest and safer than the classical pretracheal route.[26]

Cervical Bypasses

Cervical bypass grafting is an easy and safe solution for patients with isolated lesions of the CCA and/or SA, especially in those with contraindications for thoracic approach. We prefer ipsilateral carotid–subclavian or subclavian–carotid bypass to crossover bypass.

The carotid–subclavian bypass (Fig. 12–8A) is performed through a supraclavicular incision with division of the clavicular head of the sternomastoid muscle. The CCA and distal SA are dissected, respectively, on each side of the jugular vein, avoiding traction injury to the vagus and phrenic nerves. In this location we use a 7- or 8-mm Dacron or an 8-mm PTFE tube graft. After systemic heparinization the distal anastomosis is constructed first, end-to-side to the distal SA, with 6-0 monofilament. The graft is then tunneled behind the internal jugular vein and in front of the phrenic and vagus nerve. The CCA is clamped and an arteriostomy is made in its lateral wall. The distal

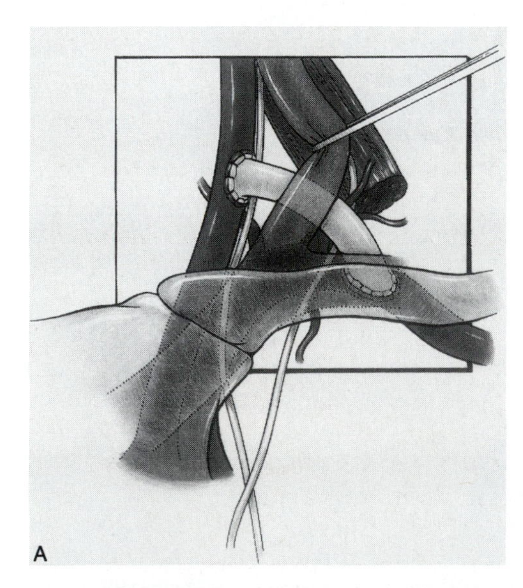

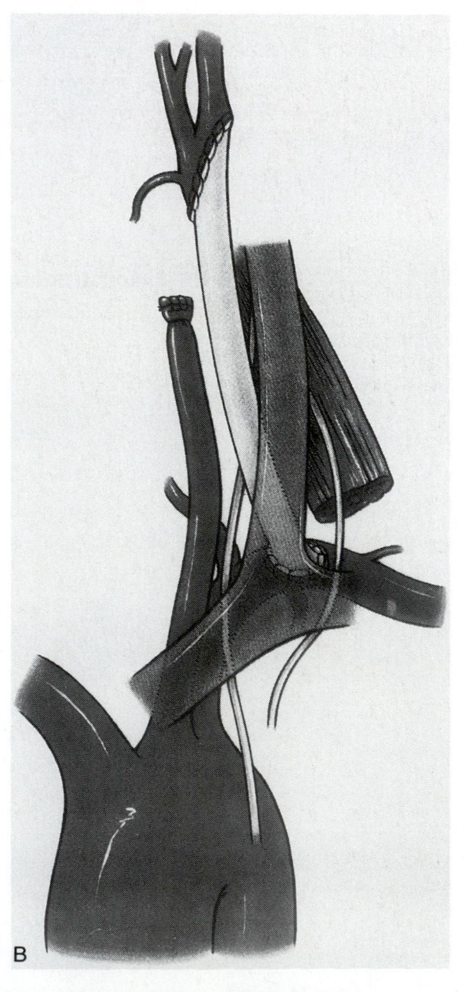

Figure 12–8. Ipsilateral cervical bypasses. **(A)** Carotid–subclavian bypass. **(B)** Subclavian–carotid bypass for extensive disease of the common carotid artery.

CCA, the proximal CCA, and then the bypass are allowed to back-bleed, with flow being resumed first into the bypass and then into the distal CCA.

The same procedure applies to the treatment of isolated lesions of the proximal CCA. In the case of extensive disease of the CCA, a presternomastoid incision is performed and the distal anastomosis is done end-to-end to the carotid bifurcation (Fig. 12–8B).

Carotid–axillary bypass is performed through separate incisions and routed behind the clavicle. The mobility of the shoulder makes a vein graft in this location preferable to a prosthesis.

We use crossover cervical bypasses (Figs. 12–9A–C) only in unusual, specific situations when other techniques cannot be used. When one of the two anastomosis involves the CCA, we prefer the retropharyngeal route, which is shorter than the pretracheal.[26] Crossover bypasses are usually constructed with prosthetic grafts.

REMOTE RECONSTRUCTIONS

In a few patients with multiple proximal lesions of the brachiocephalic vessels, a sternotomy incision may be contraindicated owing to poor cardiopulmonary reserve, previous operations on the ascending aorta (usually an aortocoronary bypass grafting procedure), previous sternal infection, or previous irradiation of the mediastinum. In such cases, an alternative is a remote reconstruction using femoro-axillary, femoro-subclavian, or femoro-carotid bypasses combined with various types of crossover cervical extension. This technique, however, is reserved for the rare elderly and debilitated patient who does not have concomitant aortoiliac occlusive disease.

Our technique of choice for good-risk patients with an inaccessible ascending aorta is a bypass originating from the descending aorta. It can be done using one of the following techniques.[21]

1. The descending aorta may be approached from the left side (Fig. 12–10). The patient is placed in the right lateral position with his neck, left arm, and left hemithorax in the field. An L-shaped cervical incision combines a presternomastoid and a supraclavicular approach, transecting the sternomastoid muscle. The descending aorta is isolated through the left fourth intercostal space. A 10-mm graft is first anastomosed end-to-side to the descending aorta and then tunneled through the pleural apex to the supraclavicular fossa, where it passes between the SA and the subclavian vein. In the neck, the graft is anastomosed first side to side to the distal SA and then end to end to the carotid bifurcation. With the chest wound closed, the patient is placed supine and revascularization of the arteries on the right side of the neck is done as indicated by a crossover cervical bypass either in front of the trachea or behind the esophagus.

2. The descending aorta may also be approached from the right side. The right chest is slightly elevated, and the descending aorta is isolated low in the thorax between the esophagus and the vertebral bodies, through an anterolateral thoracotomy in the right fifth intercostal space. Care should be taken not to open the left pleural space. After anastomosing a 10-mm graft end-to-side to the descending aorta, the graft is tunneled in the right hemithorax along the mediastinum and behind the pulmonary pedicle to the right side of the neck. Here, it can be anastomosed sequentially to the right SA and then to the right carotid bifurcation. With this right-sided approach, it is possible to do the crossover graft to the left side of the neck without having to change the patient's position.

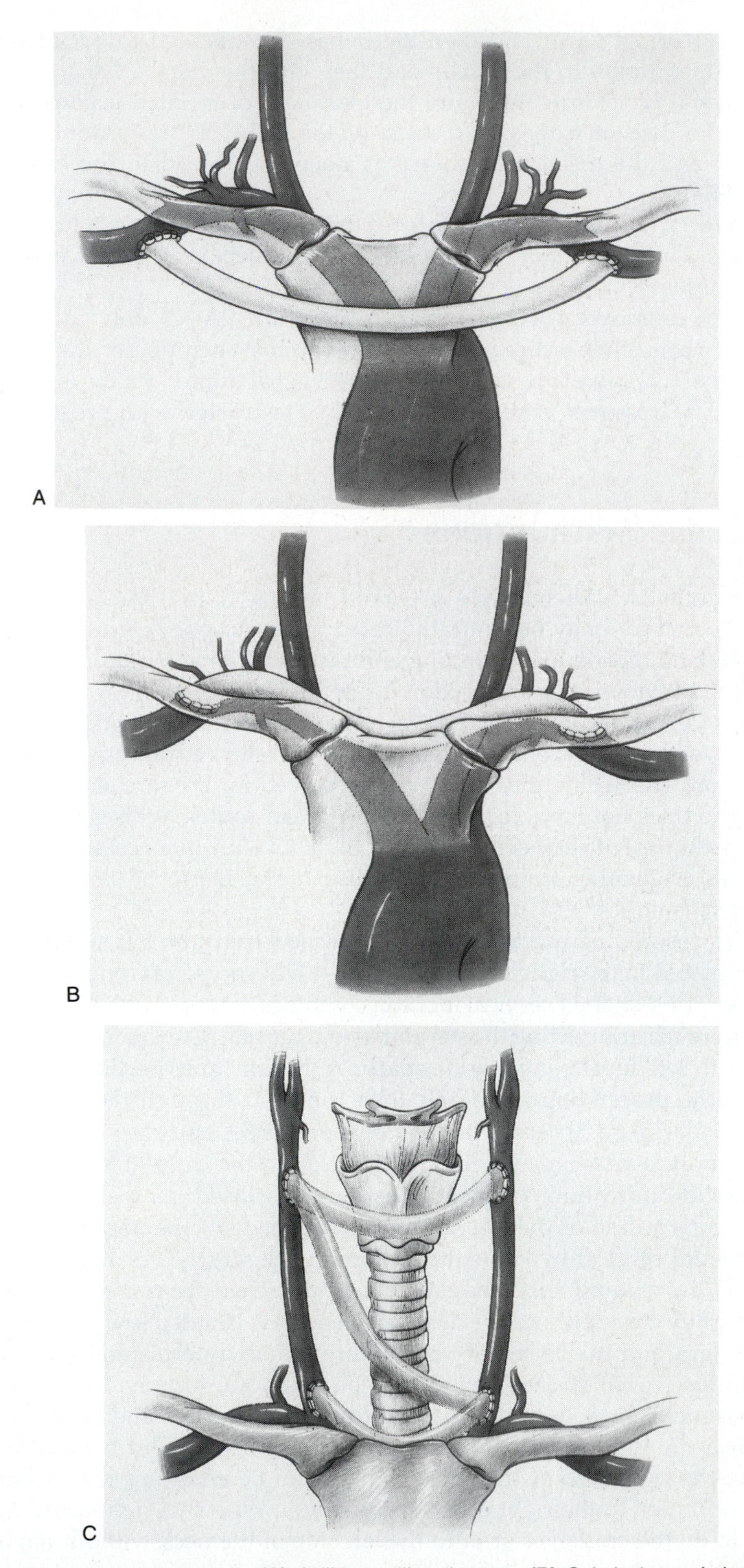

Figure 12–9. Crossover bypasses. **(A)** Axillary–axillary bypass. **(B)** Subclavian–subclavian bypass. **(C)** Various types of carotid–carotid bypass.

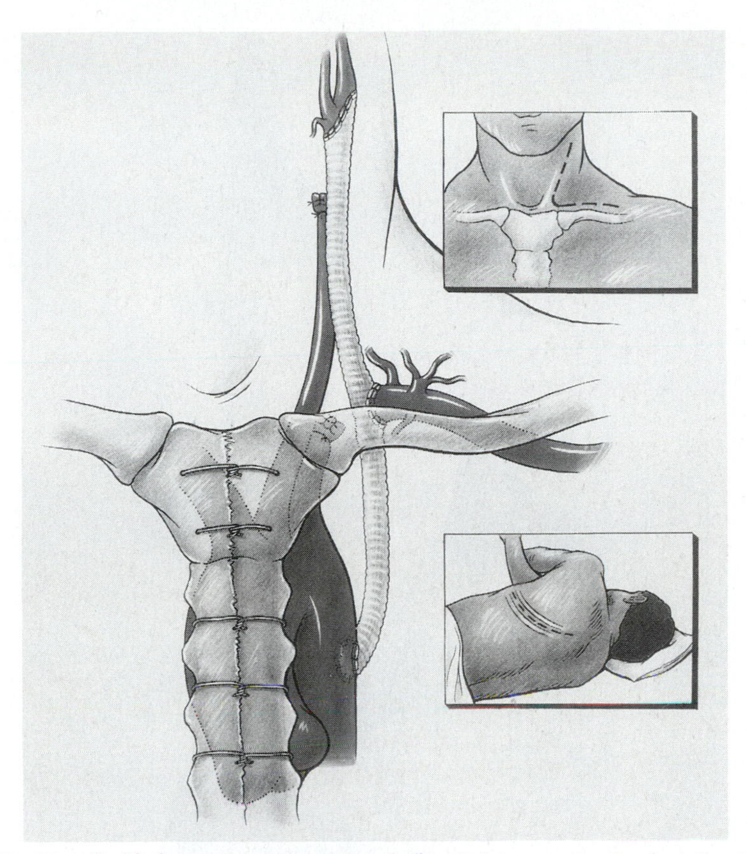

Figure 12–10. Left-sided approach to brachiocephalic arterial reconstruction from the descending aorta in a patient with an inaccessible ascending aorta.

3. The third option for bringing a bypass to the neck when the ascending aorta cannot be used is to expose the supraceliac aorta through an upper median or chevron laparotomy by dividing the crus of the diaphragm. After end-to-side anastomosis to the supraceliac aorta, the graft is tunneled to the right or left side of the neck through an intra- or extrathoracic pathway and distal anastomosis is performed to the appropriate vessel(s).

TACTICAL CHOICE

Thoracic Approach

The thoracic approach with prosthetic bypass grafting is our first choice for reconstruction of the IA and left CCA in good-risk patients.[11,17,21] This is also the best approach for multiple lesions of the brachiocephalic vessels, which are usually associated with a large atherosclerotic plaque of the transverse aortic arch. Sequential grafting (Fig. 12–11) is usually prefered to bifurcated or multiple grafting, especially in females with a narrow thoracic inlet. Transaortic endarterectomy of these multiples lesions may be done using cardiopulmonary bypass, deep hypothermia, and circulatory arrest, especially in patients requiring concomitant myocardial revascularization. However, it requires that the lesions be strictly limited to the proximal part of the great vessels in order to avoid any problem with the end of the endarterectomy.[18,27]

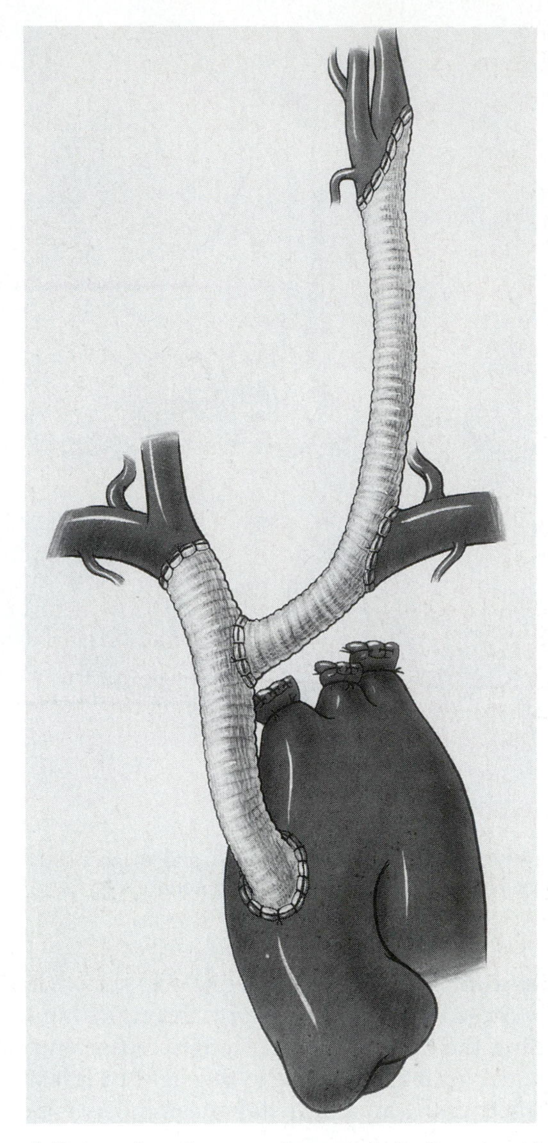

Figure 12–11. Sequential bypass from the ascending aorta to the three brachiocephalic vessels.

Endarterectomy of the IA may still be indicated in a small woman with a narrow thorax in which a prosthesis may occupy too much space; in the presence of a lesion involving the distal two-thirds of the IA; and when there has been a previous aortocoronary bypass graft, and a cervical reconstruction is not feasible.[11] The thoracic approach to the left SA is used in the rare good-risk patient with inoperable occlusion the left CCA, and in patients undergoing a concomitant operation of the descending aorta.

Cervical Approach

The transposition is the common technique for repair of isolated lesions of the SA or proximal CCA.[17,21] A bypass may, however, be preferred to a transposition in patients with morbid obesity or with a narrow thoracic inlet, where safe exposure of the proximal subclavian artery is difficult; in patients who have had myocardial revascularization using the internal mammary artery; and in patients with extensive lesions of the CCA.

ANEURYSMAL DISEASE

Resection of aneurysms of the first portion of the left SA requires a left thoracotomy. The usual technique includes partial exclusion clamping of the aorta around the origin of the left SA, lateral aortorraphy between two Teflon felt strips, and an aortosubclavian bypass (Fig. 12–12). For large aneurysms extending to the base of the neck, it may be wise to dissect the first and second portion of the SA through a supraclavicular approach first. If the VA originates low or within the aneurysm, the artery is transposed to the CCA. Preliminary transposition of the left SA to the CCA is less appealing, as it usually entails a potentially risky supraclavicular dissection of the distal part of the aneurysm. In both cases, the rest of the operation is done through a thoracotomy. The distal anastomosis is greatly facilitated by the previous supraclavicular dissection of the second portion of the SA.

If the aneurysm has a wide base of implantation in the aorta, closure of its proximal end may not be safely done by exclusion-clamping of the aorta and may require cross-clamping and closure with a patch or segmental aortic replacement. These procedures may be done by cross-clamping under pharmacologic control of proximal hypertension or by using a left atrio-femoral bypass or partial femorofemoral cardiopulmonary bypass.

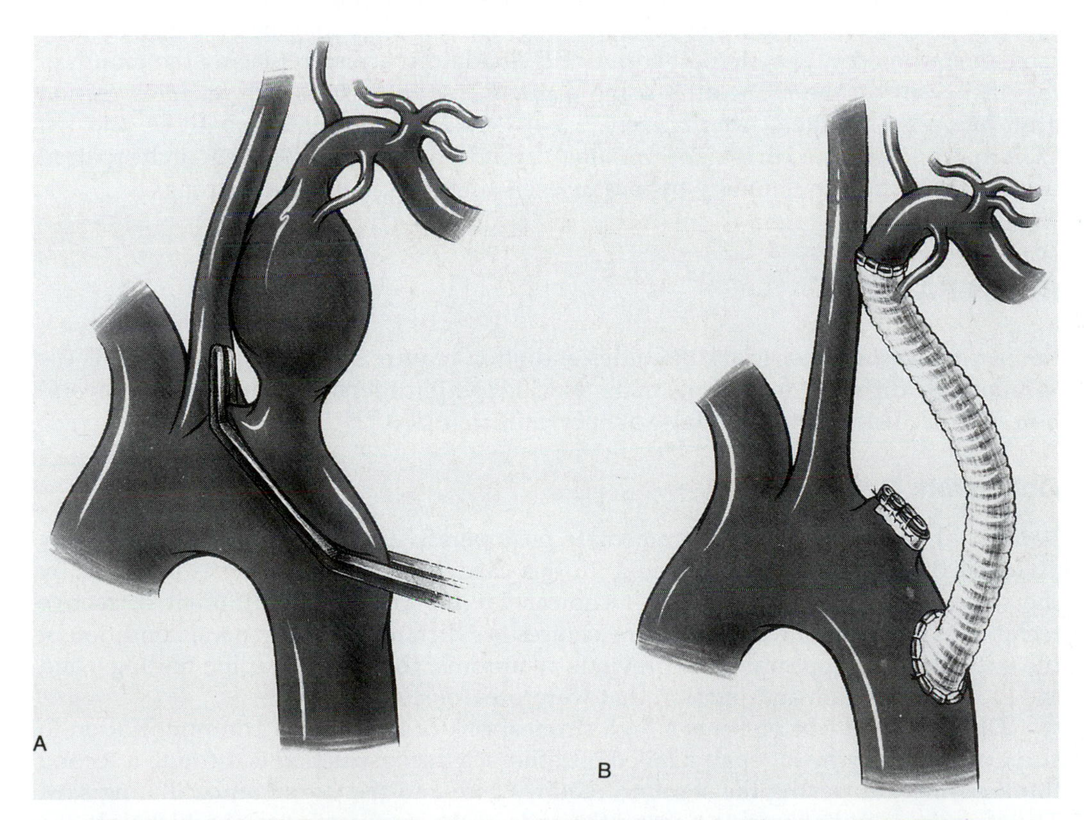

Figure 12–12 (A,B). Repair of a localized proximal aneurysm of the left subclavian artery using aortosubclavian bypass and closure of the aneurysmal neck.

All other aneurysms of the SA, including those of the proximal right SA, require an anterior approach, usually a median sternotomy. With large aneurysms, the CT scan may suggest attachment to the sternum, and in such cases it is wise to avoid the midsternotomy approach. Proximal control can be obtained through bilateral anterolateral thoracotomies, usually through the right second and left third or fourth intercostal spaces, and an oblique sternotomy. After proximal control is secured, distal arterial control is obtained in the neck through a separate incision. Once the aneurysm is isolated between clamps, the two incisions can be joined, with the upper half of the sternum being split longitudinally to gain direct access to the aneurysmal sac. A better solution to this unusual problem is femorofemoral cardiopulmonary bypass to induce deep hypothermia and circulatory arrest before opening the sternum through the midline. As soon as proximal control of the aneurysm is obtained, circulation and rewarming may be resumed rapidly unless there is some associated repair that needs to be done in the aorta itself.

Once proximal control of the trunk bearing the aneurysm has been obtained, either by clamping the artery itself or by exclusion-clamping of the aortic arch, the treatment is usually an interposition graft or a bypass graft from the neighboring aorta. Thrombus and debris are removed from within, and the wall is left in place to avoid injury to adjacent structures (e.g., the brachiocephalic vein, trachea, and esophagus). The graft suture is done from the inside, and the wall of the aneurysm is wrapped over the graft after flow is resumed. An alternative technique includes preliminary ascending aorta to distal IA bypass followed by partial exclusion clamping of the aorta around the origin of the IA and pledgetted closure of the latter.

Some aneurysms of the IA originate from large openings in the aortic arch that preclude exclusion-clamping of the aorta (Fig. 12–13). They may be best managed by median sternotomy, deep hypothermia, and circulatory arrest, replacing the mouth of the aneurysm on the aortic arch using a prosthetic patch to which an interposition graft has been attached. Alternatively, a bypass to the distal IA or both IA and left CCA may be implanted first in the proximal ascending aorta and the aortic arch repaired using partial cardiopulmonary bypass or even single aortic cross-clamping.

REOPERATIONS

Reoperations present special difficulties and often require innovative solutions. These solutions are different depending on the specific complications that prompt the reoperation (i.e., occlusion, infection, false aneurysm formation).[21,28]

Occlusion

Rarely a thrombectomy for an immediate postoperative occlusion, usually caused by a technical error, must be performed. In this case, the thrombectomy is followed by the surgeon revising the previous technical flaw or choosing a different corrective technique. With chronic occlusion, the choices are dictated by the general condition of the patient, the reappearance of previous symptoms, the arteriographic findings, and the type of operation and incision that were previously used.

Unless the patient presents a high surgical risk or some other contraindication to surgery, the best way to repair a failed intrathoracic reconstruction is through a second thoracotomy. Reopening the sternum requires care and the use of an oscillating saw. The sternum is pulled upward, using the ends of the previous wire of which only the anterior loop has been cut. When approaching the anterior portion of the aorta, it is

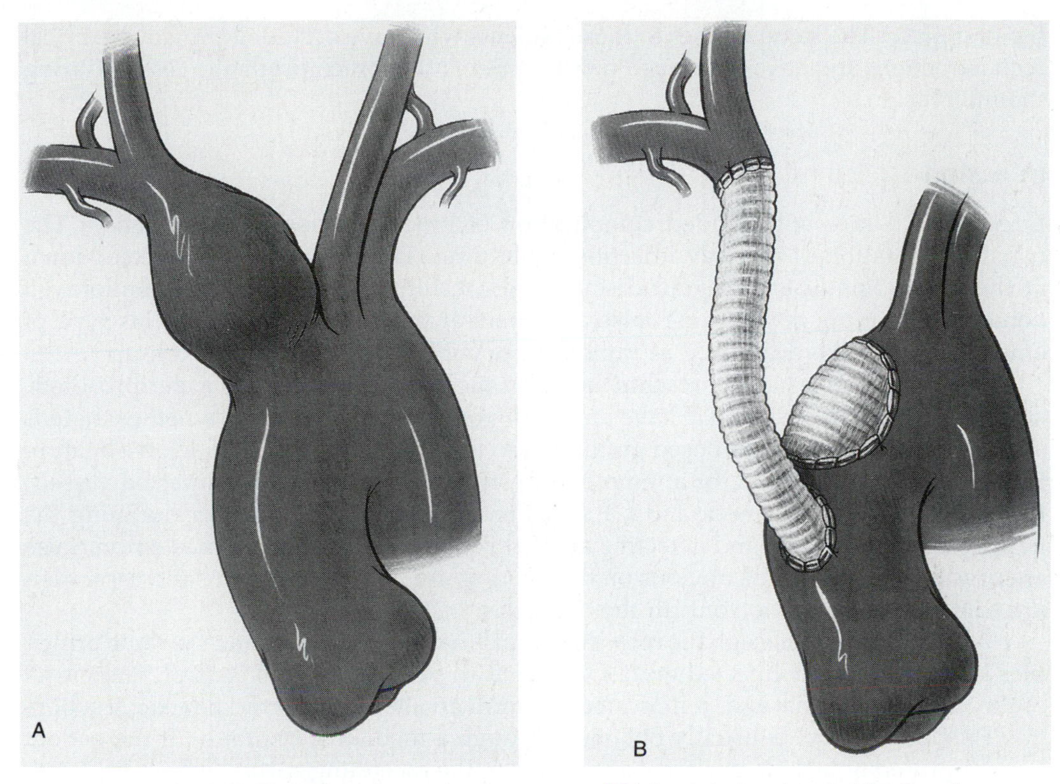

Figure 12–13 (A,B). Repair of a proximal aneurysm of the innominate artery that involves the transverse aortic arch using aortoinnominate artery bypass and patch closure of the aorta.

often helpful to enter both pleural cavities under the sternal edges to allow the heart and mediastinum to drop into the chest while the sternal edges are lifted.

If the previous operation was an endarterectomy of the IA, a good portion of ascending aorta should be available for insertion of a bypass. If the previous operation was a bypass from the ascending aorta, it is best to use the same site for proximal reimplantation. To accomplish this step, the occluded graft is transected and, using retrograde dissection, the previous anastomotic site is isolated by partial exclusion-clamping. The previous anastomosis is then excised and a new bypass inserted.

If the repeat sternotomy must be avoided because of a previous coronary vein graft or an internal mammary artery transposition, or if the patient has become a poor risk since the first operation, the alternative is a crossover cervical bypass. The latter can be done only if there is at least one patent brachiocephalic vessel that can be used as a source. If not, the alternative is an atypical reconstruction using other sources of inflow such as the descending or supraceliac aorta or even the iliac or common femoral arteries, as discussed previously.

If the thrombosis has taken place in a previous cervical repair, the repeat operation is normally done again in the neck. The specific choice of operation is dictated by what was done before. For instance, if the failed operation is a carotid–subclavian or subclavian–carotid bypass, the second operation should be an axillary–axillary or carotid–carotid bypass to avoid redissecting the supraclavicular fossa, a step fraught with a substantial rate of complications. A transthoracic approach should be considered in good-risk patients in whom failure of the cervical approach (because of disease of the inflow vessel) could have been averted had a transthoracic approach been used in the first place. The same applies to those patients who have occluded previous cervical reconstructions and have developed new lesions in other brachiocephalic vessels during the interval.

Infection

Infection is a rare but dreaded complication of brachiocephalic reconstruction. The usual presentation of an early infection is bleeding. The infected artery breaks down at the suture line or a vein graft disintegrates, resulting in a massive hemothorax, a hemomediastinum, or a leaking false aneurysm at the base of the neck. This type of emergency must be dealt with as rapidly as possible without further work-up.

Late infection usually presents as a chronic false aneurysm or a periprosthetic abscess. These patients should have an arteriogram not only to show whether there is a false aneurysm or a thrombosed graft but also to help the surgeon decide on a ligature technique versus the need for a remote reconstruction away from the infected vessels. Ultrasonography of the neck and CT scans of the chest are helpful for outlining the periprosthetic collection and detecting another proximal intrathoracic anastomotic false aneurysm that may not be obvious on the arteriogram. Needle puncture and aspiration are sometimes needed to confirm the diagnosis.

An infected brachiocephalic reconstruction is handled by following the same principles that apply to any infected graft. One needs to obtain proximal control, remove all of the infected material and, if indicated, perform an alternative arterial reconstruction.

Proximal control is usually obtained through a median sternotomy. If the patient has a ruptured or leaking proximal aneurysm on the ascending aorta, the best approach is to place the patient on cardiopulmonary bypass and deep hypothermia. Circulatory arrest is then undertaken immediately before opening the chest in order to avoid exsanguination during the repeat sternotomy incision. In most cases, however, control may be obtained without undue difficulty by using generous lateral clamping of the ascending aorta and pharmacologically induced hypotension. All prosthetic material is removed, and the gap in the ascending aorta is closed with large, interrupted, monofilament sutures buttressing the aortic wall between two fascial bands obtained from the sheath of the rectus abdominalis. If the infected mediastinum needs to be debrided, this step is followed either with continuous lavage through large drains or omentoplasty with or without primary closure of the sternum. Patients who survive often have residual sternal infection.

In the presence of infection, ligation of just one brachiocephalic vessel may result in complications. It is of course safe when the infected graft has thrombosed, and it is the only solution available when there is active bleeding associated with infection. Ligation and excision of one brachiocephalic vessel is reasonably safe in patients who have isolated SA or CCA artery reconstructions with patent arteries on the contralateral side and brisk carotid back-bleeding. However, in patients with multiple occlusive disease, the risk of stroke after ligation of just one brachiocephalic vessel is high. Patients with an infected reconstruction involving both CCAs or all three brachiocephalic vessels must have an alternative surgical reconstruction if a stroke is to be avoided.

This alternative revascularization can be performed *in situ* at the time of operation using either a fresh or cryopreserved allograft, or autogenous material such as saphenous vein graft or an arterial autograft. The latter may be fashioned from a superficial femoral artery that is either normal or was occluded and is endarterectomized at the time of the reconstruction. In the rare patient whose infected graft was originally done to correct an occlusion of the IA through a bypass from the ascending aorta to one of the branches of the IA (end-to-side) or through a crossover cervical bypass, the alternative of IA endarterectomy after excision of the infected graft should be entertained. If a patch is needed to close the arteriotomy, it can be fashioned from autogenous vein or artery.

The remote bypasses used to treat infected reconstructions of the brachiocephalic vessels include the remote cervical crossover bypasses or bypass from the descending aorta or the supraceliac aorta, iliac, or femoral arteries.

Aneurysms

Late, noninfected aneurysms following reconstruction of the brachiocephalic vessels are rare. Over a 20-year period we have seen only one patient with a noninfected false anastomotic aneurysm arising from a prosthetic bypass inserted into the ascending aorta. False aneurysms, however, have been seen at the distal anastomotic site of prosthetic aortocarotid grafts, especially when an ICA endarterectomy was performed simultaneously. They have also been seen in carotid–subclavian bypasses, on the subclavian side, probably caused by the notorious fragility of this artery and the mobility of the base of the neck. Late aneurysmal dilatation of vein grafts used for carotid–subclavian bypass has been reported. Noninfected false aneurysms in the carotid anastomosis of a prosthesis are treated by direct reconstruction. To avoid repeated dissection of the supraclavicular fossa, false aneurysms in the subclavian position are best dealt with by exclusion of the SA and use of the CCA to revascularize the VA (transposition) and as a source for a carotid–axillary artery bypass.

REFERENCES

1. Bahnson HT, Spencer FC, Quattelbaum JK. Surgical treatment of occlusive disease of the carotid artery. *Ann Surg.* 1959;149:711–720.
2. Cate WR Jr, Scott HW Jr. Cerebral ischemia of central origin: relief by subclavian–vertebral artery thromboendarterectomy. *Surgery.* 1959;45:19–31.
3. Davies JB, Grove WJ, Julian OC. Thrombotic occlusion of the branches of the aortic arch. Martorell syndrome: report of a case treated surgically. *Ann Surg.* 1956;144:124–126.
4. Hass WK, Fields WS, North RR, et al. Joint study of extracranial arterial occlusion, II: Arteriography, techniques, sites and complications. *JAMA.* 1968;203:961–968.
5. Brewster DC, Moncure AC, Darling RC, et al. Innominate artery lesions: problems encountered and lessons learned. *J Vasc Surg.* 1985;2:99–112.
6. Cherry K Jr, McCullough JL, Hallett JW Jr, et al. Technical principles of direct innominate artery revascularization: a comparison of endarterectomy and bypass grafts. *J Vasc Surg.* 1989;9:718–724.
7. Cormier F, Ward A, Cormier JM, et al. Long-term results of aortoinnominate and aortocarotid polytetrafluoroethylene bypass grafting for atherosclerotic lesions. *J Vasc Surg.* 1989; 10:135–142.
8. Crawford ES, DeBakey ME, Morris GC Jr, et al. Surgical treatment of occlusion of the innominate, common carotid and subclavian arteries: a 10-year experience. *Surgery.* 1969;65:17–31.
9. Crawford ES, Stowe CL, Powers RW Jr. Occlusion of the innominate, common carotid and subclavian arteries: long-term results of surgical treatment. *Surgery.* 1983;94:781–791.
10. Evans W, Williams T, Hayes JP. Aortobrachiocephalic reconstruction. *Am J Surg.* 1988;156:100–102.
11. Kieffer E, Sabatier J, Koskas F, et al. Atherosclerotic innominate artery occlusive disease: early and long-term results of surgical reconstruction. *J Vasc Surg.* 1995;21:326–337.

12. Najafi H, Javid H, Hunter JA, et al. Occlusive diseases of the branches of the aortic arch. In: Bergan JJ, Yao JST, eds. *Surgery of the Aorta and Its Body Branches.* New York: Grune and Stratton; 1979:191–203.
13. Reul GJ, Jacobs MJHM, Gregoric ID, et al. Innominate artery occlusive disease: surgical approach and long-term results. *J Vasc Surg.* 1991;14:405–412.
14. Schroeder T, Buchardt Hansen HJ. Arterial reconstruction of the brachiocephalic trunk and the subclavian arteries: 10 years' experience with a follow-up study. *Acta Chir Scand.* 1980;502:122–130.
15. Vogt DP, Hertzer NR, O'Hara PJ, et al. Brachiocephalic arterial reconstruction. *Ann Surg.* 1982;196:541–552.
16. Zelenock GB, Cronenwett JL, Graham LM, et al. Brachiocephalic arterial occlusions and stenoses: manifestations and management of complex lesions. *Arch Surg.* 1985;120:370–376.
17. Kieffer E. Chirurgie des troncs supra-aortiques. In: *Techniques Chirurgicales: Chirurgie Vasculaire.* Paris: Encyclopedie Medicochirurgicale;1987:1–20.
18. Thevenet A. Surgical management of atheroma of the aortic dome and origin of supra-aortic trunks. *World J Surg.* 1979;3:187–195.
19. Kieffer E, Natali J. Supraaortic trunk lesions in Takayasu's arteritis. In: Bergaı. JJ, Yao JST, eds. *Cerebrovascular Insufficiency.* New York: Grune and Stratton, 1983:395–415.
20. Kieffer E, Bahnini A, Koskas F. Aberrant subclavian artery: surgical treatment in thirty-three adult patients. *J Vasc Surg.* 1994;19:100–111.
21. Berguer R, Kieffer E. *Surgery of the Arteries to the Head.* New York: Springer-Verlag, 1992.
22. Selle JG, Cook JW, Elliott CM, et al. Simultaneous revascularization for complex brachiocephalic and coronary artery disease. *Surgery.* 1981;90:97–101.
23. Vermeulen FEE, Hamerlijnck RPHM, Defauw JJAM, et al. Synchronous operation for ischemic cardiac and cerebrovascular disease: early results and long-term follow-up. *Ann Thorac Surg.* 1992;53:381–390.
24. Carlson RE, Ehrenfeld WK, Stoney RJ, et al. Innominate artery endarterectomy: a 16-year experience. *Arch Surg.* 1977;112:1389–1393.
25. Sandmann W, Kniemeyer HW, Jaeschok R, et al. The role of subclavian–carotid transposition in surgery for supra-aortic occlusive disease. *J Vasc Surg.* 1987;5:53–58.
26. Berguer R, Gonzales JA. Revascularization by the retropharyngeal route for extensive disease of the extracranial arteries. *J Vasc Surg.* 1994;19:217–225.
27. Thevenet A, Chaptal PA, Negre E. L'arret circulatoire en hypothermie profonde dans la chirurgie des branches de la crosse aortique. *Ann Chir Thorac Cardiovasc.* 1968;7:69–71.
28. Kieffer E, Petitjean C, Bahnini A. Surgery of failed brachiocephalic reconstructions. In: Bergan JJ, Yao JST, eds. *Reoperative Arterial Surgery.* New York: Grune and Stratton, 1986:581–607.

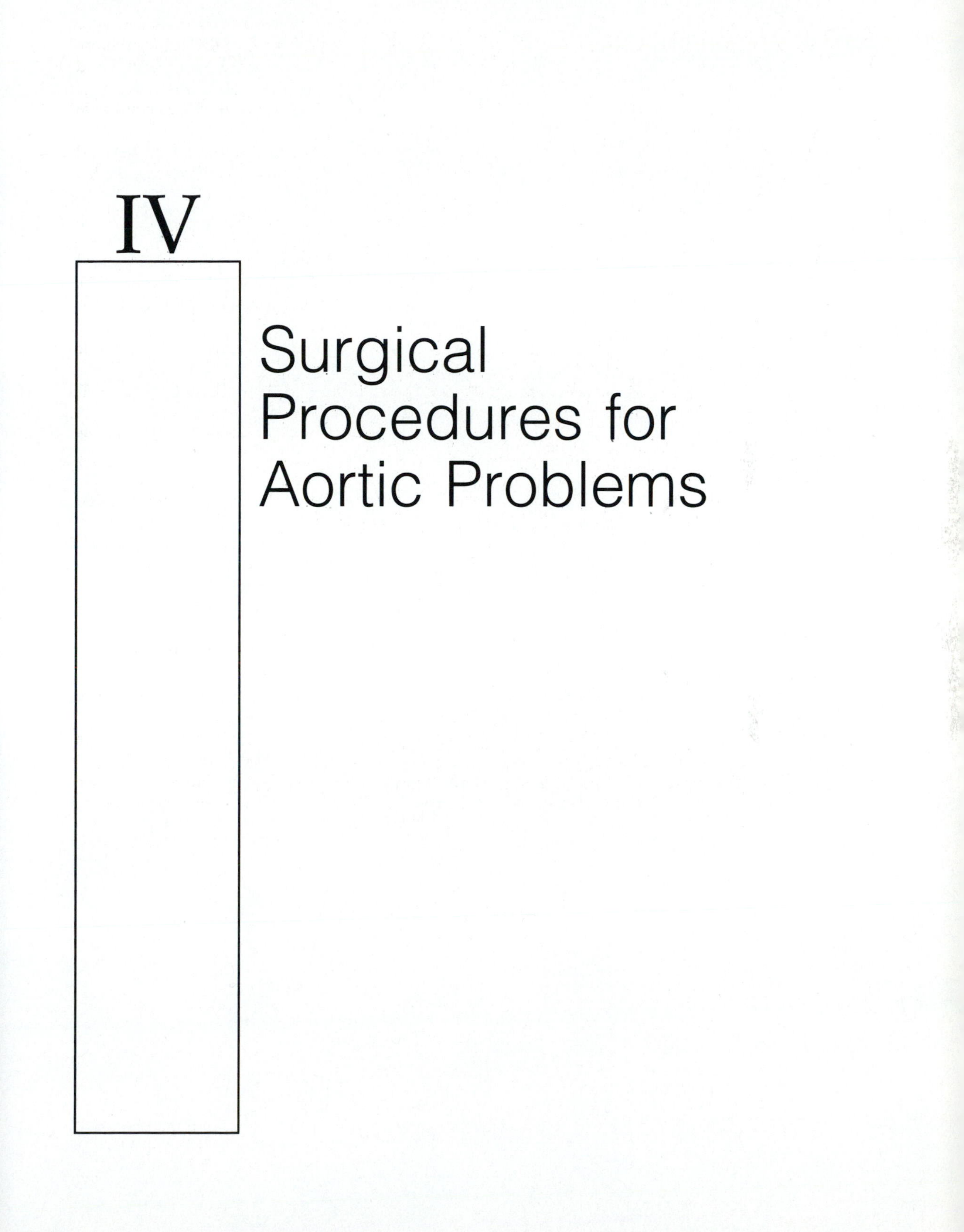

IV

Surgical Procedures for Aortic Problems

13

Transperitoneal Medial Visceral Rotation

Ronald J. Stoney, MD, Jean W. Gillon, MD, and Steven M. Santilli, MD, PhD

The traditional surgical exposure of abdominal aortic disease does not offer cephalad extension to the upper abdominal aorta and its branches because of overlying organs. A newer technique to achieve more extensive exposure of the proximal abdominal aorta permits surgical repair of both obstructive and aneurysmal disease involving this region. A number of reports describe the evolution of this method of aortic exposure. DeBakey et al., in 1956,[1] first described unrestricted access to the thoracoabdominal aorta for repair of aneurysmal disease, using left-to-right medial visceral rotation and left thoracotomy. In 1967 Shirkey et al.[2] described left medial visceral rotation anterior to the left kidney in order to expose and repair an injury to the proximal superior mesenteric artery. Subsequently, Buscaglia et al.[3] used left medial visceral rotation to obtain optimal exposure for penetrating abdominal vascular injury advocating a plane anterior to the left kidney to expose the aorta. They proposed an optional dissection plane posterior to the left kidney for exposure of the posterolateral aorta. Finally, they described right-to-left medial visceral rotation for exposure of inferior vena cava injuries, but they did not describe any experience.[4–6] These exposures have become routine in the management of abdominal vascular injuries but vascular surgeons have rarely used these exposures for upper abdominal aortic disease. Crawford[7] first used medial visceral rotation as part of a thoracoabdominal approach to complex aneurysms of the upper abdominal and thoracoabdominal aorta.

Our original approach for exposure of this portion of the abdominal aorta began with a combination of the thoracoabdominal incision described by DeBakey et al.[8] and the retroperitoneal approach first used by Dubost et al.[9] for the repair of an abdominal aortic aneurysm. Although exposure of the aorta was satisfactory, the pulmonary morbidity was increased with this two-cavity exposure. This stimulated interest in achieving unrestricted access to the proximal abdominal aorta and its branches exclusively using an abdominal approach.

Initially we evaluated a left subchondral incision with left medial rotation of the viscera in an extraperitoneal plane. Since prospective studies showed no superiority of retroperitoneal versus transperitoneal aortic exposure,[10] we adopted a traditional transabdominal midline incision combined with medial visceral rotation. The experience with transperitoneal medial visceral rotation continues to the present and has convinced us that it provides the ultimate exposure of the entire abdominal aorta and its branches. This chapter describes the anatomy, surgical techniques, and the strategies designed to meet all revascularization requirements of the entire abdominal aorta and its branches.

INDICATIONS

Transperitoneal medial visceral rotation is selected whenever the infracolic exposure of juxta- or pararenal aortic disease is inadequate and a thoracoabdominal exposure unnecessary. Occlusive and aneurysmal disease of the aorta are ideally managed using this exposure, although aneurysmal disease is the most frequent pathologic indication. Because this technique allows consistent, unrestricted aortic exposure, it has encouraged wider application of this approach in the pararenal segment of the upper abdominal aorta. This surgical exposure allows unlimited reconstruction options to manage complex aortic disease. For patients who have undergone prior aortic or other intra-abdominal procedures, transperitoneal medial visceral rotation offers a surgical route free of scar, avoiding tedious dissections and potential organ injury.

LEFT MEDIAL VISCERAL ROTATION

A standard full-length midline transabdominal incision is employed followed by a careful abdominal exploration. The small bowel is then enclosed in an intestinal bag and displaced to the right. The descending and sigmoid colon are mobilized in the standard manner by incising the lateral peritoneal reflection (Fig. 13–1). This incision is carried cephalad through the phrenocolic and lienorenal ligaments (Fig. 13–2). Using gentle dissection, a plane is developed between the pancreas and Gerota's fascia as the descending colon, pancreas, spleen, and stomach are then rotated anteromedially. The left lobe of the liver is mobilized by dividing its triangular ligament and it is gently retracted to the right while the gonadal vein, ureter, left kidney, left renal vein, and adrenal vein remain in situ (Fig. 13–3). It is imperative to remain in the correct bloodless plane during the mobilization; this will avoid pancreatic or adrenal injury as well as unwanted bleeding. The spleen, pancreas, and left lobe of the liver are protected with moistened pads and the table mounted Omni-Tract Self-Retaining Retractor System is positioned to hold all of the displaced viscera to the right. The peritoneum is reflected from the left crus of the diaphragm and the esophagogastric ligament is preserved to protect the vegas nerve. The aorta is now clearly visualized, crossed only by the left renal vein, the autonomic ganglion tissue, and proximally by the left crus of the diaphragm.

The upper abdominal aorta requires further adjuncts for complete circumferential exposure. Complete mobilization of the left renal vein from the inferior vena cava to the left renal hilus allows wide cephalad and caudad displacement of this structure over the aorta (Fig. 13–4). This maneuver facilitates the mobilization of the origin of the right renal artery and the full length of the left renal artery as needed. Lateral retraction of the inferior vena cava improves exposure of the proximal right renal artery as well.

In order to more fully expose the visceral branches, the dense autonomic ganglion tissue overlying the left anterior surface of the aorta is incised and mobilized. The

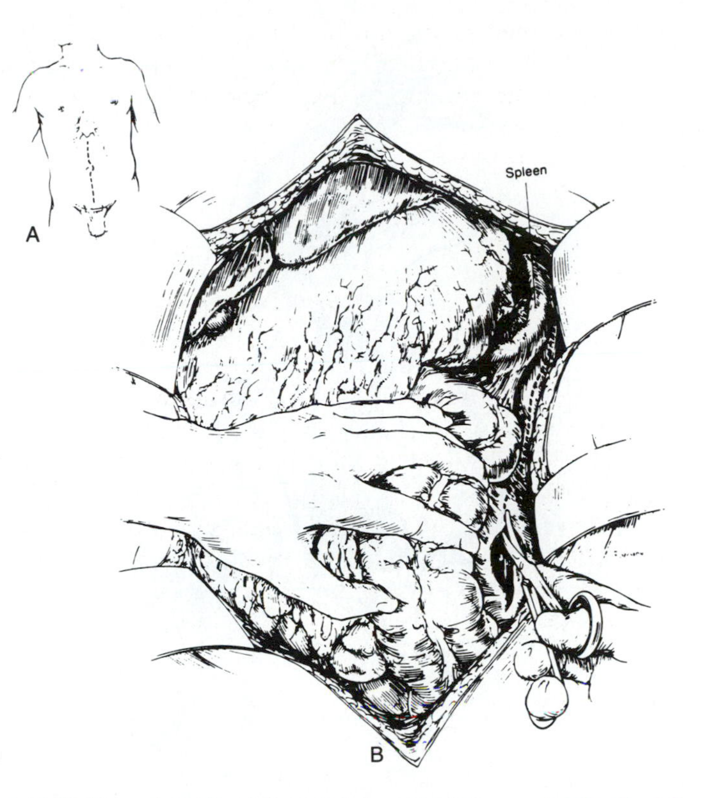

Figure 13–1 (A,B). Transabdominal left medial visceral rotation—retracting the left colon. *(Reprinted with permission from Murray SP, Kuestner LM, Stoney RJ. Transperitoneal medial visceral rotation. Ann Vas Surg. 1995;9:209–216.)*

dissection in the plane of Leriche allows the initial visualization of the upper abdominal aorta and continues with division of the arcuate ligament of the diaphragm. Separation of the muscular fibers of the left crus of the diaphragm allows exposure of the distal thoracic aorta within the lower mediastinum (Fig. 13–5).

The infrarenal abdominal aorta can be further mobilized by incising the loose areolar tissue along its left lateral surface. Reflection of this tissue to the right reveals the origin of the inferior mesenteric artery with the course of this vessel now vertical as a result of the displacement of the left colon. The aortic bifurcation and proximal iliac arteries are easily exposed if necessary. The left common and external iliac arteries as well as the right common iliac artery to its bifurcation can be exposed from a left medial visceral rotation.

The exposure provided by this approach offers a sector of view of the aorta from left of the midline rather than the vertical midline orientation often seen in infrarenal aortic surgery. This is not thought to be a disadvantage but one should recognize the angle of approach to the aorta from the left rather than from the vertical position. For the surgeon, this often means taking a position on the left side of the patient to take advantage of this orientation. The proximal limitations are the distal quarter of the thoracic aorta; the distal limitations are the left external iliac artery as it passes under the inguinal ligament and the right common iliac artery bifurcation. The right renal artery is not easily exposed beyond its origin. The aorta itself can be circumferentially mobilized from above the aortic hiatus to its bifurcation including all intervening branches.

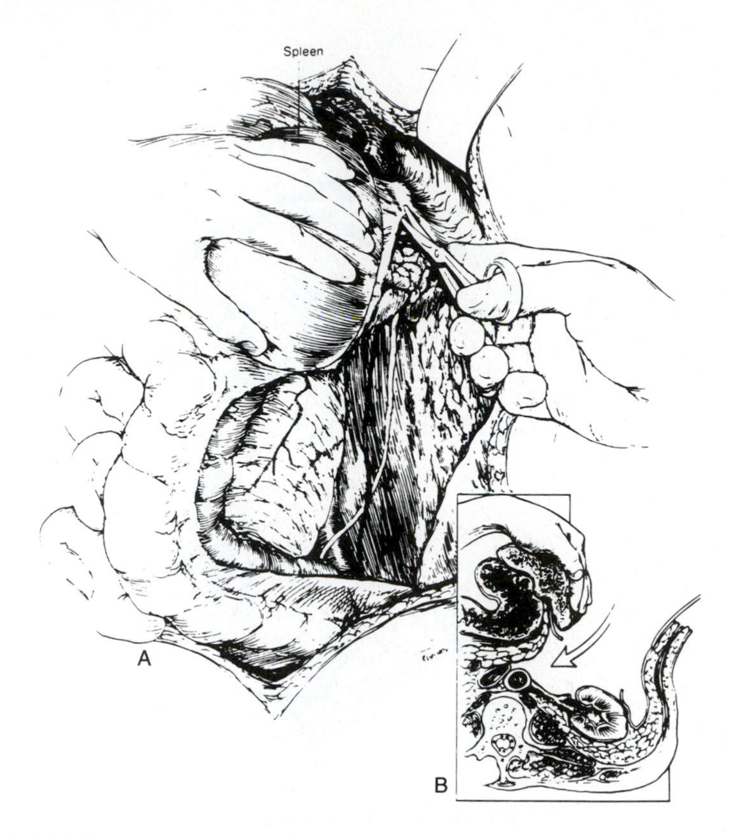

Figure 13–2 (A,B). Transabdominal left medial visceral rotation—incising the lateral peritoneum. *(Reprinted with permission from Murray SP, Kuestner LM, Stoney RJ. Transperitoneal medial visceral rotation. Ann Vas Surg. 1995;9:209–216.)*

MODIFIED LEFT MEDIAL VISCERAL ROTATION

The technique of transabdominal left medial visceral rotation can be modified according to the required level of aortic exposure and the planned revascularization. Exposure of the pararenal aorta for aneurysmal or occlusive disease can be performed in a plane posterior to the left kidney. This is particularly advantageous for large aneurysms involving the upper abdominal aorta as the exposure of the posterolateral aorta between the renal artery and the edge of the lumbar spine is simplified (Fig. 13–6).

When the proximal extent of the required aortic exposure is in the pararenal segment below the superior mesenteric artery, the medial visceral rotation can be confined to the colon leaving the pancreas, spleen, and stomach *in situ*. This results in a partial, or limited, left medial visceral rotation. The incision in the lateral peritoneal reflection extends only up to the splenic flexure dividing the phrenocolic ligament but leaving the lineorenal ligament intact. Next, the lineocolic ligament is divided, which allows the splenic flexure and descending colon to be displaced anteriorly and medially. The perirenal and infrarenal aorta can then be generously exposed as previously described.

COMPLICATIONS

Complications associated with this exposure are either anatomic or related to limitations of the mobilized aorta and its branches.

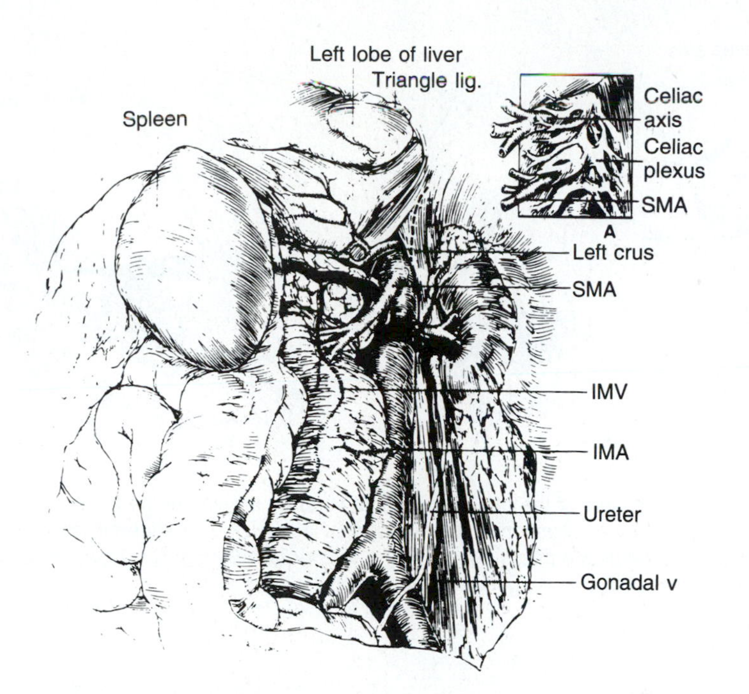

Figure 13–3. Illustration showing aortic exposure following left medial visceral rotation anterior to the left kidney. IMA = inferior mesenteric artery; IMV = inferior mesenteric vein; SMA = superior mesenteric artery. *(Reprinted with permission from Murray SP, Kuestner LM, Stoney RJ. Transperitoneal medial visceral rotation. Ann Vas Surg. 1995;9:209–216.)*

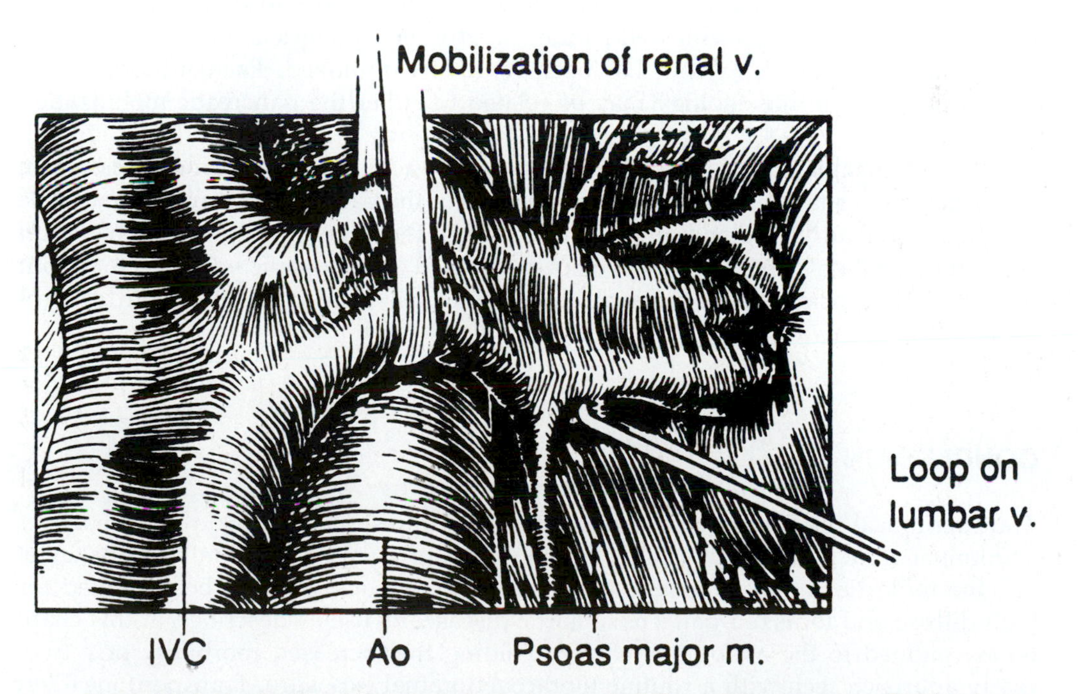

Figure 13–4. Mobilization of the left renal vein. Ao = aorta; IVC = inferior vena cava. *(Reprinted with permission from Murray SP, Kuestner LM, Stoney RJ. Transperitoneal medial visceral rotation. Ann Vas Surg. 1995;9:209–216.)*

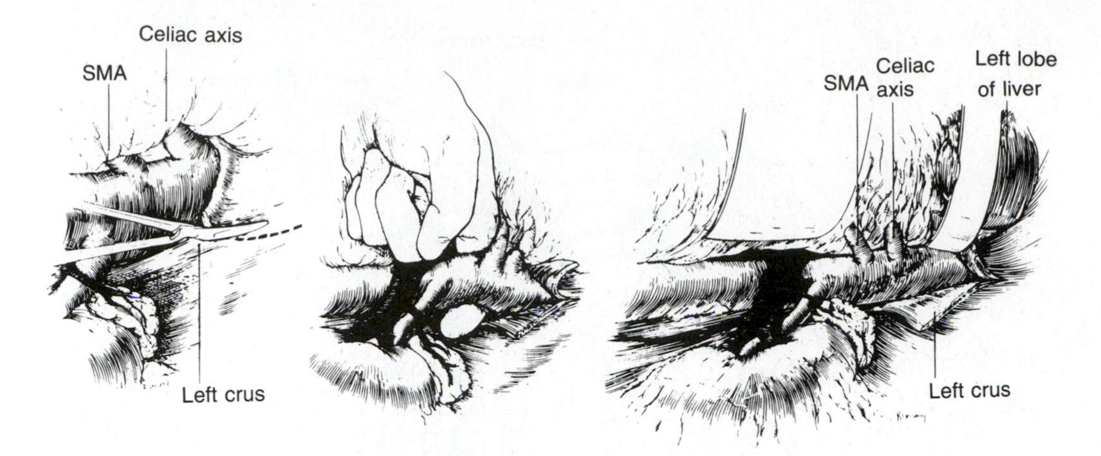

Figure 13–5. Exposure of the upper abdominal aorta by division of the left crus of diaphragm and circumferential mobilization of the suprarenal aorta. SMA = superior mesenteric artery. *(Reprinted with permission from Murray SP, Kuestner LM, Stoney RJ. Transperitoneal medial visceral rotation. Ann Vas Surg. 1995;9:209–216.)*

The spleen is the solid organ most vulnerable to operative trauma during medial visceral rotation. The spleen must be mobilized and the phrenocolic and lineocolic ligament divided so that the spleen and tail of pancreas can be mobilized and retracted medially and anteriorly. Iatrogenic splenectomy occurs in our experience in about one-fourth of patients requiring this approach.[11] The mobilization and retraction of the pancreas are necessary but are potential maneuvers that may cause pancreatic injury. Retraction of the pancreas with well-padded laparotomy sponges using the Omni-Tract Self-Retaining Retractor System has been routinely employed. Pacreatitis occurs in 2% of patients, and the etiology may be related to either the pancreatic mobilization or retraction.[11]

The adrenal gland and its venous tributaries are adjacent to the plane of dissection between Gerota's fascia and the posterior surface of the pancreas. It is usually possible to mobilize the adrenal gland and separate it from the edge of the aorta to make full aortic mobilization possible. We have not performed an iatrogenic adrenalectomy but have had two incidences of adrenal bleeding, which were controlled with electrocautery.[11]

CONCLUSION

Transperitoneal medial visceral rotation provides unrestricted exposure of the upper abdominal aorta and its major branches. Since the original description by DeBakey et al.[1], the indications and technique of medial visceral rotation have been refined for both diffuse and localized patterns of aortic disease. Its use as described in this chapter is confined to the abdominal cavity avoiding the increased morbidity of a two-cavity approach seen with a routine thoracoabdominal exposure. Transperitoneal left medial visceral rotation with the Omni-Tract Self-Retaining Retractor System provides superior exposure of the abdominal aorta for all reconstruction options required.

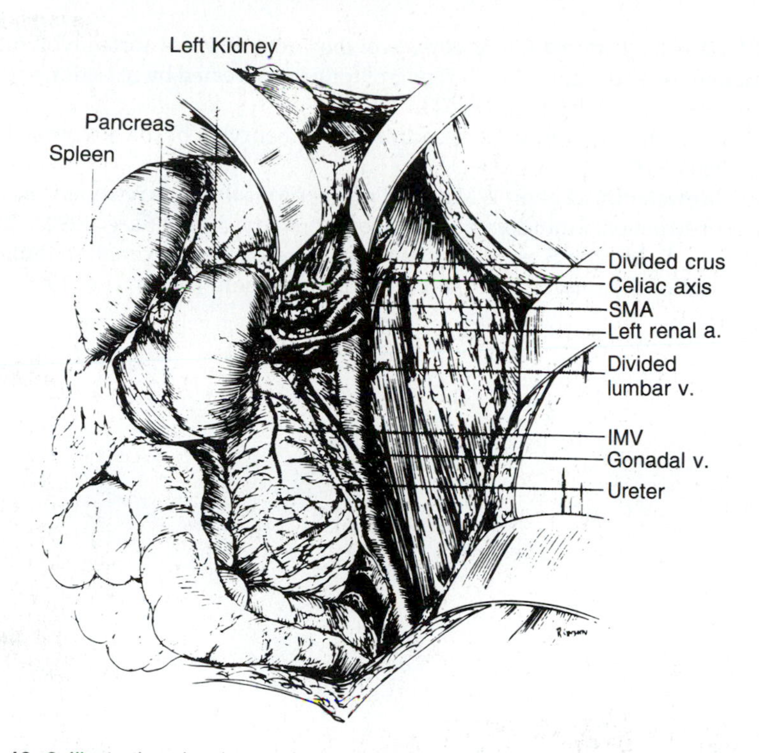

Figure 13–6. Illustration showing aortic exposure following left medial visceral rotation posterior to the left kidney. IMV = inferior mesenteric vein; SMA = superior mesenteric artery. *(Reprinted with permission from Murray SP, Kuestner LM, Stoney RJ. Transperitoneal medial visceral rotation. Ann Vas Surg. 1995;9:209–216.)*

Supported in part by the Pacific Vascular Research Foundation in San Francisco, California.

REFERENCES

1. DeBakey M, Creech OJ, Morris GJ. Aneurysm of thoracoabdominal aorta involving the celiac, superior mesenteric and renal arteries: report of four cases treated by resection and homograft replacement. *Ann Surg.* 1956;144:549–573.
2. Shirkey A, Quast D, Jordan GJ. Superior mesenteric artery division and intestinal function. *J Trauma.* 1967;7:7–24.
3. Buscaglia L, Blaisdell F, Lim RJ. Penetrating abdominal vascular injuries. *Arch Surg.* 1969;99:764–769.
4. Mattox K, McCollum W, Jordan GJ, et al. Management of upper abdominal vascular trauma. *Am J Surg.* 1974;128:823–828.
5. Hunt T, Leeds R, Wanebo H, et al. Arteriovenous fistulas of major vessels in the abdomen. *J Trauma.* 1971;11:483–493.
6. Elkins R, DeMeester T, Brawley RK. Surgical exposure of the upper abdominal aorta and its branches. *Surgery.* 1971;70:622–627.
7. Crawford E. Thoraco-abdominal and abdominal aortic aneurysms involving renal, superior mesenteric, and celiac arteries. *Ann Surg.* 1974;179:763–772.

8. DeBakey M, Creech OJ, Morris GJ. Aneurysm of thoracoabdominal aorta involving the celiac, superior mesenteric and renal arteries: report of four cases treated by resection and homograft replacement. *Ann Surg.* 1956;144:549–573.
9. Dubost C, Allary M, Osconomos N. Resection of an aneurysm of the abdominal aorta. *Arch Surg.* 1952;64:405–408.
10. Cambria RP, Brewster DC, Abbott WM, et al. Transperitoneal versus retroperitoneal approach for aortic reconstruction: a randomized prospective study. *J Vasc Surg.* 1990;11:314–325.
11. Reilly L, Ramos T, Murray S, et al. Optimal exposure of the proximal abdominal aorta: a critical appraisal of transabdominal medial visceral rotation. *J Vasc Surg.* 1994;19:375–390.

14

Surgical Techniques in the Repair of Inflammatory Aneurysms

Robert B. Rutherford, MD

Inflammatory abdominal aortic aneurysms (IAAAs) are not rare, averaging 6.1% (range 3% to 12%) in a dozen articles from the recent literature.[1-12] They have now been well characterized clinically, by many series reported in the past three decades, to have a number of typical tendencies, for example, to be larger and more frequently symptomatic (pain, weight loss) than abdominal aortic aneurysms (AAAs) without inflammatory change. Erythrocyte sedimentation rate (ESR) is often elevated, and tagged white blood cell scans may be positive without there being true infection. Ureteral involvement is not uncommon (about 25%) and in addition, duodenal, left renal vein, and iliocaval involvement in the inflammatory reaction create technical problems leading to a higher operative mortality and morbidity rate. As a result, IAAAs are considered a technical challenge, one of the foremost facing vascular surgeons today. This chapter focuses on the technical aspects of surgical repair in recognition of these difficulties; however, without belittling the challenges posed by IAAAs, it is important to point out at the outset that most of these can and should be avoided by accurate preoperative diagnosis, as well as knowledge of the technical pitfalls and their best means of avoidance. Unfortunately, IAAAs are often first experienced unexpectedly by a surgeon unprepared for the challenge, which may thereby become a strained encounter of the worst kind. Stated differently, knowing in advance that this condition exists allows even the relatively inexperienced surgeon to research, plan, and execute a safer technical approach.

PREOPERATIVE EVALUATION AND PREPARATION

Computed tomography (CT) has now replaced aortography as the preferred "routine" diagnostic study in the preoperative evaluation of AAAs. This is because most of the information obtained by aortography can be determined intraoperatively or is captured when selective indications for aortography are employed, whereas CT scan yields additional important information that might be missed by aortography and that may

This chapter is reprinted with permission from Yao JST, Pearce WH, eds. *Aneurysms: New Findings and Treatments.* Norwalk, CT: Appleton & Lange; 1994.

influence the operative approach, for example, presence of horseshoe or ectopic kidney, caval/renal vein anomalies, and, of course, inflammatory aneurysm. Ultrasound is a good test for aneurysm screening, sizing, and serial follow-up, but it only suggests the presence of IAAA in one-third or less of cases.[13] CT scan may not be as good as magnetic resonance imaging (MRI) in detecting subtler degrees of periaortic inflammation,[14] but essentially will detect all inflammatory changes sufficient to produce technical difficulties. Additional serial cuts should be obtained as needed to be sure that the extent of both the aneurysm and the inflammatory reaction is well delineated. Because the inflammatory reaction limits the surgeon's ability to palpate major branches of the abdominal aorta, aortography is helpful and should also be obtained. Furthermore, one can take advantage of the contrast medium administered for this study to obtain excretory urography at the same time and, thus, have definitive information regarding ureteral involvement. Even in the absence of ureteral involvement, however, the author prefers to have ureteral catheters placed prior to operation on IAAAs. Other aspects of preoperative evaluations and testing are generic for AAA repair and are discussed elsewhere in this issue.

TECHNICAL CONSIDERATIONS

The main difficulties encountered in the repair of IAAAs are (1) injuring the duodenum or left renal veins in dissecting them away to allow exposure of the proximal neck of the aneurysm; (2) damaging a ureter either because one is unaware that it is often drawn medially, closer to the lateral aspect of the AAA, by the inflammatory reaction, or in attempting to perform ureterolysis when it is partially obstructed; and (3) injuring the iliac veins (or ureters) while obtaining distal (iliac artery) control. Although these are potential pitfalls of any AAA repair, their likelihood is greatly magnified by the surrounding inflammatory response, which usually is not limited just to the anterior surface of the main body of the AAA. As will be apparent, the best approach is willful avoidance of these vulnerable structures, both by choice of incision and approach and by avoiding direct dissection of these structures where possible.

Choice of Incision

In most but not all instances, when the diagnosis of IAAA has been made preoperatively, a left retroperitoneal approach should be chosen, because the worst inflammatory reaction is primarily located anteriorly and, to some extent, laterally.[15] Choosing this incision allows a posterolateral approach where the inflammatory reaction is least, avoids dissection of the duodenum (which lies 180 degrees away and thus is not even seen), and allows the left renal vein to be mobilized upward with the kidney and away from the aneurysm neck. Generic contraindications to this approach, primarily those involving the need for extended right-sided exposure (e.g., to deal with a right iliac aneurysm), obviously apply to this choice of incision. If a retroperitoneal incision is contraindicated or when the standard direct frontal approach has been chosen unaware that the AAA is inflammatory in type, dissection may be continued in the usual fashion, if the inflammatory response is reasonably limited, or, if it is not, complete or partial medial visceral rotation may be used to gain advantages similar to those of the left retroperitoneal approach. The basic details of each of these approaches are well described elsewhere.[16]

Proximal Control

With medial visceral rotation or the left retroperitoneal approach, the kidney may be mobilized upward and medially with the rest of the viscera. This is preferable if the inflammatory process extends up to the left renal vein to allow safer proximal dissection and clamp placement. When a left posterolateral approach to the aneurysm and its proximal neck is used, the duodenum is far away from the line of dissection. This approach may not be necessary with lesser degrees of inflammatory reaction proximally but, if, for this or other reasons, the dissection proceeds anteriorly, no attempt should be made to dissect the duodenum away from the aorta. It should be left in place and the aorta incised away from it. Another option to avoid getting into difficulties with the duodenum and left renal vein when using a frontal approach is to expose and control the aorta at the diaphragm, approaching it through the lesser sac and opening the fibers of the left crus.

Distal Control

The extent of the aortic aneurysm, or more specifically any iliac aneurysmal component, dictates the site of distal control. With no iliac aneurysms present, and with either use of the retroperitoneal approach or mobilization of the sigmoid colon to the right, the left common iliac artery is usually readily controlled and clamped. Often, in such circumstances, the right common iliac artery is best controlled intraluminally using a Foley balloon catheter. Otherwise, the inflammatory reaction may dictate more distal exposure at the iliac bifurcation(s).

If the iliac artery orifices are too widely separated to readily be accommodated by circumferential anastomosis of the same-diameter prosthesis as fits the proximal aneurysm neck, a short-stemmed bifurcation graft can be used, even though there is no need for formal iliac reconstruction. With the direct frontal approach, distal control at the iliac bifurcations is preferable, regardless of iliac involvement with aneurysmal change, to stay well below the lower extent of the inflammatory reaction, in the face of which iatrogenic bleeding from the iliac veins would be catastrophic.

Opening the Aneurysm

After heparin administration and proximal and distal cross-clamping, the aneurysm is opened longitudinally in the usual linear fashion if one is approaching it posterolaterally (i.e., via the left retroperitoneal approach or using medial visceral rotation). The duodenum is not a problem here. But when the aneurysm is approached directly anteriorly, the duodenum must be widely skirted when the aneurysm is opened. Electrocautery is useful in dividing the vascular shell of an IAAA, applying it slowly with cutting current to the outer layers before finally entering the lumen. If the edge of the duodenum cannot be seen, the additional thickness it adds to the aortic surface can best be felt using a finger inside the lumen, inserted from below. It is safer if the aneurysm is first opened lower down on its anterior surface and the intramural clot is evacuated before proceeding upward, and then only as far as needed for exposure of the aneurysm neck, staying well to the left of the midline and away from the duodenum.

Once the aneurysm is sufficiently opened to visualize the proximal neck and distal cuff(s), and the patent (lumbar) collaterals are sutured closed, aneurysm repair proceeds in standard fashion; the prosthesis is sutured in place from within the lumen, in the universally accepted manner popularized by DeBakey. Closure of the shell is performed as completely as possible, but may be difficult considering the thickness of the aneurysm shell and the fixed position of the duodenum. Incomplete closure is not a problem with the posterolateral approach. The replaced viscera are protected. Even with an anterior approach, the duodenum may well be protected from contact with the prosthesis by its adherence to the aneurysm shell or neck, provided it is avoided during closure. Otherwise, the use of an omental pedicle may prevent the surgeon from compromising the accepted principle of avoiding contact between the prosthesis and the duodenum or other viscera.

REFERENCES

1. Leseche G, Schaetz A, Arrive L, et al. Diagnosis and management of 17 consecutive patients with inflammatory abdominal aortic aneurysm. *Am J Surg.* 1992;164:39–44.
2. Rose AG, Dent DM. Inflammatory variant of abdominal atherosclerotic aneurysm. *Arch Pathol Lab Med.* 1981;105:409–413.
3. Moosa HH, Peitzman AB, Steed DL, et al. Inflammatory aneurysms of the abdominal aorta. *Arch Surg.* 1989;124:673–675.
4. Hall RG, Coupland GA, Appleberg M. Inflammatory aneurysms of the abdominal aorta. *Aust N Z J Surg.* 1985;55:189–193.
5. Luna G, Cole CW, Choi J, et al. Inflammatory aneurysms of the abdominal aorta. *Can J Surg.* 1990;33:197–200.
6. Fiorani P, Bondanini S, Faraglia V, et al. Clinical and therapeutical evaluation of inflammatory aneurysms of the abdominal aorta. *Int Angiol.* 1986;5:49–53.
7. Boontje AH, van den Dungen JJ, Blanksma C. Inflammatory abdominal aortic aneurysms. *J Cardiovasc Surg (Torino).* 1990;31:611–616.
8. Sterpetti AV, Hunter WJ, Feldhaus RJ, et al. Inflammatory aneurysms of the abdominal aorta: incidence, pathologic, and etiologic considerations. *J Vasc Surg.* 1989;9:643–650.
9. Pennell RC, Hollier LH, Lie JT, et al. Inflammatory abdominal aortic aneurysms: a thirty-year review. *J Vasc Surg.* 1985;2:859–869.
10. Savarese RP, Rosenfeld JC, DeLaurentis DA. Inflammatory abdominal aortic aneurysm. *Surg Gynecol Obstet.* 1986;162:405–410.
11. Hill J, Charlesworth D. Inflammatory abdominal aortic aneurysms: a report of thirty-seven cases. *Ann Vasc Surg.* 1988;2:352–357.
12. Kniemeyer HW, Kolvenbach R, Rohde E, et al. Inflammatory aneurysm of the aorta: diagnosis, therapy, results. *Chirurg.* 1990;61:27–31.
13. Fitzgerald EJ, Blackett RL. Inflammatory abdominal aortic aneurysms. *Clin Radiol.* 1988;39:247–251.
14. Tennant WG, Hartnell GG, Baird RN, et al. Inflammatory aortic aneurysms: characteristic appearance on magnetic resonance imaging. *Eur J Vasc Surg.* 1992;6:399–402.
15. Metcalf RK, Rutherford RB. Inflammatory abdominal aortic aneurysm: an indication for the retroperitoneal approach. *Surgery.* 1991;109:555–557.
16. Rutherford RB. *Atlas of Vascular Surgery: Basic Techniques and Exposures.* Philadelphia: WB Saunders; 1993.

15

Management of Special Problems Associated with Abdominal Aortic Aneurysm

Spencer Galt, MD, and Walter McCarthy, MD

Abdominal aortic aneurysm (AAA) repair is most commonly performed by direct intraluminal graft replacement of the aneurysm without excision. This procedure is the standard of practice with which surgeons are well acquainted. In a majority of patients, the procedure is relatively uniform. However, there is a small but significant subset of patients in whom unusual circumstances may modify operative management. This chapter reviews some of these special circumstances, including coexistent intra-abdominal tumors, infrarenal venous anomalies, left renal vein division, supraceliac control of the aorta, and aortic surgery for patients with abdominal wall stomata.

COEXISTENT INTRA-ABDOMINAL MALIGNANCY

Patients with simultaneous AAA and other intra-abdominal pathology are not commonly encountered, but any busy surgeon is bound to face this dilemma periodically. In general, there is a paucity of literature concerning management of AAA and coexistent intra-abdominal malignancy. This is largely a reflection of the relative rarity of the situation, leaving appropriate management strategies ill defined. Naturally, no randomized trials are published. Therefore, detailed knowledge of the natural history of both the aneurysm and malignancy, along with a healthy dose of common sense, is necessary to achieve optimal outcomes. The following summarizes the available literature and conveys the philosophy followed at Northwestern University Medical School, Chicago, Illinois.

Colorectal Carcinoma

It is the rare patient who suffers simultaneous colorectal carcinoma and AAA, yet this is likely the most common simultaneous malignancy. Synchronous colorectal carcinoma is estimated to be present in 0.5% to 1.0% of all patients with AAA,[1,2] although this figure may be somewhat low, since the incidence of AAA is increasing. Historically, three patterns of diagnosis were evident: (1) that in which the diagnosis of both conditions was made preoperatively; (2) that in which the tumor was discovered at the time of aneurysm resection; and (3) that in which the aneurysm was discovered at the time of tumor resection.[1,2] In contemporary surgical practice, the last scenario is unusual, given the widespread use of CT scanning for tumor staging.

The management strategy for the patient in whom both conditions are discovered preoperatively is first guided by the presence of symptoms or the lack thereof. In general, any symptomatic lesion takes priority. Abdominal or back pain is ominous and prompt repair of the aneurysm should be undertaken, unless another source of the pain is obvious. Similarly, aneurysm tenderness demands attention. However, the colon is resected first if signs or symptoms of impending intestinal obstruction are present. Perforation is, of course, a surgical emergency requiring prompt intervention. If the colon cancer needs to be resected first, Nora et al.[1] recommend waiting 4 to 6 weeks and obtaining a barium enema, to rule out any anastomotic leek. If abscess or fistula is demonstrated, this must be resolved prior to aneurysm repair. Otherwise, the aneurysm is repaired through the retroperitoneal approach after the 4-to-6-week wait.

If neither lesion is symptomatic, the operations are staged. In general, the size of the aneurysm will dictate the sequence. Any aneurysm over 5 cm is repaired first, with colon resection following after sufficient time for recovery, as early as 2 weeks.[3] It is unlikely that this period of time will affect the cancer prognosis, but given the capricious nature of aneurysms, fatal rupture is entirely possible if the sequences were reversed. Although sporadic reports of simultaneous aneurysm repair and colon resection have been published,[1,3] this approach should be avoided as it may increase the risk of graft contamination. If widespread metastatic disease is discovered at the time of laparotomy, a less aggressive approach is warranted.

Discovery of an unsuspected colon tumor at laparotomy for aneurysm resection remains a possibility, as the CT scan is not a sensitive diagnostic modality for colorectal carcinoma. The operation proceeds as planned with aneurysm repair unless there appear to be signs of near obstruction or unless there is widespread metastatic disease. The colectomy follows after a sufficient period of recovery.

Renal Tumors

Similar to colorectal carcinoma, synchronous AAA and renal malignancy is rare. In a recent review from Northwestern University, 10 cases of concurrent renal malignancy out of 500 patients undergoing AAA repair were noted for a 2% prevalence,[4] and DeMasi et al.[5] reported on renal tumors in 2.6% of patients with AAA. Like colorectal carcinoma, since the incidence of AAA is increasing, one may anticipate diagnosing an increasing number of patients with both conditions.

With the widespread use of CT scanning, the diagnosis of both the aneurysm and the renal tumor will usually be made preoperatively, in the elective setting (Fig. 15–1). Most often, the renal tumors are occult, discovered on CT scan during AAA work-up. In the Northwestern series, eight suspicious renal masses were diagnosed serendipitously by CT scan during evaluation of a known or suspected AAA. Less frequently, CT evaluation of hematuria reveals the suspected renal neoplasm and an unsuspected AAA. Typically, the renal malignancy has a characteristically heterogeneous appearance (Fig. 15–1), leaving little doubt of the diagnosis.

For lesions that appear confined to the kidney on CT scan, no further evaluation is required; angiography is used if indicated for the aneurysm. Simultaneous nephrectomy and AAA repair is the approach of choice for most patients. The sequence of the

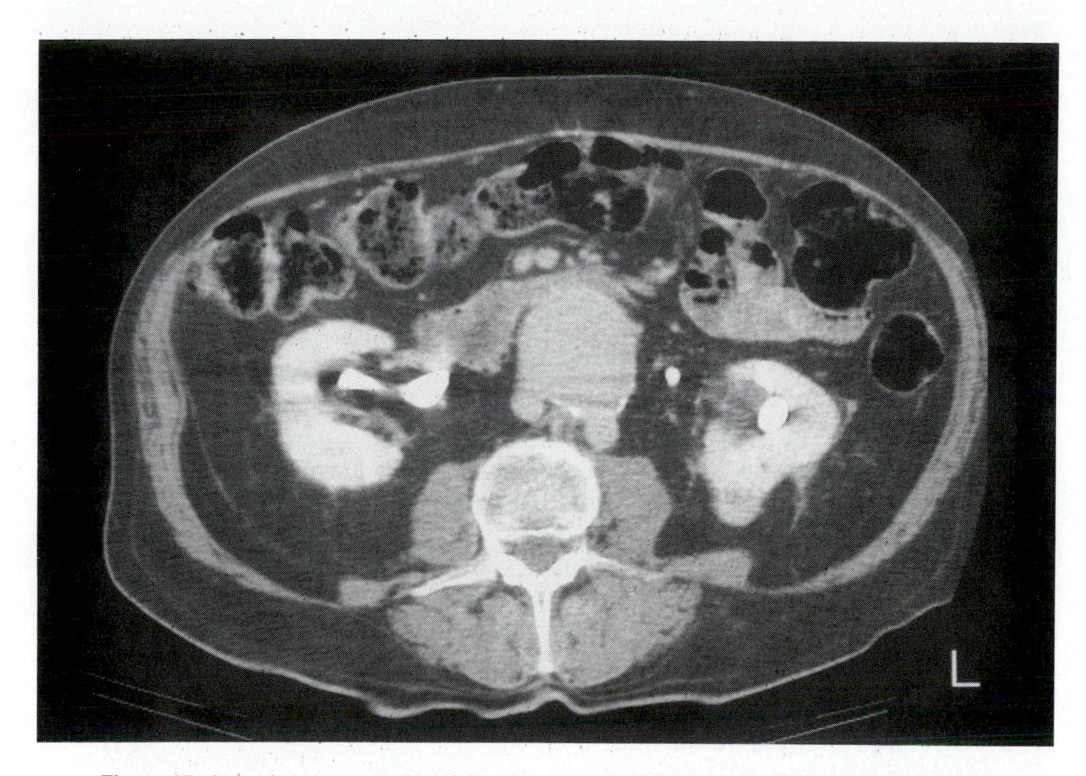

Figure 15–1. Aortic aneurysm with left renal tumor. Notice that this patient also has a duplicated vena cava, seen posterior to the aorta. *(Reprinted with permission from Galt SW, McCarthy WJ, Pearce WH, et al. Simultaneous aortic aneurysm repair with nephrectomy for neoplasm. Am J Surg. 1995;170:227–230.)*

operation should be planned as if it were to be staged; in general, the aneurysm should be repaired first, because it likely represents a greater short-term risk of mortality from rupture. If the aneurysm is small (<5 cm), nephrectomy may precede aneurysm repair, at the discretion of the surgeon.

In some circumstances, a staged approach may still be desirable. Tumor thrombus extension into the vena cava increases the magnitude of the cancer surgery substantially, so staging the aneurysm repair seems wise. Chronic urinary tract infection may increase the possibility of graft infection. Local tumor invasion into the perinephric fat and lymph nodes may prohibit long-term survival, so staging may be appropriate under these circumstances as well. Finally, the surgeon may judge that the patient is simply not a good risk for a long operation with the potential for greater blood loss.

Out of ten patients managed at Northwestern with simultaneous AAA resection and nephrectomy for renal neoplasms, there were no perioperative deaths. One patient with lymph node invasion died of metastatic tumor and three others died of unrelated causes during follow-up. Six patients remained alive and well from 1 to 4 years after surgery and none had evidence of recurrent tumor. There were no cases of graft infection. The simultaneous approach, then, seems safe and effective in appropriately selected patients.

Tumors Elsewhere in the Gastrointestinal Tract

Gastric adenocarcinoma is becoming increasingly rare in the Western hemisphere. However, it is endemic in Asia and is the most commonly surgically treated malignancy in Japan.[6] Like colorectal and renal tumors, the gastric tumor and the aneurysm must both be resected if meaningful long-term survival is to be realized. Staged operations are recommended, because of the theoretical potential for graft infection. As usual, the symptomatic lesion is addressed first. If the patient is asymptomatic, the sequence of operations is based on the degree of progression of the gastric cancer and the size of the aneurysm. Cancer thought to be advanced should be explored first and, given the poor survival of this tumor, if it is unresectable the aneurysm should be left alone unless it is in danger of imminent rupture. For early gastric tumors, the aneurysm should take precedence with gastric resection after several weeks. Simultaneous resection has been reported sporadically,[6] but, as with colon tumors, probably is best avoided if possible.

Adenocarcinoma of the pancreas is curable only if it is small and asymptomatic. Considering the usually dismal prognosis, staged procedures, starting with pancreaticoduodenectomy seems reasonable. The decision to proceed with aneurysm repair depends on its size and the best estimate of the patient's chance to survive for 2 years. Cancers of the biliary tree will likely be diagnosed when symptomatic, making chances of a cure remote. Coincidental hepatocellular carcinoma may be discovered on CT scan. If lobectomy or transplantation is contemplated, a staged approach is recommended.

VASCULAR PATHOLOGY AND VENOUS ANOMALIES ASSOCIATED WITH ANEURYSM SURGERY

Spontaneous Aorto-Left Renal Vein Fistula

Rupture of an AAA into the left renal vein results in an aorto-left renal vein fistula and was first reported by Lord et al. in 1964.[7] This situation is analogous to an aortocaval fistula but decidedly less common, occurring approximately one-tenth as often[8] and almost always into a retroaortic left renal vein. Patients with this fistula usually present with abdominal pain and flank pain, which may radiate to the groin, mimicking ureteral colic.[9,10] The aneurysm may be palpable, and most patients will have an abdominal bruit. Microscopic or gross hematuria is present in all cases and about one-half of the patients have proteinuria. Mild azotemia is usually present. The pain is similar to ureteral colic and, therefore, intravenous pyelography is often the first diagnostic test obtained; this study usually demonstrates nonvisualization of the left kidney. Contrast-enhanced CT scanning may suggest the diagnosis, where an AAA retroaortic left renal vein and nonenhancement of the left kidney are seen. Aortography will confirm the diagnosis of a fistula, although it often cannot distinguish between an aorto-left renal vein fistula and an aortocaval fistula. The hematuria supports the diagnosis of renal vein fistula, because this is much less commonly present in aortocaval fistula.[8] Duplex scanning may be helpful in confirming whether the fistula is to the cava or the left renal vein. It seems likely that spiral CT scanning would also be able to demonstrate the location of the fistula, although this is not yet known.

Knowledge of the renal vein fistula facilitates the appropriate operative approach. Control of the aorta is obtained just below the renal arteries, cephalad to the retroaortic renal vein. Control above the renal arteries may be necessary. The retroaortic left renal vein often conveniently follows an oblique course inferiorly as it joins the IVC, facilitating control of the aorta above the renal vein. Distal control is obtained in the usual fashion. Once the aorta is opened, the copious venous bleeding may be controlled with digital pressure within the aneurysm on the renal vein on the left and its confluence with the vena cava on the right. The fistula is then closed from within the aneurysm.

The aneurysm repair proceeds normally. Postoperatively, renal function may be anticipated to return to normal, although this may take weeks to months.

Venous Anomalies

Anomalies of the IVC and left renal vein are important to consider when planning AAA repair. Unanticipated venous anatomy can lead to inadvertent injury, resulting in substantial, and occasionally fatal, bleeding.[11] The various anomalies are not common, but knowledge of those pertinent to aortic surgery will facilitate a smooth intraoperative course by allowing appropriate planning of technical maneuvers. Fortunately, all of these anatomic variants may be identified by the CT scan; therefore, they are infrequently unexpectedly encountered during emergency repair. The four main venous anomalies affecting aortic surgery include vena caval duplication, left-sided (transposed) vena cava, retroaortic left renal vein, and circumaortic left renal vein.

A detailed review of the embryogenesis of the IVC is beyond the scope of this text and has been well described elsewhere,[12] but brief review will facilitate understanding. The renal and infrarenal caval system originates from the development, regression, and anastomosis of three parallel sets of primitive veins: the posterior cardinal, subcardinal, and supracardinal (Fig. 15–2). The most primitive, the posterior cardinal veins regress first and their drainage is gradually taken over by the subcardinal veins. Only caudal remnants of the posterior cardinal veins persist, forming the iliac bifurcation.[13] The subcardinal veins develop medial to the posterior cardinal vein. Similarly, the supracardinal veins develop dorsal to the subcardinal veins and medial to the posterior cardinal veins. Anastomosis between the subcardinal and supracardinal veins form the renal segment of the IVC. In the embryo, there are usually both dorsal and ventral components, which exist as a renal "collar" around the developing aorta. The right

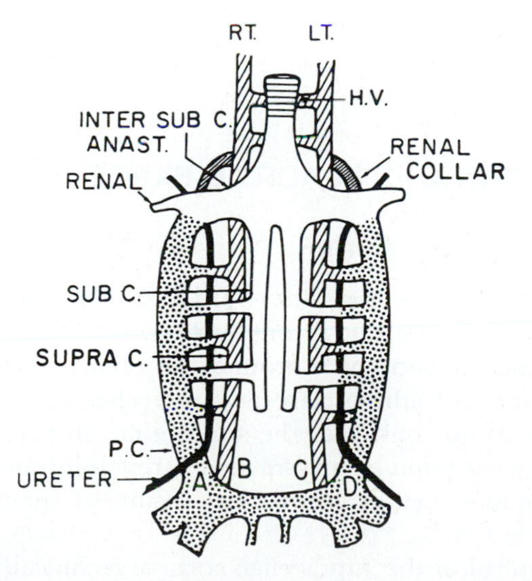

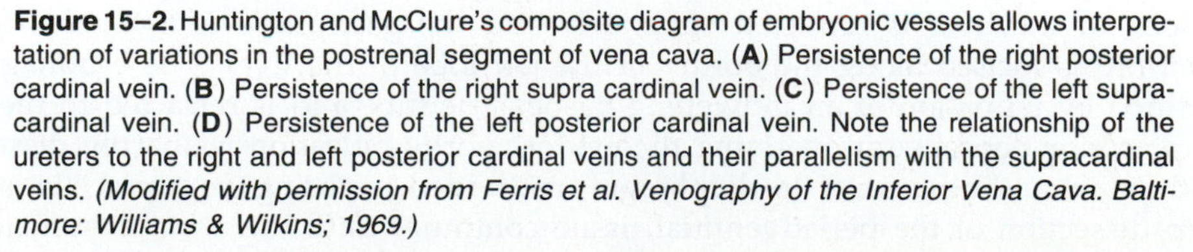
Figure 15–2. Huntington and McClure's composite diagram of embryonic vessels allows interpretation of variations in the postrenal segment of vena cava. (**A**) Persistence of the right posterior cardinal vein. (**B**) Persistence of the right supra cardinal vein. (**C**) Persistence of the left supracardinal vein. (**D**) Persistence of the left posterior cardinal vein. Note the relationship of the ureters to the right and left posterior cardinal veins and their parallelism with the supracardinal veins. *(Modified with permission from Ferris et al. Venography of the Inferior Vena Cava. Baltimore: Williams & Wilkins; 1969.)*

supracardinal vein persists caudally, becoming the normal right infrarenal IVC, and the left-sided veins regress, leaving the usual right-sided unilateral system. The dorsal part of the renal collar also regress, leaving the left renal vein anterior to the aorta.

Caval duplication or persistent left vena cava results from persistence of the left supracardinal vein (Fig. 15–2). Exposure of the aneurysm neck is usually not problematic, as the left renal vein may be divided if needed to aid exposure. Occasionally, interruption of the left cava may be required and seems to be well tolerated.[11] Posterior communicating channels may be present between the two cavas. Avoidance of injury to these is best accomplished by limiting circumferential dissection around the aorta. *Transposition of the IVC* (left-sided cava) results when, like duplication, the left supracardinal vein persists but the right side regresses. Aortic exposure in this instance may be more problematic. If the transposed cava joins the left renal vein and the latter then crosses to a right-sided suprarenal IVC, division of the right renal vein medial to its collaterals may be all that is required. However, the cava may cross anteriorly, obscuring the aneurysm neck. Division of the cava may be required.[11] Preoperative vena cavography is sometimes useful if major caval anomalies are demonstrated on CT scan.

Retroaortic left renal vein is caused by regression of the ventral, instead of dorsal, venous collar. Dissection on the anterior neck of the aorta without encountering a left renal vein suggests this possibility.[13] The aorta can safely be controlled above the renal vein, just below the renal arteries, as the retroaortic right renal vein usually drains into the cava more caudally, following an oblique course. A *circumaortic left renal vein* occurs when both the dorsal and ventral limbs of the supra- and subcardinal vein anatomies persist. In contrast to an isolated retroaortic left renal vein, control of the aorta in this circumstance is best obtained below the anomaly, where aneurysm repair then proceeds in the usual fashion. Injury of a retroaortic left renal vein may occur during dissection. This can be controlled and repaired after aortic cross-clamping by completely transecting the aorta below the infrarenal aortic clamp. Elevating the divided aortic ends allows hemostasis. Fortunately, each of these anomalies is evident on CT scan,[14] allowing appropriate operative planning. If the anatomy is unclear, cavography should be considered.

SPECIAL CONSIDERATIONS IN AORTIC EXPOSURE

Control of the Supraceliac Aorta

Supraceliac aortic clamping is a straightforward and useful technique for a variety of situations encountered during aortic reconstruction. Whenever rapid control of aortic inflow must be obtained, when space around the renal arteries is limited, or when there is abundant juxtarenal atherosclerosis, supraceliac clamping will facilitate safe repair. Therefore, obtaining control of the supraceliac aorta is a useful technique to consider when facing a ruptured aneurysm, a juxtarenal–infrarenal aneurysm, a proximal anastomotic pseudoaneurysm, a proximal recurrent aneurysm, or an aneurysm with juxtarenal atherosclerosis.[15,16]

Exposure and control of the supraceliac aorta is technically straightforward. The left lobe of the liver is retracted superiorly and the gastrohepatic ligament (lesser omentum) is incised along the border of the left lobe of the liver. The esophagus is identified by palpation of an indwelling nasogastric tube and is retracted to the left. The posterior peritoneum overlying the evident aortic pulsation is sharply dissected and the surrounding crura of the diaphragm are divided, exposing the supraceliac aorta. Sharp dissection of the periadventitial tissue continues until the aorta is sufficiently mobilized. The index and third fingers of the surgeon's left hand are insinuated on either side of the aorta, allowing placement of a DeBakey-type clamp. Complete circumferential control is both difficult and unnecessary. It should be avoided, as lumbar arteries may be damaged, causing bothersome hemorrhage.

Supraceliac aortic clamping is generally well tolerated. Upon clamp placement, intravenous nitrates may be required for afterload reduction. Vigorous volume infusion should continue during application of the clamp, as reperfusion of the viscera may cause hypotension. Gradual restoration of inflow helps blunt this response. Ischemic renal failure is obviously of concern, but Green et al.[15] found no increased incidence of renal failure with this approach when the creatinine was normal preoperatively. Similarly, Nypaver et al.[17] did not elicit an increased incidence of renal failure if the renal ischemia time was kept under 30 minutes, and if no concomitant visceral revascularization was performed. Intravenous manitol (12.5 g) may be helpful, although its use is empiric.

Colostomies, Ileostomy, or Abdominal Wall Urinary Stomata

Patients in whom fecal or urinary stomata are present on the abdominal wall require an extra measurement of preparation prior to aneurysm replacement. First, patients with abdominal wall stomata usually have undergone operation for malignancy and, therefore, careful consideration of long-term survival is essential. Second, these stomata are necessary sources of bacterial contamination and extra caution must be used to avoid graft contamination. Third, normal anatomy is obviously altered. Clear definition of anatomy preoperatively, particularly of the ureters in patients with ileourinary diversion and the colon blood supply in patients who have undergone colectomy, is critical. Nevertheless, in an otherwise acceptable candidate, an abdominal wall stoma is not a contraindication to aortic reconstruction.

Special attention should be paid to skin preparation. DeNatale et al.[18] suggest antibacterial bathing twice daily for 2 days prior to surgery with the administration of broad spectrum antibiotics starting 8 hours prior to surgery and continuing for 5 days postoperatively. Patients with colostomies should undergo a full bowel prep with both purging and oral antibiotics. A clean ostomy pouch is placed on the stoma the morning of surgery and is removed after the patient is anesthetized and the chest to upper thighs are thoroughly scrubbed with antibacterial soap, prepped with iodoform solution, and dried. A soft red rubber catheter is placed in the stoma and then run to a collection system attached to the side of the operating table. A plastic adhesive drape is then used to cover the chest, abdomen, and thighs, segregating the stoma from the line of the incision.

The approach to the aneurysm remains the choice of the surgeon and is essentially unaffected by the ostomy. For the left lower quadrant stoma, a transperitoneal approach works well. Alternatively, the aneurysm may be approached from the retroperitoneum, particularly if the ostomy is in the right lower quadrant. In patients with loop urinary diversion stomata in whom the uretral anatomy and loop ileostomy anatomy is not clear, the retroperitoneal approach is especially appealing as damage to the ureter ileal conduit may be more easily avoided. The exact location of the ureters is always problematic following ureter ileal conduit. A retroperitoneal incision with anterior reflection of the left kidney avoids this uncertainty as the left ureter is moved anteriorly by the dissection. This is also true in patients who have had multiple previous transperitoneal procedures where adhesions may cause difficulty with exposure.

DeNatale et al.[18] have summarized indications for aneurysm repair in patients with abdominal stomata. They suggest that patients with a mature stoma and healthy surrounding skin, with good control of the disease that led to the need for the stoma are reasonable candidates for the usual indications for aortic aneurysm repair. Conversely, contraindications to elective repair include uncontrolled advanced cancer and immature stomata. Stoma complications including abscesses, sinuses, skin rashes, and ulcerations are also contraindications, as are hydronephrosis, pyelonephritis, and uremia complicating malfunctioning urinary diversion procedures.

Division of the Left Renal Vein

Division of the left renal vein is a useful technique when exposure of the pararenal aorta is necessary during AAA repair. First reported on by Neal and Shearburn[19] in 1967, surgeons who employ this maneuver should be well acquainted with its safety and possible adverse consequences.

In the majority of patients, the left renal vein crosses the aorta anteriorly, where it drains into the IVC. Tributaries from the inferior phrenic, adrenal, gonadal, and ureteric veins drain directly into the left renal vein. In addition, a small proportion of renal blood flow drains through capsilar veins directly into the lumbar veins. Therefore, an extensive network of collateral venous drainage communicating into both the azygous–hemizygous system and the IVC is present from the left kidney. Owing to this collateral network, division of the left renal vein is often feasible with no demonstrated decrease in renal function, as long as the vein is divided near the renal vein–vena cava junction, preserving the collaterals.

Since Neal and Shearburn's[19] original description, both the opinions among vascular surgeons and published reports of the consequences of left renal vein division have varied. Some authors advocate that left renal vein division is harmless and should be a readily employed adjunct to aortic exposure,[20,21] but other authors have reported significant complications.[22] Abu Rahma[22a] retrospectively reviewed the records of 332 patients undergoing elective AAA repair. Left renal vein ligation was performed in 13, and there was a significantly higher incidence of postoperative azotemia in this group compared to 319 patients who did not undergo left renal vein division. Johnston and Scobie,[23] in the prospective Canadian study, likewise found that renal vein ligation was a significant independent determinant of renal damage. Rastad et al.[24] also found a higher incidence of permanent renal damage in patients with left renal vein ligation, but a significant number of patients with ruptured aneurysms were included in this study, in which postoperative renal dysfunction is more often to be expected. Other complications reported, albeit with less frequency include hematuria and hypertension. Rare reports of massive hemorrhage from venous hypertension and venous infarctions also exist.[24] As a result of potential complications, Szilagyi et al.[25] advocated routine reanastomosis of the divided left renal vein, but not all authors agree that this step is necessary.[22] At best, reanastomosis is difficult, and it is sometimes impossible because of inadequate length.

In general, division of the left renal vein should be avoided if possible. Simple mobilization and gentle retraction of the vein will often achieve the necessary extra centimeter or two of required exposure of the aorta, with no morbidity. However, if division is required to obtain the necessary exposure, this should be done, rather than compromising the safety and effectiveness of the operation. In the patient with a normal serum creatinine, this maneuver will most likely be well tolerated, and as long as the ligation is near the IVC. However, in the patient with impaired renal function, with the left kidney as the single functioning kidney, or who has suffered significant hypotension, reanastomosis of the renal vein should be considered, if technically feasible.

CONCLUSION

Although most patients with aortic aneurysms are operated on in a very routine manner, occasionally they present with complicating intra-abdominal findings. Most such situations have been well thought out by previous authors, and rules exist for their safe management. These include intra-abdominal tumors of various types, some of which are better staged, and others operated on simultaneously with aneurysm repair. Techniques of supraceliac aortic control are quite useful in many operative settings and safe management of patients with abdominal wall stoma can be accomplished with careful planning. Finally, interesting venous anomalies involving the vena cava and left renal vein may be managed in a logical fashion if their anatomy is understood ahead of time.

REFERENCES

1. Nora JD, Pairolero PC, Nivatvongs S, et al. Concomitant abdominal aortic aneurysm and colorectal carcinoma: priority of resection. *J Vasc Surg.* 1989;9:630–636.
2. Szilagyi DE, Elliott JP, Berguer R. Coincidental malignancy and abdominal aortic aneurysm: problems of management. *Arch Surg.* 1967;95:402–412.
3. Lobbato VJ, Rothenberg RE, LaRaja RD, et al. Coexistence of abdominal aortic aneurysm and carcinoma of the colon: a dilemma. *J Vasc Surg.* 1985;5:724–726.
4. Galt SW, McCarthy WJ, Pearce WH, et al. Simultaneous aortic aneursym repair with nephrectomy for neoplasm. *Am J Surg.* 1995;170:227–230.
5. DeMasi RJ, Gregory RT, Snyder SO, et al. Coexistent abdominal aortic aneurysm and renal carcinoma: management options. *Am Surg.* 1994;60:961–966.
6. Komori K, Okadome K, Funahashi S, et al. Surgical strategy of concomitant abdominal aortic aneurysm and gastric cancer. *J Vasc Surg.* 1994;19:573–576.
7. Lord JW, Vigorita J, Florio J. Fistula between abdominal aortic aneurysm and anomalous renal vein. *JAMA.* 1964;187:535–536.
8. Mansour MA, Rutherford RB, Metcalf RK, et al. Spontaneous aorto-left renal vein fistula: the "abdominal pain, hematuria, silent left kidney" syndrome. *Surgery.* 1991;109:101–106.
9. Suzuki M, Collins GM, Bassinger GT, et al. Aorto-left renal vein fistula: an unusual complication of abdominal aortic aneurysm. *Ann Surg.* 1976;184:31–34.
10. Merrill WH, Ernst CB. Aorta-left renal vein fistula: hemodynamic monitoring and timing of operation. *Surgery.* 1981;89:678–682.
11. Brener BJ, Darling RC, Frederick PL, et al. Major venous anomalies complicating abdominal aortic surgery. *Arch Surg.* 1974;108:159–165.
12. Chuang VP, Mena CE, Hoskins PA. Congenital anomalies of the inferior vena cava. Review of embryogenesis and presentation of a simplified classification. *Brit J Rad.* 1974;47:206–213.
13. Bartle EJ, Pearce WH, Sun JH, et al. Infrarenal venous anomalies and aortic surgery: avoiding vascular injury. *J Vasc Surg.* 1987;6:590–593.
14. Royal SA, Callen PW. CT evaluation of anomalies of the inferior vena cava and left renal vein. *Am J Roentgenol.* 1979;132:759–763.
15. Green RM, Ricotta JJ, Ouriel K, et al. Results of supraceliac aortic clamping in the difficult elective resection of infrarenal abdominal aortic aneurysm. *J Vasc Surg.* 1989;9:124–134.
16. Crawford ES, Beckett WC, Greer MS. Juxtarenal infrarenal abdominal aortic aneurysm: special diagnostic and therapeutic considerations. *Ann Surg.* 1986;203:661–670.
17. Nypaver TJ, Shepard AD, Reddy DJ, et al. Supraceliac aortic cross-clamping: determinants of outcome in elective abdominal aortic reconstruction. *J Vasc Surg.* 1993;17:868–876.
18. DeNatale RW, Crawford ES, Safi HJ, et al. Graft reconstruction to treat disease of the abdominal aorta in patients with colostomies, ileostomies, and abdominal wall urinary stomata. *J Vasc Surg.* 1987;6:240–247.

19. Neal HS, Shearburn EW. Division of the left renal vein as an adjunct to resection of abdominal aortic aneurysms. *Am J Surg.* 1967;113:763–765.
20. Adar R, Rabbi I, Bass A, et al. Left renal vein division in abdominal aortic aneurysm operations: effect on renal function. *Arch Surg.* 1985;120:1033–1036.
21. James EC, Fedde CW, Khuri NT, et al. Division of the left renal vein: a safe surgical adjunct. *Surgery.* 1978;83:151–154.
22. McCombs PR, DeLaurentis DA. Division of the left renal vein. Guidelines and consequences. *Am J Surg.* 1979;138:257–263.
22a. Abu Rahma AF, Robinson PA, Boland JP, Lucente FC. The risk of ligation of the left renal vein in resection of the abdominal aortic aneurysm. *Surg Gynecol Obstet.* 1991;173:33–36.
23. Johnston KW, Scobie TK. Multicenter prospective study of nonruptured abdominal aortic aneurysms, 1: population and operative management. *J Vasc Surg.* 1988;7:69–79.
24. Rastad J, Almgren B, Bowald S, et al. Renal complications to left renal vein ligation in abdominal aortic surgery. *J Cardiovasc Surg.* 1984;25:432–436.
25. Szilagyi DE, Smith RF, Elliott JP. Temporary transection of the left renal vein: a technical aid in aortic surgery. *Surgery.* 1969;65:32–40.

16

Replacement of Infected Aortic Prostheses with Lower Extremity Deep Veins

Definitive Treatment

G. Patrick Clagett, MD

Cure of aortic prosthetic infection requires removal of infected prosthetic material and restoration of adequate pelvic and lower extremity arterial blood flow. Surgical strategies to achieve these objectives are listed in Table 16–1, in which morbidity and mortality are calculated by pooling data from contemporary major series reported since 1980. The limitations in comparing approaches by pooling data in this manner are obvious: Heterogeneity of patients and conditions, differing severity and types of infections among series, inclusion in some series of many patients with aortoenteric fistulae, and widely varying time periods with limited follow-up all limit accuracy. In addition, data are woefully incomplete in many reports, and this literature suffers from a lack of reporting standards that preclude valid comparison between series. Despite these limitations, review of the data listed in Table 16–1 provides some insight into contemporary approaches.

Removal of the infected aortic prosthesis with no revascularization is usually not possible and is associated with high mortality, 36.7% (95% confidence interval [CI], 23.7% to 50.2%) and an even higher amputation rate, 45% (95% CI, 29.6% to 60.4%).[1–7] In contrast, *in situ* prosthetic replacement appears to have the lowest mortality, 13.7% (95% CI, 4.6% to 23.1%) and low amputation rate.[7–13] This is an attractive option in high-risk patients with low virulence *Staphylococcus epidermidis* infections involving one limb of an aortobifemoral bypass.[12,13] However, follow-up is limited and recurrent infection remains a risk despite long-term antibiotics. Complete prosthetic replacement of infected aortic prostheses with antibiotic-treated vascular materials and long-term antibiotic replacement has been reported with encouraging success[13]; however, long-term follow-up is lacking, and the risk of recurrent infection involving the aortic anastomosis remains a grave concern.

Currently, the most widely favored strategy is extra-anatomic bypass through uninfected tissues and removal of the aortic prosthesis. In data pooled from major

TABLE 16–1. POOLED DATA FROM SERIES OF INFECTED AORTIC PROSTHESES REPORTED SINCE 1980

		Mortality			Amputation		
Operations	***References***	***No. Pts.***	***Incidence***	***(95% CI[a])***	***No. Pts.***	***Incidence (%)***	***(95% CI[a])***
Excise prosthesis, no revascularization	1–7	18/49	36.7	(23.7–50.2)	18/48	45.0	(29.6–60.4)
In situ prosthetic replacement	7–13	7/51	13.7	(4.6–23.1)	0/22	0.0	—[b]
Extra-anatomic bypass, excise prosthesis (any sequence, with or without delay)	1–7,10,14–23	75/386	19.4	(15.5–23.3)	27/257	10.5	(0–22.1)
Autogenous reconstruction	24–30	14/72	19.4	(10.3–28.5)	11/72	15.3	(6.9–23.5)

[a] CI, confidence interval.
[b] —, no data.

contemporary series (Table 16–1), the overall mortality with this approach is 19.4% (95% CI, 15.5% to 23.3%) and the amputation rate is 10.5% (95% CI, 0% to 22.1%).[1–7,10,14–23] Most surgeons prefer staging these procedures with extra-anatomic bypass preceding removal of the infected prosthesis by a 2 to 3 day interval. However, critical analysis of the data demonstrates little difference in outcome between a staged or simultaneous operative approach. A limitation to extra-anatomic bypass and removal of the aortic prosthesis is the potential for infection of the new prosthesis and aortic stump blowout. In pooled data reported since 1980, the rate of infection of the extra-anatomic bypass is 16% (95% CI, 10% to 21%) and the incidence of fatal aortic stump blowout is 9.4% (95% CI, 6.7% to 12.1%).[1,4,7,10,14–17,19,21–23]

One of the most disappointing features of extra-anatomic bypass is the high rate of acute occlusion. This often occurs in patients with extensive vascular disease and complex extra-anatomic bypasses such as axillo-unilateral popliteal or profunda bypasses. Thrombosis of these reconstructions limited by poor outflow is usually sudden and catastrophic, and leads to amputation in a large number of cases. In a recently reported series of patients with extra-anatomic bypasses placed for aortic prosthetic infection, the primary patency rate was 43% at 3 years, and approximately one-third of all survivors required major amputation.[3]

In *in situ* autogenous reconstructions from endarterectomized arterial segments and venous conduits have proven resistant to infection.[24–30] This attractive feature has been offset by the extensive nature of these complex operations that carry a mortality and amputation rate similar to that of extra-anatomic bypass with removal of the aortic prosthesis (Table 16–1). In addition, long-term patency has been a problem with autogenous reconstructions fashioned from endarterectomized arterial segments and greater saphenous veins.[25,27,28] However, recent experience with large caliber lower extremity deep veins has documented low mortality and amputation rates (less than 10%) and excellent patency.[28,29] This experience is detailed as follows.

As alternatives to the approaches listed in Table 16–1, recent reports of *in situ* replacement of infected aortic prostheses with venous and aortic homografts appear promising.[30–32] In one large series, an operative mortality rate of 12% was reported in 43 patients in whom infected aortic prostheses were replaced with aortic homografts.[33] However, even with this approach, recurrent infection and graft rupture has occurred, and late deterioration may be expected. Another approach includes debridement of infected tissues, drainage of infection, antibiotic irrigation, and intensive systemic antibiotic therapy.[34–36] This approach may have a role in limited, extracavitary infections and in patients with reduced life expectancy. Reasonable results have even been reported for more extensive aortic prosthetic infections.[35,36] However, this more conservative approach is associated with unpredictable rates of recurrent infection, false aneurysms, and aortoenteric fistulae.

Dissatisfaction with extra-anatomic prosthetic bypass and other approaches stimulated our development of an *in situ* autologous reconstruction from major lower extremity veins. Building on the experience of others using greater saphenous veins,[25,27] we extended this approach to using the superficial femoral-popliteal veins or deep veins to reconstruct the aortoiliac femoral system.[28] For simplicity, we have termed this a *neo-aortoiliac femoral (NAIF) system.*

NEO-AORTOILIAC FEMORAL PROCEDURE

Large venous autografts are critical for successful NAIF reconstruction. It is important to assess preoperatively the size of the greater saphenous and deep veins. As experience has developed, it has become apparent that only very large saphenous veins, at least 8 mm in distended diameter, perform satisfactorily for this approach. Smaller veins are prone to develop focal stenoses and diffuse neointimal hyperplasia that has led to the need for multiple revisions and replacement procedures. We currently favor the use of the deep veins in most instances and avoid using greater saphenous veins. It is also important to image the superficial femoropopliteal veins with duplex ultrasonography prior to performing this operation. We have noted occasional anomalies, as well as areas of occlusion and recanalization in the deep veins, that preclude their successful use. The most frequent anomaly encountered, in approximately 5% of patients, is a dominant profunda system that communicates directly with the distal popliteal vein. In these circumstances, the superficial femoropopliteal vein is usually small and incomplete. Shulman has reported finding a dominant profunda venous system in approximately 7% of patients undergoing femoral-popliteal bypass with deep vein grafts.[37] Fortunately, this anomaly is most often unilateral, and one can plan a reconstruction using the normal deep vein from one extremity and a segment of greater saphenous vein from the other. It is desirable, but not an absolute necessity, to preserve the greater saphenous vein from the extremity in which the deep vein is harvested. Limb edema has occurred in circumstances where both veins are harvested from the same extremity.

The operation begins with vein harvest, and every effort is made to ensure that this remains a sterile procedure. Infected femoral wounds are excluded from the field by secure placement of adherent, iodine-impregnated plastic drapes (Ioban) over grossly infected wounds that are dressed with dry gauze sponges to absorb contaminated fluids during the course of the operation. A two-team approach is preferred, with one team harvesting veins while the other removes the infected aortic prostheses.

In harvesting deep vein autografts, the lateral border of the sartorius muscle is mobilized from the upper thigh to the knee joint (Fig. 16–1). The sartorius muscle is freed along its lateral border and reflected medially and posteriorly to preserve its blood supply, which enters the muscle belly from its inferomedial aspect. Hunter's canal is exposed, and care is taken to preserve major collateral branches of the superficial femoral and popliteal arteries, the saphenous nerve, and the ipsilateral greater saphenous vein. Saphenous neuralgia will occur if the saphenous nerve is injured, and this complication is especially troubling to patients (although usually temporary, lasting weeks to a few months). The adductor canal is opened by incising the tendinous portion of the adductor magnus muscle, and multiple branches of the superficial femoral-popliteal vein are carefully ligated and divided; large branches are doubly ligated or suture ligated. The importance of secure ligation of these branches cannot be overemphasized. Ligatures on branches are prone to be displaced when passing these large caliber conduits down through the restricted space of tunnels fashioned in the retroperitoneum to the femoral sites. The most tedious portion of this dissection occurs in the adductor canal region where there are multiple large branches, and the vein is in close apposition to the artery and the aponeurosis of the adductor magnus.

A critically important feature in preventing excessive venous hypertension is careful preservation of the junction of the profunda femoris vein with the common femoral vein (Figure 16–1). The entrance of the profunda femoris vein into the common femoral vein is identified, and the proximal superficial vein is transected and oversewn flush with this junction. The popliteal vein is mobilized distally until a length adequate for NAIF reconstruction is achieved, often requiring mobilization of this vein to the knee joint or just below.

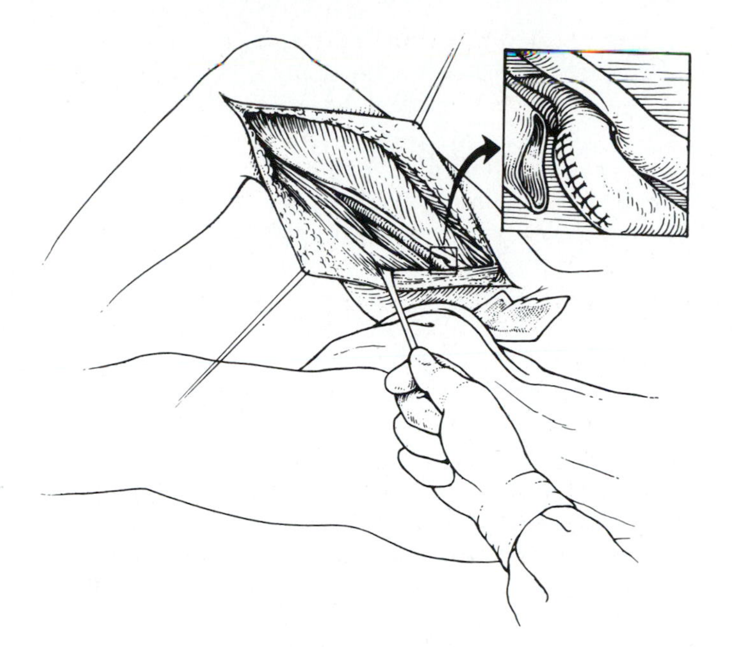

Figure 16–1. Harvest of superficial femoropopliteal vein for deep vein autograft. The profunda femoris vein is carefully preserved and the proximal end of the transected superficial vein is oversewn flush with the profunda and common femoral vein junction. *(Reprinted with permission from Clagett GP, Bowers BL, Lopez-Viego MA, et al. Ann Surg. 1993;218:239–249.)*

Vein grafts are distended with chilled, whole blood or a cold solution consisting of Ringer's lactate (1 L), heparin (5,000 units), albumin (25 g), and papaverine (60 mg). Because the largest diameter of this vein is encountered proximally, valves are fractured by retrograde passage of a Mills–Leather valvulotome so that the large caliber end can be anastomosed comfortably to the aortic stump. There are usually only three or four major valves in the long, deep vein autograft. Valves within 10 to 15 cm from either the proximal or distal end can be easily excised after exposing them by everting the graft. Vein grafts are stored in the solutions kept at 4°C until required for NAIF reconstruction. Vein harvest incisions are irrigated copiously with antibiotic solutions and closed completely.

All prosthetic material is excised and the aorta and periaortic tissues are liberally debrided to achieve a clean proximal anastomotic site for the deep vein autograft. Aortic debridement may be facilitated by suprarenal aortic control either by cross-clamping at the diaphragmatic level or intraluminal balloon control. The most favorable proximal anastomotic technique involves simply suturing the deep vein autograft end to end to the debrided aorta (Fig. 16–2). Standard, continuous polypropylene (4-0) suture technique is used, taking care to make slightly more advancement on the aorta than the venous autograft because of the greater circumference of the aorta. In our experience, we have encountered three patients with very large proximal aortas, two with dilation and the other with frank aneurysmal change. In these situations, the deep veins have been joined together and sewn to the aneurysmal aorta.

Infected femoral wounds are then opened and debrided, and all prosthetic material is removed from below. The retroperitoneal tunnels are irrigated with antibiotic solutions and mechanically debrided by pulling gauze sponges through them. Venous

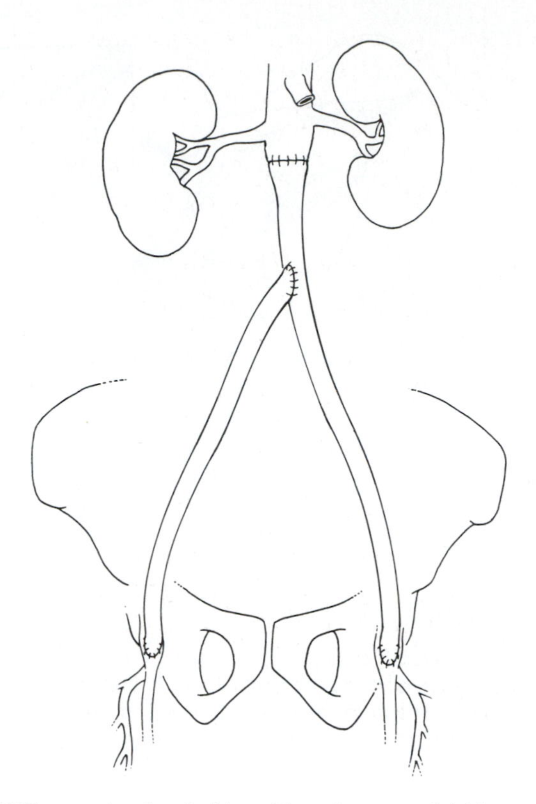

Figure 16–2. NAIF reconstruction fashioned from two superficial femoropopliteal veins.

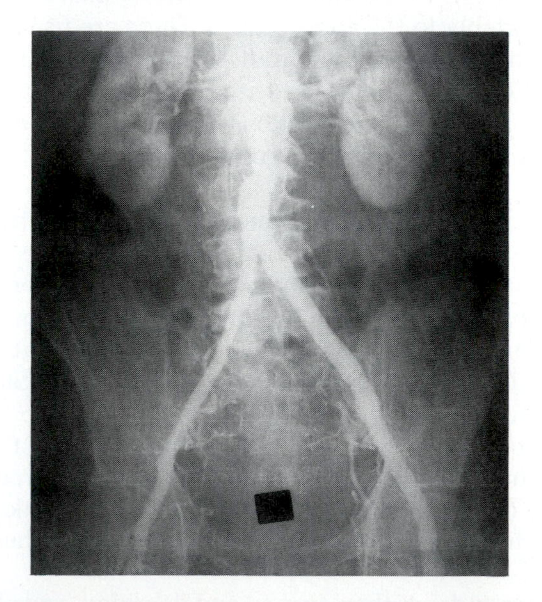

Figure 16–3. Angiogram of NAIF reconstruction fashioned from two superficial femoropopliteal veins as depicted in Figure 16–2. The deep vein used for the right limb was slightly smaller than that used on the left.

grafts are brought through the old tunnels and anastomosed directly to the debrided femoral vessels. Venous autografts are brought through the old tunnels in an undistended state avoiding twisting and kinking. Creation of new tunnels is difficult because of limited space and retroperitoneal inflammation and scarring. We frequently dilate the old, fibrotic tunnels by simple finger insertion or passage of large caliber graft-passer. This is important because portions of the deep vein graft have a larger diameter than the tunnel.

The operation proceeds by anastomosing a deep vein autograft to the terminal aorta and to a femoral or iliac artery. A second deep vein autograft is anastomosed end to side to the autograft in place and then passed through a retroperitoneal tunnel to the contralateral femoral vessel. Another configuration is to use the second deep vein autograft as a femoral crossover bypass. These reconstructions are illustrated in Figures 16–2 through 16–8. Distal anastomoses have been fashioned to the common femoral artery, the profunda femoris artery, and the superficial femoral artery with relatively equal frequency. At the completion of NAIF reconstruction, the debrided subcutaneum of the femoral wounds is closed over the venous autografts and the skin loosely approximated or left open. It has not been necessary to cover the venous autografts with muscle flaps. Drainage is rarely employed and antibiotics are discontinued within 5 to 7 days after operation. These patients are prone to deep venous thrombosis, which is engendered by stasis in the residual distal popliteal vein. An important adjunct to prevent this complication is intermittent pneumatic compression combined with low-dose heparin prophylaxis.

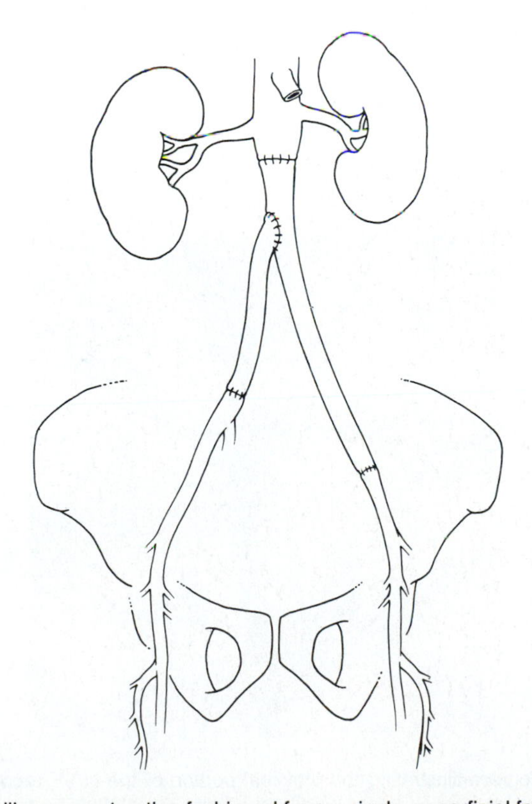

Figure 16–4. Aortoiliac reconstruction fashioned from a single, superficial femoropopliteal vein.

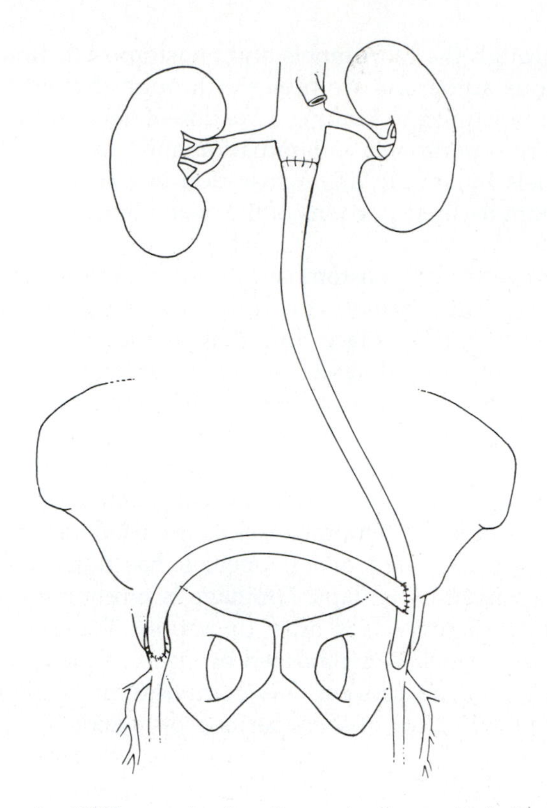

Figure 16–5. Alternative NAIF reconstruction. Deep veins are used to fashion an aorto-unilateral femoral bypass with a crossover extension to the contralateral femoral artery.

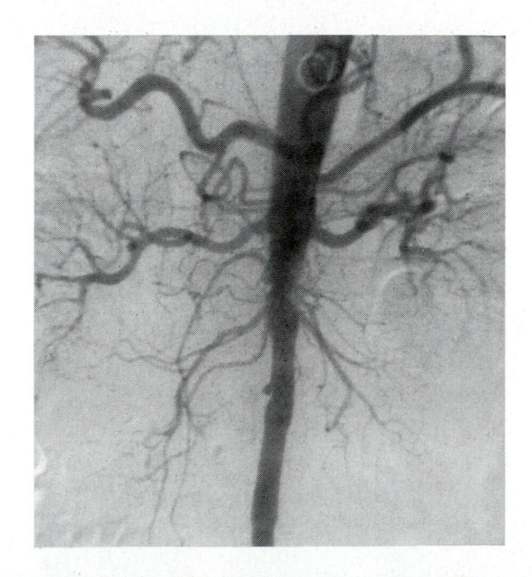

Figure 16–6. Angiogram illustrating the proximal portion of the NAIF reconstruction drawn in Figure 16–5.

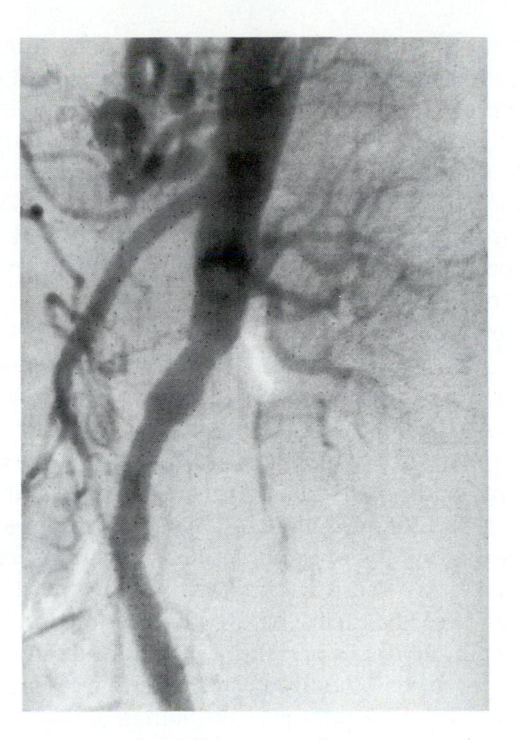

Figure 16–7. Lateral view of proximal NAIF reconstruction depicted in Figure 16–5.

UNIVERSITY OF TEXAS SOUTHWESTERN MEDICAL CENTER EXPERIENCE

Our early experience with the NAIF reconstruction has been reported,[28] and an update will now be provided. Thirty-four patients have undergone this procedure at the University of Texas Southwestern Medical Center. Twenty-six patients underwent NAIF reconstruction because of aortic prosthetic infection (26 infected aortobifemoral by-

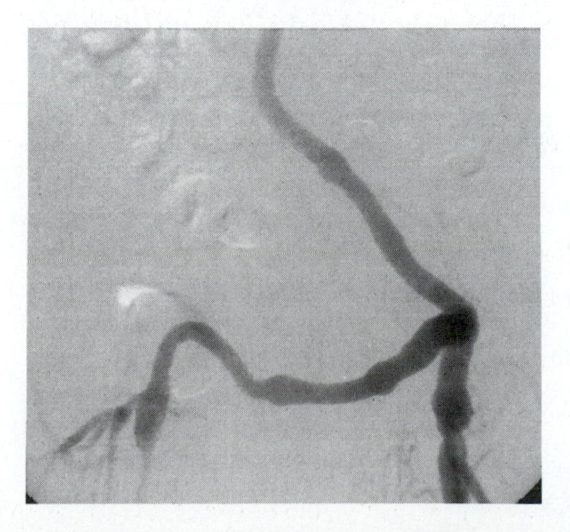

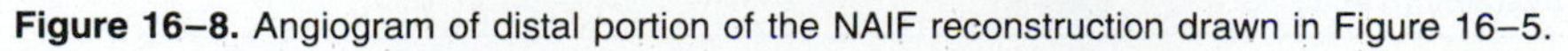

Figure 16–8. Angiogram of distal portion of the NAIF reconstruction drawn in Figure 16–5.

passes, 2 aortoenteric fistulae, and 1 aortoenteric erosion). Eight patients had this operation because of complex aortic problems. These included patients who had contraindications to standard prosthetic reconstruction because of ongoing regional infections (e.g., advanced perineal, scrotal, and pubic hydradenitis suppurativa or gastrointestinal fistulae) that could not be cleared in a timely fashion. These patients also had failed attempts at interventional radiologic approaches to achieve revascularization. Other patients in this category of complex aortic problems included those with multiple recurrent prosthetic aortobifemoral bypass thromboses from exuberant anastomotic neointimal hyperplasia or severely restricted outflow that would not support prosthetic reconstruction. Our experience in this latter group of patients suggests that severely restricted outflow, along with exceedingly small aortoiliac vessels, leads to an unacceptable rate of occlusion with a standard aortobifemoral prostheses.[38]

Among the patients with infected prostheses, 19 had paninfected aortobifemoral bypasses or aortoiliac prostheses with pus surrounding the body and limbs of the prostheses and 7 patients had a single aortobifemoral bypass limb involvement. The majority of these patients had infected, knitted Dacron prostheses, most of which were placed for occlusive disease, but 3 had expanded polytetrafluoroethylene (ePTFE) limb replacements that subsequently became reinfected. The mean (±SD) interval between original aortic operation and diagnosis of prosthetic infection was 68 ± 54 months (range, 4 to 192 months) and modes of presentation included femoral abscesses, chronic draining groin sinuses, infected femoral anastomotic aneurysms, fever, anemia, and gastrointestinal bleeding. Almost all patients complained of malaise and chronic fatigue. Risk factors for prosthetic infection included multiple femoral reoperations after initial aortic procedure (mean, 3 ± 2; range, 0 to 10), usually for anastomotic aneurysms, limb thromboses, or wound complications. Other risk factors in single patients included renal failure requiring dialysis, immunosuppressive therapy with cytoxan for an autoimmune disorder, and multiple chronically infected cutaneous squamous cell carcinoma lesions.

At least one-half of the patients in this series had failure of more conservative local procedures. These included removal of single aortobifemoral bypass limb with extra-anatomic bypass (obturator bypass, axillofemoral superficial femoral bypass, and axillopopliteal bypass), continuous irrigation with antibiotic solutions coupled with multiple debridements, muscle flap coverage, and debridement with *in situ* replacement with ePTFE. All of these patients were treated with prolonged oral or parenteral antibiotics and had healing of femoral wounds before developing signs of recurrent, more extensive infections. Organisms cultured from excised prosthetic material or pus surrounding prostheses are shown in Table 16–2. Consistent with most contemporary

TABLE 16–2. NAIF RECONSTRUCTION

Infected AFBs, Organisms
S. epidermidis (*n* = 10)
S. aureus (*n* = 5)
Pseudomonas aeruginosa (*n* = 2)
E. Coli (*n* = 1)
β-hemolytic *streptococcus* (*n* = 1)
Enterobacter aerogenes (*n* = 1)
Bacteroides bivius (*n* = 1)
Proteus mirabilis (*n* = 1)
Serratia marcescens (*n* = 1)
Propionibacterium acnes (*n* = 1)
Candida albicans (*n* = 1)

reports, gram-positive organisms, especially *Staph epidermidis*, predominated; however, there were also gram-negative infections that included *Pseudomonas aeruginosa*, *Escherichia coli*, and *Proteus mirabilis*.

Veins harvested for NAIF reconstruction included bilateral saphenous veins (7 patients), deep veins and greater saphenous veins from opposite limbs (3 patients), bilateral deep veins (12 patients), and unilateral deep veins (12 patients). The mean operative time was 6.5 ± 1.8 hours (range, 4.5 to 10 hours) and intraoperative blood transfusion requirement was 4 ± 4 units (range, 0 to 9 units). When two teams were used, operative time was less than 5 hours. Supraceliac aortic control has been required in 5 patients.

There have been no immediate operative deaths. However, three patients died at prolonged intervals (greater than 30 days after operation) from peritonitis, sepsis, and multisystem organ dysfunction. Interestingly, all of these patients presented with aortoenteric fistula or erosion. There were two acute amputations in survivors for an overall procedure-related mortality and amputation rate of 9% and 6%, respectively. Other major morbidity included gastrointestinal complications with peritonitis in four patients that were of great interest because they demonstrated the ability of the deep veins to resist infection. Peritonitis developed in these patients from a perforated duodenal diverticulum with septic pancreatitis, ischemic small bowel necrosis, acute cholecystitis, and gangrene of the gallbladder. Three of these patients had diffuse peritonitis with deep vein autografts bathed in polymicrobial pus (*Enterobacter aerogenes*, *Pseudomonas maltophilia*, and *Candida albicans*). These vein grafts were inspected when patients were explored on multiple occasions and deep vein grafts and anastomoses remained intact and uninfected. Deep venous thrombosis has occurred in two patients and one sustained major pulmonary embolism. The site of deep vein thrombosis was on the side of deep vein harvest in both cases.

The mean follow-up time has been 32 ± 23 months (range, 2 to 90 months). There have been four deaths related to cardiac disease and none directly attributable to the NAIF reconstruction. One patient required amputation for progression of distal disease.

An interesting finding was the difference in behavior of greater saphenous vein and deep vein autografts on long-term follow-up. Three patients with a greater saphenous vein NAIF developed total occlusion within 1 year from progressive, diffuse, neointimal hyperplasia documented by angiography and biopsy at reexploration. One of these patients underwent secondary prosthetic extra-anatomic bypass and the remaining two patients have noncritical lower extremity ischemia with severe claudication. However, they have no desire for further intervention. Four patients developed focal stenoses in greater saphenous vein autografts and three required reoperation with patch angioplasty or femoral crossover limb replacement. Small greater saphenous veins were particularly prone to failure; in contrast, large saphenous veins had sustained patency. Discrete stenoses were likely to develop at areas of kinking and at valve sites. Aortic anastomoses with greater saphenous vein were also prone to develop problems. All failures were apparent within the first year after operation and were manifested by falling ankle pressure indices, changes on duplex surveillance (decrease in luminal caliber and focal areas of jet flow velocity), and onset of intermittent claudication. Despite the high failure rate of greater saphenous veins, no amputations have been required. In contrast, all NAIF reconstructions from larger caliber deep vein autografts have remained patent and free of stenoses. The overall failure rate (defined as occlusion or stenosis requiring reintervention) of greater saphenous vein NAIF was 64% in comparison to 0% for deep vein NAIFs ($p = 0.01$).

Because of the tendency of greater saphenous vein grafts used for NAIF reconstruction to develop focal stenoses, as well as diffuse intimal hyperplasia, it is important to survey these vein grafts with frequent duplex ultrasound examinations and clinical assessment, especially in the first year after placement. Focal stenoses can be corrected by timely reintervention. Despite this limitation, greater saphenous vein NAIF occlusion is more gradual than the sudden thrombotic occlusion experienced by patients with extra-anatomic bypasses who frequently present with profound, irreversible limb ischemia. The slowly progressive occlusion in our patients with greater saphenous vein NAIF reconstructions has allowed for early detection, reintervention, and, possibly, development of collateral circulation.

We currently favor deep vein autografts for NAIF reconstructions and rarely use greater saphenous veins unless they are large (≥8 mm in diameter). We have not observed focal or diffuse intimal hyperplasia in deep vein autografts. The superficial femoropopliteal vein has a diameter of 1.0 to 1.5 cm, which allows end-to-end anastomosis to a normal-caliber aorta with relative ease. Another advantage of the deep vein autografts is that minor kinks and areas of intimal hyperplasia at valve sites do not produce hemodynamic disturbances to the degree that similar-size defects would produce in small caliber greater saphenous vein grafts. The potential for aneurysmal dilation of deep vein grafts is a serious concern. We have not observed this to date but continue to monitor all of the patients with serial duplex ultrasonography, CT, and, in some cases, repeat angiography.

Of the 27 patients (39 limbs) who had unilateral or bilateral deep vein harvest, only 4 (15%) have had significant chronic limb edema requiring compression stockings. These patients either had ipsilateral venous thrombosis with resulting valvular dysfunction or prior harvest of the ipsilateral greater saphenous vein, usually for a prior distal bypass. The absence of significant limb edema has been gratifying. This has also been the experience of Shulman et al.[39], who pioneered the use of the deep vein autograft for femoral-popliteal reconstructions. Schanzer et al.[40] reported mild calf enlargement along with a pattern on strain gauge plethysmography indicative of venous outflow obstruction in the majority of patients who had deep vein harvest for femoropopliteal bypass. Despite this, clinically significant edema requiring compression stockings was rare, and there was no functional disability. This is in agreement with the findings of Masuda, Kistner, and Ferris,[41] who studied the long-term hemodynamic and clinical outcomes in patients who had ligation of the superficial femoral vein. These investigators concluded that there was no correlation between physiologic obstruction of this vein and the presence or absence of limb edema. They further observed that obstruction is well tolerated when the profunda femoris and ipsilateral greater saphenous veins are intact. Although Schulman et al.[39] did not find significant edema in limbs from which both greater saphenous and deep veins were removed, we caution against this. We also believe that preservation of the profunda femoris vein is critical in preserving sufficient venous collateral flow to prevent excessive venous hypertension.

CONCLUSION

Venous autografts resist infection when used for NAIF reconstructions. Small greater saphenous veins are prone to failure from development of focal stenoses and intimal hyperplasia. In contrast, deep veins perform well, anastomose comfortably with the proximal aorta, and have sustained patency. This favorable experience has been reported by others.[29] Furthermore, deep vein harvest is well tolerated with no functional disability and minimal problems with limb edema, as long as the profunda and common femoral veins remain intact and the ipsilateral greater saphenous vein is preserved.

Finally, we believe that the NAIF reconstruction is a successful option in patients with aortic prosthetic infections and other complex aortic problems. Freedom from reinfection and sustained patency make this a definitive treatment.

REFERENCES

1. Ricotta JJ, Faggioli GL, Stella A, et al. Total excision and extra-anatomic bypass for aortic graft infection. *Am J Surg.* 1991;162:145–149.
2. Reilly LM, Stoney RJ, Goldstone J, et al. Improved management of aortic graft infection: the influence of operation sequence and staging. *J Vasc Surg.* 1987;5:421–431.
3. Quinones-Baldrich WJ, Hernandez JJ, Moore WS. Long-term results following surgical management of aortic graft infection. *Arch Surg.* 1991;126:507–511.
4. Schellack J, Stewart MT, Smith RB, et al. Infected aortobifemoral prosthesis—a dreaded complication. *Am Surg.* 1988;54:137–141.
5. Lorentzen JE, Nielsen OM, Arendrup H, et al. Vascular graft infection: an analysis of sixty-two graft infections in 2411 consecutively implanted synthetic vascular grafts. *Surgery.* 1985;98:81–86.
6. Casali RE, Tucker WE, Thompson BW, et al. Infected prosthetic grafts. *Arch Surg.* 1980;115:577–580.
7. Sharp WJ, Hoballah JJ, Mohan CR, et al. The management of the infected aortic prosthesis: a current decade of experience. *J Vasc Surg.* 1994;19:844–850.
8. Walker WE, Cooley DA, Duncan JM, et al. The management of aortoduodenal fistula by *in situ* replacement of the infected abdominal aortic graft. *Ann Surg.* 1987;205:727–732.
9. O'Mara CS, Williams GM, Ernst CB. Secondary aortoenteric fistula, a 20 year experience. *Am J Surg.* 1981;142:203–209.
10. Yeager RA, Moneta GL, Taylor LM, et al. Improving survival and limb salvage in patients with aortic graft infection. *Am J Surg.* 1990;159:466–469.
11. Robinson JA, Johansen K. Aortic sepsis: is there a role for *in situ* graft reconstruction? *J Vasc Surg.* 1991;13:677–684.
12. Towne JB, Seabrook GR, Bandyk D, et al. *In situ* replacement of arterial prosthesis infected by bacterial biofilms: long-term follow-up. *J Vasc Surg.* 1994;19:226–235.
13. Torsello G, Sandmann W, Gehrt A, et al. *In situ* replacement of infected vascular prostheses with rifampin-soaked vascular grafts: early results. *J Vasc Surg.* 1993;17:768–773.
14. Yeager RA, McConnell DB, Sasaki TM, et al. Aortic and peripheral prosthetic graft infection: differential management and causes of mortality. *Am J Surg.* 1985;150:36–43.
15. Bacourt F, Koskas F, and the French University Association for Research in Surgery. Axillobifemoral bypass and aortic exclusion for vascular septic lesions: a multicenter retrospective study of 98 cases. *Ann Vasc Surg.* 1992;6:119–126.
16. O'Hara PJ, Hertzer NR, Beven EG, et al. Surgical management of infected abdominal aortic grafts: review of a 25-year experience. *J Vasc Surg.* 1986;3:725–731.
17. Trout HH, Kozloff L, Giordano JM. Priority of revascularization in patients with graft enteric fistulas, infected arteries, or infected arterial prostheses. *Ann Surg.* 1984;6:669–682.
18. Olah A, Vogt M, Laske A, et al. Axillo-femoral bypass and simultaneous removal of the aortofemoral vascular infection site: is the procedure safe? *Eur J Vasc Surg.* 1992;6:252–254.
19. Schmitt DD, Seabrook GR, Bandyk DF, et al. Graft excision and extra-anatomic revascularization: the treatment of choice for the septic aortic prosthesis. *J Cardiovasc Surg.* 1990;31:327–332.
20. Turnipseed WD, Berkoff HA, Detmer DE, et al. Arterial graft infections: delayed v. immediate vascular reconstruction. *Arch Surg.* 1983;118:410–414.
21. Leather RP, Darling RC III, Chang BB, et al. Retroperitoneal in-line aortic bypass for treatment of infected infrarenal aortic grafts. *Surg Gynecol Obstet.* 1992;175:491–494.
22. Lehnert T, Gruber HP, Maeder N, et al. Management of primary aortic graft infection by extra-anatomic bypass reconstruction. *Eur J Vasc Surg.* 1993;7:301–307.

23. Kuestner LM, Reilly LM, Jicha DL, et al. Secondary aortoenteric fistula: contemporary outcome with use of extraanatomic bypass and infected graft excision. *J Vasc Surg.* 1995;21:184–196.
24. Quinones-Baldrich WJ, Gelabert HA. Autogenous tissue reconstruction in the management of aortoiliofemoral graft infection. *Ann Vasc Surg.* 1990;4:223–228.
25. Ehrenfeld WK, Wilbur BG, Olcott CN, et al. Autogenous tissue reconstruction in the management of infected prosthetic grafts. *Surgery.* 1979;85:82–92.
26. Lorentzen JE, Nielsen OM. Aortobifemoral bypass with autogenous saphenous vein in treatment of paninfected aortic bifurcation graft. *J Vasc Surg.* 1986;3:666–668.
27. Seeger JM, Wheeler JR, Gregory RT, et al. Autogenous graft replacement of infected prosthetic grafts in the femoral position. *Surgery.* 1983;93:39–45.
28. Clagett GP, Bowers BL, Lopez-Viego MA, et al. Creation of a neo-aortoiliac system from lower extremity deep and superficial veins. *Ann Surg.* 1993;218:239–249.
29. Nevelsteen A, Lacroix, H, Suy R. Autogenous reconstruction with the lower extremity deep veins: an alternative in the treatment of prosthetic infection after reconstructive surgery for aortoiliac disease. *J Vasc Surg.* 1995;22:129–134.
30. Hakaim AG, Hertzer NR, O'Hara PJ, et al. Autogenous vein grafts for femorofemoral revascularization in contaminated or infected fields. *J Vasc Surg.* 1994;19:912–915.
31. Bahnini A, Ruotolo C, Koskas F, et al. *In situ* fresh allograft replacement of an infected aortic prosthetic graft: eighteen months' follow-up. *J Vasc Surg.* 1991;14:98–102.
32. Snyder SO, Wheeler JR, Gregory RT, et al. Freshly harvested cadaveric venous hemografts as arterial conduits in infected fields. *Surgery.* 1987;101:283–291.
33. Kieffer E, Bahnini A, Koskas F, et al. *In situ* allograft replacement of infected infrarenal aortic prosthetic grafts: results in forty-three patients. *J Vasc Surg.* 1993;17:349–356.
34. Calligaro KD, Veith FJ, Schwarz ML, et al. Selective preservation of infected prosthetic arterial grafts: analysis of a 20 year experience with 120 extracavitary infected grafts. *Ann Surg.* 1994;220:461–471.
35. Morris GE, Friend PJ, Vassallo DJ, et al. Antibiotic irrigation and conservative surgery for major aortic graft infection. *J Vasc Surg.* 1994;20:88–95.
36. Gordon A, Conlon C, Collin J, et al. An eight year experience of conservative management for aortic graft sepsis. *Eur J Vasc Surg.* 1994;8:611–616.
37. Schulman ML, Schulman LG, Lledo-Perez AM. Unusual autogenous vein grafts. *Vasc Surg.* 1992;26:257–264.
38. Valentine RJ, Hansen ME, Myers SI, et al. The influence of sex and aortic size on late patency following aortofemoral revascularization in young adults. *J Vasc Surg.* 1995;21:296–306.
39. Schulman ML, Badhey MR, Yatco R. Superficial femoral-popliteal veins and reversed saphenous veins as primary femoropopliteal bypass grafts: a randomized comparative study. *J Vasc Surg.* 1987;6:1–10.
40. Schanzer H, Chiang K, Mabrouk M, et al. Use of lower extremity deep veins as arterial substitutes: functional status of the donor leg. *J Vasc Surg.* 1991:14:624–627.
41. Masuda EM, Kistner RL, Ferris EB III. Long-term effects of superficial femoral vein ligation: thirteen-year follow-up. *J Vasc Surg.* 1992;16:741–749.

17

Aortocaval Fistula

William H. Baker, MD

Arteriovenous fistulae between the aorta and its adjacent veins is a subject that does indeed belong in a book concerned with the "management of challenging problems." Due to the central location and large size of the blood vessels involved, flow through these fistulae may be massive, and the associated clinical conditions and complications are usually dramatic. The patients present with severe, refractory congestive heart failure rather than the usual rales in the lungs. Massive venous congestion and hypertension may occur suddenly. Hemorrhage through the unexpected fistula that is not controlled is perhaps the most dramatic of these situations.

Fortunately for patients and surgeons alike, these fistulae do not occur often. Nonetheless, the surgeon who operates on the aorta and vena cava must be well acquainted with the disorder in order to avoid or deal with the potentially morbid complications.

ETIOLOGY

As are all fistulae, aortovena caval fistulae are classified as congenital or acquired. Congenital fistulae in this position are the less common, and are adequately treated in pediatric textbooks. Acquired fistulae may be due to trauma or most often are the result of a ruptured aortic abdominal aneurysm (AAA) into the adjacent inferior venal cava (IVC).[1,2] Rarer causes are the erosion of false aneurysms of any cause, as well as specific aortitides. Aortocaval fistulae in general do not occur secondary to tumors, although hypernephromas have led to arterial venous fistulae between the renal artery and vein.[3]

Trauma, both iatrogenic as well as trauma from usual sources, may be a major cause of arteriovenous fistulae (Fig. 17–1). High-velocity missiles will cause immediate exsanguination and, thus, these patients do not present with fistula. Low-velocity missiles, especially knife wounds, may damage adjacent arteries and veins, yet be small enough to allow for spontaneous containment within a false aneurysm and the eventual formation of a fistula. Surgeons have unwittedly caused such fistulae. Neurosurgeons, during disc operations, may penetrate the anterior longitudinal ligament with their rongeurs. The major blood vessels that are anchored by their lumbar tributaries or branches may be injured and fistula formation may result. The aorta and IVC are most

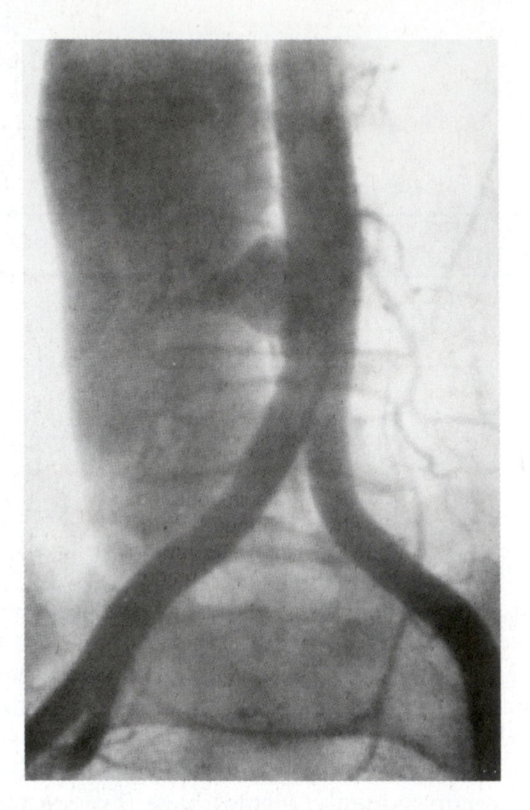

Figure 17–1. This patient had a lumbar discectomy approximately 6 months prior to the above arteriogram. A fistula can easily be seen. Not the extremely large IVC.

often injured opposite the L4-L5 disc space, whereas the iliac vessels are injured opposite the L5-S1 disc space. Complete discectomy is no longer the neurosurgical standard. Thus, the neurosurgeon is less apt to attempt complete extirpation of the disc and therefore less apt to cause penetration of the ligament, creating a fistula.

DIAGNOSIS

Diagnosis requires an accurate history and physical examination, as well as a keen awareness of the condition. The trauma patient with a thrill or a bruit in the abdomen must be carefully evaluated. Patients with AAAs who have a bruit that is present in both systole and diastole must likewise be considered to have an aortocaval fistula. Those patients who have the sudden onset of congestive heart failure following abdominal trauma or in association with large aneurysms should be investigated for an A-V fistula. The associated venous hypertension may cause a variety of conditions including hematuria, renal failure, sudden onset of venous insufficiency of the legs, or even rectal bleeding. Patients with aortocaval fistulae theoretically could steal blood so that leg ischemia would result, but the author has never seen this clinical situation.

All patients may not have a bruit heard over the fistula. This is especially true in those patients who have atherosclerotic AAAs. These aneurysms are lined with thrombotic material. The aneurysm may rupture into the IVC, and this thrombotic material may extend from time to time over the fistula. Thus, the fistula may be partially, completely, or intermittently occluded with this clot. Accordingly, signs and symptoms may come and go. Thus, there may be no way for the operating surgeon to diagnosis such a condition until he or she removes the clot in the operating room.

Noninvasive testing is useful in these patients to establish a baseline of distal arterial flow. Pulsatile venous signals may be recorded. Direct catheterization may be utilized to measure central and peripheral venous pressures, as well as pulmonary artery (wedge) pressures. A catheter may be passed in the vein past the fistula to measure the changing oxygen content of the arterialized venous blood at the site of the fistula. Such a test, however, is usually unnecessary. Arteriography is clearly the most precise method to localize the fistula. This is an examination that should be performed in all patients who present more or less electively to the surgeon. Obviously, it is an examination that will not be obtained in patients who present in shock with a ruptured aneurysm.

Since the carefully planned treatment of a patient with an aortocaval fistula depends on the proper recognition of the problem, the importance of a proper diagnosis cannot be overemphasized. Physician awareness is the key to many of these diagnostic dilemmas. The surgeon must spend the extra few minutes to examine the patient completely. The stethoscope should diagnose most aortocaval fistulae if, indeed, a bruit is present. Patients with an aneurysm or trauma should be examined for distended leg veins. Hematuria cannot be blamed on prostatism. The rather sick, elderly patient who has the sudden onset of congestive heart failure must be thoroughly evaluated for an aortocaval fistula.

THERAPY

Once the diagnosis has been established, therapy should begin immediately. Patients with a functioning fistula will be hyperdynamic and fluid overloaded. Thus, vigorous fluid administration prior to the closure of the fistula is contraindicated. However, patients who have an acute fistula may have pulsating veins. If, indeed, they have an associated retroperitoneal hematoma, they may be hypovolemic despite these pulsating veins. Such patients are clearly a conundrum for the surgeon and anesthesiologist alike.

A central venous pressure monitoring line should be established. The central venous pressure will, obviously, be abnormally elevated in a patient with aortocaval fistula. A Swan-Ganz catheter, particularly one that measures cardiac output, may facilitate fluid management. Transesophageal echography will help the anesthesiologist to assess left ventricular function. The modern surgical team should employ the methodologies that are well known to them so that fluid management can be facilitated.

These patients should not be transferred to the medical floor for "tuning up." These patients with congestive heart failure in all likelihood will have a high output cardiac failure. That is, their myocardium is working to full capacity, but the system is overloaded. To treat these patients with ionotrophic drugs is usually foolhardy. These patients need urgent operative control of their fistula. Once the fistula has been controlled, preload will be decreased, cardiac function will appear improved, and diuresis will correct their congestive heart failure. It is during this latter stage of treatment, after the fistula has been controlled, that judicious treatment with drugs, including diuretics, is advised. Most patients will correct themselves within a matter of hours to days.

In the operating room, the patient is prepped and draped to allow for a generous exposure. Most of the aortocaval fistulae will involve the infrarenal abdominal aorta. The aorta should be controlled in the usual and customary location. Occasionally these fistulae will involve the left renal vein and the aorta. Almost all of these patients will have a retroaortic left renal vein. The surgical incision, therefore, must be placed in such a manner so that the vascular surgeon can control the aorta proximal to the fistula. This control may have to be obtained in the suprarenal position under the dissected pancreas or at the diaphragmatic hiatus in the lesser sac. The author has not had the opportunity to repair one of these fistulae through the retroperitoneal approach and, thus, must confine his comments to transabdominal repair through a midline incision.

Blood loss during one of these repairs may be excessive. Therefore, the blood bank should be alerted to the impending problem. Autotransfusion devices should be ready from the start of the case.[4] Large fistulae could be managed with the patient on bypass. Total circulatory arrest has also been successfully used in these patients.[5]

The aorta is approached in the usual way by framing the incision with the colon and retracting the small intestines to the right. A hand placed upon the aorta should localize the fistula. Assuming the fistula to be in the terminal aorta, the proximal aorta under the renal arteries should be controlled. The surgeon should be warned that small veins, which are ordinarily just a nuisance, become a major problem when they are arterialized. Dissection may be facilitated by intermittently clamping the aorta, thereby reducing the pressure in the surrounding veins. In general, this will not be necessary. Distal control is obtained in the usual manner.

Once the arteries are controlled, no attempt is made to control the veins. Instead, sponge sticks or other devices are readied for venacaval and iliac vein compression (Fig. 17–2). The aorta is opened widely, and the surgeon's finger is usually sufficient to control the venous bleeding from the vena cava. Once all the thrombus has been removed from the aneurysm and the exact site of the fistula identified, the posterior aortic wall is closed with running monofilament suture. This can usually be performed with a large needle under the occluding finger or using compression. In some patients, it will be necessary to visualize the fistula using a rapid suction device from the autotransfuser. Once venous control has been accomplished, the operation proceeds as would any aneurysmectomy or aortic repair.

Why not attempt to control the IVC? In the author's experience, this procedure is fraught with hazard because of venous bleeding. The IVC is enlarged and turgid, making dissection quite difficult. Although intermittent clamping of the abdominal aorta may facilitate this dissection, the author does not find that the benefits of the dissection outweigh the risks of continued hemorrhage. Clearly, distal control of the iliacs should not be attempted, lest entry into the presacral venous plexus creates a major problem of hemorrhage.

Once the fistula has been controlled, the anesthesiologist must be alerted. The patient who has been hyperdynamic and hypervolemic up to this point in the operation may now show signs of hypovolemia. Careful communication at this point is essential. In addition, the various compressive maneuvers of the IVC may decrease cardiac return and temporarily be responsible for systemic hypotension.

Aortovena caval fistulae that are associated with AAAs may, in addition, have a special problem. These aneurysms are all lined with thrombotic material. If, indeed, any of this thrombotic material becomes loosened it may embolize through the fistula to become a pulmonary embolus (Fig. 17–3). The author has had one patient who had rhythm disturbances in the midst of an operation that were believed to be due to this mechanism.[1] The aorta may rupture into the underlying retroaortic renal vein. By necessity the aorta will have to be controlled proximal to the renal arteries. Once the fistula is identified and controlled, the operation proceeds as usual. Prolonged renal ischemia time should not be a problem. Alternatively, the left renal vein could be isolated between ligatures, thus

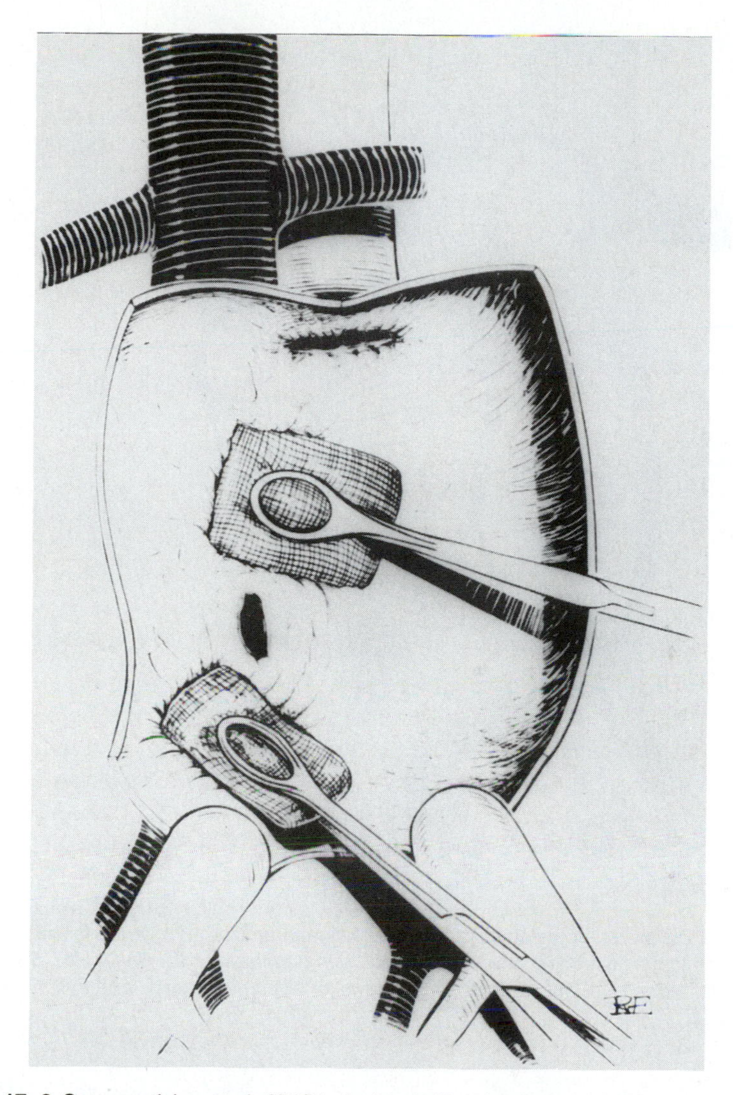

Figure 17–2. Sponge stick control of IVC is depicted. *(Reprinted with permission from Baker WH, Sharzer LA, Ehrenhaft JL. Aortocaval fistula as a complication of abdominal aortic aneurysms. Surgery. 1972;72:993.)*

effectively controlling the fistula. A graft may then be placed at some point proximal to the fistula, but in the infrarenal position. Under these circumstances, the gonadal and/or adrenal veins should be preserved for venous collateral.

CONCLUSION

Aortovena cava fistula is a dramatic surgical event, which may be lethal. The importance of a correct preoperative diagnosis cannot be overemphasized. When comparing a later series from the Massachusetts General Hospital[2] with an earlier series from The University of Iowa, one is impressed that the mortality rates are much different (10% vs. 50%). In the more recent series, most patients were diagnosed appropriately preoperatively. Thus, these patients benefited from an orderly controlled operation. In the

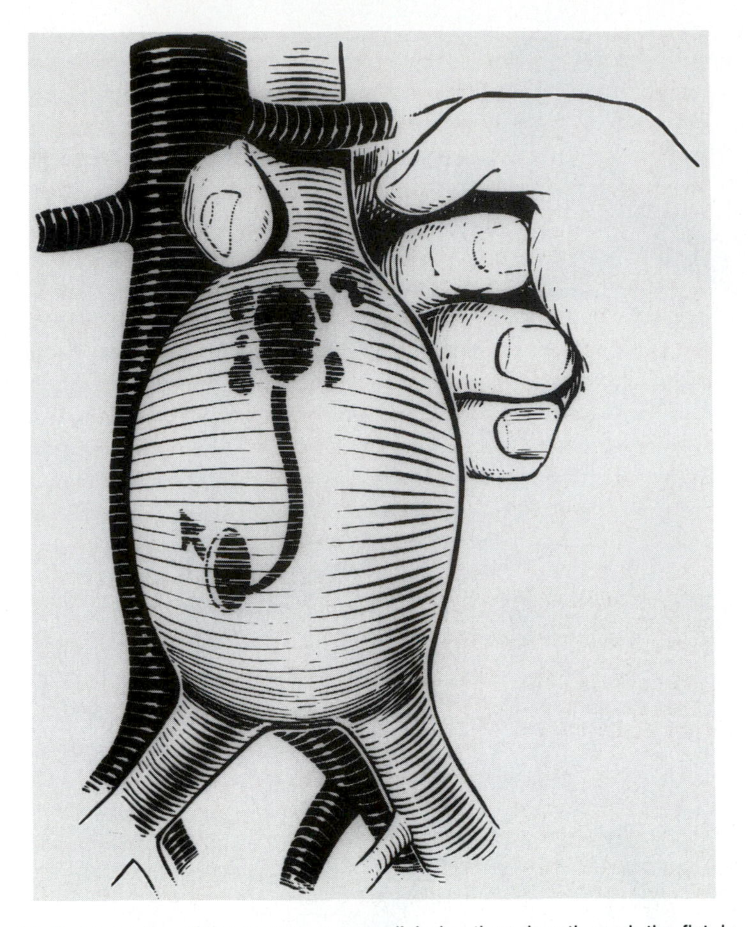

Figure 17–3. Dissection of the aneurysm may dislodge thrombus through the fistula, which will then embolize to the pulmonary artery. *(Reprinted with permission from Baker WH, Sharzer LA, Ehrenhaft JL. Aortocaval fistula as a complication of abdominal aortic aneurysms. Surgery. 1972;72:993.)*

older series, most patients were diagnosed in the operating room once the aneurysm was opened. Thus, those patients who survived did so despite excessive blood loss and wide swings in blood pressure.

All vascular surgeons should be prepared mentally for that day when they encounter a previously undiagnosed aortovena cava fistula in the midst of an aneurysm repair. Bleeding should be controlled by placing a finger (the thumb, typically) in the fistula. Bleeding may be massive, but it is from a low pressure venous source and is usually controllable. The author prefers sponge stick compression of the vena cava while repairing the fistula. Other surgeons might use another technique to achieve the same purpose. The surgeon who does not have a plan to address this sudden, critical situation, may have a patient that does not fare well. Aortovena cava fistula is truly a challenging surgical problem.

REFERENCES

1. Baker WH, Sharzer LA, Ehrenhaft JL. Aortocaval fistula as a complication of abdominal aortic aneurysms. *Surgery*. 1972;72:933.

2. Brewster DC, Cambria RP, Moncure AC, et al. Aortocaval and iliac arteriovenous fistulas: recognition and treatment. *J Vasc Surg*. 1991;13:253.
3. Crawford ES, Turrell DJ, Alexander JK. Aorto-inferior vena caval fistula of neoplastic origin. *Circulation*. 1963;27:414.
4. Doty DB, Wright CB, Lamberth WC, et al. Aortocaval fistula associated with aneurysm of the abdominal aorta: current management using autotransfusion techniques. *Surgery*. 1978;84:250.
5. Griffin LH Jr, Fishback ME, Galloway RF, et al. Traumatic aortorenal vein fistula: repair using total circulatory arrest. *Surgery*. 1977;81:840.

18

Aortoenteric Fistula

Steven M. Santilli, MD, PhD, and Jerry Goldstone, MD

Development of a fistula between the aorta and the intestine is a rare complication of aortic reconstructive surgery and an even rarer complication of untreated abdominal aortic aneurysms (AAAs). Aortoenteric fistulae (AEF) are difficult to manage for even the most experienced vascular surgeons and are usually encountered under urgent or emergency conditions. Without the prompt institution of appropriate diagnosis and treatment, the outcome is uniformly fatal.

AEF are classified as either primary or secondary. *Primary aortoenteric fistulae* are usually due to the erosion of an AAA into a segment of intestine, usually of the duodenum.[1–3] These were first described in 1927 by Sir Astley Cooper[4] as a naturally occurring complication of an AAA. The etiology of primary AEF is varied and also includes tuberculosis, syphilis, and other mycotic aortic infections.[5–7] However, in most series the most common etiology is erosion of an atherosclerotic AAA into a viscus with the duodenum being involved in more than 80% of cases.[1–7]

Secondary aortoenteric fistulae are due to the erosion of a vascular prosthesis or suture line into a loop of bowel. It is the most lethal complication of aortic reconstruction. Brock (1953) first described a case of a secondary AEF that occurred 1 year following aortic replacement with a homograft; Clayton (1956) reported the first AEF following the placement of a synthetic graft. The first successful treatment of this condition was reported by McKenzie in 1958. Because of several modest-sized studies from large medical centers, the incidence, pathogenesis, clinical presentation, diagnosis, and management of this condition can now be described reasonably well.[8–11]

SECONDARY AORTOENTERIC FISTULA

The incidence of secondary aortoenteric fistulae is difficult to determine from the literature because of its relative rarity, as well as the long time interval from graft implantation to the subsequent presentation of graft infection or fistula. In addition, patients are often not treated by the same surgeons for the complications as those who implanted their original graft. At the University of California, San Francisco, the average interval between the definitive treatment of the AEF and the original aortic graft placement was 6.1 years.[12] Aortic graft infection is estimated to develop in 1% to 2% of patients who have prosthetic aortic reconstructions and most estimates place the development of an AEF at about one-third of these cases. Utilizing these numbers, the estimated incidence of an AEF occurring after a primary prosthetic aortic graft placement is from 0.4% to 2%.[1,12,13]

Pathogenesis

Although there is no definitively known pathogenesis for an AEF, it is believed that infection or mechanical erosion of the graft into the bowel are the primary causes of fistula formation. Most prosthetic aortic grafts that become infected are thought to be contaminated at the time of implantation; hematogenous seeding probably accounts for very few aortic graft infections. A frequent association with aortic graft infection is reoperations on graft limbs due to stenosis, thrombus, or false aneurysm formation. Graft contamination presumably occurs during these secondary procedures. Reilly et al.[13] and Goldstone and Moore[14] reported these graft limb reoperations contributed to subsequent aortic graft infections in 40% to 46% of cases.

Following graft contamination, infection spreads along the graft, eventually involving perigraft tissues and the graft–artery anastomosis leading to the formation of a pseudoaneurysm. As the pseudoaneurysm enlarges, it erodes into the previously mobilized, scarred, and fixed duodenum, producing a fistula. Another postulated contributing factor is the anteriorly oriented "whiskers" of the suture used for the graft–artery anastomosis. These fistulae between the aortic suture line and the bowel are considered *anastomotic AEF,* and most frequently involve the third or fourth portions of the duodenum. Occasionally the cecum, sigmoid colon, and appendix are sites of fistula formation because of their proximity to the right and left iliac artery–graft anastomoses. Another form of AEF is a *periprosthetic aortoenteric erosion.* This occurs when a graft lies in direct contact with and erodes into a loop of bowel some distance from the suture lines. These fistulae appear to be primarily mechanically induced although infection may also play an important role in their pathogenesis.[16,17]

In our recent series[12] of secondary AEF, the initial aortic grafting was prompted by either aneurysmal or occlusive disease with equal frequency. Approximately one-half were aortofemoral and half aortoiliac grafts. Tube (aorto-aortic) grafts were very rare. End-to-end anastomoses were found to be twice as common as end-to-side anastomoses. Additional factors that may have contributed to the development of a graft infection and fistula formation were present in 67% of cases. These included emergency aortic reconstruction, subsequent reoperations on an aortic graft, and various perioperative complications.[12]

CLINICAL PRESENTATION

An AEF may present with a wide spectrum of symptoms varying from minimal discomfort to sudden exsanguinating hemorrhage in a septic patient. The clinical manifestations of an AEF are more variable than a perigraft infection without fistula. An AEF is, in general, a more unstable, more septic, and more deadly clinical entity. In our recent report, the most frequent presenting symptoms and findings were GI bleeding (66.7%, fever (66.7%), positive blood and/or wound cultures (78.3%, fever and chills (60.6%), and malaise (36.4%).[12]

The clinical presentation is dependent upon the type of AEF; either an anastomotic fistula or a periprosthetic aortic erosion. For example, we have previously reported that GI bleeding was found in 14 of 15 patients with an anastomotic AEF but in only

50% of patients with aortoenteric paraprosthetic erosion.[16] These data also reinforce the fact that an AEF can occur without any detectable GI bleeding at all.

Clinical suspicion remains the cornerstone of successful evaluation and treatment of patients with either type of AEF. We have found that patients with infected aortic grafts who are clinically septic are more likely to have a fistula than just perigraft infection. Therefore, profound sepsis in a patient with an infected aortic graft should lead to the search for an AEF. The possibility of an AEF should also be aggressively evaluated in all patients with aortic prosthetic grafts who exhibit GI bleeding, but it must be remembered that GI bleeding in patients with aortic graft infections may be due to septic stresses such as peptic ulcer disease, gastritis, or stress erosions. Previous widespread beliefs that (1) all graft AEFs bleed, (2) graft infections without bleeding exclude the possibility of an AEF, and (3) the demonstration of another etiology for GI bleeding excludes the diagnosis of an AEF have all be shown to be not true. In our recent series only 66.7% of patients with proven AEF presented with GI bleeding (48.5% of these patients had acute bleeding, 15% had chronic blood loss, and 6.1% had occult blood loss).[12]

Most patients with an AEF will have signs and symptoms of sepsis but be hemodynamically stable. In our series only 12% of patients presented with hemodynamic instability due to hemorrhage and required emergency diagnosis and treatment.[12]

DIAGNOSIS

Untreated AEF is a uniformally fatal clinical condition and therefore should be placed high on the list of possible diagnoses in any patient with GI bleeding at any time following an aortic operation, especially those involving placement of a prosthetic graft. This diagnosis should not be discarded until there is clear proof that this pathologic process is not present. Unfortunately, the preoperative diagnosis of an AEF is infrequent, being made preoperatively in only about one-third of patients with this disorder.[1,2,4,12] The remainder of patients are diagnosed in the operating room. This was true in our recent series in which the diagnosis was made preoperatively in 33.3% of patients.[12] It was suspected and confirmed during operation in 51.5% of patients and unsuspected but encountered during operations in 15.2%.[12]

The diagnosis of an AEF is dependent on a good history and physical examination followed by preoperative assessment, which should include esophagogastroduodenoscopy (EGD), computed tomography (CT) of the abdomen and pelvis, and angiography. Unfortunately, the only reliable physical finding, which is rarely encountered, is a pulsatile abdominal mass when a pseudoaneurysm is present.

EGD is the most important diagnostic test. It can be performed in the intensive care unit while the patient is undergoing resuscitation and prepared for operation. EGD should be performed by an experienced endoscopist with the surgeon in attendance, and an operating room should be prepared if the patient is actively bleeding. A thorough examination of the distal duodenum frequently requires the use of a longer endoscope (colonoscope). AEF are typically found in the third and fourth portions of the duodenum but have no typical appearance. They can appear as ragged mucosa or simply as a red spot. Very rarely graft material may be seen protruding through the bowel wall, and this clearly establishes the diagnosis (Fig. 18–1). In some cases ongoing bleeding from an uncertain source in the third or fourth portion of the duodenum is the only abnormality found. EGD is also useful for establishing the etiology of other upper gastrointestinal (GI) bleeding sources, such as esophagastric varices and gastric or duodenal ulcers or

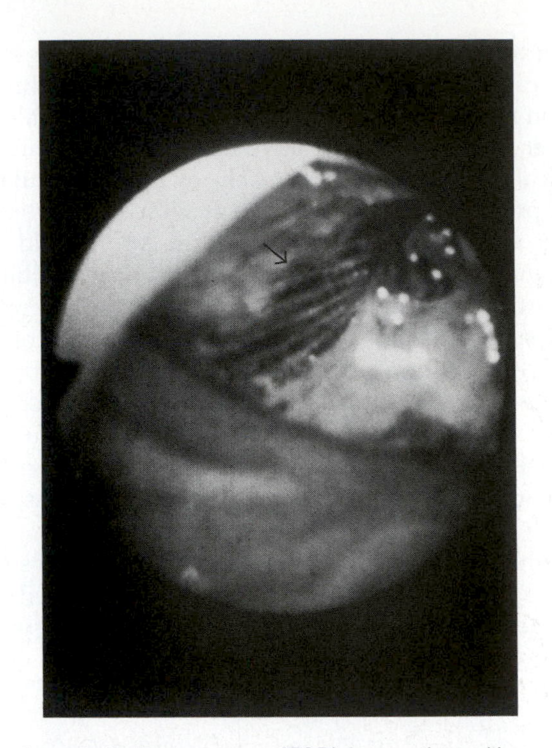

Figure 18–1. Esophagogastroduodenoscopy (EGD) in a patient with an aortoenteric fistula demonstrates the graft clearly visible in the third portion of the duodenum. The graft's black stripes (*arrow*) are visible within the lumen of the small bowel.

erosions. The presence of a nonfistulous upper GI bleeding pathology does not rule out an AEF. Although a source of upper GI bleeding may be found in the first and second portions of the duodenum, the endoscopist must complete the examination through the fourth portion of the duodenum. The diagnosis of an AEF is established when the fistula is seen or a bleeding site is identified in the distal duodenum with an entirely normal esophagus, stomach, and proximal duodenum. Using these criteria to establish a diagnosis, our recent series found that EGD was abnormal in more than one-half the patients who had a secondary AEF; however, it was diagnostic of a fistula in only two cases where graft material was seen. The false negative rate was 47.1%. This may in part be due to the fact that endoscopy to the fourth portion of the duodenum was only documented in 6 of 33 patients.[12]

CT scan with contrast is another primary test for the diagnosis of AEF. It directly assesses the retroperitoneum, perigraft space, and the relationship between the duodenum or other bowel and the graft. Findings that strongly suggest the diagnosis of an AEF include: (1) perigraft fluid or gas more than 2 to 3 months after aortic surgery, (2) an increase in perigraft soft tissue, (3) pseudoaneurysm formation, (4) loss of the continuous aneurysm wrap around the graft, (5) thickening of the adjacent bowel wall, or (6) prosthetic graft erosion into the lumen[1,12,18,19] (Fig. 18–2). Normal CT findings do not rule out the presence of an AEF. In our series, CT scans were abnormal in all cases, although they were diagnostic of a fistula in only 8 of 33 cases.[12] Magnetic resonance imaging (MRI) may be an even more highly reliable diagnostic technique for demonstrating perigraft infection, even though experience with MRI is less extensive.

Aortography is not an important study for the diagnosis of an AEF because it is rare to find extravasation of dye into the intestinal lumen.[20] In our series angiography

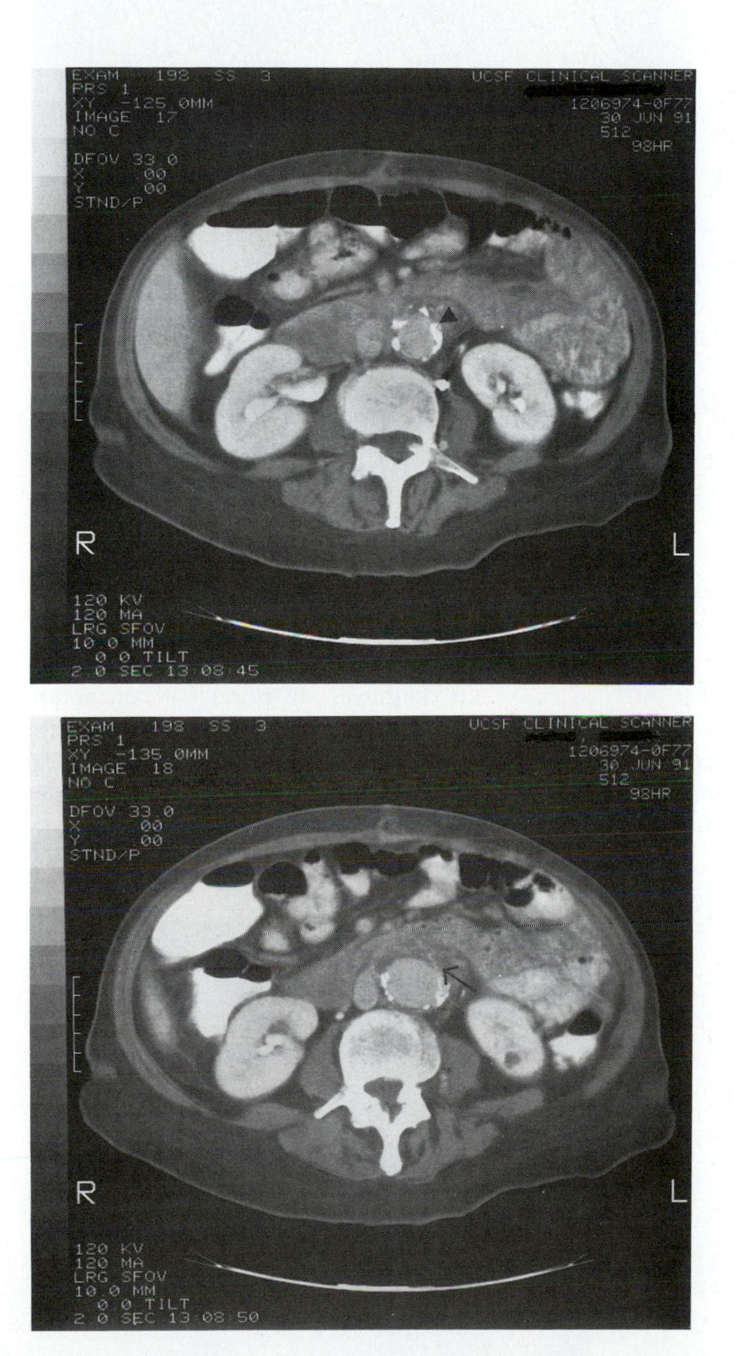

Figure 18–2. CT scan of a patient with an aortoenteric fistula demonstrates a dilated aortic graft that appears partially thrombosed (*bold arrow*). There is a loop of bowel surrounding the graft with no fat plane separating these two structures (*large arrow*) and indistinctness and streaking of the fat in mesentery surrounding the graft (*small arrow*). These findings are highly suggestive of an aortoenteric fistula.

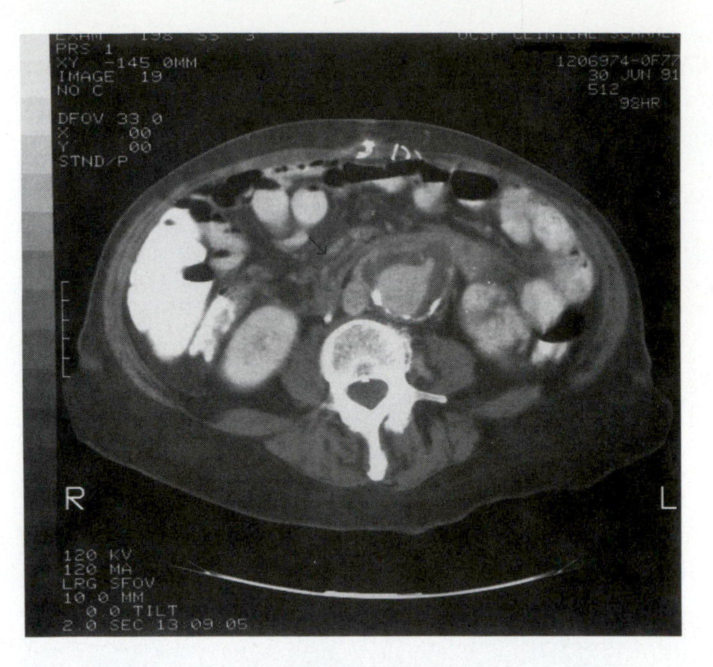

Figure 18–2. (*continued*)

was abnormal in 40% of cases but diagnostic in none.[12] When abnormal, it is most likely to show a normal aortic lumen or an anastomotic false aneurysm (Fig. 18–3). However, arteriography is critical for planning a well thought out, carefully executed vascular reconstruction, and for this purpose it should visualize the entire abdominal aorta, the aortic graft, native vessels, and runoff into the lower extremities.

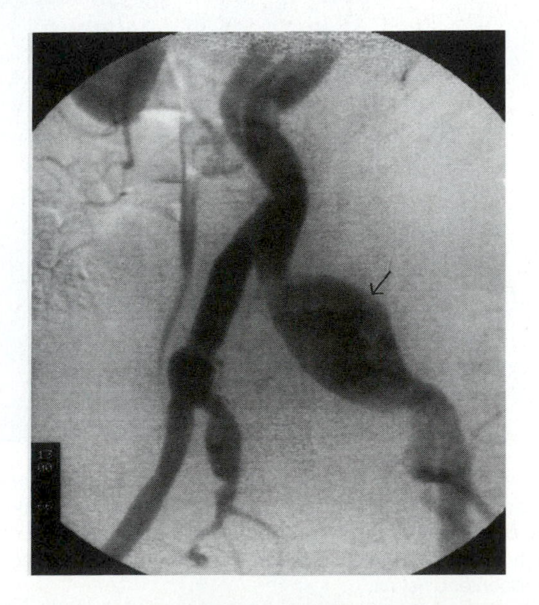

Figure 18–3. Arteriogram of a patient with aortoenteric fistula demonstrating a pseudoaneurysm at the anastomosis between the left limb of the aortobi-iliac graft and the left common iliac artery (*arrow*).

The diagnostic workup in a patient with a suspected AEF should proceed at a rapid pace. EGD, CT (or MRI), and aortography can usually be accomplished within a few hours after admission and while the patient is being prepared for operation with fluid resuscitation, placement of appropriate invasive monitors, and preparation of the operating room. In our series, the typical elapsed time between the onset of symptoms and definitive operative treatment was 84.8 days.[12] Most of this time was the delay in referral to our hospital. Despite this relatively long diagnostic delay, only 12.1% of patients required emergency treatment of their AEF.[12]

Numerous other studies have been used in the evaluation of patients with a suspected AEF, including ultrasound, contrast sinography, lower and upper GI contrast series, and radionuclide labeled white blood cell scans.[20–26] All are occasionally helpful but are not recommended as a part of the routine preoperative assessment of patients with this condition.

TREATMENT

Preoperative Preparation

Once the diagnosis of an AEF is strongly suspected or confirmed, prompt surgical treatment should follow. Appropriate pre- and intraoperative monitoring is necessary to maximize the patient's physiologic status. Hematologic resuscitation with blood products should be guided by preoperative and ongoing laboratory evaluation. Some patients will be quite emaciated due to their long illness and may require nutritional support, but operations should not be delayed for this purpose. All patients require broad-spectrum antibiotic coverage, which should be instituted when the diagnosis is suspected. The antibiotics should be effective against gram-positive (including *Staphylococcus epidermidis*, the most common organism responsible for vascular prosthetic graft infections),[1,4,9,12,16] gram-negative, and other enteric bacteria. The selected antibiotics should also cover any organism that has been cultured from draining wounds, aspirated perigraft fluid collections, or positive blood cultures. There is often a poor correlation between preoperative cultures and intraoperative gram stain results so antibiotic coverage should remain quite broad until definitive intraoperative culture and sensitivity data are available. Antibiotic treatment can then be tailored to the particular case.

Reconstructive Options

Treatment of an AEF requires the surgeon to take into account the hazards of revascularization through infected or contaminated fields. Autogenous tissue is the only material that can be safely used reliably when the vascular repair or reconstruction must pass through an infected field. Saphenous vein or endarterectomized superficial femoral artery are most often used as patches for repair of partial arterial wall defects (only possible with end-to-side anastomoses). Occasionally autogenous reconstruction can be performed by endarterectomizing previously bypassed native vessels, such as the aortic bifurcation and iliacs following an aortofemoral bypass for occlusive disease. Autograft replacement of infected arteries may also be accomplished using either the saphenous vein, which can be fashioned into a large caliber by sewing segments together in a side-to-side or spiral manner, the superficial femoral vein, or a segment of endarterectomized superficial femoral artery.

Prosthetic materials should only be used outside of all infected fields. This will most commonly require axillobifemoral revascularization of the lower extremities. Our preference is to utilize externally supported polytetrafluoroethylene (PTFE) for this purpose. A completely prosthetic revascularization is possible when the infected graft was placed in the aortic or aortoiliac position. If the femoral vessels are involved in the infectious process the axillofemoral limb of the graft must be tunneled out of the infected field to the profunda femoral artery or mid-to-distal superficial femoral artery if it is patent, and a cross-femoral graft constructed out of autogenous tissue utilizing either greater saphenous vein, superficial femoral vein, or endarterectomized, previously occluded, superficial femoral artery. These groin reconstructions can be extremely challenging and technically difficult. We do not routinely perform angiographic assessment of the axillary or subclavian arteries as donor vessels for axillobifemoral bypass instead relying on bilateral arm blood pressures to prevent placing the axillary anastomosis distal to a subclavian stenosis.

There are many options for the operative treatment of the AEF itself. Controversy remains over the optimal method because of the continued publication of series with high mortality, amputation, and aortic stump disruption rates.[27–31] The surgeon must choose an operative plan that is appropriate to the urgency and seriousness of the patient's manifestations of fistula and infection. The goal of treatment is to first prevent death due to hemorrhage, and sepsis, and then limb loss because of ischemia.

Treatment Options

The operative treatment of a secondary AEF has two distinct components: (1) excision of the infected graft and repair of the fistula, and (2) revascularization. The *traditional* treatment plan consists of removal of the infected graft, repair of the fistula, and then immediate extra-anatomic bypass for revascularization of the lower extremities. Recently this traditional approach has been challenged and the sequence has been reversed with extra-anatomic bypass being performed first followed by the transabdominal removal of the infected graft and repair of the fistula. This results in less lower extremity ischemia. The time interval between lower extremity revascularization and infected graft excision may be immediate or *staged*. A third treatment option, which has been recently proposed for selected patients by several groups, is *in situ* reconstruction immediately following the removal of the infected graft and repair of the enteric fistula.

All of these treatment schemes involve lengthy, complex operations that stress not only the patient but also the surgical team. All phases of the procedure are difficult, technically demanding, and unforgiving of mistakes. This is one of the major reasons why we prefer a staged treatment plan. Although some surgeons have advocated infected graft removal and lower extremity revascularization only when necessary, most patients will require revascularization of the lower extremities following removal of the infected graft and delays often lead to profound ischemic problems. However, revascularization may not be necessary in patients who have had previous amputations or chronically occluded graft limbs with viable extremities.

The choice of operative therapy is primarily dictated by the clinical status of the patient. Treatment priorities are: (1) resuscitation of the unstable patient, (2) control of bleeding, (3) control of sepsis, and (4) infected graft removal and revascularization of the lower extremities. If the patient is actively bleeding and hemodynamically unstable, transabdominal control of the aorta must be accomplished first accompained by graft removal and fistula repair. Extremity revascularization then follows using fresh instruments and drapes. The staged treatment sequence in this circumstance is contraindicated. However, as we have recently reported, this is an unusual event occurring in only 12% of patients in our series.[12] Most patients will present in a stable clinical state and the method of operative treatment, be it traditional or reversed, staged or not staged, is dependent on surgeon preference. The presence of an AEF does not make the staged approach unfeasible since in our experience one-third of patients with fistulas had no evidence of bleeding at all and only one patient ruptured an aortic false aneurysm in the interval between extra-anatomic bypass[12] and removal of the infected aortic graft.

The overall mortality rates for the traditional approach to the treatment of an AEF remain greater than 50% with an associated amputation rate of 8% to 10%. The rate of aortic stump disruption averages 21.6%.[27–31] These outcomes are based on small series that accumulate patients over long periods of time. Due to various reporting techniques and operative procedures, pooling these data do not reveal clear information regarding the current outcomes that can be achieved with one consistent treatment approach. However, these data do suggest unacceptably high morbidity and mortality rates following the traditional approach to repair of an AEF.

We recently reported our more contemporary series of patients with secondary AEF treated, when possible, with the reversed staged approach, that is, extra-anatomic bypass (axillobifemoral) first, followed several days later by infected graft excision and closure of the fistula. Our results were: 18.2% periopertive death rate, 6% incidence of aortic stump disruption, 9% incidence of late deaths related to the aortic graft infection, and 9% amputation rate. Cummulative survival rates in our series were 74.5% at 1 year, which stabilized and remained constant at 70% at 3 years. This is essentially the cure rate. There were six failures of the extra-anatomic bypass, two perioperatively, and four during late follow-up, an incidence of 18.2%. Only one patient required a late amputation. The cumulative 4-year primary patency rate was 71%, while the secondary patency rate was 89.6%.[12]

In situ reconstruction for secondary AEF has been reported in several small studies.[32–36] Only two studies used *in situ* prosthetic graft replacement exclusively, and only one of these contained more than 10 patients.[34,36] The reported morbidity and mortality rates were 30.4% while the overall cure rate was 56.5%. There were additional treatment failures from false aneurysm formation or re-infection of the newly placed grafts. This is a relatively new approach, which requires further consideration and study. The advent of coated Dacron grafts with bonded antibiotics for slow, delayed release may make *in situ* graft replacement a more successful option in the future.

Not all patients are candidates for our preferred reversed staged procedure of extra-anatomic bypass followed by infected graft removal and fistula repair. Obviously, a patient who presents with active bleeding that cannot be controlled or stabilized is one example. Such patients must be taken immediately to the operating room, the bleeding controlled, and the graft removed, followed by revascularization. The course of bleeding is unpredictable and the treatment plan for a patient who presents with active bleeding must be carefully individualized. Stable patients with active bleeding that stops can be considered for the reversed stage approach. The timing between extra-anatomic bypass and infected graft removal will vary depending on the clinical situation. The length of staging interval should be kept as short as the patient's condition will allow, and over time we have progressively shortened this interval. Usually, extra-anatomic bypass can be followed within the next 1 to 3 days by removal of the infected graft and repair of the fistula. Even a delay this short allows the patient to recover physiologically from the first operation and contributes to the lower morbidity and mortality rates with this technique.[12] In patients who present with active bleeding and significant hemodynamic instability but who then stop bleeding with a high degree of concern for rebleeding, the extra-anatomic bypass should be followed immediately by infected graft removal and fistula repair in a single operation. In our series only two patients died in the interval between extra-anatomic bypass and infected graft removal, and one was due to a myocardial infarction.[12]

Principals of Extra-anatomic Bypass

Axillobifemoral bypass is the most practical and reliable method for restoring circulation to the lower extremities in the presence of an AEF. When an aortobi-iliac graft is involved in the infectious process, the groins are usually unaffected and the axillofemoral limb of the revascularization is placed to the common femoral artery. A 6- to 8-mm externally reinforced PTFE graft has become our preference for this purpose. The site of origin is from as far medial as possible on the axillary artery. The right side is preferred unless there is a proximal subclavian stenosis. The absence of groin sepsis allows the cross-femoral limb to also be a synthetic conduit. Occasionally the common iliac arteries can be sewn together to form an *in situ* autogenous femoral–femoral bypass. Specific techniques of reconstruction have been described in several previous vascular surgery texts.

In the presence of an infected aortobifemoral graft with involvement of one or both femoral regions, the reconstruction must be modified to avoid contamination of the axillofemoral graft. This is accomplished by routing the graft out of the contaminated groin, usually laterally, to the mid-profunda femoris artery or superficial femoral artery if it is patent. An autogenous cross-femoral graft, constructed out of saphenous vein, superficial femoral vein, or endarterectomized, previously occluded superficial femoral artery can then originate and terminate on the common femoral arteries.

Principals of Aortoenteric Fistula Repair and Infected Graft Removal

The abdomen is opened through a full-length midline incision (xiphoid to pubis). Proximal aortic control is obtained at the supraceliac level via a transcrural approach but cross-clamping at this level is performed only when needed. After establishing adequate inflow control the distal graft limbs are dissected and control obtained. The next operative goal is to dissect the graft from the adherent segment of the GI tract thereby gaining control of the fistula. For an aortoduodenal fistula the entire duodenum must be reflected away from the graft to allow a tension-free duodenal repair. A large defect in the duodenum may require serosal patching and in some cases primary duodenal resection with an end-to-end anastomosis or a duodenojejunostomy. In most patients, a feeding jejunostomy is placed to allow early postoperative enteral feeding while protecting the duodenal repair.

Following vascular control and fistula repair, the infected aortic graft is removed. The entire infected prosthesis should always be completely removed with segments submitted for bacteriologic analysis. The most critical feature of aortic graft removal is the technique for handling the aortic stump. A leading cause of perioperative death and late mortality from the treatment of AEF is dehiscence of the aortic stump.[12,27–31] Survival from this event is rare. In our recent series there was a 6% incidence of aortic stump disruption with 100% mortality.[12] Adequate debridement of the aortic stump is critically important for a secure and durable closure. The aortic wall must be debrided back to healthy tissue even if it means relocating one or both renal arteries. Proximal portions of the debrided aortic wall should be sent for culture, sensitivity, and Gram's stain. The aorta must be closed without tension using a double row of nonabsorbable, monofilament sutures; one horizontal mattress and one simple running placed into healthy tissue. Temporary cross-clamping of the suprarenal or supraceliac aorta is usually required to ensure adequate infrarenal aortic tissue to sew. There are various methods of aortic stump reinforcement, including jejunal serosal patch, anterior spinal ligament patch, or an omental pedicle. These techniques may be helpful but have not yet proven beneficial in reducing the incidence of stump disruption and are no substitute for proper aortic debridement and closure.

The retroperitoneal tissue should be debrided and drainage considered in all cases where gross pus is present. Drains should be soft sump drains carefully placed to avoid direct contact with either the aortic stump or the duodenal repair. Infected femoral wounds also require very careful management. At the time of graft removal, all necrotic and infected tissue should be excised and the wounds packed open with antibiotic-soaked dressings. When there is an autogenous conduit in the femoral area, noninfected subcutaneous tissue can be loosely approximated over the graft and the remainder of the wound left open. In cases where the infection requires extensive debridement leaving vessels exposed, wound closure utilizing rotated or free muscle flaps is used to prevent drying and erosion of exposed vessels as well as to ensure wound healing.

Long-Term Follow-Up

Late infections can occur in patients who have had an infected graft removed and an AEF repaired. These late infections usually involve prosthetic portions of the extra-anatomic reconstruction used to revascularize the lower extremities. In our experience, most new graft infections occurred in the midportions of the axillofemoral graft where a counter-incision had been made to facilitate subcutaneous tunneling.[15] We subsequently have abandoned the use of the counter-incision and axillofemoral graft infections have occurred in only 2 of the last 33 patients.[12] These new graft infections occasionally result in limb loss but are not associated with death. For these reasons patients should be periodically reevaluated for the remainder of their lives.

Those patients who have had positive proximal aortic wall cultures require appropriate imaging studies at regular intervals. CT or MRI scans of the abdomen are recommended to identify persistent infection in or about the aortic stump or the formation of a pseudoaneurysm. In addition, antibiotics should be continued for a least 3 to 6 months postoperatively.

Summary

Secondary AEF is a highly lethal, yet rare, complication of aortic reconstructions. It can present with a wide variety of symptoms, and the diagnosis is only firmly established in about one-third of patients prior to operation. We have treated a large contemporary series of patients using a reversed, staged operative repair, consisting of extra-anatomic bypass first, followed by infected graft removal and repair of the fistula.[12] Utilizing this approach, the morbidity and mortality rates associated with this highly lethal condition have been reduced significantly.

PRIMARY AORTOENTERIC FISTULA

Primary AEF is a rare clinical condition. Less than 200 cases have been reported in the English language literature.[1–7,37–41] The most common cause is erosion or rupture of an AAA into an adjacent, adherent segment of bowel, usually the duodenum. Most contemporary series suggest that the diagnosis can be established based on characteristic CT scan findings of the duodenum stretched over an aortic aneurysm that is associated with retroperitoneal air. As many as one-third of patients with a primary AEF die within the first 6 to 12 hours after the onset of symptoms. It is essential to consider the diagnosis and to initiate treatment immediately. The majority of these patients will present with major upper GI hemorrhage resulting in hemodynamic instability. This clinical situation limits the use of diagnostic studies and precludes the use of reversed, staged treatment protocol as described for a secondary AEF. In this setting, repair of the enteric fistula and *in situ* prosthetic aortic grafting is considered appropriate treatment. Anecdotally, long-term results appear to be satisfactory.

REFERENCES

1. Bunt TJ. Synthetic vascular graft infections. Secondary graft enteric erosions and graft enteric fistulas. *Surgery*. 1983;94:1.
2. Reckless JPD, McColl I, Taylor GW. Aortoenteric fistulae: an uncommon complication of abdominal aortic aneurysms. *Br J Surg*. 1972;59:458.
3. Thompson WM, Jackson DC, Johnsrude IE. Aortoenteric and paraprosthetic-enteric fistulae. Radiologic findings. *Am J Roentgenol*. 1976;127:235.
4. Cooper A. *The Lectures of Sir Astley Cooper on the Principles and Practice of Surgery with Additional Notes and Cases by Tyrell F.* 5th ed. Philadelphia: Haswell, Barrington, and Haswell; 1939.
5. Walker WE, Cooley DA, Duncan JM, et al. The management of aortoduodenal fistula by *in situ* replacement of the infected abdominal aortic graft. *Ann Surg*. 1987;205:727.
6. Sweeney MS, Godacz TR. Primary aortoduodenal fistula: manifestations, diagnosis, and treatment. *Surgery*. 1984;96:492.
7. TenEyck FW, Wellman WE. Salmonellosis associated with abdominal aortic aneurysm and edema of lower extremities. Case report. *Postgrad Med*. 1954;26:334.
8. Goldstone J, Effeney DJ. Prevention of arterial graft infections. In: Bernhard VM, Towne JB eds. *Complications in Vascular Surgery*. New York; Grune and Stratton; 1985:487.
9. Bergqvist D. Arterioenteric fistula. *Acta Chir Scand*. 1987;153:81–86.
10. Connolly JE, Kwaan JHM, McCart PM, et al. Aortoenteric fistula. *Ann Surg*. 1988;194:402.
11. O'Mara CS, Williams GM, Ernst CB. Secondary aortoenteric fistula: a 20-year experience. *Am J Surg*. 1981;142:203.
12. Kuestner LM, Reilly LM, Jicha DL et al. Secondary aortoenteric fistula: contemporary outcome with use of extraanatomic bypass and infected graft excision. *J Vasc Surg*. 1995;21:184.
13. Reilly LM, Altman H, Lusby RJ, et al. Late results following surgical management of vascular graft infection. *J Vasc Surg*. 1984;1:36.
14. Goldstone J, Moore WS. Infection in vascular prostheses: clinical manifestation and surgical management. *Am J Surg*. 1974;128:228.
15. Reilly LM, Goldstone J, Ehrenfeld WK, et al. Gastrointestinal tract involvement by prosthetic graft infection: the significance of gastrointestinal hemorrhage. *Ann Surg*. 1985;202:342–348.
16. Macbeth GA, Rubin JR, McIntyre KE Jr, et al. The relevance of arterial wall microbiology to the treatment of prosthetic graft infections: graft infection vs. arterial infection. *J Vasc Surg*. 1984;1:750.
17. Busuttil RW, Reese W, Baker JD, et al. Pathogenesis of aortoduodenal fistula. Experimental and clinical correlates. *Surgery*. 1979;85:1–10.
18. Harris KA, Kozak R, Carrol SF, et al. Confirmation of infection of an aortic graft. *J Cardiovasc Surg*. 1989;30:230.
19. Low RN, Wall SD, Jeffrey RB Jr, et al. Aortoenteric fistula and perigraft infection: evaluation with CT. *Radiology*. 1990;175:157.
20. Kleinman LH, Towne JB, Bernhard VM. A diagnostic and therapeutic approach to aortoenteric fistulas: clinical experience with twenty patients. *Surgery*. 1979;86:868.
21. Reilly LM, Ehrenfeld WK, Goldstone J, et al. Gastrointestinal tract involvement of prosthetic graft infection. The significance of gastrointestinal hemorrhage. *Ann Surg*. 1985;202:342.
22. O'Mara CS, Williams GM, Ernst CB. Secondary aortoenteric fistula. A 20-year experience. *Am J Surg*. 1981;142:203.
23. Ferris EJ, Koltay MRS, Koltay OP, et al. Abdominal aortic and iliac graft fistulae: unusual roentgenographic findings. *Am J Roentgenal*. 1965;94:416.
24. La Muraglia GM, Fischman AJ, Strauss HW, et al. Utility of the indium^{111}-labeled human immunoglobulin G scan for the detection of focal vascular graft infection. *J Vasc Surg*. 1989;10:20.

25. Lawrence PF, Dries DJ, Alazraki N, et al. Indium[111]-labeled leukocyte scanning for detection of prosthetic graft infection. *J Vasc Surg.* 1985;2:165.
26. Alfrey EJ, Stanton C, Dunnington G, et al. Graft appendiceal fistulas. *J Vasc Surg.* 1988;7:814.
27. O'Hara PJ, Hertzer NR, Beven EG, et al. Surgical management of infected abdominal aortic grafts: review of a 25-year experience. *J Vasc Surg.* 1986;3:725–731.
28. Plate G, Hollier LA, O'Brien P, et al. Recurrent aneurysms and late vascular complications following repair of abdominal aortic aneurysms. *Arch Surg.* 1985;120:590–594.
29. Bergeron P, Espinoza H, Rudondy P, et al. Secondary aortoenteric fistulas: value of initial axillofemoral bypass. *Ann Vasc Surg.* 1991;5:4–7.
30. Champion MC, Sullivan SN, Coles JC, et al. Aortoenteric fistula. Incidence, presentation, recognition and management. *Ann Surg.* 1982;195:314–317.
31. Trout HH III, Kozloff L, Giordano JM. Priority of revascularization in patients with graft enteric fistulas, infected arteries, or infected arterial prostheses. *Ann Surg.* 1984;199:669–683.
32. Jacobs MJHM, Reul GJ, Gregoric I, et al. In-situ replacement and extra-anatomic bypass for the treatment of infected abdominal aortic grafts. *Eur J Vasc Surg.* 1991;5:83–86.
33. Gozzetti G, Poggioli G, Spolaore R, et al. Aorto-enteric fistulae: spontaneous and after aortoiliac operations. *J Cardiovasc Surg.* 1984;5:420–426.
34. Sorensen S, Lorentzen JE. Recurrent graft-enteric fistulae: case report. *Eur J Vasc Surg.* 1989;3:583–585.
35. Vollmar JF, Kogel H. Aorto-enteric fistulas as postoperative complication. *J Cardiovasc Surg.* 1987;28:479–484.
36. Walker WE, Cooley DA, Duncan JM, et al. The management of aortoduodenal fistula by in situ replacement of the infected abdominal aortic graft. *Ann Surg.* 1986;205:727–732.
37. Evans DM, Webster JHH. Spontaneous aortoduodenal. *Br J Surg.* 1972;59:368.
38. Foster JH, Vetto RM. Aortic intra-aneurysmal abscess caused by sigmoid-aortic fistula. *Am J Surg.* 1962;104:850.
39. Frosch HL, Horowitz W. Rupture of abdominal aorta into duodenum (through a sinus tract created by a tuberculous mesenteric lymphadenitis). *Ann Intern Med.* 1944;21:481.
40. Reckless JPD, McColl I, Taylor GW. Aortoenteric fistulae: an uncommon complication of abdominal aortic aneurysms. *Br J Surg.* 1972;59:458.
41. Thompson WM, Jackson DC, Johnsrude IE. Aortoenteric and paraprosthetic-enteric fistulae. Radiologic findings. *Am J Roentgenol.* 1976;127:235.

19

Surgical Technique, Preoperative and Intraoperative Management of Thoracoabdominal Aortic Aneurysm

Joseph S. Coselli, MD

Thoracoabdominal aortic aneurysms are those that involve both the thoracic and the abdominal aorta in continuity. Despite substantial improvements in anesthetic management, operative technique, and perfusion technology, treatment of these aneurysms continues to present a significant challenge to the vascular surgeon. With the general aging of our population and increased availability of diagnostic modalities, recognition of this entity is occurring with increased frequency. Bahnson[1] in 1952 reported on the successful repair of a saccular thoracoabdominal aortic aneurysm by lateral resection and aortorrhaphy. Ellis and colleagues[2] at the Mayo Clinic reported the first repair of an aneurysm involving a visceral artery, the renal artery, by resection and graft replacement in 1955. The first more complex thoracoabdominal aneurysm repair, including celiac axis and superior mesenteric artery, was reported in 1955 by Etheredge and colleagues.[3] DeBakey and colleagues[4] reported the successful repair of a thoracoabdominal aortic aneurysm involving all the visceral arteries—the celiac, superior mesenteric, and both renals—in 1956. Subsequently, DeBakey's group devised a technique for aneurysm replacement utilizing a permanent Dacron bypass graft with visceral arterial reattachment to appropriately positioned sidearm grafts. In 1965 they reported a 26% mortality in 42 patients operated on using this approach.[5] Crawford revolutionized and simplified the surgical treatment of thoracoabdominal aortic aneurysm by employing an inclusion technique substantially reducing morbidity and mortality.[6–8] Patients undergoing surgical treatment for thoracoabdominal aortic aneurysms continue to suffer morbidity associated with postoperative renal insufficiency or failure and/or neurologic deficits including paraplegia or paraparesis.[9,10] In this chapter, current concepts and technical modifications are addressed with emphasis on techniques to reduce the frequency and severity of distal organ ischemic injury.

NATURAL HISTORY

Thoracoabdominal aortic aneurysms are probably not as rare as many vascular surgeons maintain. Certainly they are the result of a degenerative process in the aortic wall with mechanical stress factors leading to progressive aneurysmal enlargement and ultimately rupture. Larger aneurysms are at increased risk of rupture consequent to the direct relationship between aortic wall tension and the diameter of the aorta (LaPlace's Law). Ingoldby et al.[11] found 78 of 338 (23%) deaths due to aortic aneurysms to be from thoracic or thoracoabdominal aneurysms in a population-based study. Crawford and DeNatale reported on 94 patients who did not undergo aneurysm repair and found a 2-year survival rate of only 24%, with half of the deaths due to aneurysmal rupture. The overall 5-year survival was only 19%.[12] Bickerstaff et al.[13] identified similar survival rates, noting a 2-year actuarial survival rate of 28.5% in patients with untreated thoracic aortic aneurysms. Again, rupture was the most common cause of death. It is now, of course, abundantly clear that surgical intervention has favorable impact on the expected survival in patients treated for thoracoabdominal aortic aneurysms with 2-year survival approximating 70%, and 5-year, 60%.[9,10,14]

PREOPERATIVE EVALUATION PREPARATION

In addition to direct aortic evaluation, all patients are thoroughly examined with particular focus placed upon cardiac, pulmonary, and renal parameters. All patients undergo transthoracic echocardiography to evaluate biventricular and valvular function. Patients with a history of angina or ejection fraction of 30% or less undergo cardiac catheterization and coronary artery study. Patients with severe cardiac disease and asymptomatic thoracoabdominal aortic aneurysms may require surgical correction of cardiac pathology prior to undergoing aneurysm replacement. All patients undergo pulmonary function testing. Borderline pulmonary function may frequently be improved with cessation of smoking, treatment of bronchitis, weight loss, and a general exercise program for a period of 1 to 3 months preoperatively. Preoperative serum BUN and creatinine levels to evaluate renal function are established in all patients. Intravenous hydration with 1 L of lactated Ringer's solution and 50 mg of Mannitol is administered prior to aortography in all patients. Operation in symptomatic patients and patients with large aneurysms has not been withheld from patients despite poor pulmonary function. Patients with preoperative renal failure and an established hemodialysis program have no more morbidity than patients with normal renal function. Patients with severely impaired renal function, not on chronic hemodialysis, frequently require transient hemodialysis in the early postoperative period allowing treatment in patients with symptomatic aneurysms. Most patients with severe renal occlusive disease, treated at operation with endarterectomy or bypass grafting, are substantially improved regarding renal function.

OPERATIVE TECHNIQUES

The essentials of operative repair for the treatment of thoracoabdominal aortic aneurysms have been reported on previously in detail (Fig. 19–1).[14–16] The combined efforts of an anesthesiologist and perfusion technologist with interest and experience in aortic surgery is essential. In all patients a double lumen endotrachial tube is utilized to allow

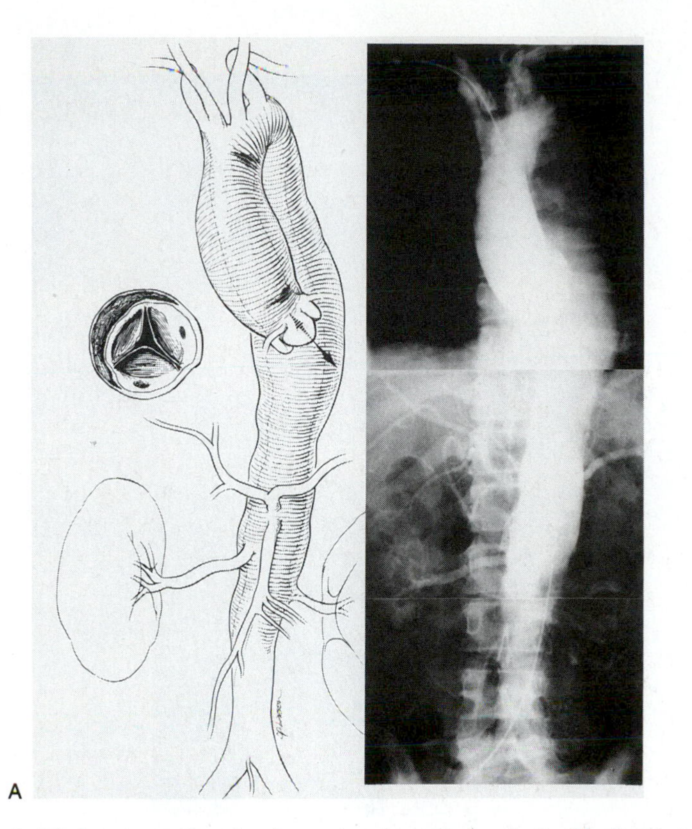

Figure 19–1. (**A**) A preoperative drawing and aortogram of patient with chronic type I aortic dissection. Ascending aortic aneurysm and aortic valvular insufficiency are secondary to proximal dissection with commissural disruption. In addition, thoracoabdominal aortic aneurysm, Crawford extent II, is present.

complete deflation of the left lung and selective right lung ventilation to facilitate exposure and repair without cardiac compression and pulmonary trauma. A Swan-Ganz pulmonary artery catheter is routinely placed, and lines for intraoperative monitoring of arterial blood pressure, central venous pressure, arterial blood gases, electrolytes, temperature, and electrocardiogram are placed. In patients with a significant history of cardiac disease, known impaired cardiac function, or cardiac valvular disease, a transesophageal echocardiography probe is inserted. I have not employed cerebrospinal fluid drainage nor used intrathecal papaverine.

Patients are positioned in a right lateral decubitus position using a bean bag apparatus to maintain the shoulders and upper thorax at 60° and the hips more supine at about 30°. In patients in whom the aneurysm has a proximal extent in the superior aspect of the thorax (Crawford extents I and II), the upper portion of the thoracoabdominal incision is through the sixth intercostal space or the bed of the resected sixth rib. With aneurysm of lower aortic involvement (Crawford extent III or IV), an incision through the seventh, eighth, or ninth interspace is employed, depending on the desired level of exposure.

Abdominal dissection is carried out via transperitoneal exposure with the retroperitoneum entered lateral to the left colon. An open abdominal approach allows for direct examination of the bowel and abdominal viscera and their blood supply following the completion of aortic repair. An entirely retroperitoneal approach is used in patients

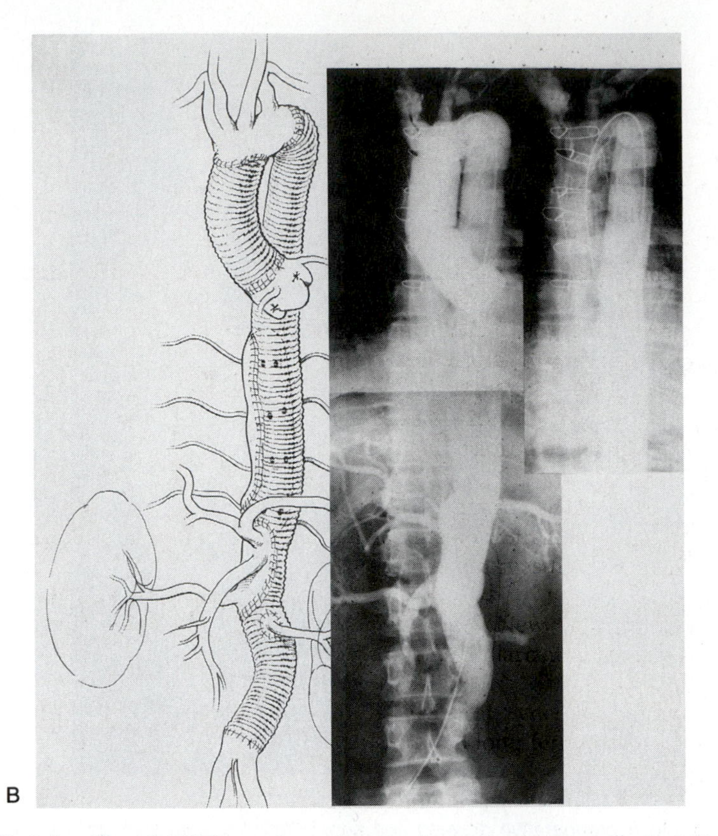

Figure 19–1. (*continued*) (**B**) The postoperative drawing and aortogram following initial resection and graft replacement of ascending aorta and aortic valve resuspension and subsequent resection and replacement of all of the thoracoabdominal aorta with reattachment of intercostal, visceral, and renal arteries.

with multiple prior abdominal surgeries, particularly if there is a history of extensive adhesions or peritonitis, the so-called "hostile" abdomen. The perioperative fluid requirements and pulmonary morbidity are no different for the retroperitoneal or transperitoneal exposure. A dissection plane is developed in the retroperitoneum to the aorta anterior to the psoas muscle and posterior to the left kidney. The diaphragm is divided in a circumferential fashion preserving the maximum amount of muscle, leaving a rim of 1 to 2 cm of diaphragm laterally on the chest wall.

The left crus of the diaphragm is divided and the left renal, superior mesenteric, and celiac arteries are identified but not encircled. Intravenously, heparin, 1 mg/kg, is administered prior to the initiation of bypass and/or aortic clamping.

In patients with extensive thoracoabdominal aortic aneurysm (Crawford extents I and II), particularly those with dissection, that is, patients at greatest risk for postoperative paraparesis/paraplegia, distal aortic perfusion during proximal aortic repair has been employed using left atrium to femoral artery (usually left) bypass, using an inline centrifugal pump (Biomedicus, Medtronic, Inc., Eden Prairie, MN) (Fig. 19–2A). Bypass flows are adjusted to maintain a distal arterial pressure of 70 mm Hg. No inline heat exchanger is used; the patient is allowed to drift down to a rectal temperature of 32°C to 33°C. The proximal anastomosis is carried out between aortic clamps isolating the proximal extent of the aneurysm with the distal clamp placed at the level of T_4 to T_7. The vagus, recurrent laryngeal, and phrenic nerves are identified and protected. The

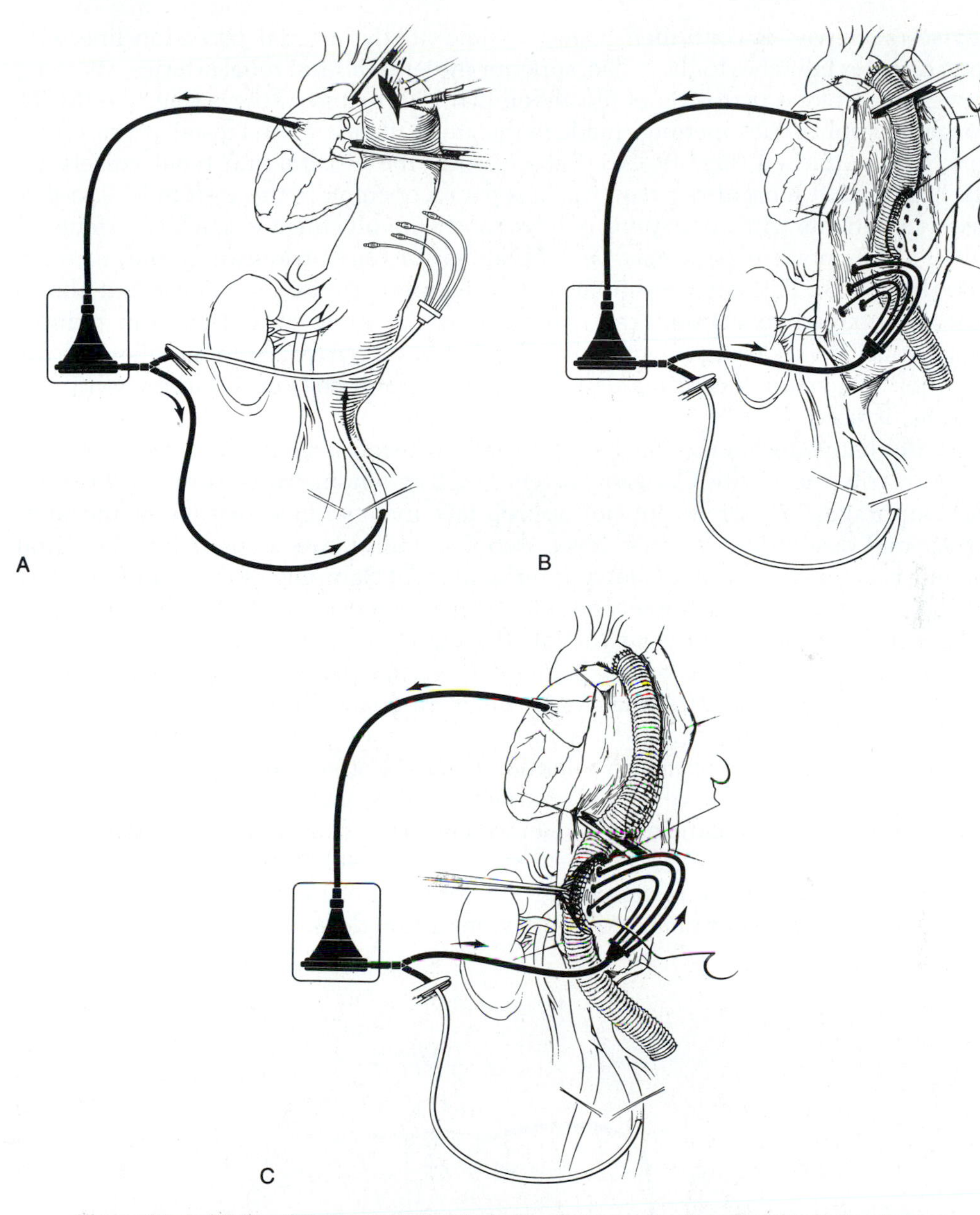

Figure 19–2. (**A**) Drawing demonstrating technique for extensive thoracoabdominal aortic aneurysm repair utilizing proximal aortic isolation with distal aortic perfusion employing left atrial to left common femoral artery bypass with centrifugal pump. (**B**) Following completion of proximal anastomosis, visceral and renal arteries are perfused with oxygenated blood from bypass circuit during intercostal arterial reattachment. (**C**) Prior to completion of distal reconstruction, visceral and renal perfusion is continued during their reattachment to the aortic graft. Sequential clamping consequently allows for intercostal perfusion.

aorta is completely transected prior to suturing the proximal anastomosis (3-0 Prolene) to allow for full thickness suturing of the aortic wall without possibility of injury to the esophagus. In patients with reduced cardiac or renal function, the distal aortic clamp is sequentially moved to a position proximal to the renal arteries. Alternatively, atriofemoral bypass is discontinued and the aneurysm opened to its distal extent.

Atriovisceral bypass is continued using a Y-line off the arterial perfusion line with balloon catheter branches to the celiac, superior mesenteric, and renal arteries, allowing for oxygenated blood perfusion of the abdominal viscera and kidneys (Fig. 19–2B). To one or more appropriate openings made in the graft, all patent intercostal arteries from T_7 to L_2 are reattached (Fig. 19–2C). Subsequently the visceral and renal vessels are reattached, the left renal artery requiring a separate opening in the graft in 30% to 40% of cases. In patients with aneurysms of lower aortic involvement (Crawford extents III and IV), atriofemoral bypass may be supplanted for only atriovisceral and/or renal bypass (Fig. 19–3). This latter technique avoids femoral arterial cannulation but allows for cardiac preload reduction, renal parenchymal ischemic protection, and reduces post-clamp acidosis. During the period of distal ischemic cross-clamping following the termination of bypass, a continuous intravenous drip of sodium bicarbonate (3 mm Eq/kg/hr) is used.

An alternative technique for distal arterial perfusion is employed in selected patients, primarily those with Crawford extent I or II in whom cross-clamping the aorta at the diaphragm is feasible but not appropriate for anatomic reasons at the mid- or upper-mid-descending thoracic level. Atriofemoral bypass is used but the distal anastomosis is carried out first, allowing for sequential clamping of the graft following initial visceral arterial reattachment and subsequent intercostal reattachment (Fig. 19–4).

After the completion of reconstruction, the aneurysm wall is wrapped around the graft using 2-0 Prolene. Direct suture hemostasis is achieved at all suture lines prior to closure; consequently, using the aneurysm wall to tamponade bleeding is not necessary. Routinely, a collagen-impregnated Dacron graft is employed. As a result, bleeding through interstices is nonexistent. Protamine sulfate is given to reverse the heparin. All shed blood in the operative field is returned to the patient using a rapid cell saving device. Blood product transfusion, packed red cells, fresh frozen plasma, platelets, and cryoprecipitate are employed to achieve a satisfactory level of hemostasis.

Two chest tubes and one closed suction retroperitoneal drain are placed prior to closure in layers. To stimulate renal function, a low-dose dopamine drip of 2 to 3

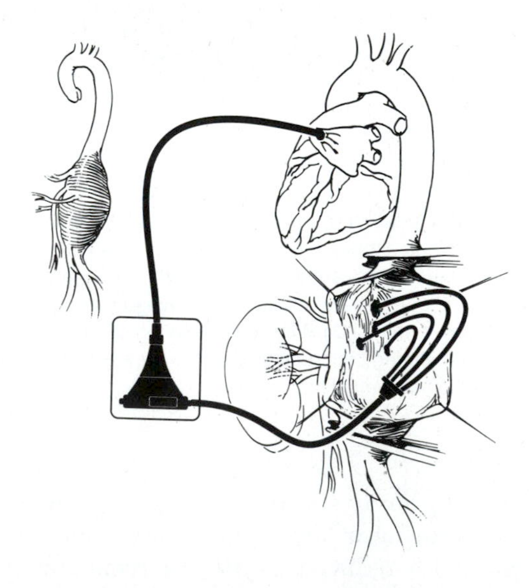

Figure 19–3. Drawing of patient with Crawford type IV thoracoabdominal aortic aneurysm with visceral and renal oxygenated blood perfusion from left atrium during reconstruction.

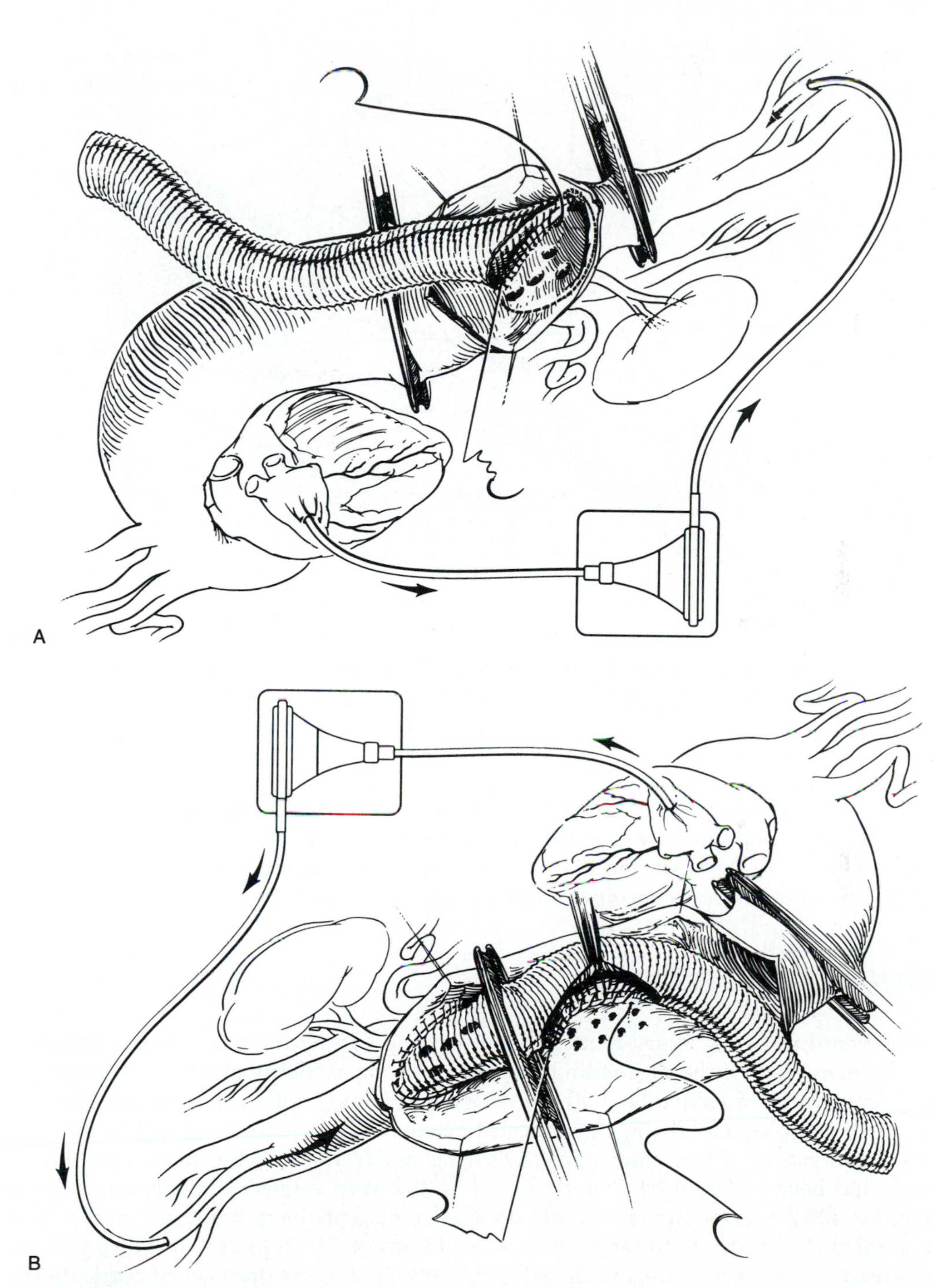

Figure 19–4. (**A**) Drawing of patient with extent I thoracoabdominal aortic aneurysm, using atriofemoral bypass, with distal anastomosis carried out first and including visceral and renal arterial reattachment. (**B**) Sequential clamping of graft allows for renal and visceral perfusion during reattachment of intercostal arteries.

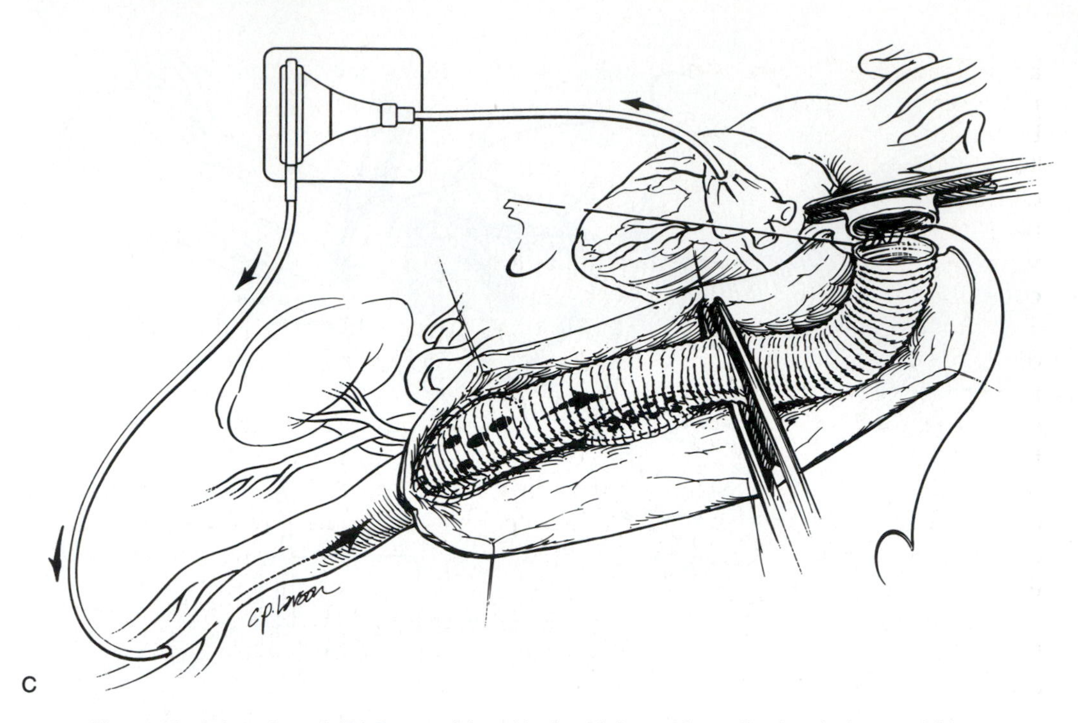

Figure 19–4. (*continued*) (**C**) Sequential positioning of clamp allows distal perfusion to additionally include the reattached intercostal arteries during proximal aortic anastomosis.

mg/kg/min is used for 48 hours. Patients are weaned from the respirator over night and extubated the following morning. Blood pressure is closely monitored and maintained at the patient's preoperative levels. Drains are removed and antibiotics discontinued at 48 hours. Ambulation is encouraged by the third postoperative day.

SPINAL CORD STRATEGIES

Spinal cord ischemic injury remains a devastating complication in patients operated on for aneurysm of the descending thoracic or thoracoabdominal aorta. The reported incidence varies considerably with the extent and etiology of aorta replaced. The incidence of paraplegia following repair of aortic coarctation is quite low (0.41% to 1.5%).[17,18] The incidence of spinal cord injury following replacement of the thoracoabdominal aorta has been reported by Crawford et al. in the most extensive aneurysms to be as high as 40%.[9,19] More current reports on similar patients have found an incidence of paraplegia/paraparesis to range from a maximum of 13.5% to 28% in those patients at greatest risk for neurological deficit.[14,20,21] Consistently, the presence of aortic dissection has been associated with an increased incidence of postoperative neurologic deficit when compared to fusiform medial degenerative disease without dissection.[9,19,20]

The most frequently noted etiologies for spinal cord ischemia have been the duration of aortic clamping, the ligation of cortical blood supply to the cord (artery of Adamkiewicz), and increased cerebrospinal fluid (CSF) pressure. The increase in CSF pressure following cross-clamping of the aorta has been shown to be dependent primarily on the central venous pressure (CVP).[22] With increasing CVP the CSF pressure rises and results in increased outflow resistance in the spinal cord circulation for any given arterial pressure. Theoretically, drainage of CSF with resultant decrease in CSF pressure produces an increase in spinal cord perfusion. In animal studies, drainage of CSF has been shown to improve neurologic outcome in some[23,24] and in others it has not.[25] The only reported prospective randomized trial addressing this issue was unable to demonstrate a difference in neurologic outcome, drawing into question a clear clinical benefit of CSF drainage in human subjects.[26] Virtually all reported clinical experiences with CSF drainage have included one or another form of distal arterial perfusion, complicating the distinction.

Rationally, the sacrifice of intercostal or lumbar arteries that are critical to the direct blood supply of the cord is an important factor in the development of postoperative spinal cord injury. Crawford et al.[9] were unable to demonstrate that a beneficial effect resulted from the reimplantation of these arteries in an attempt to employ this technique to reduce the incidence of paraplegia in patients undergoing resection of thoracoabdominal aortic aneurysms. In their analysis of variables associated with spinal cord ischemic injury, the reattachment of intercostal and lumbar arteries was a significant independent variable; however, it was inseparable from stronger factors such as extent, clamp time, and aortic dissection. The arteria radicularis magna or artery of Adamkiewicz in humans arises from an intercostal artery between T_9 and T_{12} 75% of the time. Consequently, the author has continued to aggressively reattach all segmental arteries from T_7 to L_2.

That hypothermia is protective of organ function during periods of ischemia is well established. Rokkas et al.[27] in a baboon model demonstrated that profound systemic hypothermia protected the spinal cord during periods of ischemia lasting 60 minutes. The protective effect of hypothermia was associated with a blunting of the hyperemic response of spinal cord blood flow in the lower thoracic and lumbar segments of the spinal cord after unclamping of the aorta. Crawford et al.[28] reported on the clinical use of cardiopulmonary bypass using hypothermic circulatory arrest with posterolateral exposure in the treatment of 25 patients with thoracic aortic aneurysms. There were 21 early survivors, cerebral protection was satisfactory, and 2 (11%) of 18 patients at risk for ischemic cord dysfunction had paraplegia immediately following operation. The latter could be attributed to the sacrifice of critical intercostal arteries. The more recent evaluation of elective hypothermic cardiopulmonary bypass and circulatory arrest for spinal cord protection during thoracic aortic surgery was reported by Kouchoukos et al.[29] They treated five patients judged to be at high risk for the development of spinal cord ischemic injury requiring replacement of the entire descending thoracic aorta and upper abdominal aorta (Crawford thoracoabdominal extent I) employing total cardiopulmonary bypass with periods of hypothermic circulatory arrest (temperatures of 15° to 19°C). They encountered only one hospital mortality, and none of the four survivors suffered spinal neurologic deficit or renal or cardiac dysfunction.

Williams' group has reported upon a technique where partial bypass is employed using only moderate hypothermia for organ protection during the ischemic period.[30] The advantage of moderate over deep hypothermia is that an intrinsic cardiac rhythm may be maintained, thus eliminating the need for full cardiopulmonary bypass. They reported upon a series of 20 patients undergoing thoracic or thoracoabdominal aortic aneurysm resection with moderate (30°) hypothermia with a left heart bypass circuit and a heat exchanger. Their hospital mortality was 10% and there was no incidence of paraplegia. Atrial fibrillation developed in only three patients.

Colon et al.[31] described a technique for hypothermic regional perfusion for protection of the spinal cord during the ischemic period of aortic cross-clamping in the pig model. Oxygenated arterial blood from the distal aortic arch was diverted through a

TABLE 19–1. 500 CONSECUTIVE PATIENTS TREATED WITH GRAFT REPLACEMENT FOR THORACOABDOMINAL AORTIC ANEURYSMS

Extent	No. of Pts.	30-Day Survival	In-Hospital Survival	Paraparesis/Paraplegia	Renal Failure	Post-op Bleeding
I	181	170 (94.4%)	165 (91.2%)	8 (4.4%)	5 (2.8%)	5 (2.8%)
II	139	131 (92.2%)	127 (91.4%)	16 (11.5%)	14 (10.1%)	5 (3.6%)
III	92	88 (95.7%)	89 (96.7%)	3 (3.3%)	7 (7.6%)	0 (0.0%)
IV	88	83 (94.3%)	79 (89.8%)	2 (2.3%)	11 (12.5%)	1 (1.1%)
Total	500	472 (94.4%)	460 (92.0%)	29 (5.8%)	37 (7.4%)	11 (2.2%)

heat exchanger, cooled to a mean temperature of 25.5°C ± 3.75°C, and reinfused into the thoracic and upper lumbar aorta isolated between clamps for a period of 30 minutes. Ten animals were able to walk after 30 to 45 minutes of ischemia.

Epidural cooling for regional spinal cord hypothermia has been found to be effective in preventing paraplegia following aortic cross-clamping in the dog model by a number of investigators.[32–34] Davison et al.[35] reported on a clinical trial of epidural cooling in eight patients undergoing thoracoabdominal aortic replacement for aneurysm and found the technique to provide a satisfactory method of achieving regional spinal cord hypothermia. They encountered no postoperative neurologic deficits in their small series. The devastating complication of spinal cord injury is a multifactorial problem that will continue to require a multimodality approach and extensive further investigation.

RESULTS OF TREATMENT

During the period between January 11, 1986, and January 13, 1995, the author operated on a consecutive series of 500 patients for the treatment of aneurysm of the thoracoabdominal aorta (Table 19–1). There were 276 (55%) male and 222 (45%) female patients. Their mean age was 64.7 years (median 67.0 years) with a range from 21 to 85 years. One hundred and twenty-seven patients (25%) had either acute aortic dissection (18 patients, 14%) or chronic aortic dissection (109 patients, 86%), while 373 patients (75%) were treated for medial degenerative fusiform aneurysm or other nondissection etiology. Marfan syndrome was present in 40 patients (8%), and 47 patients (9.4%) were treated for rupture. Extent of aortic replacement based on the Crawford classification included 181 patients (36.2%) in extent I, 139 patients (27.8%) in extent II, 92 patients (18.4%) in extent III, and 88 patients (17.6%) in extent IV (Table 19–1). The overall 30-day survival rate was 94.4%, for dissection 95.3% and for nondissection 94.1%. The overall rate of postoperative neurologic deficit involving the lower extremities was 29

TABLE 19–2. 422 THORACOABDOMINAL AORTIC ANEURYSM REPAIRS PERFORMED WITHOUT ATRIOFEMORAL BYPASS

Extent	No. of Pts.	30-Day Survival	In-Hospital Survival	Paraparesis/Paraplegia	Renal Failure	Post-op Bleeding
I	155	145 (93.5%)	141 (91.0%)	7 (4.5%)	4 (2.6%)	3 (1.9%)
II	91	86 (94.5%)	84 (92.3%)	15 (16.5%)	7 (7.7%)	4 (4.4%)
III	89	85 (95.5%)	86 (96.6%)	3 (3.4%)	7 (7.9%)	0 (0.0%)
IV	87	82 (94.3%)	79 (90.8%)	2 (2.3%)	10 (11.5%)	1 (1.1%)
Total	422	398 (94.3%)	390 (92.4%)	27 (6.4%)	28 (6.6%)	8 (1.9%)

TABLE 19–3. 78 THORACOABDOMINAL AORTIC ANEURYSM REPAIRS PERFORMED WITH ATRIOFEMORAL BYPASS

Extent	No. of Pts.	30-Day Survival	In-Hospital Survival	Paraparesis/Paraplegia	Renal Failure	Post-op Bleeding
I	26	25 (96.2%)	24 (92.3%)	1 (3.8%)	1 (3.8%)	2 (7.7%)
II	48	45 (93.8%)	43 (89.6%)	1 (2.1%)	7 (14.6%)	1 (2.1%)
III	3	3 (100.0%)	3 (100.0%)	0 (0.0%)	0 (0.0%)	0 (0.0%)
IV	1	1 (100.0%)	0 (0.0%)	0 (0.0%)	1 (100.0%)	0 (0.0%)
Total	78	74 (94.9%)	70 (89.7%)	2 (2.6%)	9 (11.5%)	3 (3.8%)

out of 500 (5.8%). Fourteen patients (2.8%) developed paraparesis, while 15 patients (3.0%) developed postoperative paraplegia. Postoperative renal failure with a postoperative increase in creatinine to greater than 3.0 mg/dl or the need of transient or permanent hemodialysis developed in 37 patients (7.4%). Only 11 patients (2.2%) of the 500 patients were returned to the operating room for postoperative bleeding.

Four hundred and twenty-two patients (84.4%) were operated upon without the use of distal aortic perfusion (i.e., atriofemoral bypass) (Table 19–2). Of these, paraparesis or paraplegia developed in 27 (6.4%), and renal failure developed in 28 patients (6.6%). Atriofemoral bypass for distal aortic perfusion using a Biomedicus pump (Medtronic, Inc., Eden Prairie, MN) was utilized as an operative adjunct in 78 patients (15.6%) (Table 19–3). These included 26 patients with extent I, 48 patients with extent II, 3 patients with extent III, and 1 patient with extent IV. Of these 78 patients, only 2 patients (2.6%) developed paraplegia or paraparesis, 9 patients (11.5%) developed postoperative renal insufficiency, and 3 patients (3.8%) were returned to the operating room for postoperative bleeding.

Thirty-six preoperative, operative, and postoperative variables were analyzed for their influence on the development of postoperative neurologic deficit and early (30-day) mortality. Univariate analysis found extent II, rupture, and renal complications to be associated with paraplegia/paraparesis, while male sex, cardiac, and renal complications were associated with early death.

At least in this series of 500 patients, atriofemoral bypass from the left atrium to a common femoral artery with an incircuit to centrifugal pump for distal aortic perfusion as an adjunct to graft replacement of the thoracoabdominal aorta appeared to have a substantial favorable impact by reducing the postoperative complication of paraplegia and/or paraparesis. Distal aortic perfusion, however, had no significant influence on the development of postoperative renal failure or early survival.

REFERENCES

1. Bahnson HT. Definitive treatment of saccular aneurysms of the aorta with excision of sac and aortic suture. *Surg Gynecol Obstet*. 1953;96:383.
2. Ellis FH Jr, Helden RA, Hines EA Jr. Aneurysm of the abdominal aorta involving the right renal artery: report of case with preservation of renal function after resection and grafting. *Ann Surg*. 1955;142:992.
3. Etheredge SN, Yee J, Smith JV, et al. Successful resection of a large aneurysm of the upper abdominal aorta and replacement with homograft. *Surgery*. 1955;38:1071.
4. DeBakey ME, Creech O Jr, Morris GC Jr. Aneurysm of thoracoabdominal aorta involving the celiac, superior mesenteric, and renal arteries: report of four cases treated by resection and homograft replacement. *Ann Surg*. 1956;144:549.

5. DeBakey ME, Crawford ES, Garrett HE. Surgical considerations in the treatment of aneurysm of the thoraco-abdominal aorta. *Ann Surg*. 1965;162:650.
6. Crawford ES. Thoraco-abdominal and abdominal aortic aneurysms involving renal, superior mesenteric, and celiac arteries. *Ann Surg*. 1974;179:763.
7. Crawford ES, Snyder DM, Cho GC, et al. Progress in treatment of thoracoabdominal and abdominal aortic aneurysms involving celiac, superior mesenteric, and renal arteries. *Ann Surg*. 1978;188:404.
8. Coselli JS. Contribution of E. Stanley Crawford in thoracoabdominal aortic aneurysms. In: Yao JST, Pearce WH, eds. *Aneurysms: New Findings and Treatment*. Norwalk, CT: Appleton & Lange; 1993:173–194.
9. Crawford ES, Crawford JL, Safi HJ, et al. Thoracoabdominal aortic aneurysms: preoperative and intraoperative factors determining immediate and long-term results of operations in 605 patients. *J Vasc Surg*. 1986;3:389–404.
10. Svensson LG, Crawford ES, Hess KR, et al. Experience with 1509 patients undergoing thoracoabdominal aortic operations. *J Vasc Surg*. 1993;17:357–370.
11. Ingoldby CJH, Wijanto W, Mitchell JE. Impact of vascular surgery on community mortality from ruptured aortic aneurysms. *Br J Surg*. 1986;73:551–553.
12. Crawford ES, DeNatale RW. Thoracoabdominal aortic aneurysm: observations regarding natural course of the disease. *J Vasc Surg*. 1986;3:578–582.
13. Bickerstaff LIC, Pairolero PC, Hollier LH, et al. Thoracic aortic aneurysms: a population-based study. *Surgery*. 1982;92:1103–1108.
14. Coselli JS. Thoracoabdominal aortic aneurysms: experience with 372 patients. *J Card Surg*. 1994;9:638–647.
15. Coselli JS. Suprarenal aortic reconstruction: perioperative management: patient selection, patient workup, operative management, and postoperative management. *Sem Vasc Surg*. 1992;5:146–156.
16. Coselli JS. Suprarenal aortic reconstruction: endovascular repair. *Sem Vasc Surg*. 1992;5:180–191.
17. Lerberg DB, Hardesty RG, Siewers RD, et al. Coarctation of the aorta in infants and children and 25 years of experience. *Ann Thorac Surg*. 1982;3:159–170.
18. Pennington DG, Liberthson RR, Jacobs MJ, et al. Critical review of experience with surgical repair of coarctation of aorta. *J Thorac Cardiovasc Surg*. 1979;77:217–229.
19. Svensson LG, Crawford ES, Hess KR, et al. Experience with 1509 patients undergoing thoracoabdominal aortic operations. *J Vasc Surg*. 1993;17:357–370.
20. Schepens MAAM, Defauw JJAM, Hamerlijnck RPHM, et al. Surgical treatment of thoracoabdominal aortic aneurysms by simple crossclamping: risk factors and late results. *J Thorac Cardiovasc Surg*. 1994;107:134–142.
21. Cox GS, OHara PJ, Hertzer NR, et al. Thoracoabdominal aneurysm repair: a representative experience. *J Vasc Surg*. 1992;15:780–788.
22. Wadouh F, Arndt CF, Oppermane, et al. The mechanism of spinal cord injury after simple and double aortic crossclamping. *J Thorac Cardiovasc Surg*. 1986;92:121–127.
23. McCullough J, Hollier L, Nugent M. Paraplegia after thoracic aortic occlusion: influence of cerebrospinal fluid drainage. *J Vasc Surg*. 1988;7:153–168.
24. Bower T, Murry M, Gloviezki P, et al. Effects of thoracic aortic occlusion and cerebrospinal fluid on regional spinal cord blood flow in dogs: correlation with neurologic outcome. *J Vasc Surg*. 1988;9:135–144.
25. Wadouh F, Lindemann EM, Arndt CF, et al. The arteria radicularis magna anterior as a decisive factor influencing spinal cord damage during aortic occlusion. *J Thorac Cardiovasc Surg*. 1984;88:1–10.
26. Crawford ES, Svensson LG, Hess KR, et al. A prospective randomized study of cerebrospinal fluid drainage to prevent paraplegia after high-risk surgery on the thoracoabdominal aorta. *J Vasc Surg*. 1991;13:36–46.
27. Rokkas CK, Sundaresan S, Shuman TA, et al. Profound systemic hypothermia protects the spinal cord in a primate model of spinal cord ischemia. *J Thorac Cardiovasc Surg*. 1993;106;1024–1035.

28. Crawford ES, Coselli JS, Safi HJ. Partial cardiopulmonary bypass, hypothermic circulatory arrest, and posterolateral exposure for thoracic aortic aneurysm operation. *J Thor Cardiovasc Surg*. 1987;94:824–827.
29. Kouchoukos NT, Wareing TH, Izumoto H, et al. Elective hypothermic cardiopulmonary bypass and circulatory arrest for spinal cord protection during operations on the thoracoabdominal aorta. *J Thorac Cardiovasc Surg*. 1990;99:659–664.
30. Frank SM, Parker SD, Rock P, et al. Moderate hypothermia, with partial bypass and segmental sequential repair for thoracoabdominal aortic aneurysm. *J Vasc Surg*. 1994;19:687–697.
31. Colon R, Frazier OH, Cooley DA, et al. Hypothermic regional perfusion for protection of the spinal cord during periods of ischemia. *Ann Thorac Surg*. 1987;43:639–643.
32. Berguer R, Porto J, Fedoronko B, et al. Selective deep hypothermia of the spinal cord prevents paraplegia after aortic cross-clamping in the dog model. *J Vasc Surg*. 1992;15:62–72.
33. Marsala M, Vanicky I, Galik J, et al. Panmyelic epidural cooling protects against ischemic spinal cord damage. *J Surg Res*. 1993;55:21–31.
34. Wisselink W, Becker MO, Nguyen JH, et al. Protecting the ischemic spinal cord during aortic clamping: the influence of selective hypothermia and spinal cord perfusion pressure. *J Vasc Surg*. 1994;19:788–796.
35. Davison JK, Cambria RP, Vierra DJ, et al. Epidural cooling for regional spinal cord hypothermia during thoracoabdominal aneurysm repair. *J Vasc Surg*. 1994;20:304–310.

20

Endoluminal Repair of Complex Abdominal Aortic Aneurysms

James May, MS, FRACS, FACS, Geoffrey H. White, FRACS, Weiyun Yu, BSc (Med), MB, BS, Timothy J. McGahan, FRACS (Vasc), Richard Waugh, FRACR, Michael S. Stephen, FRACS, and John Preston Harris, MS, FRACS, FACS

Endoluminal repair of abdominal aortic aneurysms (AAAs) in human beings was first reported by Parodi,[1] who treated five patients with AAA by transfemoral intraluminal Dacron grafts anchored by modified stainless steel stents. These aneurysms were all of the fusiform variety, with a discrete proximal neck between the renal arteries and the proximal extent of the aneurysm and a distal neck between the distal extent of the aneurysm and the aortic bifurcation. Not all aneurysms, however, are suitable for this type of endoluminal tube-graft repair. We have previously reported the outcome of endoluminal tube-graft repair in these aneurysms, which we have designated Type I.[2] These aneurysms have a proximal neck of length 2 cm or greater, a distal neck of length 1.5 cm or greater, and nontortuous iliac arteries of diameter 8 mm or greater. The more complex aneurysms that do not meet one or more of these criteria we have designated Type II. The most common reason for an aneurysm to be classified as Type II is lack of a distal neck. We have also drawn attention to the more favorable outcome associated with Type I aneurysms than with Type II.[3]

These complex AAAs may be managed by either a combination of endoluminal and extraluminal repair or entirely by the endoluminal method. In this chapter, we present our experience with both methods.

MATERIAL AND METHODS

Between May 1992 and March 1995, endoluminal repair of AAA was undertaken in 72 patients at the Royal Prince Alfred Hospital. Of these, 39 conformed to Type I criteria and 33 to Type II. This latter group, which forms the basis of this report, was divided into two subgroups, the first consisting of 28 patients whose AAA lacked a distal neck. Six of these had iliac aneurysms in addition to the aortic one, and 1 had a dissection of the thoracic aorta in addition to the aortic aneurysm.

TABLE 20–1. MEDICAL COMORBIDITIES

Comorbidity	No. of Instances
Poor left ventricular function (3 with renal impairment also)	8
Chronic Obstructive Airways Disease (COAD)	2
Chronic hepatitis	1
Hostile abdomen	3
Total	**14**

The second subgroup of 5 patients had a distal neck and were thus suitable for an endoluminal tube-graft repair but were classified as Type II due to narrow and/or tortuous iliac arteries.

Fourteen of these 33 patients had medical comorbidities, which led to them being rejected for open repair of their AAA at other medical centers. The comorbidities are listed in Table 20–1.

Repair by a Combination of Endoluminal and Extraluminal Methods

Twenty-four patients were treated by combined endoluminal and extraluminal methods (Table 20–2). Nineteen of these had endoluminal tapered aortofemoral or aortoiliac grafts combined with extraluminal crossover grafts and interruption of the contralateral common iliac artery to exclude the aneurysm. The remaining five patients were suitable for and had an endoluminal tube graft repair but required the use of a temporary extraluminal Dacron conduit for access (Fig. 20–1). This method was devised by Parodi and has been described in detail by the authors.[4] Access for 12 of the 19 patients treated by endoluminal tapered grafts was also via a Dacron conduit to the common iliac artery. Following deployment of the endoluminally placed tapered graft, the conduit was transected together with the coaxially placed tapered graft within it (Fig. 20–2). Both common iliac arteries were interrupted to exclude the AAA, and circulation restored to the lower limbs by means of an extraluminal extraperiotoneal bifurcated graft (Fig. 20–3). The patient with dissection of the thoracic aorta and fusiform AAA was treated in this manner. The dissection originated in the infrarenal aorta and extended proximally in a retrograde manner (Fig. 20–4). This patient has been reported in detail previously, following successful endoluminal repair of both lesions.[5] Femoral artery access was used for the remaining 7 of 19 patients treated with an endoluminal tapered graft. In 3 of these, the tapered endoluminal graft

TABLE 20–2. SUMMARY OF ENDOLUMINAL TREATMENT OF TYPE II AAA

Treatment	No. of Instances
Combination of Endoluminal and Extraluminal Repair	
Tapered endoluminal graft	
Femoral access and extraluminal femoro–femoral crossover	7
Iliac access and extraluminal extraperitoneal bifurcated graft	12
Tube endoluminal graft	
Iliac access via temporary conduit	5
Entirely Endoluminal Repair	
Bifurcated graft	
One-piece graft	7
Three-piece graft	2

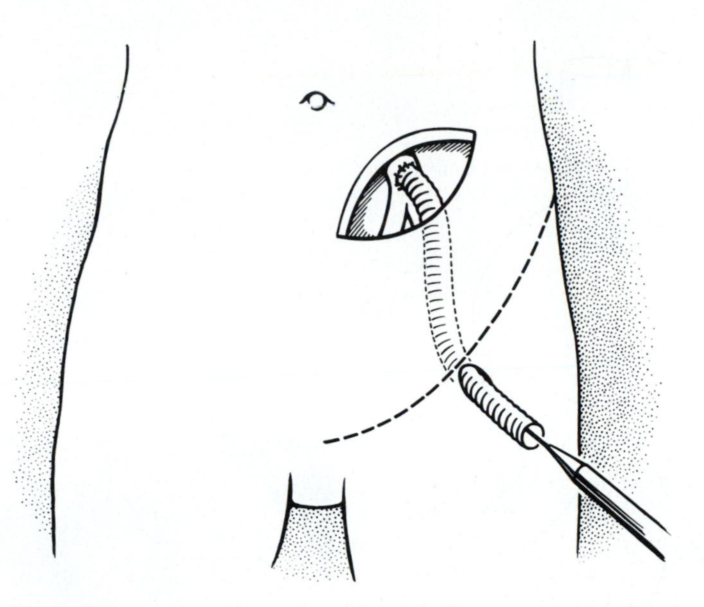

Figure 20–1. Extraluminal extraperitoneal Dacron tube graft used as a conduit to gain access to the aorta.

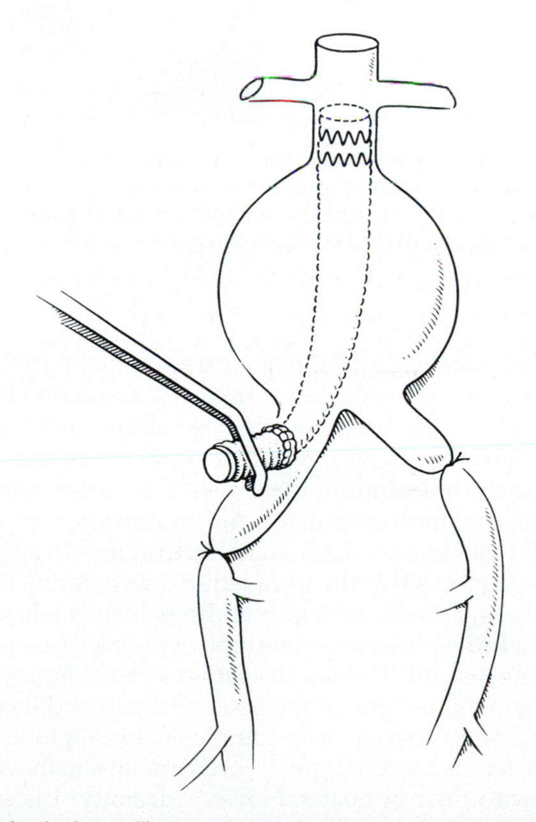

Figure 20–2. Endoluminal aortoiliac tapered graft delivered via and lying within the Dacron conduit. Note AAA has been isolated by ligation of common iliac arteries.

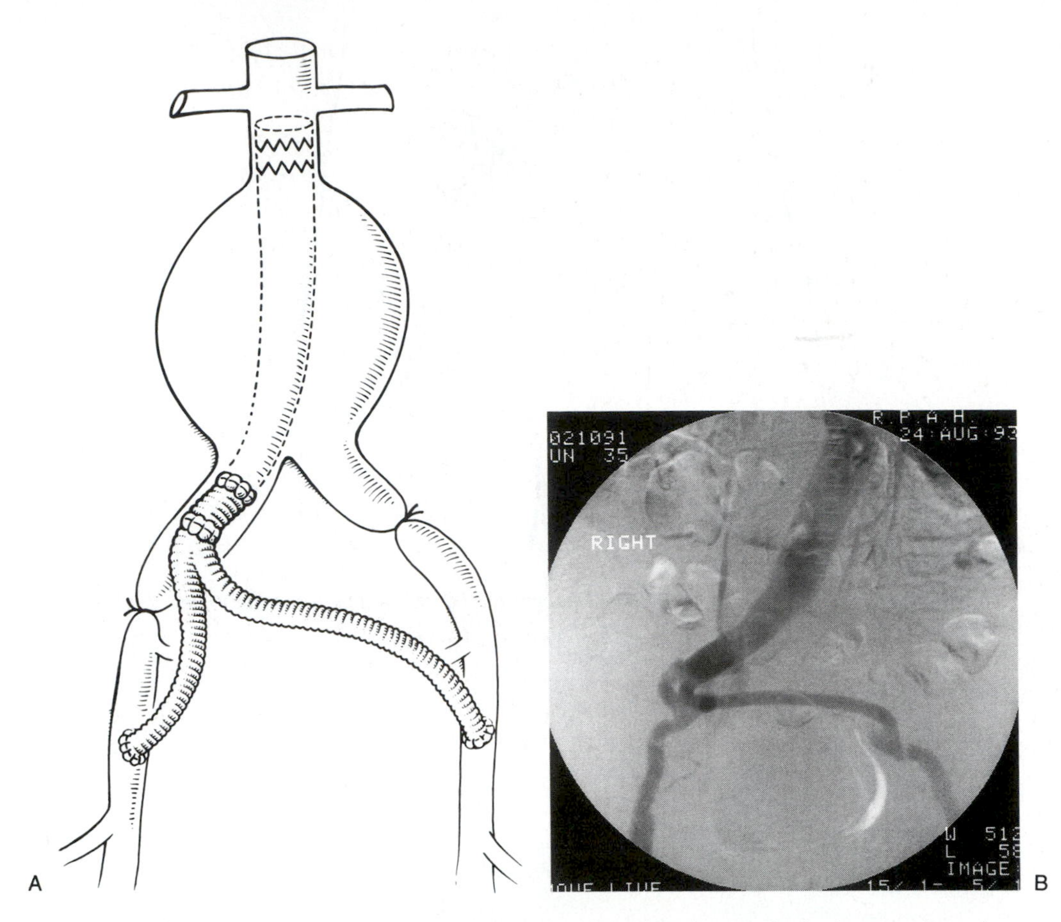

Figure 20–3. (**A**) Revascularization of both lower extremities by extraluminal extraperitoneal graft. *(From May J, White GH, Yu W, et al. Endoluminal repair of atypical dissecting aneurysm of the descending thoracic aorta and fusiform aneurysms of the abdominal aorta. J Vasc Surg. 1995;22:163. With permission.)* (**B**) Postoperative aortogram of patient with repair by technique depicted in A.

ran from the aorta immediately below the renal arteries down to the femoral access site (Fig. 20–5). Following interruption of the contralateral common iliac artery, the circulation to the contralateral lower limb was restored by extraluminal femoro–femoral crossover graft. In the remaining 4 patients in which femoral artery access was used for treatment with a tapered endoluminal graft, the graft was inserted in two parts (Fig. 20–6). A bifurcated graft with one limb amputated and oversewn at its origin was deployed immediately below the renal arteries. The remaining ipsilateral limb was cut short enough so that the limb remained free within the aorta rather than entering the proximal common iliac artery. The introducing sheath with its mandril was then reinserted over the guidewire and passed up inside the remaining open limb of the previously deployed endograft. Following removal of the mandril, a second endograft was deployed with its proximal end within and overlapping the limb of the first endograft and its distal end within the common iliac artery. The procedure was completed by deploying a blind endograft through a contralateral femoro-arteriotomy to interrupt flow in the contralateral common iliac artery. Blood flow to the contralateral lower extremity was achieved by way of a femoro–femoral crossover graft using the previously formed arteriotomies for the anastomotic sites.

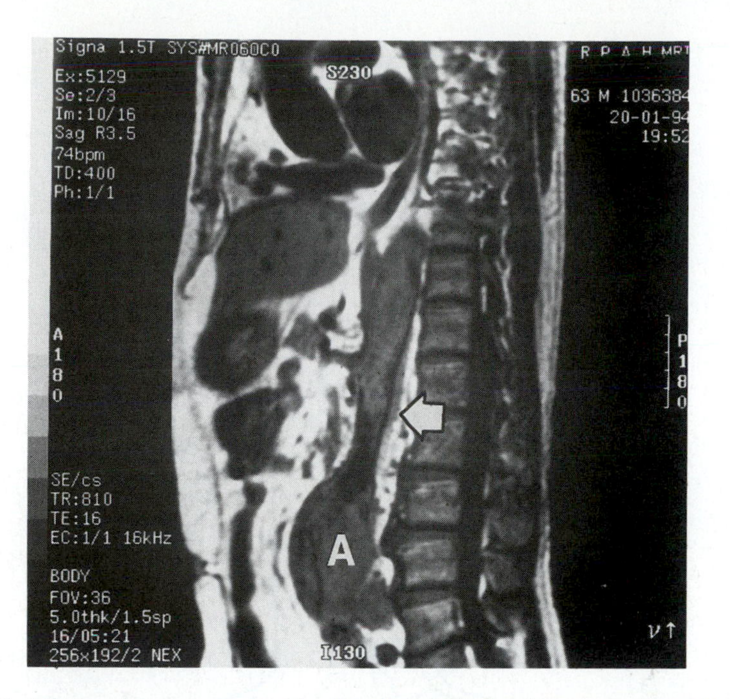

Figure 20–4. Magnetic resonance imaging (saggital view) of patient with fusiform AAA (A) and thoracic aortic dissection originating below the renal arteries (*arrow*). *(From May J, White GH, Yu W, et al. Endoluminal repair of atypical dissecting aneurysm of the descending thoracic aorta and fusiform aneurysms of the abdominal aorta. J Vasc Surg. 1995;22:163. With permission.)*

Entirely Endoluminal Method

An entirely endoluminal method of repairing Type II aneurysms requires some form of endoluminal bifurcated graft to avoid the need for the extraluminal component to ravascularise the contralateral lower extremity. In the study group of 33 patients, a bifurcated graft has been attempted in 9 (Table 20–2). In 7 of these, a one-piece bifurcated graft was used. This involved delivering the contralateral limb across the aortic bifurcation into the contralateral common iliac artery in the manner described by Chuter.[6] In the remaining 2 patients, a three-piece bifurcated graft was used. This involved a modification of the technique depicted in Figure 20–6.

All procedures were elective and performed in the operating room with the patient draped for a standard open repair in the event of failed endoluminal repair. Endovascular repair of aneurysms, with materials currently used in vascular surgery, is approved by the institutional review board. Informed consent was obtained from each patient. Laboratory and clinical experience in the use of intraluminal grafts for treatment of aneurysms has previously been reported by the aurthors.[7–14]

RESULTS

Endoluminal grafts were successfully deployed in 24 patients. In the remaining 9 patients, the endoluminal repair was abandoned in favor of an open repair. Five of these failures occurred with attempts to deploy a bifurcated graft. One of these was a failure due to access but the remaining four were due to technical problems involved in using a demanding method. A postoperative arteriogram of one of the

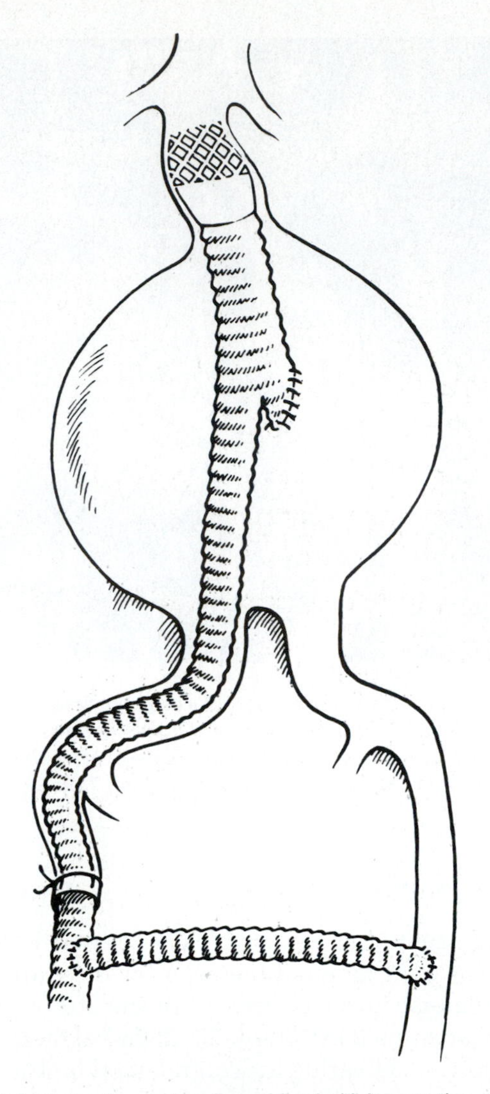

Figure 20–5. Endoluminal aortofemoral graft combined with interruption of contralateral common iliac artery and extraluminal crossover graft between the femoral arteries. Interruption of contralateral iliac artery not shown. *(From May J, White GH, Waugh W, et al. Treatment of complex abdominal aortic aneurysms by a combination of endoluminal and extraluminal aortofemoral grafts. J Vasc Surg. 1994;19:930. With permission.)*

four successful endoluminal grafts is shown in Figure 20–7. Four failures occurred in patients in which a nonbifurcated technique was used. One of these was a failure of access, and two were due to stent displacement produced by inadvertent traction on the tapered endograft on withdrawal of the balloon catheter. The remaining failure was due to graft thrombosis resulting from inadvertent administration of dilute heparin.

Complications

Complications have been classified according to the Ad-hoc Committee on Reporting Standards Recommendations.[15] The local/vascular complications are shown in Table 20–3. The patient with iliac artery perforation was repaired with an iliofemoral bypass graft, which was then used for access for his endoluminal tube-graft repair and to revascularise the lower extremity. The patient with external iliac artery dissection

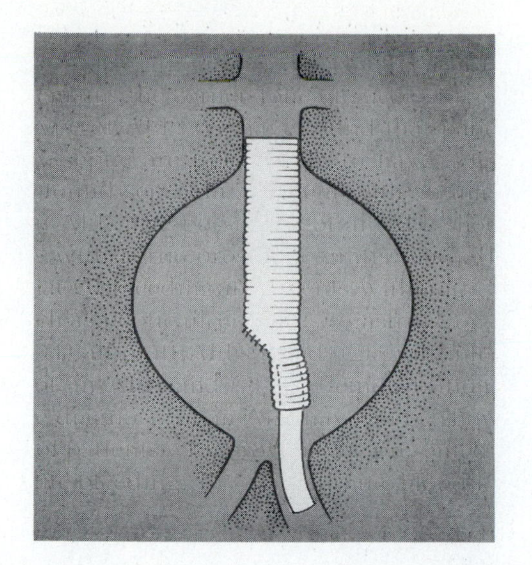

Figure 20–6. Two-piece tapered endoluminal graft. Note this procedure requires interruption of contralateral common iliac artery and extraluminal crossover graft (not shown).

occurred 3 hours after successful endoluminal tapered graft repair. This complication was corrected by endoluminal placement of a stent at the proximal entry point of the dissection 3 cm below the distal end of the tapered graft. There were no instances of microembolization.

The remote systemic complications included three patients with renal impairment due to contrast medium and one patient with a stroke. The latter recovered strength in the affected side but died from cardiac causes 3 months after operation.

Mortality

Two patients died within 30 days of operation, giving a mortality of 6% for the group. Both were procedure related. There were four late deaths not procedure related, 2 due to cardiac causes and 2 due to liver failure.

DISCUSSION

Considering the number of patients with serious medical comorbidities, the mortaility rate of 6% in the first 30 days is acceptable. When the 10 (30%) patients with local/vascular complications are added to the 9 (27%) patients with complications leading to failure of endoluminal repair and conversion to open operation it can be seen that the total of 19 or 57% of patients with complications directly attributable to the endoluminal technique is considerable. This morbidity, however, should be seen in the context that these patients survived the complications, and that many patients were treated who would not otherwise have been accepted for standard open repair.

It may reasonably be asked whether the iliac approach involving the combination of endoluminal and extraluminal repair has any advantage over a standard retroperitoneal open repair of a AAA. We have found that the smaller wound in the iliac fossa, well away from the upper abdomen and chest, allows a quicker recovery with less need for intensive care than the standard retroperitoneal approach for AAA.

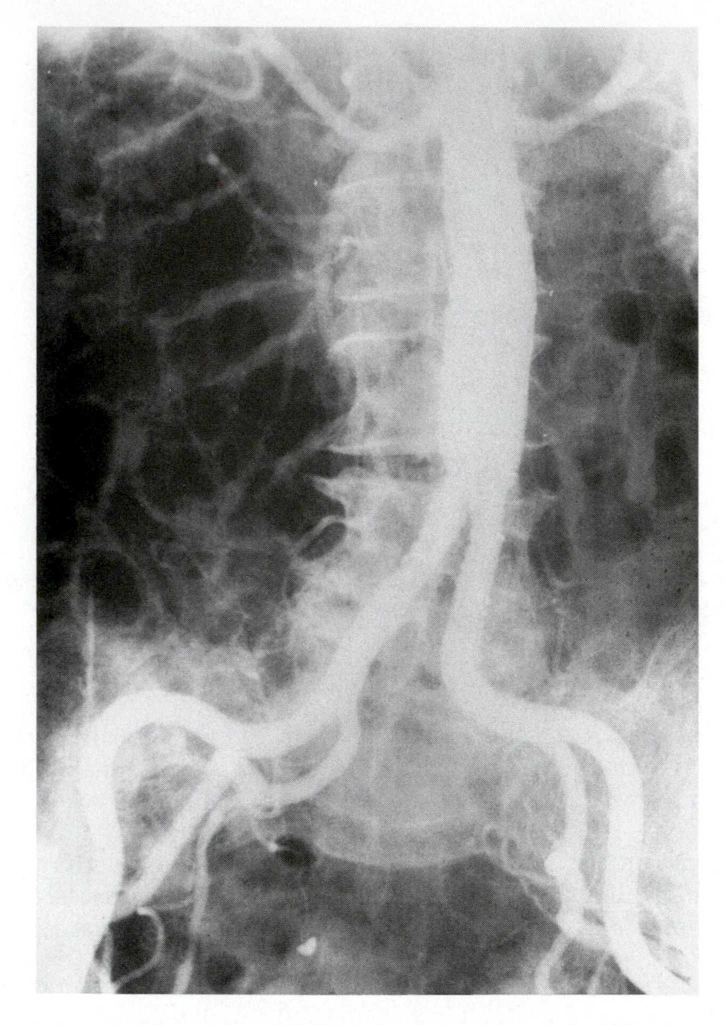

Figure 20–7. Postoperative aortogram following endoluminal repair by EVT bifurcated graft.

The high failure rate for endoluminal bifurcated grafts reflects the more complex nature of this type of repair. Chuter has reported occlusion in five graft limbs in his early experience of endoluminal bifurcated grafts. He now routinely deploys two additional wall stents in the limbs of his bifurcated grafts to minimize this problem.

TABLE 20–3. LOCAL/VASCULAR COMPLICATIONS

Complication	No. of Instances
Iliac artery perforation	1
Iliac artery dissection	1
Graft stenosis	2
Fever and back pain	2
Bleeding (return to OR 1 and hematoma 1)	2
Wound infection/lymph fistula	2
Total	**10 (30%)**

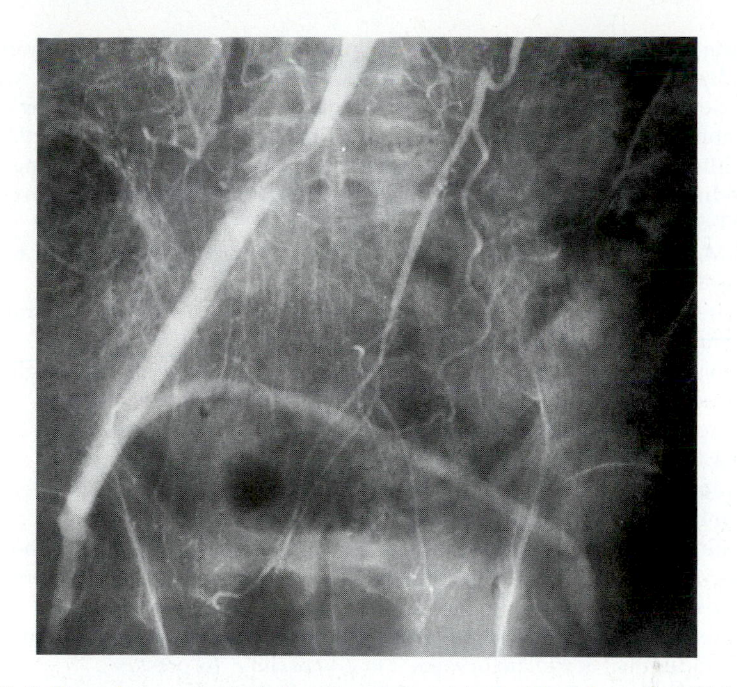

Figure 20–8. Stenosis occurring in that section of an endoluminal aortofemoral graft lying within the origin of the right common iliac artery.

We have found early experience with the three-piece endoluminal bifurcated graft to be more encouraging than with the one-piece graft. Early experience with the Endovascular Technologies, Inc. (EVT) endoluminal bifurcated graft has also been encouraging. In the Food and Drug Administration approved study of this device, there were only two failures in 10 patients.[16]

The endoluminal aortofemoral graft performed through a femoral arteriotomy was attractive in theory. In practice, we experienced problems placing standard thickness grafts within arteries of the same diameter. Invagination occurred, and this was not picked up by uniplanar post procedure angiography but caused symptoms in the first 2 weeks due to progressive stenosis (Fig. 20–8). We have found the two-piece endoluminal tapered graft depicted in Figure 20–6 to be more reliable. The graft lies only within a short section of the iliac artery, and patency is encouraged by the presence of graft attachment devices in this section that minimize invagination.

Further careful evaluation is required to determine the long-term outcome of endoluminal repair of AAA. If it can be shown that the aneurysmal process is arrested or reversed, there is the prospect that AAA may be picked up and treated endoluminally at the stage where they conform to Type I criteria. If this could be achieved, the evolution to Type II AAA would be prevented and the problems of treating these complex aneurysms avoided.

REFERENCES

1. Parodi JC, Palmaz JC, Barone HD. Transfemoral intraluminal graft implantation abdominal aortic aneurysms. *Ann Vasc Surg*. 1991;5:491–499.
2. May J, White GH, Yu W, et al. Results of endoluminal grafting of abdominal aortic aneurysms. *Cardiovasc Surg*. 1994;2:649.

3. May J, White GH, Yu W, et al. Results of endoluminal grafting of abdominal aortic aneurysms are dependent on aneurysm morphology. *Vasc Surg*. In press.
4. May J, White G, Yu W, et al. Treatment of complex abdominal aneurysms by a combination of endoluminal and extraluminal aorto-femoral grafts. *J Vasc Surg*. 1994;19:924–933.
5. May J, White GH, Yu W, et al. Endoluminal repair of atypical dissecting aneurysm of the descending thoracic aorta and fusiform aneurysm of the abdominal aorta. *J Vasc Surg*. 1995;22:163–172.
6. Chuter TAM, Green RM, Ouriel K, et al. Transfemoral endovascular aortic graft replacement. *J Vasc Surg*. 1993;18:185–197.
7. May J, White G, Waugh R, et al. Transluminal placement of a prosthetic graft-stent device for treatment of subclavian aneurysm. *J Vasc Surg*. 1993;18:1056–1059.
8. White GH, Yu W, May J, et al. A new non-stented endoluminal graft for straight or bifurcated repair of aneurysms. *J Endovasc Surg*. 1994;1:16–24.
9. May J, White GH, Waugh R, et al. Endoluminal repair of abdominal aortic aneurysm. *Med J Aust*. 1994;161:541–543.
10. May J, White GH, Yu W, et al. Endoluminal grafting of abdominal aortic aneurysms: causes of failure and their prevention. *J Endovasc Surg*. 1994;1:44–52
11. May J, White GH. Specialized endovascular techniques: combined surgical and endovascular approaches. In: RA White, TJ Fogarty, eds. *Peripheral Endovascular Interventions*. St. Louis, MO: Mosby–Year Book. 1994.
12. May J, White GH, Yu W, et al Surgical management of complications following endoluminal grafting of abdominal aortic aneurysms. *Eur J Vasc Surg*. In press.
13. White GH, May J, Yu W. Development of a clinical program of endoluminal aneurysm grafting: experience in 60 patients. In: Parodi JC, Veith FJ, Marin ML, eds. *Endovascular Grafting Techniques*. St. Louis, MO: Quality Medical Publishers, 1994.
14. White GH, May J, Yu W. Stented and non-stented grafts for aneurysmal disease: the Sydney experience. In: Chuter T, Donayre C, White R, eds. *Endoluminal Vascular Prostheses*. Boston: Little, Brown and Co. 1994:107–152.
15. Rutherford RB, Flanigan DP, Gupta SK, et al. Suggested standards for reports dealing with lower extremity ischaemia. *J Vasc Surg*. 1986;4:80–94.
16. Bernhard V. Personal communication.

21

Management of Peripheral Artery Complications in Patients with Aortic Dissection

David C. Brewster, MD

The term *aneurysme dissequant*—dissecting aneurysm—was first introduced by Laennec in 1819 and has often been used to describe the disease process since that time. However, it is actually a misnomer because although the aorta is frequently somewhat enlarged in the acute phase of the condition, it is rarely aneurysmal. The process is more accurately described as an intramural hematoma that dissects secondary to arterial pressure. Hence, the term *acute aortic dissection* is a more appropriate depiction of the disorder and is more common today.[1]

Although significant advances in the diagnosis and treatment of aortic dissection have occurred since the 1950s, the condition remains a relatively frequent and highly morbid clinical event. Indeed, acute aortic dissection is the most common lethal catastrophe involving the aorta, with an incidence at least twice that of ruptured abdominal aortic aneurysm (AAA).[2,3] While some debate remains in regard to the pathophysiology of the process, it is generally accepted that the initiating mechanism is a tear in the aortic intima through which blood surges into the media, separating the layers of the vessel wall. Dissections usually propagate from the site of the intimal entry point distally in the aorta, although retrograde extension can occasionally occur. The origin of any arterial branch arising from the dissected segment of aorta may be compromised or the aortic valve may be rendered incompetent. Blood in the false channel can reenter the true lumen anywhere along the course of the dissection process, or external rupture of the aortic adventitia forming the wall of the false channel may occur. Rupture of the aorta, the most common cause of death, occurs most frequently into the pericardial space or left pleural cavity.

Since the initial introduction of surgical repair by DeBakey and colleagues in 1955,[4] the evolution of thought and experience in the treatment of aortic dissection has gradually shifted toward definitive central repair of the aortic tear by cardiothoracic surgeons with increasingly successful results.[5–9] Nonetheless, vascular surgeons may still become important members of the team of physicians and surgeons caring for patients with aortic dissection, both in initial diagnosis of the basic condition and in primary or adjunctive management of peripheral vascular complications of aortic dissection.[10]

PERIPHERAL VASCULAR COMPLICATIONS

It is well established that the major risk of early death from acute aortic dissection relates to central complications of the proximal dissection process itself. Such events include acute rupture of the aorta into the mediastinum or left pleural cavity, rupture into the pericardium producing acute tamponade, acute aortic valvular insufficiency with compromise of left ventricular function, or interference with coronary artery blood flow causing myocardial infarction. However, occlusion or obstruction of major aortic branch vessels commonly occurs as a consequence of distal propagation of the dissection process, thereby causing ischemic manifestations in these vascular beds or vital organs. Indeed, such aortic branch occlusions may be appropriately considered peripheral vascular complications of aortic dissection and may sometimes constitute the principle mode of presentation, or become the primary focus of treatment, in some patients.[3,11–13]

Mechanism of Aortic Branch Obstruction

The most common mechanism of vessel obstruction involves extrinsic compression of the true arterial lumen by the bulging dissected false lumen, thereby compromising or obstructing flow to the vascular territory perfused by the branch vessel.[3,11,14] This process may be circumferential at a branch vessel orifice or it may extend for varying distances into the particular branch (Fig. 21–1). On other occasions, the ostium of a branch vessel may be obstructed by disrupted intimal flaps or intussusception of

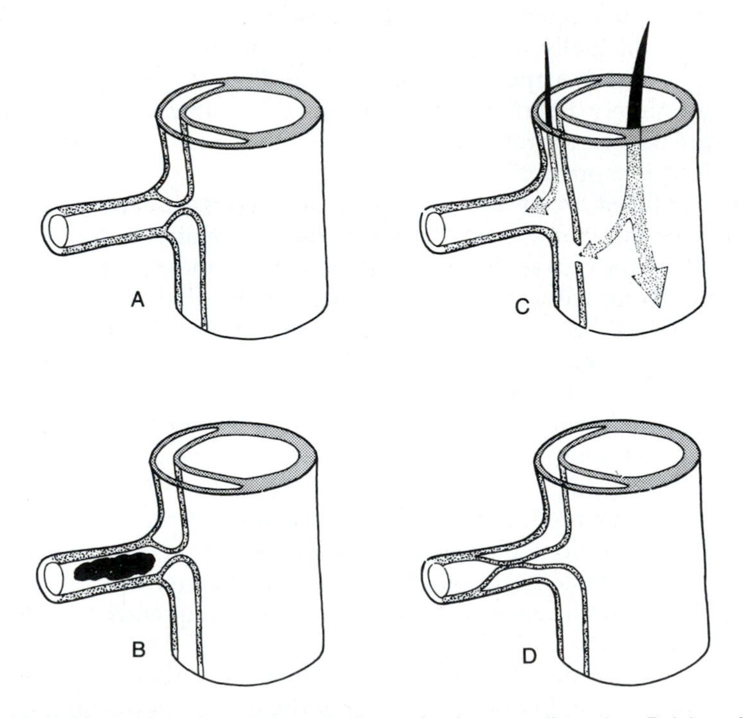

Figure 21–1. Mechanism of aortic branch obstruction in acute dissection. Bulging of the false lumen can produce occlusion at the branch orifice (**A**), and subsequent thrombosis may occur distally (**B**). Intimal detachment at the branch orifice may occur with perfusion largely via the false channel (**C**). The dissection process may also proceed into the branch, causing obstruction beyond the actual branch orifice (**D**). *(Reprinted with permission from Cambria RP, Brewster DC, Gertler J, et al. Vascular complications associated with spontaneous aortic dissection. J Vasc Surg. 1988;7:199–209.)*

detached intima into the proximal aspect of the branch artery.[15] Rarely, embolic occlusion of vessels remote from the dissection process may occur secondary to discharge of clot from the false lumen.[16] Such embolic material may originate at either the site of the initiating intimal tear or at a more distal point of reentry.

In addition to possible compromise of branch vessel origins by the dissection, if branch vessel flow obstruction is complete *in situ* thrombosis formation distal to the point of occlusion may occur secondary to stasis. In these circumstances, branch obstruction may persist despite correction of the dissection by proximal thoracic aortic repair. Similarly, continued obstruction of branch orifices by persistent intimal flaps or remote embolization may persist despite redirection of flow into the true lumen by initial central repair. These circumstances explain why primary aortic repair may not always relieve the peripheral vascular complications of aortic dissection, and they emphasize that additional methods of revascularization may occasionally be required for a successful outcome.

Spontaneous reentry of the false lumen (Fig. 21–2) may relieve obstruction in the true lumen and account for the fluctuating clinical picture of visceral or peripheral ischemic manifestations often noted in patients with acute dissection.[1] Reentry commonly occurs at points where aortic tributaries are sheared off or may occur spontaneously at one or more points where aortic tributaries are sheared off or may occur spontaneously at one or more points along the extent of the dissection. Reentry provides communication between the true and false lumens, and allows the potential for double-channel distal perfusion or continues adequate perfusion of certain aortic branches solely from the false lumen. Indeed, this concept provides the rationale for the surgical procedure of fenestration, to be discussed subsequently.

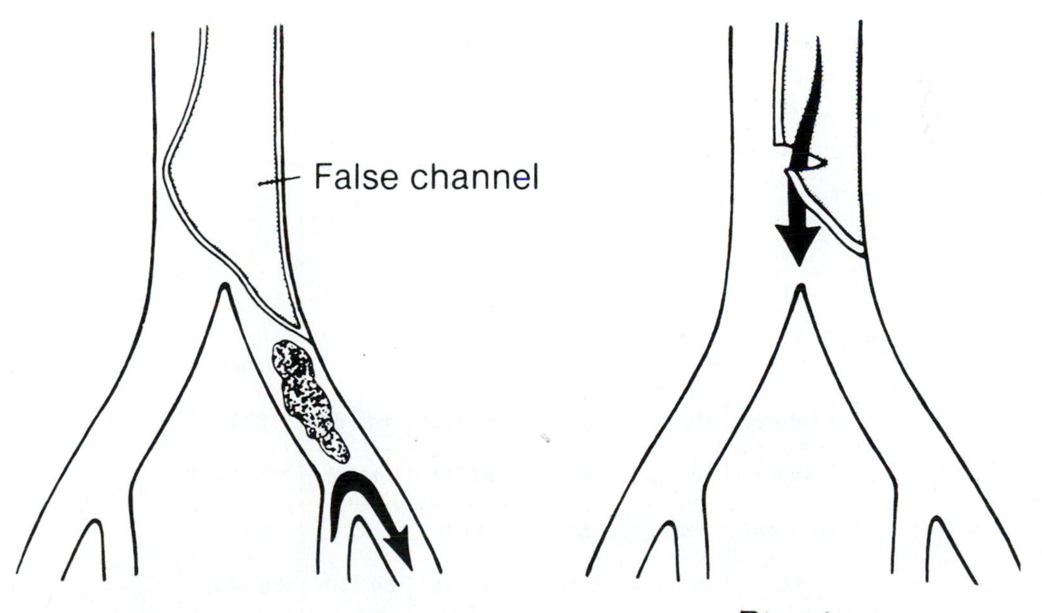

Figure 21–2. Compromise of true lumen by dissection channel producing distal aortic obstruction. This may be complicated by distal thrombosis or relieved by spontaneous (or surgical) reentry. *(Reprinted with permission from Brewster DC, Cambria RP. Role of the vascular surgeon in the management of dissecting aortic aneurysms. In: Veith FJ, ed. Current Critical Problems in Vascular Surgery. St. Louis, MO: Quality Medical Publishing Inc; 1989:291–302.)*

Incidence

Peripheral vascular complications of aortic dissection are relatively common, noted in from 20% to 50% of patients with acute aortic dissection in various series in the literature.[3,5,11,12,14,16,17] The frequency of branch vessel obstruction will vary, depending on both the distribution and extent of dissection and the method of diagnosis. If one employs the commonly utilized classification of DeBakey et al.,[5] peripheral vascular complications are understandably more common with more extensive type I and IIIb dissections, which involve areas of the aorta from which major visceral or extremity branches originate, as opposed to dissections confined to the ascending or descending thoracic aorta (DeBakey type II and IIIa), which potentially involve only intercostal and spinal arteries. Thus, in our report of the Massachusetts General Hospital experience,[11] peripheral vascular complications were noted in 33% of all 345 patients with aortic dissection, but occurred in approximately 50% of patients with types I and IIIb dissections in contrast to only 10% with types II and IIIa lesions (Fig. 21–3).

Similarly, evolution and changes in diagnostic methods employed in evaluation of patients with suspected aortic dissection will influence the incidence of documented peripheral vascular complications. For example, the recently reported review from Hughes et al.[16] at Emory cited a 21% incidence of peripheral vascular complications in 86 cases of aortic dissection, substantially less that the approximately 30% incidence noted in several other large series focusing primarily on this topic.[11,12] As the Emory group acknowledges, however, angiography was used to diagnose or define the extent of dissection in only 22% of cases in their recent 5-year series. Transesophageal echocardiography (TEE), the most frequently (52%) employed technique in their series, may

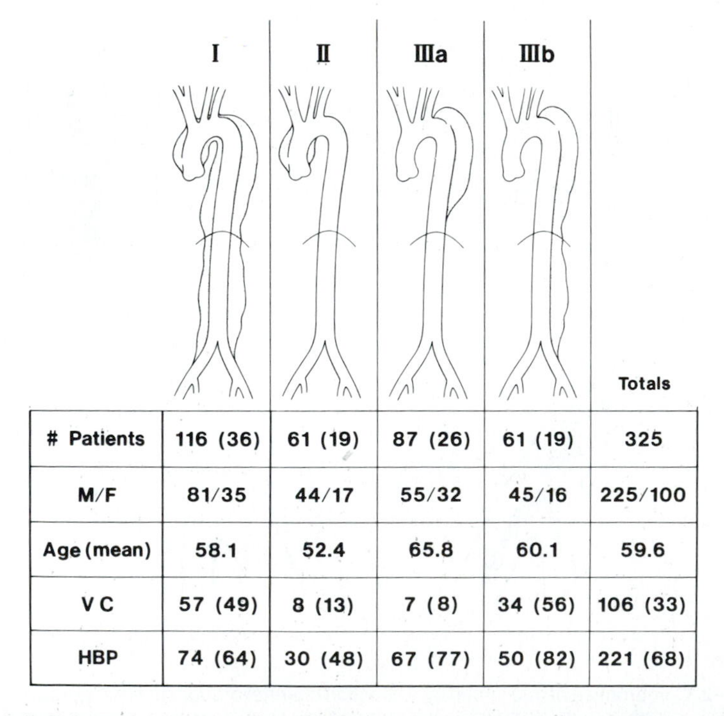

	I	II	IIIa	IIIb	Totals
# Patients	116 (36)	61 (19)	87 (26)	61 (19)	325
M/F	81/35	44/17	55/32	45/16	225/100
Age (mean)	58.1	52.4	65.8	60.1	59.6
VC	57 (49)	8 (13)	7 (8)	34 (56)	106 (33)
HBP	74 (64)	30 (48)	67 (77)	50 (82)	221 (68)

Figure 21–3. Schematic representation of DeBakey classification and findings of Massachusetts General Hospital study with demographic features, incidence of hypertension (HBP), and vascular complications (VC) for each type of dissection. Numbers in parentheses are percentages. *(Reprinted with permission from Cambria RP, Brewster DC, Gertler J, et al. Vascular complications associated with spontaneous aortic dissection. J Vasc Surg. 1988;7:199–209.)*

be more expeditious and highly accurate in diagnosis of the condition, but does not examine the abdominal aorta or its branches. Likewise, MRI or CT scanning is not likely as sensitive for detection and demonstration of branch vessel involvement as is angiography.[16] Hence, the incidence of peripheral vascular lesions may be underestimated with these diagnostic modalities.

Clinical Manifestations

Although the clinical picture of classic aortic dissection is well described and recognized, patients may vary considerably in their mode of presentation and clinical course. The variable origin and extent of the dissection process, with widely different resultant anatomic and physiologic ramifications, may cause a wide spectrum of clinical problems and sometimes diagnostic uncertainty. Indeed, the condition has often been referred to as "the great clinical masquerader."[3,14]

In most cases, a history of typical chest or back pain, long-standing hypertension, murmur of aortic insufficiency, widened mediastinum on chest radiograph, or symptoms referable to occlusion of aortic branch vessels will suggest the proper diagnosis. On occasion, however, atypical presentation with primarily manifestations of a peripheral vascular complication may cause the vascular surgeon to be the first physician to evaluate the patient. For example, painless aortic dissection presenting with an acutely ischemic limb mimicking acute thromboembolic arterial occlusion is well recognized.[1,18-22] The proper diagnosis may only be suspected after unsuccessful attempts to restore extremity circulation by catheter thromboembolectomy or findings of dissection at the arteriotomy site. Hence it is important to emphasize that the general or vascular surgeon may have the first opportunity to make the correct diagnosis so that definitive diagnostic evaluation and therapy can be rapidly instituted. The importance of timely diagnosis lies in the fact that the early mortality for patients with untreated acute aortic dissection is extremely high, approximately 1% per hour for the first 48 hours in the Stanford experience.[3,8] Other studies have confirmed this poor prognosis, with approximately 50% of patients dying within the first several days, 66% by 1 week, and 80% to 90% by 1 month.[23-25]

A wide variety of both early and late vascular and complications may affect the aorta or its major branches as a consequence of the initial aortic dissection (Table 21–1). Based on a large autopsy series, iliac artery compromise is most common, followed in descending order by innominate, left common carotid, left subclavian, renal, superior mesenteric, and celiac involvement.[24,26] The site of aortic branch occlusion and related clinical events in our series from the Massachusetts General Hospital of peripheral vascular complications associated with aortic dissection is shown in Figure 21–4.[11]

Lower Extremity Ischemia

The vascular surgeon is most likely to encounter a patient manifesting acute lower extremity ischemic symptoms caused by compromise of flow in the abdominal aorta

TABLE 21–1. PERIPHERAL VASCULAR COMPLICATIONS OF AORTIC DISSECTION

Aortic or iliac artery obstruction with lower extremity ischemia
Upper extremity ischemia
Neurologic ischemic events
Mesenteric ischemia
Renal ischemia
Late aortic aneurysm formation

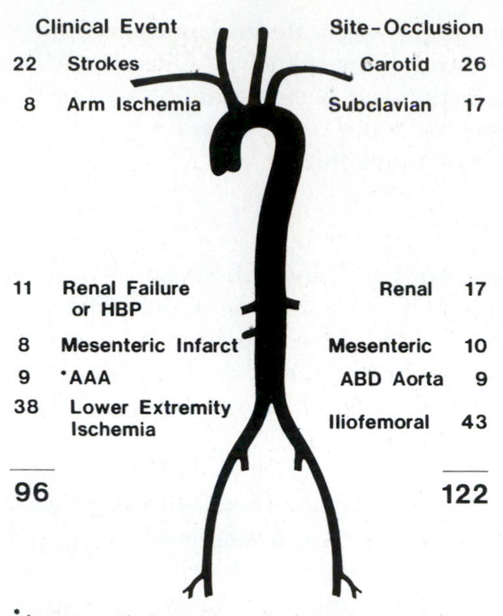

Figure 21–4. Sites and distribution of peripheral vascular complications and related clinical events of Massachusetts General Hospital study. Disparity between occlusions and clinical events reflects asymptomatic occlusions. *(Reprinted with permission from Cambria RP, Brewster DC, Gertler J, et al. Vascular complications associated with spontaneous aortic dissection. J Vasc Surg. 1984;7:199–209.)*

or iliac arteries (Fig. 21–5). DeBakey et al.[5] noted that 7% of their 527 patients with surgically treated dissection had lower extremity ischemia. Iliac artery involvement was found in Hirst's classic report[24] to be the most common complication of aortic dissection, found in 132 of 505 autopsy cases for an incidence of 26%. Indeed, the very first surgical approach to aortic dissection was described in 1935 by Gurin and colleagues[27] who performed an iliac fenestration to treat an ischemic leg caused by acute dissection. Similarly, Shaw[28] reported early effective results of aortic fenestration for lower extremity ischemia secondary to acute aortic obstruction in the acute phases of the disease.

Because pulse deficits and distal perfusion are influenced by systemic blood pressure, the presence or absence of distal reentry, and movement or oscillation of an intimal flap, typically physical findings and patient symptoms may wax and wane in the initial phases of acute dissection.[1] If the diagnosis of aortic dissection is not initially suspected and angiography carried out to evaluate acute lower extremity ischemia, it is important that characteristic arteriographic features of the process be recognized, thereby enabling a correct diagnosis to be established. As an aortic dissection progresses caudally from its thoracic origin, the false lumen tends to spiral around the long axis of the aorta, causing varying degrees of compression of the true lumen and resulting in a variable and often complex pattern of major aortic branches arising from either the true or false channels. Depending on placement of the arteriographic catheter tip and filming sequence, the narrowed true lumen may be the only vascular channel opacified, especially when dissection has extended to the iliofemoral region. Recognition may hinge on characteristic angiography findings, which in addition to actual visualiza-

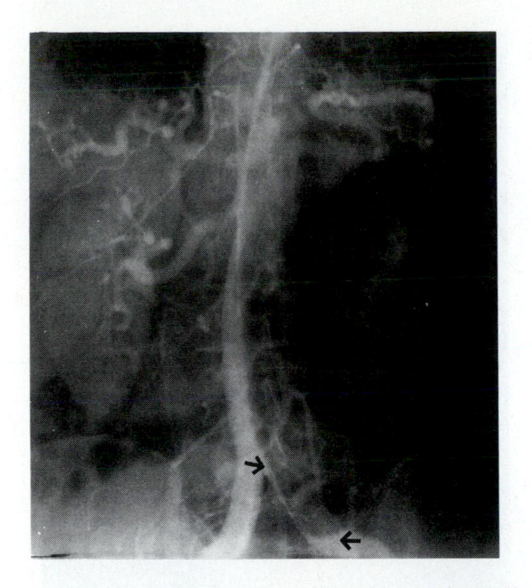

Figure 21–5. Aortogram demonstrating marked narrowing of infrarenal aorta and near total occlusion of left common iliac artery (*arrows*) in patient with Type I dissection. Ascending aortic repair restored left femoral pulse. *(Reprinted with permission from Brewster C, Cambria RP. Role of the vascular surgeon in the management of dissecting aortic aneurysms. In: Veith FJ, ed. Current Critical Problems in Vascular Surgery. St. Louis, MO: Quality Medical Publishing Inc; 1989:291–302.)*

tion of an intimal flap or double lumen include several indirect signs suggestive of aortic dissection, such as: (1) relatively small size of the opacified aortic lumen relative to that of the iliac arteries, (2) the absence of one or more lumbar vessels usually arising from the posterolateral abdominal aorta, or (3) the fusiform tapering of iliac or femoral arteries to a point of occlusion.[20] The last feature is particularly noteworthy because acute thrombotic or embolic occlusion usually results in abrupt vessel occlusion angiographically, whereas dissection typically produces a long, fusiform, tapered narrowing of the vessel proximal to the occlusion.

Upper Extremity Ischemia

Compromise of upper extremity circulation secondary to innominate or subclavian artery involvement by the dissection is also a relatively common observation (Fig. 21–6). Indeed, asymmetry of upper extremity pulses and/or blood pressure is one of the classic physical findings suggesting the diagnosis of acute aortic dissection. As with other etiologies of upper extremity arterial stenosis or occlusion, arm or hand ischemia is frequently not severe and often well tolerated because of availability of abundant collateral circulation.

Neurologic Events

Neurologic manifestations of aortic dissection most commonly represent transient ischemic attacks (TIAs) or stroke secondary to impairment of cerebral perfusion as a consequence of dissection. Syncope, a fairly frequent initial symptom of acute dissection, may be caused by hypotension or cardiac tamponade, whereas the mechanism of TIA or stroke may be related to discharge of thromboemboli from the proximal intimal tear, aortic arch, or at a reentry point in the carotid artery itself.[14,29,30] Nonetheless, most

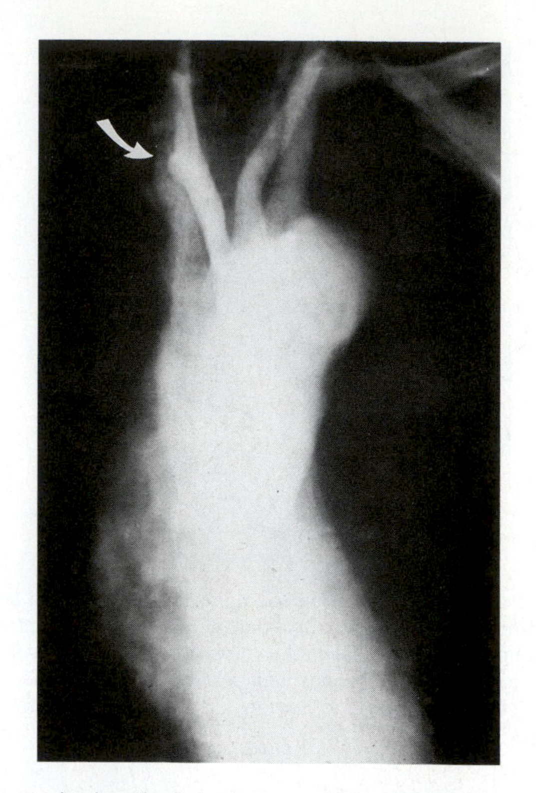

Figure 21–6. Acute proximal aortic dissection extending into innominate artery and producing occlusion of right subclavian artery at its origin (*arrow*). *(Reprinted with permission from Brewster DC, Cambria RP. Role of the vascular surgeon in the management of dissecting aortic aneurysms. In: Veith FJ, ed. Current Critical Problems in Vascular Surgery. St. Louis, MO: Quality Medical Publishing Inc; 1989:291–302.)*

acute cerebrovascular events are attributable to obstruction of the true lumen of the innominate or carotid branches of the aortic arch by the dissection (Fig. 21–7). DeBakey et al.[5] reported that 14% of patients in their extensive experience with Type I dissections had a history of syncopy and that, on admission, 6% still had clinical evidence of a central neurologic deficit.

In addition to stroke or TIAs, lower extremity neurologic manifestations may result from spinal cord injury or ischemic insult to peripheral nerves. Ischemic injury to the spinal cord, aside from its possible occurrence as a postoperative complication of direct surgical repair, may occur as a primary presenting event in a small percentage of patients with acute aortic dissection and can be of diagnostic importance.[5,31,32] Earlier autopsy studies suggested a higher incidence, but these data are obscured by the frequent coexistence of severe vascular insufficiency of the lower extremities, potentially causing an ischemic peripheral neuropathy, and/or motor deficits of extremities attributable to hemispheric strokes.[33]

Renal or Mesenteric Ischemia

Autopsy or arteriographic data reveal that approximately 10% of patients with acute aortic dissection will have impaired perfusion of major visceral or renal arteries.[5,11,12,24] Clinically evident sequelae of such impaired perfusion is less common, however, with only 5% to 6% of patients demonstrating clinically significant intestinal or renal is-

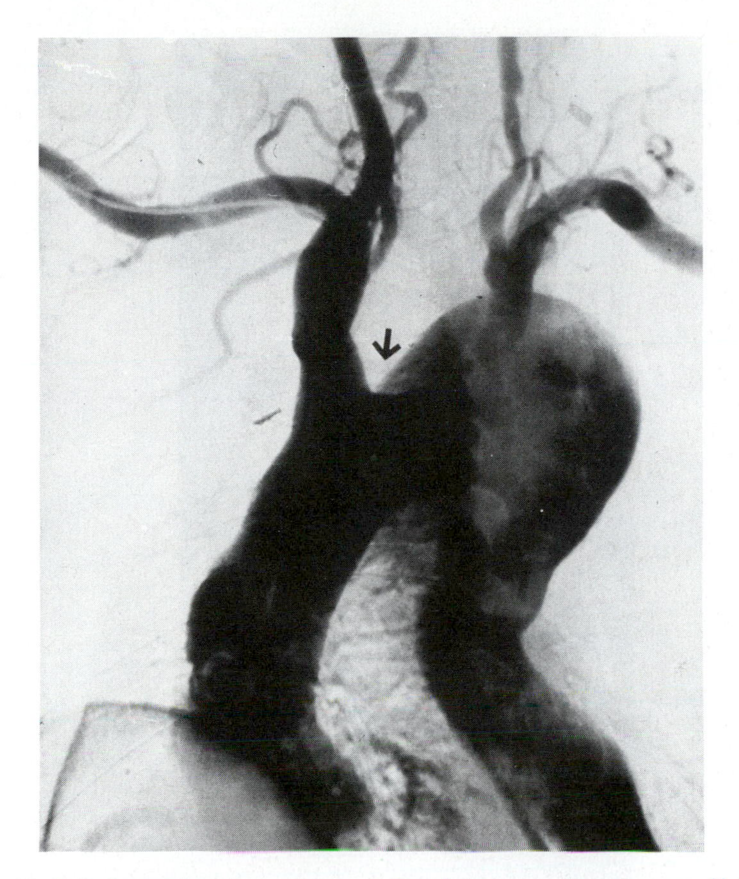

Figure 21–7. Aortogram in patient with chronic Type I dissection. Note absence of left common carotid artery (*arrow*) and aneurysm of distal arch and proximal descending thoracic aorta. This patient sustained recurrent left hemispheric watershed infarcts and was treated with a right-to-left carotid–carotid bypass before aneurysm resection. *(Reprinted with permission from Cambria RP, Brewster DC, Gertler J, et al. Vascular complications associated with spontaneous aortic dissection. J Vasc Surg. 1988;7:199–209.)*

chemia. This is fortunate, for both of these vascular complications of acute dissection are highly significant determinants of poor outcome.[8,11,12,34,35] Despite successful definitive central aortic repair of the dissection, death often results from irreversible mesenteric infarction or acute renal failure.

Abdominal pain out of proportion to physical findings, as typically noted with acute mesenteric ischemia, should suggest probable involvement of the celiac and/or superior mesenteric artery in the acute aortic dissection (Fig. 21–8), and requires urgent attention. Renal artery involvement may be considerably more difficult to recognize. Several factors may cloud evaluation of potential renal artery compromise: (1) renal function abnormalities may be preexistent and unrelated to obstruction coincident with dissection; (2) a single renal artery occlusion, not recognized as adequate function, is maintained by a normally perfused contralateral kidney (Fig. 21–9); (3) renal arteries may be perfused from true or false lumens, or both, requiring contrast opacification of both channels to verify patency or obstruction; (4) renal artery obstruction may be incomplete, producing significant hypertension without infarction or ischemic nephropathy and renal failure; and (5) developing renal insufficiency or low urinary output

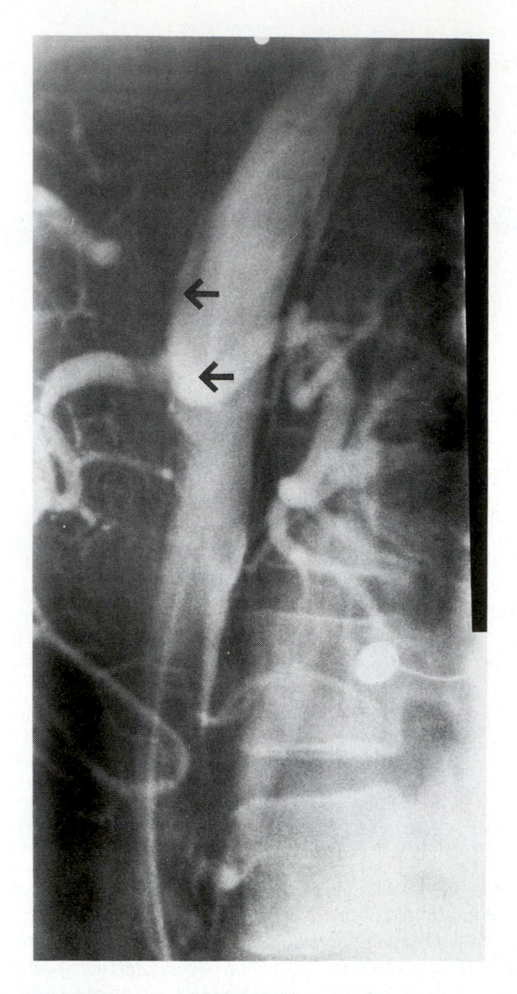

Figure 21–8. Lateral aortogram demonstrating occlusion of celiac axis origin (*upper arrow*) and compromise of proximal superior mesenteric artery (*lower arrow*) by acute Type I dissection. Note reconstitution of celiac. Patient succumbed to mesenteric infarction. *(Reprinted with permission from Brewster DC, Cambria RP. Role of the vascular surgeon in the management of dissecting aortic aneurysms. In: Veith FJ, ed. Current Critical Problems in Vascular Surgery. St. Louis, MO: Quality Medical Publishing Inc; 1989:291–302.)*

may be more a consequence of systemic hypotension than mechanical interference with renal artery blood flow.

Oliguria, flank pain, or hematuria are of possible diagnostic importance and should prompt immediate investigation.[36] It must be emphasized that diagnostic modalities such as TEE or aortic CT and MRI studies may not elucidate the status of renal artery blood flow, and contrast arteriography may often be required in these circumstances. When renal artery compromise occurs in acute aortic dissection and is sufficient to cause acute functional deterioration, resultant mortality is quite high, similar to that with acute mesenteric ischemia.[11] Thus, urgent corrective measures are required to preserve renal function and avoid a poor outcome.

Late Aneurysm Formation

Although acute aneurysmal change of the aorta and false lumen is rarely seen, subsequent frank aneurysmal dilation of the thoracoabdominal or infrarenal aorta (Fig. 21–10)

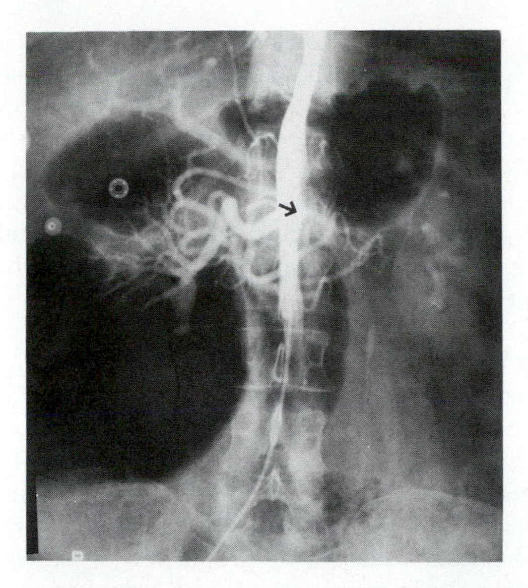

Figure 21–9. Aortogram demonstrating right renal artery perfusion from true lumen injection and scalloped defect (*arrow*) where left renal artery orifice has been detached by dissection process. *(Reprinted with permission from Brewster DC, Cambria RP. Role of the vascular surgeon in the management of dissecting aortic aneurysms. In: Veith FJ, ed. Current Critical Problems in Vascular Surgery. St. Louis, MO; Quality Medical Publishing Inc; 1989:291–302.)*

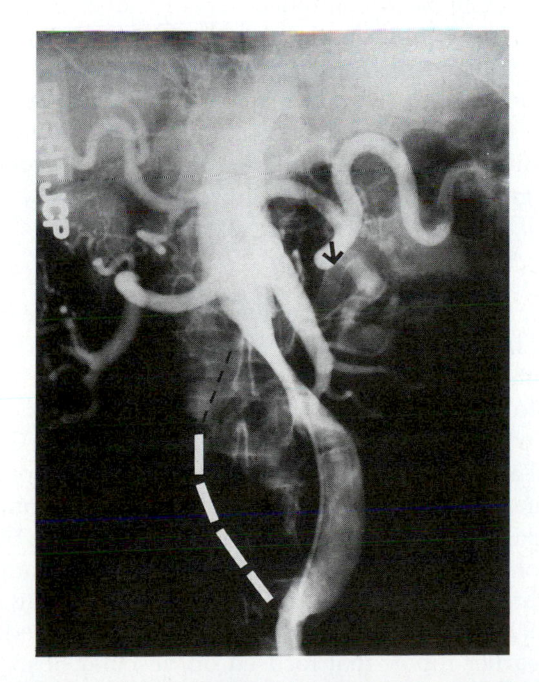

Figure 21–10. Large abdominal aortic aneurysm that developed 4 years after proximal dissection. The extent of the aneurysm (*dotted outline*) is not appreciated by this injection in the true lumen. Note faint opacification of left renal artery (*arrow*), which fills from the false lumen. *(Reprinted with permission from Brewster DC, Cambria RP. Role of the vascular surgeon in the management of dissecting aortic aneurysms. In: Veith FJ, ed. Current Critical Problems in Vascular Surgery. St. Louis, MO: Quality Medical Publishing Inc; 1989:291–302.)*

to a degree requiring consideration for delayed surgical repair is not uncommon.[5–7,37–39] Indeed, 15% to 30% of late deaths occuring in patients with prior aortic dissection is due to late rupture of the involved segment or another part of the aorta.[1] Such progressive aneurysmal dilation may occur in the aorta distal to even previously successful proximal graft repair of acute dissection, as many studies have indicated that the false lumen often remains patent via multiple points of distal reentry or by continued perfusion at the ostia of severed branches in a high percentage (approximately 85%) of patients.[40] Hence, careful lifelong follow-up by serial imaging studies of the aorta is imperitive. In addition, careful medical supervision and blood pressure control is essential. For example, DeBakey et al.[15] noted that later aneurysms of the thoracic, thoracoabdominal, or abdominal aorta developed in 45% of patients with poor blood pressure control, but in only 17% of those with well-controlled hypertension. Similar findings have been emphasized by Neya et al.[41]

Thus, vascular surgeons may become involved with repair of such late aneurysmal lesions. Operation is generally considered when symptoms occur or when progressive enlargement of the dissected aorta exceeds 6 cm in diameter in asymptomatic patients.[3,6] Chronic dissections constitute a reasonable proportion of patients undergoing thoracoabdominal aneurysm repair in many series,[6,7] and more localized repair of infrarenal aneurysms or even iliac aneurysms secondary to chronic dissections have been reported.[16,41,42]

TREATMENT

Controversy remains regarding management of peripheral vascular complications of acute aortic dissection. Much of the continued debate relates to the question of whether or not all types of aortic dissection should be treated by emergent direct repair, and to the issues of treatment priority with initial correction of vascular ischemic complications possibly taking precedence over central repair in certain patients. Although definitive data are not available to settle these questions for all patients with aortic dissection, and many surgeons and centers have their own management preferences, experience has provided certain guidelines and options for care.

Involvement of the Vascular Surgeon

It is clear that vascular surgeons may be actively involved in the treatment of patients with aortic dissection in certain situations.[10] First, aortic branch vessel occlusion may persist in some patients even following successful proximal aortic graft repair, which reestablishes flow into the true lumen, due to persistent aortic flaps or secondary thrombus formation, which continues to obstruct branch flow.[13] Or, obliteration of the false lumen by central aortic repair may actually be harmful to some patients in whom perfusion of vital branch vessels is dependent on the false channel, particularly if no distal reentry point exists.[40] Although relatively infrequent, the Stanford experience[12] documented that 8% of patients had persistent vascular complications following repair of the thoracic aorta, and in a recent report from Emory detailing results of the 5-year period from 1989 to 1994, 20% required a revascularization procedure following initial aortic repair.[16] In an earlier report that focused on vascular obstruction in dissection, Shumaker et al.[13] reported that 5 of 33 (15%) surgically treated patients required early or delayed revascularization procedures for persistent lower extremity ischemia.

Second, peripheral vascular complications may become the main treatment priority if the aortic dissection itself is judged to be best managed medically. With recognition that the principle causes of acute mortality in patients with acute dissections involving the ascending aorta (DeBakey types I and II, Stanford type A) relate to complications involving the proximal aorta (rupture, tamponade, aortic valve incompetence, or coronary obstruction), there is general consensus that the primary focus of treatment in patients with dissection involving the ascending aorta should be prompt central surgical repair. This offers the best chance of survival for patients with dissections in this location, and in most instances immediate aortic repair will suffice to alleviate or correct associated peripheral vascular compromise. However, many authorities continue to favor initial medical management of dissections originating in the descending thoracic aorta (DeBakey type III, Stanford type B), emphasizing that survival and other outcome parameters are more favorable with such treatment as opposed to immediate surgical repair.[1,2,39,40,43,44] Or, a patient may be considered an excessive risk for emergency direct aortic repair. In either case, the vascular surgeon may be called on to relieve vascular complications, with intention to manage the primary dissection itself nonoperatively.

Finally, and most controversial, is possible treatment of immediate life-threatening peripheral vascular complications by urgent primary intervention, with later semi-elective repair of the dissected aorta itself, if this is believed to be advisable. Circumstances that suggest that this treatment strategy might be considered are seen in patients with acute mesenteric or renal ischemia, or those with catastrophic advanced bilateral lower extremity ischemia due to acute aortic obstruction. In these instances, it can be argued that these complications represent even a greater risk of early lethal outcome than the primary dissection itself, as long as rupture or tamponade do not exist, and therefore should be logically addressed first: a so-called complication-specific approach.[45]

Options for Revascularization

Several methods of revascularization are available to the vascular surgeon in the management of vascular complications of aortic dissection. A fenestration procedure has been well described and documented to effectively restore lower extremity circulation in many reports and lead to acceptable long-term survival as the only treatment modality.[11,41,45–47] Similarly, by establishing effective communication between true and false lumens, it may also often successfully restore perfusion of compromised renal or visceral arteries to treat acute renal or mesenteric or renal ischemia. The principle appeal of fenestration is that it offers potential correction of life- or limb-threatening vascular complications of dissection, by means of a procedure that is most likely safer and less morbid as it does not entail thoracic aortic clamping, require any form of cardiopulmonary bypass, or expose the patient to the possibility of ischemic spinal cord injury.[45,46]

The procedure is usually carried out in the infrarenal aorta, by a retroperitoneal approach if desired. The aorta is divided, and a portion of the proximal septum between the true and false lumens is excised, providing a reentry point and free communication of flow between the two channels (Fig. 21–11). Most often, segmental graft insertion is carried out, although primary reanastomosis of the divided aorta may be done. Proximally, the suture line involves all three layers of the normal aortic wall in the portion of the aortic circumference uninvolved with dissection (true lumen) and only the aortic adventitia in that portion representing the false lumen. Use of pledgeted sutures may obviate many of the acknowledged problems of anastomosis involving such friable aortic tissue. Distally, the graft anastomosis may reapproximate both true and false lumens by incorporating both layers of the aortic wall in the distal suture line, or a distal anastomosis may be constructed more distally into nondissected portions of the iliac or femoral vessels.

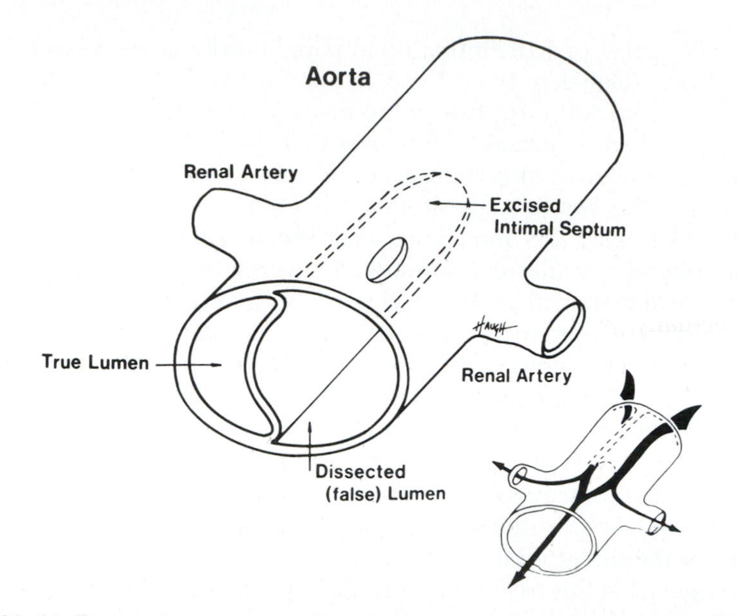

Figure 21–11. Fenestration procedure. Aorta is divided distal to renal arteries, with true and false lumens evident. Ellipse or "window" of dissected intima is excised, and then graft is sutured end to end to composite lumen. *(Reprinted with permission from the American Medical Association as it appears in: Hunter JA, Dye WS, Javid H, et al. Abdominal aortic resection in thoracic dissection. Arch Surg. 1976;111:1258–1262.)*

For lower extremity ischemia involving only one limb secondary to unilateral iliac obstruction, femoro–femoral grafts offer an expedient and effective treatment, particularly in patients with otherwise uncomplicated distal (type III or B) dissections who may be treated preferentially by medical management.[11,16,19] Use of axillobifemoral grafts has been described by Laas and colleagues[47] for patients with bilateral lower extremity ischemia associated with compromise of the aortic lumen due to more chronic dissections. Extra-anatomic grafts may also be extremely useful in other locations as well, for example correction of persistent upper extremity ischemia following repair of proximal dissection by means of an axillo-axillary bypass.[11] On occasion, carotid–carotid or subclavian–carotid bypass may be employed for cerebral ischemia persisting after aortic repair, or if the existence of an acute neurologic deficit is believed to preclude immediate direct operation.[11,48]

Relief of acute mesenteric or renal ischemia, either following initial aortic repair that fails to adequately restore flow to these branches or in selected patients as a primary intervention, may be accomplished by either a fenestration procedure or direct bypass grafting. Grafts to the visceral or renal vessels may originate from the lower aspect of the infrarenal aorta if uninvolved with the dissection, or, more commonly, from an uninvolved iliac artery. Alternatively, an aortic graft inserted as part of a fenestration procedure may serve as an origin for such bypass grafts to renal or visceral arteries if the surgeon does not feel confident enough that fenestration alone will adequately restore bowel or kidney perfusion.[49] Renal artery reconstruction may also be readily achieved by hepatorenal or splenorenal bypass grafts if the celiac origin is spared by the dissection.[50] Use of renal autotransplantation has also been reported as a method of renal salvage in aortic dissection.[51]

Endovascular Methods

The continued high morbidity and mortality of aortic dissection, particularly when associated with peripheral vascular complications, has spawned interest in development of alternative forms of therapy that may perhaps be less morbid and more expedient than conventional surgical approaches. This is particularly true of dissections complicated by ischemia of the kidneys and/or abdominal visceral in which irreversible and often lethal renal or bowel infarction may occur within hours of onset.

In recent years, a number of reports have described percutaneous catheter-based endovascular approaches and their potential application and appeal in management of both acute and chronic dissections.[52–58] Balloon dilatation catheters may be used percutaneously to either enlarge small reentry points that are providing ineffective flow to end organs being exclusively perfused from the false channel, or in some instances to actually establish *de novo* a point of reentry when these are absent by fenestrating the septum between the true and false lumens, thereby providing satisfactory flow and alleviating ischemic manifestations. As with surgical fenestration, this approach can also be employed to decompress the false lumen if it is encroaching significantly on the true aortic lumen, thereby improving antegrade flow to the lower extremities. Similarly, endovascular stents have been employed to treat the site of initiating intimal tear itself, improve a compromised true aortic lumen, or improve flow in compromised major aortic branches.[52,54–57]

Such techniques may be applied for vascular complications of subacute or chronic dissections, but perhaps have their greatest appeal as emergent therapies performed at the time of diagnostic angiography.[55] In this fashion, they could potentially serve as valuable adjunctive measures by minimizing critical organ ischemic time and thereby improving the patient's prognosis for definitive thoracic aortic repair, or represent definitive therapy in some instances where nonoperative treatment of the dissection is judged preferable. In the largest experience reported to date, Slonim et al.[52] from Stanford reported results of balloon fenestration or endovascular stenting in a series of 22 patients with lower extremity, renal, or visceral ischemic complications of acute or chronic aortic dissection. Percutaneous treatment of such peripheral complications was used in 12 type A (5 acute, 7 chronic) and 10 type B (9 acute, 1 chronic) dissections. Ten patients had leg, 13 had renal, and 6 had visceral ischemia. Technically successful revascularization with clinical success was achieved in all 22 patients with a low complication rate. Persistent relief of clinical symptoms at a mean follow-up of 13.7 months was reported for 19 patients. Although current clinical experience is obviously quite limited, such techniques appear to hold considerable promise and interest as a potential treatment option in the management of certain complex high-risk patients.

CONCLUSION

Peripheral vascular complications occur in approximately one-third of aortic dissections, as a consequence of compromise of major branch vessel flow by the dissection process. A variety of ischemic manifestations may occur, most often involving lower extremity ischemia but also potentially affecting the upper extremities, central nervous system, or circulation to the kidneys or intestines. Although direct thoracic repair of the dissection itself often corrects or alleviates the peripheral vascular complications, vascular surgical procedures may be necessary if branch vessel obstruction persists following thoracic aortic repair or if the dissection is felt preferentially treated by nonoperative management. In some patients, critical renal, mesenteric, or advanced lower extremity ischemia may assume treatment priority. A variety of reconstruction options are available. Newer endovascular treatment modalities appear to hold promise in the treatment of some of these complications.

REFERENCES

1. DeSanctis RW, Doroghazi RM, Austen WG, et al. Medical progress: aortic dissection. *N Engl J Med.* 1987;317:1060–1067.
2. Wheat MW Jr, Palmer RF. Dissecting aneurysms of the aorta. *Curr Probl Surg.* 1971:1–43.
3. Walker PJ, Sarris GE, Miller DC. Peripheral vascular manifestations of acute aortic dissection. In: Rutherford RD, ed. *Vascular Surgery.* Philadelphia: WB Saunders; 1995:1087–1102.
4. DeBakey ME, Cooley DA, Creech O Jr. Surgical considerations of dissecting aneurysm of the aorta. *Ann Surg.* 1955;142:586–612.
5. DeBakey ME, McCollum CH, Crawford ES, et al. Dissection and dissecting aneurysms of the aorta: twenty-year follow-up of five hundred twenty-seven patients treated surgically. *Surgery.* 1982;92:1118–1134.
6. Crawford ES, Svensson LG, Coselli JS, et al. Aortic dissection and dissecting aortic aneurysms. *Ann Surg.* 1988;208:254–273.
7. Svensson LG, Crawford ES, Hess KR, et al. Dissection of the aorta and dissecting aortic aneurysms. *Circulation.* 1990;82(suppl 4):IV–24–IV–38.
8. Miller DC, Mitchell RS, Oyer PE, et al. Independent determinants of operative mortality for patients with aortic dissections. *Circulation.* 1984;70(suppl 1):I–153–I–164.
9. Miller DC. Surgical management of aortic dissections: indications, perioperative management, and long-term results. In: Doroghazi RM, Slater EE, eds. *Aortic Dissection.* New York: McGraw-Hill; 1983:193–243.
10. Brewster DC, Cambria RP. Role of the vascular surgeon in the management of dissecting aortic aneurysms. In: Veith FJ, ed. *Current Critical Problems in Vascular Surgery.* St. Louis, MO: Quality Medical Publishing Inc; 1989:291–302.
11. Cambria RP, Brewster DC, Gertler J, et al. Vascular complications associated with spontaneous aortic dissection. *J Vasc Surg.* 1988;7:199–209.
12. Fann JI, Sarris GE, Mitchell RS, et al. Treatment of patients with aortic dissection presenting with peripheral vascular complications. *Ann Surg.* 1990;212:705–713.
13. Shumaker HB, Isch JH, Jolly WW. Stenotic and obstructive lesions in acute dissecting thoracic aortic aneurysms. *Ann Surg.* 1975;181:662–669.
14. Slater EE, DeSanctis RW. The clinical recognition of dissecting aortic aneurysm. *Ann J Med.* 1976;60:625–633.
15. DeBakey ME, Lawrie G. Intimal intussusception: unusual complication of dissecting aneurysm. *J Vasc Surg.* 1984;1:566–568.
16. Hughes JD, Bacha EA, Dodson TF, et al. *Peripheral vascular complications of aortic dissection.* Presented at the 23rd Annual Symposium of the Society for Clinical Vascular Surgery; March 23, 1995; Ft. Lauderdale, FL.
17. Jamieson WRE, Munro AI, Miyagishima RT, et al. Aortic dissections: early diagnosis and surgical management are the keys to survival. *Can J Surg.* 1982;25:145–149.
18. Amer NC, Schaeffer HC, Domingo RT, et al. Aortic dissection presenting as iliac-artery occlusion. *N Engl J Med.* 1962;266:1040–1042.
19. Shah PM, Clauss RH. Dissecting hematoma presents as acute lower extremity ischemia: diagnostic patient profile and management. *J Cardiovasc Surg.* 1983;24:649–653.
20. White TJ, Pinstein ML, Scott RL, et al. Aortic dissection manifested as leg ischemia. *Am J Roentgenol.* 1980;135:353–356.
21. Young JR, Dramer J, Humphries AW. The ischemic leg: a clue to dissecting aneurysm. *Cardiovasc Clin.* 1975;7:201–205.
22. Schoon IM, Holm J, Sudow G. Lower-extremity ischemia in aortic dissection. *Scand J Thorac Cardiovasc Surg.* 1985;19:93–95.
23. Anagnostopoulos CE, Prabhakar MJS, Kittle CF. Aortic dissections and dissecting aneurysms. *Am J Cardiol* 1972;30:263–273.
24. Hirst AE, Johns VJ, Kime SW. Dissecting aneurysms of the aorta: a review of 505 cases. *Medicine.* 1958;37:217–279.

25. Lindsay J, Hurst JW. Clinical features and prognosis in dissecting aneurysms of the aorta. *Circulation.* 1967;35:880–888.
26. Hirst AE Jr, Gore I. The etiology and pathology of aortic dissection. In: Doroghazi RM, Slater EE, eds. *Aortic Dissection.* New York, McGraw-Hill; 1983:13–54.
27. Gurin D, Bulmer JW, Derby R. Dissecting aneurysm of the aorta—diagnosis and operative relief of acute arterial obstruction due to this cause. *N Y State J Med.* 1935;35:1200–1202.
28. Shaw RS. Acute dissecting aortic aneurysm: treatment by fenestration of internal wall of the aneurysm. *N Engl J Med.* 1955;253:331–333.
29. Chase TN, Rosman NP, Puce DL. The cerebral syndromes associated with dissecting aneurysm of the aorta. A clinicopathologic study. *Brain.* 1966;91:173–189.
30. Zirkle PK, Wheeler JR, Gregory RT, et al. Carotid involvement in aortic dissection diagnosed by duplex scanning. *J Vasc Surg.* 1984;1:700–703.
31. Gerber O, Heyer EJ, Vieux U. Painless dissections of the aorta presenting as acute neurologic syndromes. *Stroke.* 1986;17:644–647.
32. Zull DN, Cydulka R. Acute paraplegia: a presenting manifestation of aortic dissection. *Am J Med.* 1988;84:765–770.
33. Weisman AD, Adams RD. Neurologic complications of dissecting aortic aneurysm. *Brain.* 1944;67:69–92.
34. Wolfe WG. Acute ascending aortic dissection. *Ann Surg.* 1980;192:658–666.
35. Pinet F, Froment JC, Guillot M, et al. Prognostic factors and indications for surgical treatment of acute aortic dissections: a report based on 191 observations. *Cardiovasc Intervent Radiol.* 1984;7:257–266.
36. Mulder DG, Kaufman JJ. Acute dissection of the thoracic aorta presenting as renal artery occlusion. *J Thorac Cardiovasc Surg.* 1968;56:184–188.
37. Haverich A, Miller DC, Scott WC, et al. Acute and chronic aortic dissections—determinants of long-term outcome for operative survivors. *Circulation.* 1985;72(suppl 2):II–22–II–34.
38. Miller DC. Improved follow-up for patients with chronic dissections. *Semin Thorac Cardiovasc Surg.* 1991;3:270–288.
39. Glower DD, Speier RH, White WD, et al. Management and long-term outcome of aortic dissection. *Ann Surg.* 1991;214:31–41.
40. da Gama AD. The surgical management of aortic dissection: from uniformity to diversity, a continuous challenge. *J Cardiovasc Surg.* 1991;32:141–153.
41. Neya K, Omoto R, Kyo S, et al. Outcome of Stanford type B acute aortic dissection. *Circulation.* 1992;86(suppl 2):II–1–II–7.
42. Hunter JA, Dye WS, Javid H, et al. Abdominal aortic resection in thoracic dissection. *Arch Surg.* 1976;111:1258–1262.
43. Wheat MW Jr, Palmer RF, Bartley TD, et al. Treatment of dissecting aneurysms of the aorta without surgery. *J Thorac Cardiovasc Surg.* 1965;50:364–373.
44. Doroghazi RM, Slater EE, DeSanctis RW, et al. Long-term survival of patients with treated aortic dissection. *J Am Coll Cardiol.* 1984;3:1026–1034.
45. Elefteriades JA, Hartleroad J, Gusberg RJ, et al. Long-term experience with descending aortic dissection: the complication-specific approach. *Ann Thorac Surg.* 1992;53:11–21.
46. Elefteriades JA, Hammond GL, Gusberg RJ, et al. Fenestration revisited: a safe and effective procedure for descending aortic dissection. *Arch Surg.* 1990;125:786–790.
47. Laas J, Heinemann M, Schaefers H-J, et al. Management of thoracoabdominal malperfusion in aortic dissection. *Circulation.* 1991;84(suppl 3):III–20–III–24.
48. Walterbusch G, Oelert H, Borst HG. Restoration of cerebral blood flow by extraanatomic bypass in acute aortic dissection. *Thorac Cardiovasc Surg.* 1984;32:381–382.
49. Cogbill TH, Gundersen AE, Travelli F. Mesenteric vascular insufficiency and claudication following acute dissecting thoracic aortic aneurysm. *J Vasc Surg.* 1985;2:472–476.
50. Moncure AC, Brewster DC, Darling RD, et al. Use of splenic and hepatic arteries for renal revascularization. *J Vasc Surg.* 1986;3:196–203.

51. Adib K, Belzer FO. Renal autotransplantation in dissecting aortic aneurysm with renal artery involvement. *Surgery*. 1978;84:686–688.
52. Slonim SM, Dake MD, Semba CP, et al. Aortic dissection: percutaneous management of ischemic complications with endovascular stents and balloon fenestration. Presented at the 49th Annual Meeting of the Society for Vascular Surgery; June 11, 1995; New Orleans, LA.
53. Williams DM, Brothers TE, Messina LM. Relief of mesenteric ischemia in Type III aortic dissection with percutaneous fenestration of the aortic septum. *Radiology*. 1990;174:450–452.
54. Saito S, Arai H, Kim K, et al. Percutaneous fenestration of dissecting intima with a transseptal needle: a new therapeutic technique for visceral ischemia complicating acute aortic dissection. *Cathet Cardiovasc Diagn*. 1992;26:130–135.
55. Walker PJ, Dake MD, Mitchell RS, et al. The use of endovascular techniques for the treatment of complications of aortic dissection. *J Vasc Surg*. 1993;18:1042–1051.
56. Akaba N, Ujiie H, Umezawa K, et al. Management of acute aortic dissections with a cylinder-type balloon catheter to close the entry. *J Vasc Surg*. 1986;3:890–894.
57. Trent MS, Parsonnet VP, Schoenfeld R, et al. A balloon-expandable intravascular stent for obliterating experimental aortic dissection. *J Vasc Surg*. 1990;11:707–717.
58. Shimshak TM, Giorgi LV, Hartzler GO. Successful percutaneous transluminal angioplasty of an obstructed abdominal aorta secondary to a chronic dissection. *Am J Cardiol*. 1988;61:486–487.

22

Para-Anastomotic Aneurysms of the Aorta

Diagnosis and Management

Alan B. Lumsden, MB, ChB, Robert C. Allen, MD, and Robert B. Smith, III, MD

Replacement of the abdominal aorta for both aneurysmal and occlusive disease is a common procedure. Its widespread use is a testimony to the high patency rate of replacement grafts and a low complication rate.[1] Dacron grafts are the most commonly selected prostheses, but in recent years there has been increasing use of expanded polytetrafluoroethylene (PTFE) grafts. After the immediate peri-implantation period, graft limb thrombosis is the most frequent complication; however, graft infection, aortoenteric fistulae (AEF), and anastomotic aneurysms are challenging developments. Whereas anastomotic aneurysms involving the femoral or iliac arteries at the distal anastomosis are common, and their management extensively discussed,[2,3] para-anastomotic aneurysms involving the abdominal aorta (PAA) are less common, more technically challenging, and less widely reported. Their incidence, however, may be underestimated since routine screening after aortic grafting is presently not the standard of care,[4–6] and unlike groin pseudoaneurysms, proximal anastomotic pseudoaneurysms are less likely to be clinically detected because of their location within the retroperitoneum.

PAA may follow bypass for occlusive or aneurysmal disease, may occur early or late, and may be classified as a pseudoaneurysm or true aneurysm. Detection of PAA is usually a result of increasing size, symptom development, or serendipity.[4,6,7] They carry the same risk of rupture, with its dire consequences, as did the primary aneurysm. Consequently, optimal management is surgical repair prior to development of symptoms. PAA, when detected prior to appearance of complications, can be repaired with an acceptable risk.[4,6,7]

DEFINITION

Aneurysmal disease after bypass grafting of the abdominal aorta is defined radiographically as a focal dilatation juxtaposed to the aortic suture line or an adjacent aortic diameter that is greater than or equal to 4.0 cm.[5] True aneurysms are defined as a smoothly enlarging dilatation of the aorta originating from the area of the suture line (Fig. 22–1). Pseudoaneurysms are seen as a focal bulge of the aortic lumen at the anastomosis (Fig. 22–2). Early aneurysmal disease is defined as occurring within 5 years from the time of the original aortic grafting procedure.

Perhaps a new addition to these classifications is necessary due to the introduction of endovascular grafting. Devices that are too short to completely exclude the entire length of an aneurysm engage in aneurysmal wall, leaving a para-attachment system aneurysm, which may be prone to further expansion on follow-up (Fig. 22–3). The introduction of bifurcated devices may reduce the likelihood that such aneurysms will develop because of the technical difficulty in deploying the distal attachment system sufficiently close to the aortic bifurcation to exlude all of the distal aneurysm.

INCIDENCE

A review of the recent literature reveals an apparent increase in the reported incidence (varying from 0.2% to 15%) of PAA after bypass grafting for abdominal aorta aneurysms (AAAs) or aortoiliac occlusive disease.[6,8,9] This increase in incidence seems paradoxic in light of advances in surgical technique and suture/graft material. However, patients with prostheses are living longer, and those with complicated vascular disease are receiving better medical care for their comorbid problems. Edwards and colleagues[5] have demonstrated, using life table analysis, an incidence of PAA up to 27% at 15 years after grafting. This figure could be even higher since most patients receive no routine evaluation for development of a PAA after bypass grafting.[4–7]

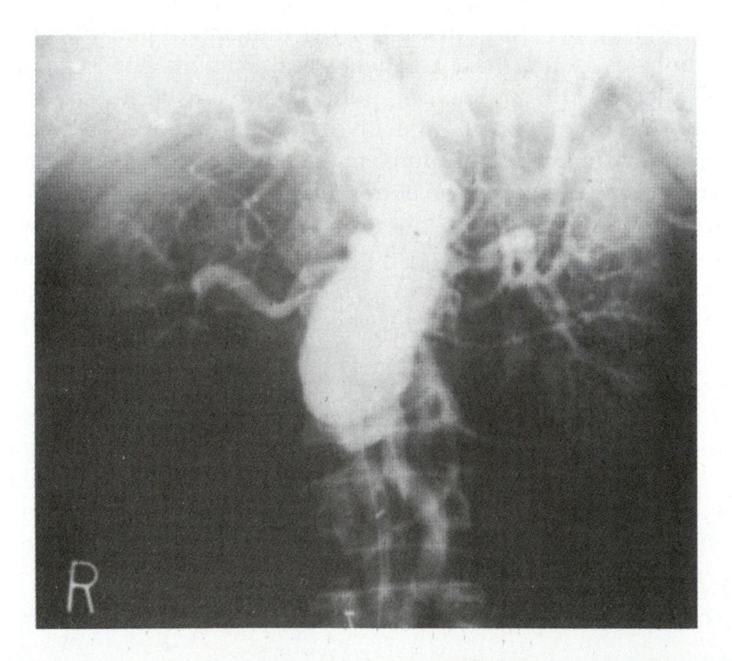

Figure 22–1. True aneurysm arises from proximal suture line with symmetric dilation and smooth taper to normal aorta. *(Reprinted with permission from Allen RC, Schneider J, Longenecker L, et al. Paraanastomotic aneurysms of the abdominal aorta. J Vasc Surg. 1993;18:424–432.)*

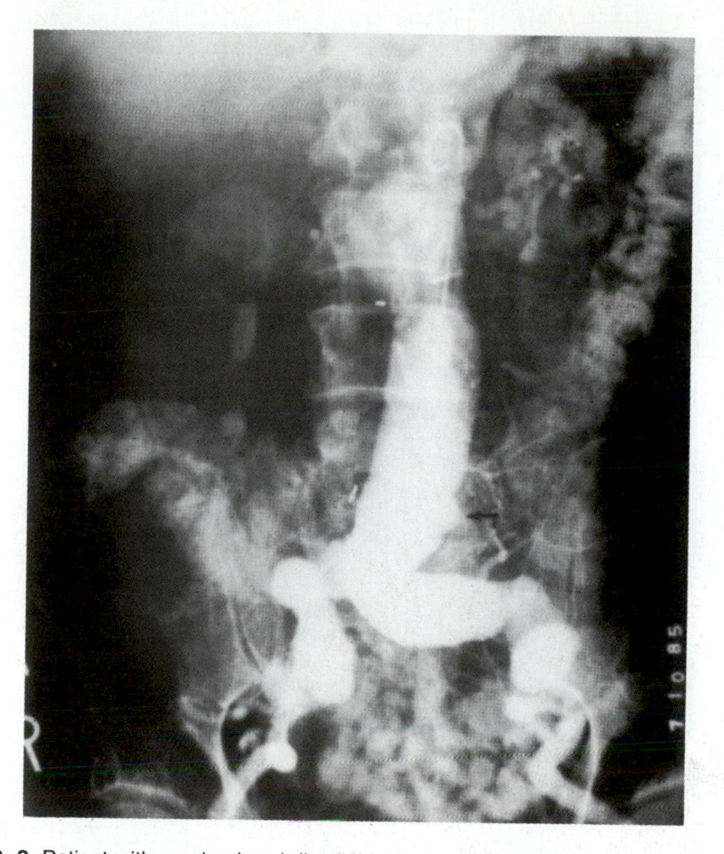

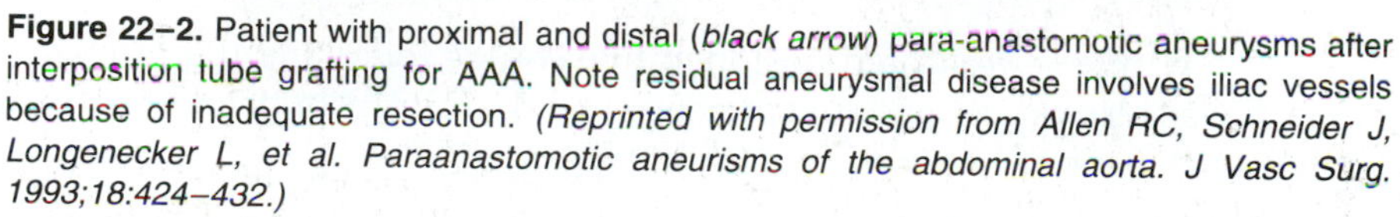
Figure 22–2. Patient with proximal and distal (*black arrow*) para-anastomotic aneurysms after interposition tube grafting for AAA. Note residual aneurysmal disease involves iliac vessels because of inadequate resection. *(Reprinted with permission from Allen RC, Schneider J, Longenecker L, et al. Paraanastomotic aneurisms of the abdominal aorta. J Vasc Surg. 1993;18:424–432.)*

ETIOLOGY

The etiology of an anastomotic aneurysm is speculative and probably multifactorial.[10,11] It is important to distinguish true versus false aneurysms and to identify early versus late aneurysmal development. In our series at Emory University Hospital, true aneurysms (19%) were much less common than false aneurysms (81%). True aneurysms usually occur after bypass grafting for aneurysmal disease[4,5,7] and develop for the same reasons as primary aneurysms, namely atherosclerosis, inherited collagen defect, and hemodynamic factors.[12,13] Inadequate resection of the infrarenal aorta at the time of the initial operation predisposes the defective residual wall to aneurysm development. Aneurysms occur most commonly at the proximal anastomosis but occasionally involve the distal anastomosis.

False aneurysms develop due to chronic dehiscence of the prosthesis from the underlying artery and may develop as a consequence of defects in the artery, suture, or graft. Defects in any or all of these components therefore predispose to pseudoaneurysm formation. Factors implicated in their development include choice of suture material (silk, braided polyester), prosthesis dilatation (Dacron), type of anastomosis (end to side), severity/progression of atherosclerosis (multilevel disease), vessel versus graft compliance mismatch, and infection (periprosthetic, AEF).[10,11] Early PAA formation has

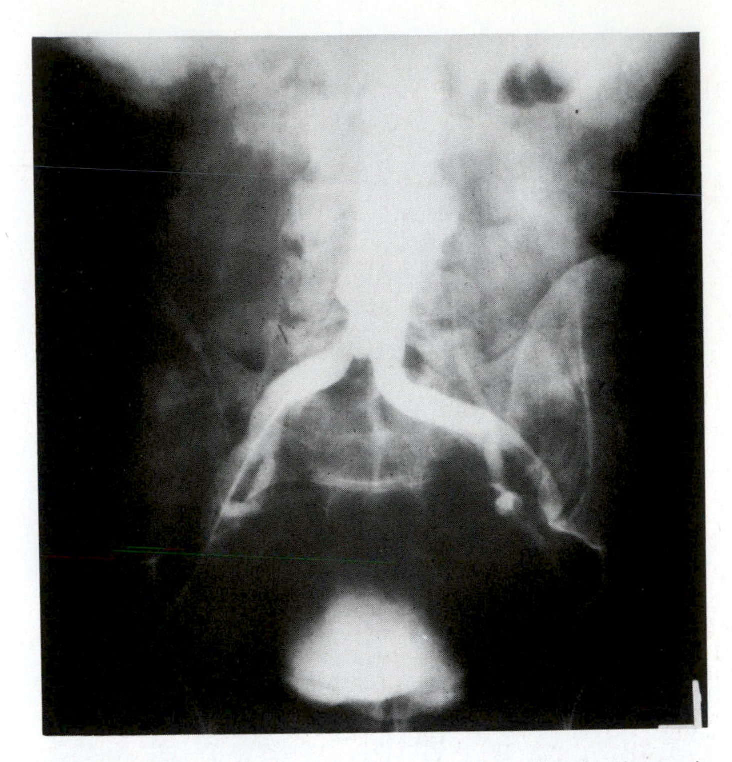

Figure 22–3. Juxta-attachment system aneurysm in a patient with an endovascular prosthesis.

been associated with a complicated postoperative course following the primary aortic procedure.[5] It was also linked in our experience to α-1 antitrypsin deficiency, recurrent PAA, and graft infection.[7]

PRESENTATION

The clinical symptoms associated with PAA are varied and nonspecific. Unfortunately, most patients are totally asymptomatic, with the PAA being detected by chance. For example, two patients in our series were diagnosed incidentally on abdominal computed tomography (CT) and intravenous pyelogram examinations. Symptoms, when present, include abdominal pain, back pain, or pain developing from compression of adjacent organs. Physical examination may reveal a pulsatile mass in nonobese patients. However, testimony to their asymptomatic nature is the fact that the majority of PAAs are detected late and, consequently, are large when detected, with an average size of approximately 7 cm.[7]

The mean interval from the time of the primary aortic procedure to PAA diagnosis is 8 to 10 years. During this interval, the patient usually has been followed and reviewed with regular physical examination. Despite this, PAAs often remain undetected and will have increased until very large. The finding of a pulsatile swelling on physical examination clearly establishes the diagnosis; however, the general inability to plapate most PAAs supports the recommendation that interval ultrasound or CT scanning be part of routine follow-up after aortic graft placement.[4,5,6]

A femoral artery false aneurysm is an associated finding in approximately 25% of patients with a PAA and should be an indication to intensify surveillance.[4,5,6,14] In contrast, approximately 15% of patients with a femoral pseudoaneurysm will have an associated PAA.[11] This figure is even higher when bilateral femoral pseudoaneurysms are detected, and in our practice, has mandated the performance of abdominal CT scanning.

Rupture of a PAA is associated with a high mortality rate.[14,15] Two patients in our study complaining of abdominal and back pain had a contained rupture of a false aneurysm early after bypass grafting.

The development of a proximal anastomotic pseudoaneurysm also predisposes to development of AEF. All three patients in our series who presented with gastrointestinal (GI) bleeding had AEF. Any patient with an aortic graft and PAA on CT scanning who develops GI bleeding probably has an AEF. Surgical intervention is warranted based on these findings alone. The characteristic presentation of AEF is a herald bleed and abdominal/black pain in a patient with a history of bypass grafting of the abdominal aorta. This classic triad was found in all three of our patients having a PAA and associated AEF.[7]

DIAGNOSTIC STUDIES

A high index of suspicion is required for diagnosis of PAA in patients after abdominal aortic bypass grafting if routine screening is not employed. Ultrasonography (US) can be helpful diagnostically, and several academic centers have documented its high accuracy.[16,17] However, this examination is operator dependent, and results are variable between institutions.[16,17,18,19] CT scanning is also effective in evaluating patients for complications after bypass grafting of the abdominal aorta.[17,19,20] It demonstrates PAA size and extent of involvement, as well as synchronous disease processes in the abdomen. Proper preoperative evaluation of PAA patients prior to operative intervention is essential because of their frequently advanced age and multiple medical problems. Aortography, the gold standard for defining the aneurysm and associated anatomy, facilitates planning of the operative approach and selection of the appropriate surgical procedure. Magnetic resonance imaging (MRI) or spiral CT angiography will have an increasing role in the diagnosis of PAA in the future and may supplant standard angiography.[21]

MANAGEMENT

The same general rules about the indications for intervention of primary AAA apply to PAA. Elective surgical management of PAA lesions is the treatment of choice since these lesions progressively increase in size and may rupture with time.[15] Morbidity and mortality rates are acceptable in asymptomatic patients undergoing elective repair, as reported in our series and those by other authors.[4,6,7]

The approach to repair is determined largely by the location of the aneurysm. When the para- and suprarenal aorta is dilated, a thoracoabdominal repair is recommended. Operative management of PAA involving the renal and/or visceral vessels is more challenging, and a thoracoabdominal approach gives excellent proximal exposure and expedites repair. If the PAA represents dilation of residual infrarenal aorta, a transabdominal approach is possible. An attempt should be made to replace as much of the infrarenal aorta as is technically feasible without suprarenal cross-clamp. This type of repair frequently involves excising the diseased segment of the artery and adjacent graft, with placement of an interposition prosthesis. An end-to-side proximal anastomosis in patients with occlusive disease has been implicated as a causative factor of operative failure, but the importance of preserving the pelvic circulation must not be ignored.[6,9,22] A bifurcated graft can be used if iliofemoral aneurysmal disease or generalized graft fatigue is present.

Operative complications are common and increase in the urgent setting or if other aortic graft complications are present (e.g., AEF, graft infection).[3,4,14,23] Likewise, surgical mortality in these complicated reoperations is substantially higher than that associated with the initial aortic reconstruction (21% in our series of 29 patients).[7] It is imperative to obtain operative cultures in every case, even if the index of suspicion for a graft infection is low. The clinical judgment of an experienced vascular surgeon is crucial in the management of these frequently elderly and frail patients. Observation with US surveillance should be considered as an option for patients with small asymptomatic PAA or for high-risk patients with an asymptomatic PAA who are poor operative candidates.

SURVEILLANCE

Several recent reports clearly show PAA to be an important problem, and each makes a plea for increased surveillance.[4–7] However, the method and frequency of follow-up are still unclear, and there is not enough detailed information, either short- or long-term, after bypass grafting of the abdominal aorta to make informed recommendations. Several pieces of information are available. These include the observations that most PAAs occur late after aortic grafting (average 8 to 10 years) and that early PAA development is associated with a complicated postoperative course following the primary aortic procedure.[4,5] US and CT scanning appear to be the most effective diagnostic modalities, but each has advantages and disadvantages. US is inexpensive and quick, but the results obtained are variable depending on the operator/institution, CT scanning is accurate and reproducible, but expensive and time consuming. US may be the preferred study in this era of cost containment, given the substantially reduced cost ($300 for US versus $850 for CT in our center). The authors believe that US is the diagnostic technique of choice, provided a track record of accuracy in abdominal US scanning has been established in that institution.

The data from our study and those from Curl, Edwards, and Gautier lend support to the proposal for routine screening.[4–7] Our follow-up protocol in the past has been purely clinical without routine radiographic surveillance. Presently, we recommend a US examination at 5 years from the time of the original aortic prosthetic reconstruction and subsequently every 2 to 3 years. High-risk patients for an early PAA should be followed more closely, with a US examination every 2 years. The presence of risk factors for aneurysm formation, such as associated ileofemoral aneurysms or possible graft infection, requires increased surveillance. Abdominal US should also be performed in patients who develop groin anastomotic pseudoaneurysms and in patients with new abdominal or back pain.

The pattern of late presentation and increased incidence over time, as evidenced by life table analysis, argues for lifetime surveillance.[4–6] Early detection and elective operative repair of PAA are essential to minimize morbidity and mortality.

REFERENCES

1. Crawford ES, Bomberger RA, Glaeser DH, et al. Aortoiliac occlusive disease: factors influencing survival and function following reconstructive operation over a 25-year period. *Surgery.* 1981;90:1055–1066.

2. Van den Akker PJ, Brand R, van Schlifgaarde R, et al. False aneurysms after prosthetic reconstructions for aortoiliac obstructive disease. *Ann Surg.* 1989;210:658–666.
3. Dennis JW, Littooy FN, Greisler HP, et al. Anastomotic pseudoaneurysms: a continuing late complication of vascular reconstructive procedures. *Arch Surg.* 1986;121:314–317.
4. Curl GR, Faggioli GL, Stella A, et al. Aneurysmal change at or above the proximal anastomosis after infrarenal grafting. *J Vasc Surg.* 1992;16:855–860.
5. Edwards JM, Teeffey FA, Zierler RE, et al. Intraabdominal paraanastomotic aneurysms after aortic bypass grafting. *J Vasc Surg.* 1992;15:344–353.
6. Gautier C, Borie H, Lagneau P. Aortic false aneurysms after prosthetic reconstruction of the infrarenal aorta. *Ann Vasc Surg.* 1992;6:413–417.
7. Allen RC, Schneider J, Longenecker L, et al. Paraanastomotic aneurysms of the abdominal aorta. *J Vasc Surg.* 1993;18:424–432.
8. Mehigan DH, Fitzpatrick B, Browna HI, et al. Is compliance mismatch the major cause of anastomotic arterial aneurysms? *J Cardiovasc Surg.* 1985;26:147–150.
9. Mikati A, Marache P, Watel A, et al. End-to-side aortoprosthetic anastomoses: long-term computed tomography assessment. *Ann Vasc Surg.* 1990;4:584–591.
10. Briggs RM, Jarstfer BS, Collins GJ. Anastomotic aneurysms. *Am J Surg.* 1983;146:770–773.
11. Gaylis H, Dewar G. Anastomotic aneurysms: facts and fancy. *Surg Ann.* 1990;22:317–340.
12. Deak SB, Ricotta JJ, Mariani TJ, et al. Abnormalities in the biosynthesis of type III procollagen in cultured skin fibroblasts from two patients with multiple aneurysms. *Matrix.* 1991;12: 92–100.
13. Tilson MD, Seashore MR. Fifty families with abdominal aortic aneurysms in two or more first order relatives. *Am J Surg.* 1984;147:551–553.
14. Plate G, Hollier LA, O'Brien P, et al. Recurrent aneurysms and late vascular complications following repair of abdominal aortic aneurysms. *Arch Surg.* 1985;120:590–594.
15. Sladen JG, Gerein AS, Miyagishima RT. Late rupture of prosthetic aortic grafts. *Am J Surg.* 1987;4153:453–458.
16. Gooding GA, Effeney DJ, Goldstone J. The aortofemoral graft: detection and identification of healing complications by ultrasonography. *Surgery.* 1981;89:94–101.
17. Hilton S, Megibow AJ, Naidich DP, et al. Computed tomography of the postoperative aorta. *Radiology.* 1982;145:403–407.
18. Turnipseed WD, Acher CW, Detmer DE, et al. Digital subtraction angiography and B-mode ultrasonography for abdominal and peripheral aneurysms. *Surgery.* 1982;92:619–626.
19. Mark A, Moss AA, Lusby R, et al. CT evaluation of complications of abdominal aortic surgery. *Radiology.* 1982;145:403–407.
20. Nevelsteen A, Suy R. Anastomotic false aneurysms of the abdominal aorta and iliac arteries. *J Vasc Surg.* 1989;10:595.
21. Guinet C, Buy JN, Ghossain MA, et al. Aortic anastomotic pseudoaneurysms: US, CT, MR, and angiography. *J Comput Assist Tomogr.* 1992;16:182–188.
22. Melliere D, Labasttie J, Bequemin JP, et al. Proximal anastomosis in aortobifemoral bypass: end-to-end or end-to-side? *J Cardiovasc Surg.* 1990;31:77–80.
23. Treiman GS, Weaver FA, Cossman DV, et al. Anastomotic false aneurysms of the abdominal aorta and the iliac arteries. *J Vasc Surg.* 1988;8:268–273.

23

Mycotic Thoracoabdominal Aortic Aneurysms

Robert Y. Rhee, MD, Kenneth J. Cherry, Jr., MD, and Thomas C. Bower, MD

Infection anywhere in the arterial circulation, whether primary or following reconstructive surgery, is a difficult problem. Management of aortic infection is particularly challenging since no generally satisfactory infection-resistant autogenous conduits of proper length and size exist, although some authors have had success with use of the deep veins of the lower extremity as aortic replacements.[1] The use of allografts has also been reported.[2] The traditional approach has been to treat primary or secondary aortic infections with aggressive antibiotic therapy, resection of the infected aorta or graft, wide surgical debridement and extra-anatomic bypass through noninfected tissue planes.[3–5] This approach, with its many modifications, works well for most infrarenal aortic and lower extremity arterial infections. Infections of the paravisceral or thoracoabdominal aorta, however, are not satisfactorily treated by this established approach, as blood flow to the viscera must be maintained or restored by direct reconstructive techniques.

Management of mycotic or infected aortic aneurysms remains controversial.[2,5–16] Most surgeons have favored the classic approach of antibiotics, debridement, excision of the infected aneurysm, and a remote bypass either preceding or subsequent to excision of the aneurysm for abdominal aortic infections.[3–5,12] Recently, the concept of *in situ* or direct repair of the infected abdominal aorta has gained proponents,[2,13,16] and *in situ* repair of the thoracic aorta is usually recommended for infected aneurysms and grafts in that location.[14,15] Resection of the infected aorta and extra-anatomic reconstruction does not readily address the problems attendant to infections of the thoracoabdominal aorta. Direct *in situ* repair is indicated for treatment of these mycotic aneurysms, because of the absolute need to maintain gastrointestinal, renal, and—perhaps—spinal cord blood flow.[14,17–19] In order to evaluate the management of this complex vascular surgical problem, we reviewed the literature and, in addition, identified 15 patients treated at our institution between 1976 and 1994 having primary mycotic thoracoabdominal aortic aneurysms (TAAA) (Table 23–1).

TABLE 23–1. MYCOTIC SUPRARENAL AND THORACOABDOMINAL AORTIC ANEURYSMS AS REPORTED IN STUDIES

Author (year)	No. Patients	Reconstruction I = *in situ* E = extra-anatomic	Outcome S = survived D = dead	Organism
Morris (1962)	1	I	D	*Salmonella*
Mundth (1969)	1	I	D	*UK*
James (1977)	1	I	S	*Salmonella*
Johanson (1983)	1	I	S	*Salmonella*
Ewart (1983)	1	NA	D (preop)	*Salmonella*
Atlas (1984)	1	E	S	*Salmonella*
Bitseff (1987)	2	I NA	S D (in OR)	*Salmonella* *Salmonella*
Yao (1988)	1	I	D	*M. Tuberculosis*
Atnip (1989)	1	I	S	*Klebsiella*
Chan and Crawford (1989)	11	I	S	*Unspecified*
Reddy (1991)	3	I (1) E (2)	S (1) D (3)	*Staphylococcus* (2) *B. fragilis* (1)
Gomes (1992)	1	I	S	*L. monocytogenes*
Hollier (1993)	6	I	S (3) D (3[a])	*Salmonella* (1) *Staphylococcus* (1) *Mycobacterium* (1) *E. coli* (1) *Candida* (1) *UK* (1)
Rhee, Cherry, and Bower (1995)	15[b]	I (14) E (1)	S (7) D (8[c])	*Salmonella* (4) *Staphylococcus* (4) *E. coli* (1) *Pseudomonas* (1) *Pneumococcus* (1) *Mycobacterium* (1) *UK* (3)
TOTALS	44	I (38) E (4) NA (2)	S (27) D (17)	*Salmonella* (12) *Staphylococcus* (7) *Others* (9) *UK* (16)

[a] 2 of 3 patients died from unrelated causes.
[b] Includes 2 patients reported previously by Hollier et al.[19]
[c] 3 of 8 patients died from unrelated causes.

The average age of these patients was 65 years. Nine men and six women were identified.

PRESENTATION AND DIAGNOSIS

Mycotic TAAA may be insidious at the time of presentation. There are few characteristics allowing initial differentiation of mycotic TAAA from nonvascular systemic infections. All patients with a documented TAAA and *unexplained* fever or infection should be regarded as having an infected aorta until proven otherwise. As patients with fever of unknown etiology invariably have chest radiographs and frequently undergo computed tomography (CT) scanning, the presence of infected TAAA is often first diagnosed at this presentation. Most series report fever, pain, pulsatile mass, leukocytosis, and positive blood cultures as the most common clinical markers for infected aortic aneurysms.[7,11] In a study by Mundt et al.,[3] fever and pain were present in 94%, leukocytosis in 77%, palpable aneurysm in 65%, and positive blood culture in 53%. In some patients, there may be a history of a recent febrile illness or a nonarterial infection such as gastroenteritis, cholecystitis, endocarditis, or pancreatitis, or of recent arterial catheterization.[8,20] In our group of 15 patients, 67% had a fever (average temperature: 38.3°C), 67% had leukocytosis (WBC $> 10 \times 10^9$/L, average: 13.9×10^9/L), and 53% had pain. Only 13% had positive preoperative blood cultures.

Arteriography may demonstrate an atypical configuration or location of the TAAA. Eccentric aneurysms, saccular aneurysms, or pseudoaneurysms of the aorta are all findings that are suggestive of and consistent with the diagnosis of mycotic aneurysm (Fig. 23–1). However, in most patients, aortography cannot be reliably used to differentiate an infected aorta from a noninfected one. CT has become the test of choice in diagnosing infected aortic aneurysms.[8,11,12,21,22] Findings on CT that suggest an infected aortic aneurysm are: inflammatory appearing tissues or fluid on the periaortic region, retroperitoneal edema, air-fluid levels, prominent periaortic lymphadenopathy, and evidence of rupture such as a hematoma (Fig. 23–2). In addition, accelerated expansion of a TAAA on serial CT scanning may indicate the presence of an ongoing aortic infection. Ultrasound does not appear to have sufficient specificity for infected tissue to be useful in this context. Nuclear medicine imaging studies such as the Indium-111 labeled white cell scan may be helpful to confirm CT findings but should not be used alone to diagnose an infected TAAA.

ETIOLOGY

The bacteriology of mycotic aneurysms has changed in the last 50 years. In the pre-antibiotic era, typical organisms that infected the aorta were those associated with endocarditis (e.g., *streptococcus* or *staphylococcus)* and most of these unfortunate

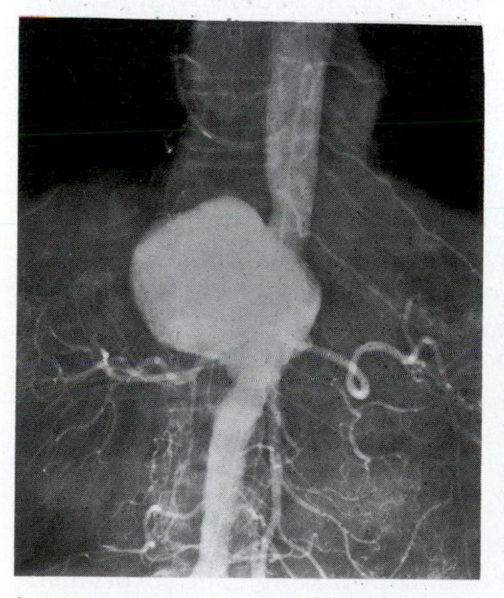

A

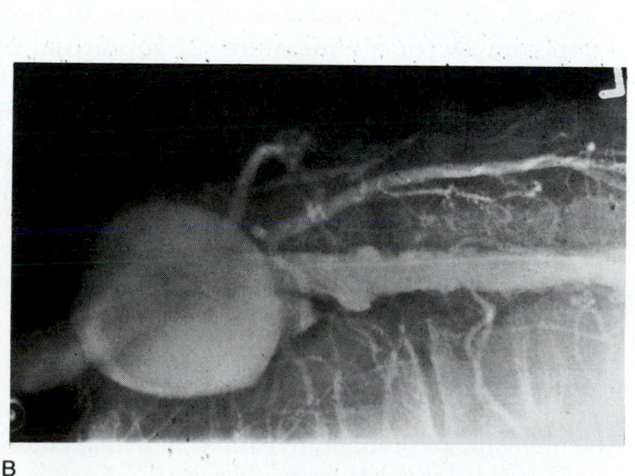

B

Figure 23–1. Aortogram of a 77-year-old male patient with a type IV mycotic thoracoabdominal aneurysm. Note the abnormal location of the saccular aneurysm. Anteroposterior view (**A**), lateral view (**B**).

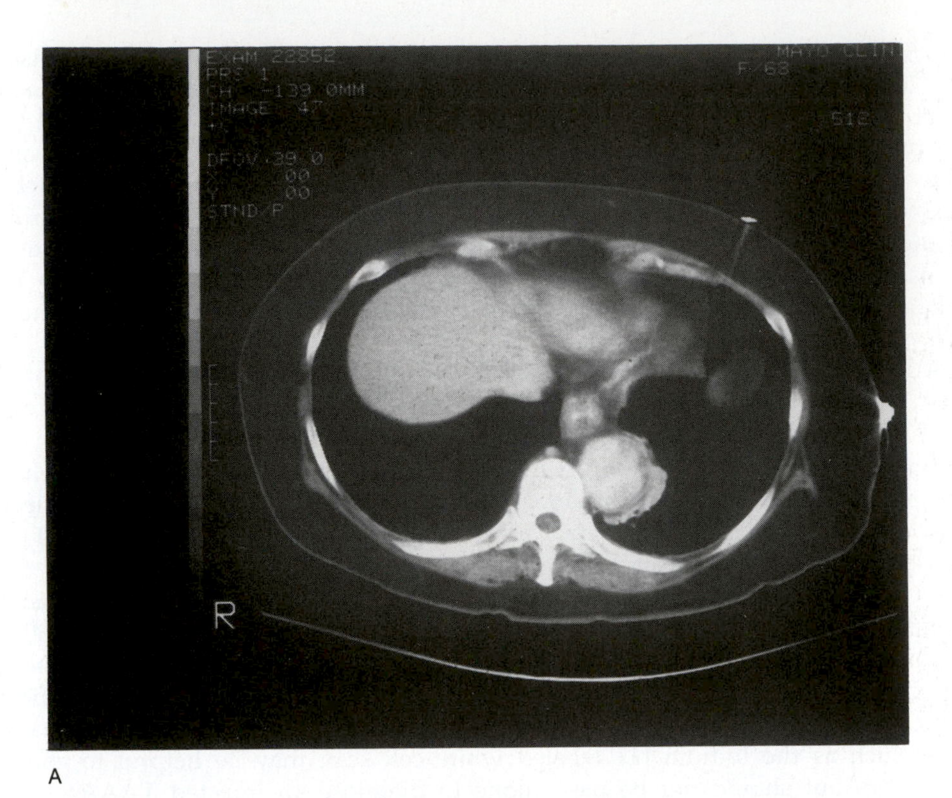

A

Figure 23–2. Computed tomography of the lower thoracic (**A**) and upper abdominal aorta (**B**) in a 68-year-old female patient with a type II mycotic thoracoabdominal aortic aneurysm. Note the inflammatory appearing tissues and fluid in the peri-aortic region, retroperitoneal edema, and an abnormal hematoma-like mass on the descending thoracic aorta.

patients died from rupture.[20] Recently, although *staphylococcus* is still the most prevalent organism when mycotic aneurysms from all arterial locations are considered,[12,20] *salmonella* is the most common pathogen isolated from patient with mycotic suprarenal and TAAAs.[18,23–25] In our series, *salmonella* and *staphylococcus* were identified in four patients each, comprising 67% of all culture positive mycotic aneurysms (Table 23–1). The responsible organisms in three patients could not be identified. Atnip's review of the literature (22 suprarenal mycotic aneurysms) reported a 57% incidence of salmonellosis with the majority of the rest also due to gram-negative bacteria.[18] Mendelowitz et al.[25] reviewed aortic salmonellosis and found a significant 77% mortality rate. Other reports, both clinical[3,18] and experimental,[26] have confirmed the extraordinary virulence of gram-negative organisms in the pathogenesis of aortic infections. Hence, mycotic aneurysms of the suprarenal and thoracoabdominal aorta are not only technically difficult operative problems but are, unfortunately, often associated with highly virulent gram-negative organisms (Table 23–1).

TREATMENT

The mainstay of preoperative medical management of unruptured mycotic aortic aneurysms is intensive antibiotic therapy.[3–5,7–10] After control of sepsis and optimization of fluids, electrolytes, and hemoglobin counts, the patients should undergo prompt *in situ* aortic reconstruction.[11,12,18,19] Most of our patients, however, presented with either

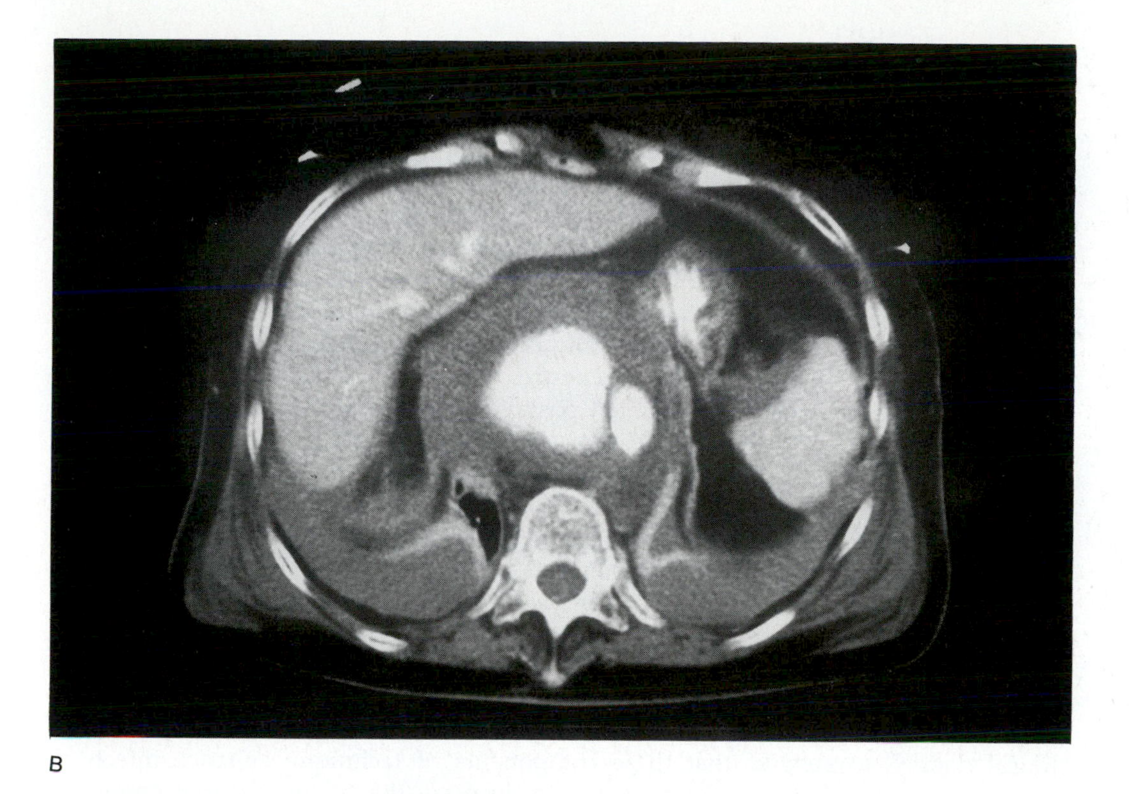

B

Figure 23–2. (*continued*)

rupture (53%) or sepsis (33%), necessitating urgent or emergent repair. Only 2 of our 15 patients underwent elective operation.

Negative blood cultures should not delay treatment. As stated earlier, we and others have found a low incidence of positive blood cultures preoperatively. Broad-spectrum intravenous antibiotics should be initiated as soon as the clinical diagnosis is suspected.[18,19] If a specific organism is isolated from the blood or any other obvious source (e.g., gallbladder, heart valve), the antibiotic coverage should be narrowed appropriately. Most authors[3,11,12,19,23] have advocated lifelong oral antibiotic treatment for patients who undergo *in situ* repair. We place all our surviving patients on lifelong oral antibiotics and obtain serial CTs in follow-up. In two of our patients, abscesses found on follow-up CTs were drained percutaneously with satisfactory results.

The extent of operative repair is dictated in part by the extent of the TAAA. In our series, there were five Crawford Type I, 6 Type II, 2 Type III, and 2 Type IV TAAAs. Whether the aneurysm is fusiform or saccular, true or false may also influence the type and extent of repair. Clearly all obviously infected aortic tissue should be excised. "Resection" in these cases indeed means "excision," in contrast to its usage in reference to elective abdominal aortic aneurysm (AAA) repairs in which reconstructive aneurysmorrhaphies are performed. For example, in the patient with a pseudoaneurysm of the paravisceral aorta demonstrated in Figure 23–1, the repair included resection of all the grossly infected aorta, not just the immediate region of the aneurysm. The aorta was replaced from the distal descending thoracic aorta to the aortic bifurcation because of the clinical extent of that infection. Although numerous reports on peripheral or infrarenal mycotic aneurysm repair[6,7,20] have cited high mortalities with *in situ* reconstruction, there is increasing evidence that, *in situ* reconstruction may be performed in selected cases with an acceptable mortality rate.[2,12–16,19] The amputation rate for *in situ* repair is impressively low.[2,12–16,19] Although the concept of placing a synthetic graft in close proximity to or in the bed of a resected infected aortic segment is certainly not intrinsically appealing, the consequences of leaving a visceral artery unrevascularized or revascularized with a long, compromised graft are significant, and usually unacceptable.[14] Ultimately, when treating patients with mycotic TAAAs, the realistic goal of management frequently becomes control of the infection, not its eradication.

Intraoperative microbacteriologic evaluation of infected aortic aneurysms to determine extent of resection has generally been of little practical help. Reports that have investigated the significance of cultures taken from aortic thrombus during elective AAA repair have demonstrated positive cultures in 14% to 43% of patients. These findings appear to be of little clinical significance.[27,28] The utility of obtaining intraoperative cultures or gram stains to determine the extent of the resection is questionable at best. Once the infected arterial contents and tissue have been manipulated, it is impossible to obtain a negative gram stain or to expose a noninfected contiguous area for anastomosis. In essence, the entire field, however well debrided and irrigated, must be considered infected. We believe that the safest and most reasonable approach is to resect those segments of the aorta that appear grossly infected. Consequently, reconstruction should always be accompanied by wide tissue debridement, copious amounts of antibiotic irrigation, and placement of suction-irrigation catheters in the infected bed.[15,19] Although there are only scant clinical data[29,30] to suggest that these components of technique enhance infection-free survival, all efforts should be made to decrease the tissue bacterial counts to levels that can be managed with chronic antibiotics. Soaking the graft with antibiotics may further decrease the bacteria count at the level of the anastomosis.[24] No specific prosthetic material has established superiority over others in resisting infection. We have used mostly polyester grafts (14 of 15) in our reconstructions, but there is no reason to believe that expanded polytetrafluoroethylene (PTFE) grafts would not be as satisfactory. Although arterial allografts have long been dismissed as a viable conduit,[31] a favorable recent report by Kieffer et al.[2] may reintroduce this technique as an alternative for selected cases. Some recent studies have shown success with the use of deep veins from the lower extremity as infrarenal aortic conduits.[1]

Fourteen of our 15 patients have been treated by the *in situ* technique. The average cross-clamp time for these patients was 49 minutes. One patient was reconstructed with a combination of *in situ* and extra-anatomic techniques because of an abscess adjacent to the infrarenal aorta that could not be adequately drained or debrided. A right axillobifemoral bypass was performed in conjunction with a suprarenal *in situ* reconstruction. Unfortunately, the suprarenal graft ultimately became infected, and the patient died of persistent sepsis.

OUTCOME

The mortality and morbidity associated with operative repair of mycotic TAAA is high (Tables 23–1 and 23–2). Persistent sepsis and bleeding were significant postoperative problems and occurred in 60% of our patients. Renal failure occurred in 3 patients with 1 patient eventually requiring dialysis. There were no limbs lost. There were no cases of paraplegia. One patient sustained embolization to the superior mesenteric artery and required bowel resection. In a review of the literature by Atnip,[18] of 22

TABLE 23–2. MORTALITY RATES OF 15 PATIENTS WITH MYCOTIC THORACOABDOMINAL AORTIC ANEURYSM TREATED AT THE MAYO CLINIC 1976–1994

	No. Patients	No. Deaths	30-Day Mortality (%)	Mortality Rate (%)
Crawford Type				(Mean f/u = 40.8 months)
I	5	2	40	40
II	6	3	17	50
III	2	1	0	50
IV	2	2	50	100
Presentation				
Rupture	8	6	38	75
Symptomatic	5	2	20	40
Elective	2	0	0	0

patients with mycotic aneurysms of the suprarenal aorta, there were 16 survivors, of which 11 were from the Houston group.[14] In Hollier's series[19] of 6 patients who underwent direct repair, 3 patients survived, 1 patient with a persistent, chronic infection. In our series of 15 patients with mycotic TAAA, the 30-day mortality rate was 27% with an overall mortality of 53% (average follow-up period: 40.8 months). Of the 8 patients who died in our group, 4 died of bleeding complications related to the original operation, 1 from persistent sepsis, and 3 from unrelated causes.

CONCLUSION

In summary, the management of patients with mycotic TAAA is a formidable challenge. Improved imaging techniques have allowed earlier diagnosis but unfortunately, most patients present urgently with significant sepsis or rupture. The operative treatment of choice is a one stage *in situ* aortic reconstruction with prosthetic graft and direct reconstruction of the mesenteric and renal arteries. The reconstruction should be accompanied by *en bloc* resection of the aneurysm, wide debridement of surrounding infected tissue, and adequate postoperative irrigation and drainage of the affected areas. Patients should be maintained on appropriate intravenous antibiotics perioperatively and lifelong oral antibiotics thereafter. Serial physical examinations and CT scans are necessary to detect abscesses, pseudoaneurysms, and other manifestations of recurrent or uncontrolled infection. Although morbidity and mortality remain high, an approximately 50% 3-year survivorship may be achieved.

REFERENCES

1. Clagett GP, Bowers BL, Lopez-Viego MA, et al. Creation of a neo-aortoiliac system from lower extremity deep and superficial veins. *Ann Surg*. 1993;218:239–249.
2. Kieffer E, Bahnini A, Koskas F, et al. *In situ* allograft replacement of infected infrarenal aortic prosthetic grafts: results in forty-three patients. *J Vasc Surg*. 1993;17:349–356.

3. Mundth ED, Darling RC, Alvarado RF, et al. Surgical management of mycotic aneurysms and the complications of infection in vascular reconstructive surgery. *Am J Surg.* 1969;117:460–470.
4. Taylor LM, Deitz DM, McConnell DB, et al. Treatment of infected abdominal aneurysms by extraanatomic bypass, aneurysm excision, and drainage. *Am J Surg.* 1987;155:655–658.
5. Reilly LM, Stoney RJ, Goldstone J, et al. Improved management of aortic graft infection: the influence of operation sequence and staging. *J Vasc Surg.* 1987;5:421–431.
6. Bennett DE, Cherry JK. Bacterial infection of aortic aneurysms—a clinicopathologic study. *Am J Surg.* 1967;113:321–326.
7. Anderson CB, Butcher HR, Ballinger WF. Mycotic aneurysms. *Arch Surg.* 1974;109:712–717.
8. Ewart JM, Burke ML, Bunt TJ. Spontaneous abdominal aortic infections: essentials of diagnosis and management. *Am Surg.* 1983;49:37–50.
9. Johansen K, Devin J. Mycotic aortic aneurysms: a reappraisal. *Arch Surg.* 1983;118:583–588.
10. Bitseff EL, Edwards WA, Mulherin JL, et al. Infected abdominal aortic aneurysms. *South Med J.* 1987;80:309–312.
11. Reddy DJ, Shepard AD, Evans JR, et al. Management of infected aortoiliac aneurysms. *Arch Surg.* 1991;126:873–879.
12. Gomes MN, Choyke PL, Wallace RB. Infected aortic aneurysms: a changing entity. *Ann Surg.* 1992;215:435–442.
13. Fichelle JM, Tabet G, Cormier P, et al. Infected infrarenal aortic aneurysms: when is *in situ* reconstruction safe? *J Vasc Surg.* 1993;17:635–645.
14. Morris GC, Crawford ES, Cooley DA, et al. Revascularization of the celiac and superior mesenteric arteries. *Arch Surg.* 1962;84:95–107.
15. Chan FY, Crawford ES, Coselli JS, et al. *In situ* prosthetic graft replacement for mycotic aneurysm of the aorta. *Ann Thor Surg.* 1989;47:193–203.
16. Walker WE, Cooley DA, Duncan JM, et al. The management of aortoduodenal fistula by *in situ* replacement of the infected abdominal aortic graft. *Ann Surg.* 1987;205:727–732.
17. James EC, Gillespie JT. Aortic mycotic abdominal aneurysm involving all visceral branches: excision and Dacron graft replacement. *J Cardiovasc Surg.* 1977;18:353–356.
18. Atnip RG. Mycotic aneurysms of the suprarenal aorta: prolonged survival after *in situ* aortic and visceral reconstruction. *J Vasc Surg.* 1989;10:635–641.
19. Hollier LH, Money SR, Creely B, et al. Direct replacement of mycotic thoracoabdominal aneurysms. *J Vasc Surg.* 1993;18:447–485.
20. Brown SL, Busuttil RW, Baker JD, et al. Bacteriologic and surgical determinants of survival in patients with mycotic aneurysms. *J Vasc Surg.* 1984;1:541–547.
21. Atlas SW, Volgelzang RL, Bressler EL, et al. CT diagnosis of a mycotic aneurysm of the thoracoabdominal aorta. *J Comp Assist Tomogr.* 1984;8:1211–1212.
22. Yao JST, McCarthy WJ. Contained rupture of a thoracoabdominal aneurysm. *Contemp Surg.* 1988;33:47–51.
23. Oz MC, Brener BJ, Buda JA, et al. A ten-year experience with bacterial aortitis. *J Vasc Surg.* 1989;10:439–449.
24. Meade RH, Moran JM. Salmonella arteritis—preoperative diagnosis and cure of Salmonella aortic aneurysm. *N Engl J Med.* 1969;281:310–312.
25. Mendelowitz DS, Ramstedt R, Yao JST, et al. Abdominal aortic salmonellosis. *Surgery.* 1979;85:514–519.
26. Geary KJ, Tomkiewicz ZM, Harrison HN, et al. Differential effects of a gram-negative and gram-positive infection on autogenous and prosthetic grafts. *J Vasc Surg.* 1990;11:339–347.
27. McAuley CE, Steed DL, Webster MW. Bacterial presence in aortic thrombus at elective aneurysm resection: is it clinically significant? *Am J Surg.* 1984;147:322–324.
28. Macbeth GA, Rubin JR, McIntyre KE, et al. The relevance of arterial wall microbiology to the treatment of prosthetic graft infections: graft infection vs. arterial infection. *J Vasc Surg.* 1984;1:750–756.

29. Lord JW, Rossi G, Daliana M. Intraoperative antibiotic wound lavage: an attempt to eliminate postoperative infection in arterial and clean general surgical procedures. *Ann Surg.* 1977;185:634–640.
30. Cherry KJ, Roland CF, Pairolero PC, et al. Infected femorodistal bypass: is graft removal mandatory? *J Vasc Surg.* 1992;15:295–305.
31. Foster JH, Berzins T, Scott HW. An experimental study of arterial replacement in the presence of bacterial infection. *Surg Gynecol Obstet.* 1959;108:356–364.

24

Endovascular Techniques for Treatment of Complications of Aortic Dissection

Suzanne M. Slonim, MD, D. Craig Miller, MD, and Michael D. Dake, MD

Aortic dissection is a complex catastrophe of the aorta that often extends into branch vessels and causes ischemic complications. Peripheral vascular ischemic symptoms occur in approximately 30% of patients.[1-3] Most of these symptoms will be relieved by surgical repair of the dissection.[1,4] However, in patients who do not undergo surgical repair of the dissection or in patients who have persistent ischemia following the repair, the appropriate treatment of these complications is not well defined. This problem is critical because there is a high mortality rate in patients with dissections complicated by ischemia involving the renal, mesenteric, and lower extremity vasculature.[1,2,5,6]

Endovascular stenting and balloon fenestration of the intimal flap are promising techniques that can safely and effectively relieve ischemic symptoms related to aortic dissection. Endovascular techniques may provide the treatments of choice for the management of these challenging problems.

DIAGNOSTIC INFORMATION

Before embarking on the treatment of ischemic complications of aortic dissection, the extent of the dissection must be fully evaluated. Clinical suspicion of ischemic areas can help direct the initial imaging studies. It is important to know whether there is flow in both the true and false lumen. The lumen that supplies each of the abdominal branch vessels must be known, even if the areas are not symptomatic. This is because any planned endovascular intervention may alter the dynamics of both the true and false lumen. It can be helpful to localize any existing natural fenestrations. Extension of the dissection flap into any branch vessel should be ascertained.

In the acute setting, all this information may be acquired during angiographic evaluation. When the patient is stable or has chronic ischemia, computed tomography (CT) or magnetic resonance imaging (MRI) of the aorta may be performed. These imaging modalities can be useful in the planning of where to gain endovascular access and in the planning of the types of interventions that may be indicated. They can help minimize the amount of contrast material that is necessary during angiography. Despite the large amount of information that can be gained from CT and MRI, most patients require angiographic evaluation of both the true and false lumen before endovascular interventions are performed. In patients with renal ischemia, a portion of the study can usually be performed with carbon dioxide in order to minimize the load of iodinated contrast material.

Intravascular ultrasound is also routinely performed during the arteriographic procedure since it is extremely helpful in the evaluation of the complex anatomy of aortic dissections. It provides detailed accurate information about the involvement of branch vessels as well as precise measurements of vessel diameter.

MANAGEMENT PLAN

After a complete understanding of the extent of the dissection and the branch vessel involvement is gained, endovascular management can be undertaken. Because of the complexity of the disease process, the appropriate management is usually unique to each case.

In general, ischemic complications arise when the lumen supplying a branch vessel (the tributary lumen) is compromised by thrombosis, extrinsic compression from the other lumen, obstruction of flow due to a flap, or poor inflow due to compression of the tributary lumen upstream in the aorta. Each of these situations must be dealt with differently.

If ischemia is due to thrombosis of the branch vessel tributary lumen proximally but there is distal flow through collateral vessels, the proximal thrombosed segment can be stented open. This will restore antegrade flow and compress the thrombus against the vessel wall. If the entire lumen supplying the compromised branch vessel is thrombosed but there is distal flow within the vessel, the stent can be placed across the thrombosed lumen to connect the branch vessel to the lumen with flow in it. If there is no distal flow within the branch vessel, usually the vascular bed cannot be salvaged.

When ischemia is due to compression of the tributary lumen by the other lumen, the usual treatment is to stent the tributary lumen. With this technique, the compromised lumen is expanded with the stent to compress or obliterate the false lumen (Fig. 24–1). When this situation arises in the iliac arteries, balloon fenestration of the flap between the two lumens may be an alternative or adjunctive treatment (Fig. 24–2). This technique relieves the constriction on the tributary lumen by allowing decompression of the other lumen. After this procedure, the blood supply to the leg is through both the true and false lumen. This technique can only be used if there is definite flow in both lumens. Otherwise, creation of a fenestration may cause distal embolization of thrombus.

When ischemia is due to a flap within the branch vessel that is compromising flow, the treatment of choice is stenting of the flap against the wall of the vessel to maintain a widely patent true lumen.

When the ischemic symptoms are due to generalized poor inflow because of upstream compression of the aortic tributary lumen, treatment may be either with stenting or balloon fenestration. The severely compressed tributary lumen of the aorta can be stented open along its course. Alternatively, a fenestration can be created within the intimal flap proximal to the ischemic vessels to allow an enhanced admixture of

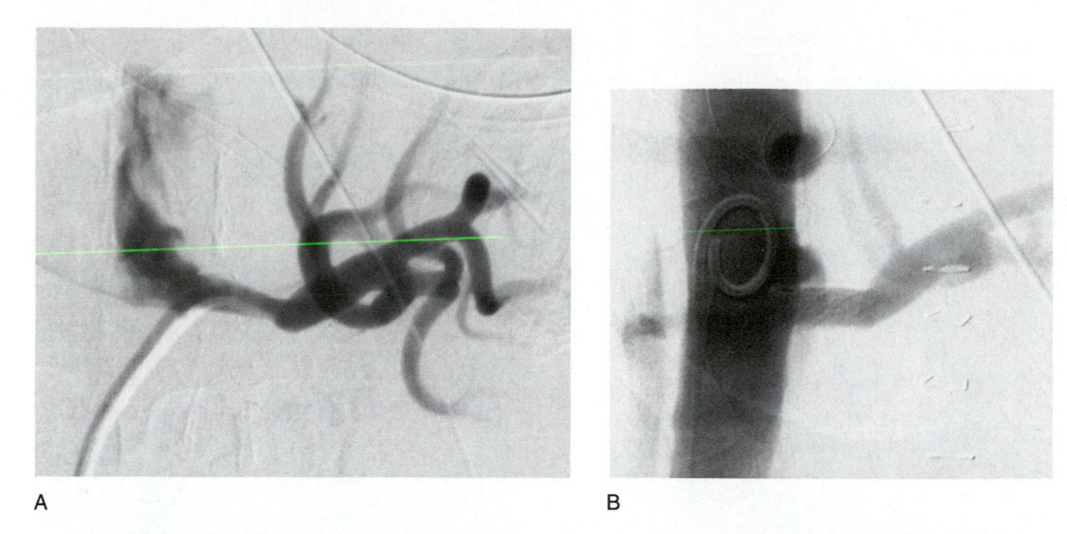

Figure 24–1. Selective left renal arteriogram from the true lumen (**A**) demonstrates concentric proximal narrowing due to extrinsic compression from the nonopacified false lumen. Aortogram (**B**) after deployment of a stent in the renal artery demonstrates a widely patent vessel. The false lumen has been obliterated.

blood flow between the two lumens. This technique will take the pressure off of the larger lumen, allowing it to decompress and decrease the constriction of the smaller lumen. Simultaneously, the inflow into the smaller lumen will be increased.

In some instances, optimal treatment involves the combination of balloon fenestration and stenting. Patients may have several branch vessels involved with the dissection, and the most suitable management for each vessel may be different. In cases in which the lumen of the aorta supplying several branch vessels is compressed upstream, there is often ischemia involving several branch vessels despite the fact that none actually have a flap extending into them.

INTERVENTIONAL PROCEDURES

Endovascular Stenting

Endovascular stents are usually deployed through either 7 or 9 French angiographic sheaths. Initially most patients will have an 8 French sheath in place to accommodate the intravascular ultrasound probe. Stent size is chosen based on measurements from a high-quality spiral CT scan with thin section collimation, angiographic measurement, or measurement using intravascular ultrasound. Balloon expandable Palmaz stents (Johnson and Johnson Interventional Systems, Warren, NJ) and/or self-expanding Wallstents (Schneider, Plymouth, MN) may be used, although the greater radial strength of the Palmaz stent is often necessary to resist the compressive force of a high-pressure lumen encroaching on a lower-pressure lumen that supplies significant branch vessels. In our experience, the smallest stents have been 10 to 15 mm in length dilated to 6 to 7 mm diameter (P104, P154) for the renal artery. The largest stent has been 50 mm in length dilated to 25 mm diameter for the aorta. The Wallstents have ranged from 42 to 96 mm in length and 10 to 12 mm diameter.

The balloon expandable stent is placed onto an appropriately sized balloon catheter. It is crimped onto the balloon to prevent premature dislodgment and advanced through

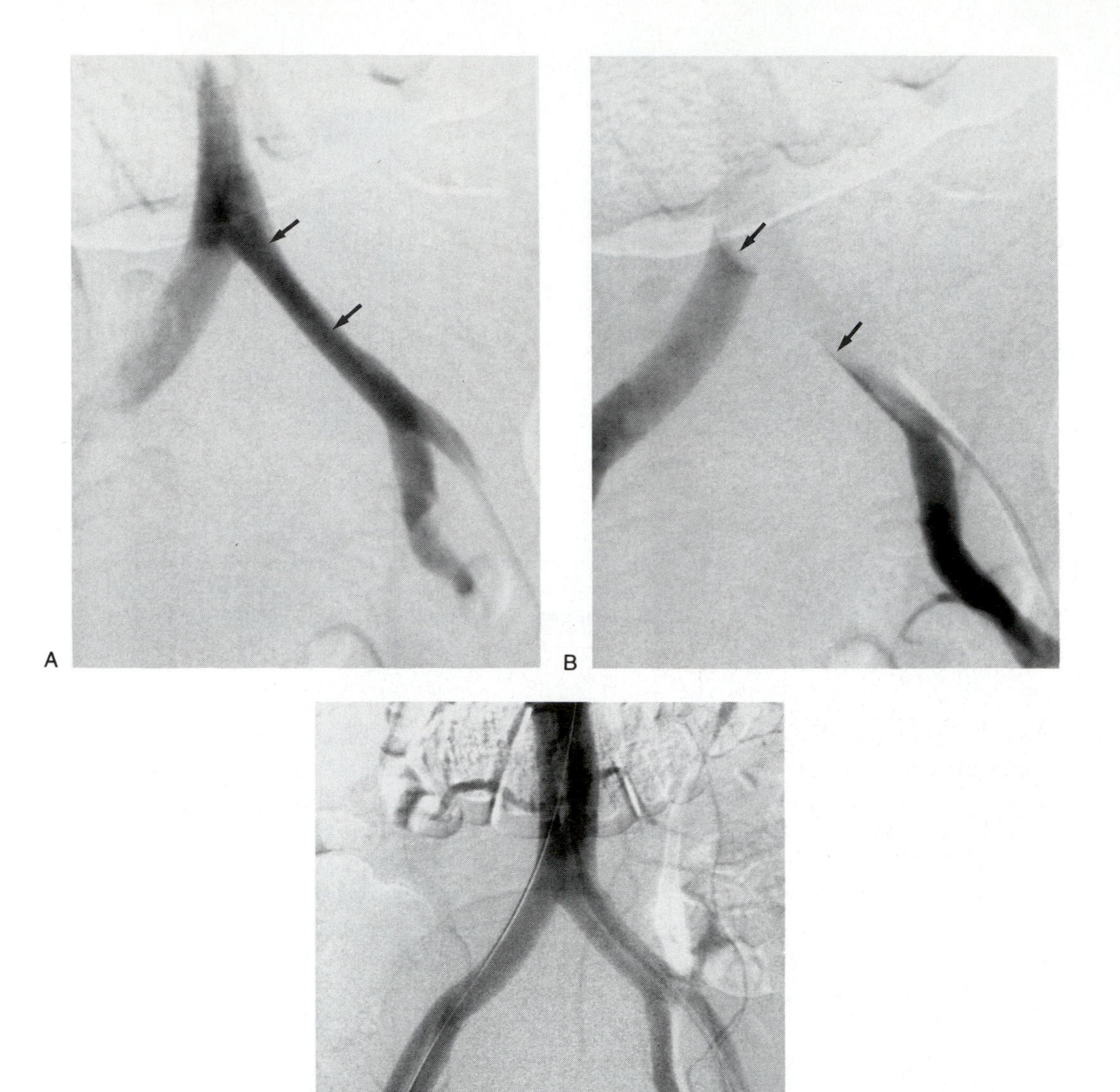

Figure 24–2. Images from an arteriogram during diastole (**A**) and systole (**B**) demonstrate an intimal flap (*arrows*) extending from the aorta into the left iliac artery. During systole, with expansion of the high-pressure false lumen, the intimal flap obstructs the true lumen of both the left and right iliac arteries. After balloon fenestration of the intimal flap in the distal aorta (**C**), the flap no longer obstructs the true lumen. Both the true and false lumen now contribute no blood supply to both legs.

the sheath to the desired location over a guide wire. The sheath is pulled back to uncover the stent, and it is deployed by inflation of the balloon.

The self-expanding stents are advanced over a guide wire to the desired location. Because these stents shorten significantly during deployment, the markers on the delivery system identifying the ends of the stent are usually centered around the desired location. The outer plastic covering over the stent is withdrawn, allowing the stent to expand and shorten.

In each situation, angiography is performed following deployment of the stent to evaluate its effectiveness and determine the need for further treatment.

Balloon Fenestration

Fenestration is performed using either intravascular ultrasound or fluoroscopic guidance. When using intravascular ultrasound guidance (Fig. 24–3), the probe is usually

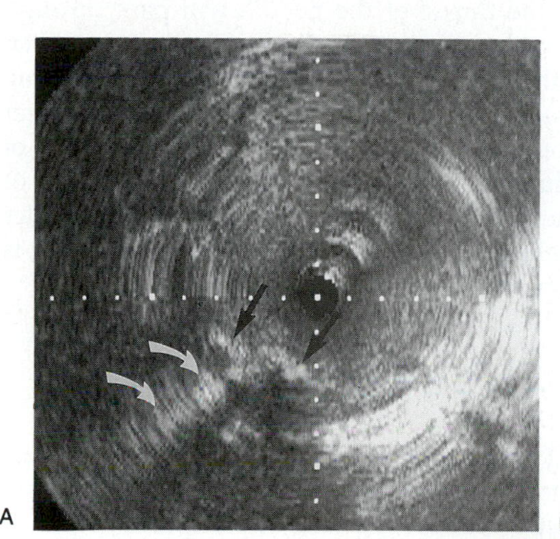

A

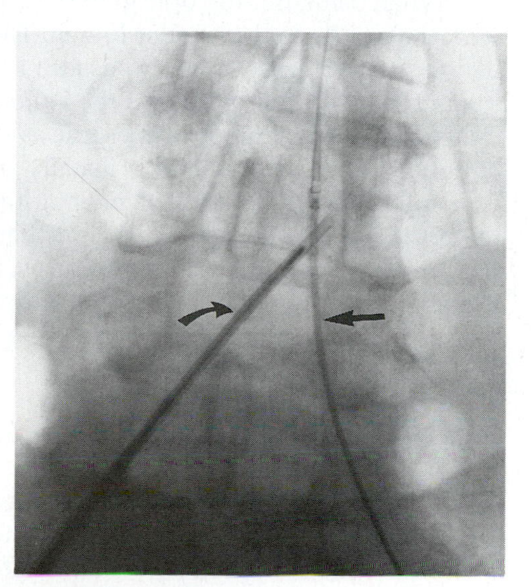

B

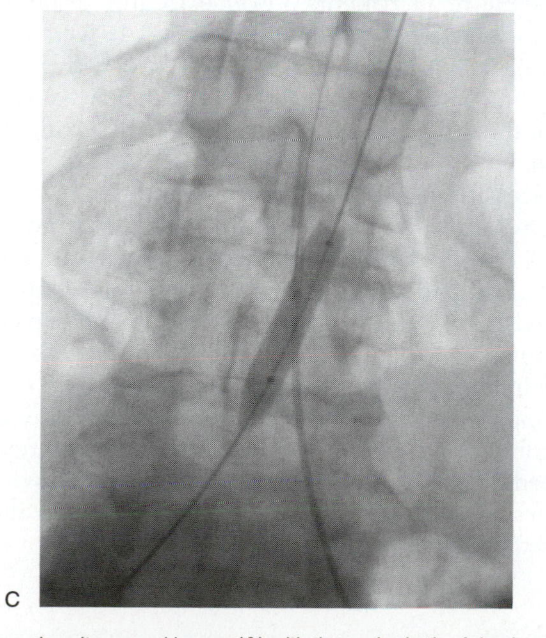

C

Figure 24–3. Intravascular ultrasound image (**A**) with the probe in the false lumen demonstrates the intimal flap between the lumens (*straight arrows*) and the bright echoes from the needle in the true lumen (*curved arrows*). Fluoroscopic image (**B**) demonstrates the ultrasound probe (*straight arrow*) in the false lumen and the needle (*curved arrow*), which has been passed across the intimal flap from the true into the false lumen. (**C**) The needle is exchanged over a guide wire for an angioplasty balloon catheter, which is used to dilate the fenestration in the intimal flap.

placed in the larger lumen, while a long curved needle or metallic cannula is placed in the smaller lumen. The needle or cannula is pointed directly at the intravascular ultrasound probe during real-time imaging to assure that the throw of the needle will be made through the middle of the intimal flap and not toward a free wall of the aorta. A smaller needle is then passed through the intimal flap, and a guide wire is passed through it into the opposite lumen. A balloon catheter is then exchanged for the needle and passed over this guide wire to dilate the fenestration in the intimal flap under ultrasound monitoring.

When using fluoroscopic guidance, a balloon catheter is placed in the larger lumen, with the needle in the smaller lumen. The tip of the needle is aligned with the inflated balloon at 90-degree angles to assure that the throw of the needle will pass through the intimal flap into or toward the balloon rather than toward a free wall of the aorta. Otherwise, the technique is the same as with intravascular ultrasound guidance. Using either technique, the needle is usually passed from the smaller lumen into the larger lumen so there is less risk of passing through the lumen out of the opposite wall of the aorta. In some instances, the smaller lumen is too small to allow safe passage of the puncture needle. In these instances, the inflated balloon is placed into the smaller lumen in an attempt to enlarge it and make it a bigger target as the needle pass is made. In our experience, no puncture of an aortic free wall has occurred.

PRELIMINARY EXPERIENCE

We have performed endovascular stenting and or balloon fenestration in 22 patients (16 men, 6 women; mean age 52 years) who had ischemic complications of 15 acute (6 Stanford type A, 9 type B) and 7 chronic (6 type A, 1 type B) aortic dissections. Symptoms included renal ischemia in 13 patients, lower extremity ischemia in 10 patients, and mesenteric ischemia in 6 patients. Of these 22 patients, 16 were treated with endovascular stenting, including 11 patients with renal stents, 6 with lower extremity stents, 2 with an SMA stent, and 2 with aortic stents. Four patients were treated with balloon fenestration of the intimal flap, and 2 were treated with a combination of stenting and balloon fenestration.

Technically successful revascularization with intial clinical success was achieved in all 22 patients. Two patients had to be brought back for further endovascular management of persistent ischemic symptoms between 6 days and 2 months following the initial procedure. A third patient required additional intervention when new ischemic symptoms developed after spontaneous recanalization and expansion of his previously thrombosed false lumen. One patient died 3 days following the procedure of peritonitis likely related to prolonged bowel ischemia. One patient died of unrelated causes 13.4 months following the procedure. One patient is lost to follow-up. The mean follow-up time is 14.6 months. No patient has required surgical revascularization for an ischemic vascular bed. The only complication has been a guide wire induced perinephric hematoma, which was treated with endovascular coil embolization. This complication has no long-term sequelae.

CONCLUSION

Endovascular techniques, including stenting and balloon fenestration, are safe and effective in treating the peripheral ischemic complications of aortic dissection. Although further study is necessary, preliminary results suggest that this endovascular approach provides a promising method for the management of these very challenging vascular problems.

REFERENCES

1. Fann JI, Sarris GE, Mitchell RS, et al. Treatment of patients with aortic dissection presenting with peripheral vascular complications. *Ann Surg.* 1990;212:705–713.
2. Cambria RP, Brewster DC, Gertler J, et al. Vascular complications associated with spontaneous aortic dissection. *J Vasc Surg.* 1988;7:199–209.
3. DeBakey ME, McCollum CH, Crawford ES, et al. Dissection and dissecting aneurysms of the aorta: twenty-year follow-up of five hundred twenty-seven patients treated surgically. *Surgery.* 1982;92:1118–1134.
4. Shumacker HB, Isch JH, Jolly WW. Stenotic and obstructive lesions in acute dissecting thoracic aortic aneurysms. *Ann Surg.* 1975;181:662–669.
5. Doroghazi RM, Slater EE, DeSanctis RW, et al. Long-term survival of patients with treated aortic dissection. *J Am Coll Cardiol.* 1984;3:1026–1034.
6. Miller DC, Mitchell RS, Oyer PE, et al. Independent determinants of operative mortality for patients with aortic dissections. *Circulation.* 1984;70(suppl I):I-153–1-164.

V

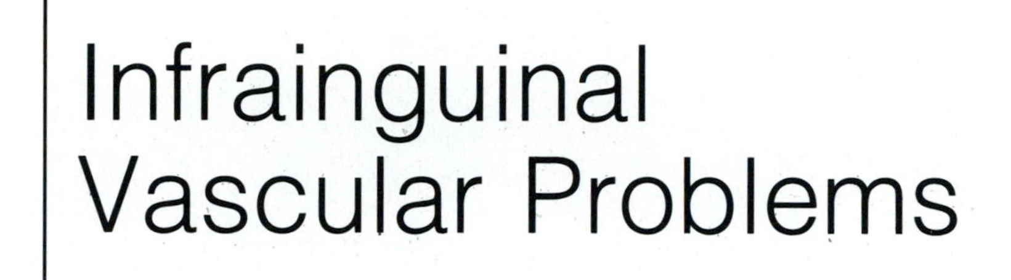

Infrainguinal Vascular Problems

25

Infected Pseudoaneurysm of the Femoral Artery

Robert W. Hobson II, MD, and
Frank T. Padberg, Jr., MD

Mycotic or infected aneurysms have been reported in virtually every artery in the body. However, involvement of the femoral artery probably accounts for 10% to 12% of cases.[1] Some controversy exists regarding the classification and nomenclature of infected aneurysms. The original term, *mycotic aneurysm,* referred to infection of fungal etiology and was described as a complication of bacterial endocarditis.[2] At times, "mycotic aneurysm" has been used to describe any arterial aneurysm caused by fungal or bacterial infection. However, a revised classification of spontaneous arterial infection (Table 25–1) has clarified the issues surrounding etiology of these lesions and their terminology.[3]

During recent years, several centers have reported results on the surgical management of infected pseudoaneurysms of the femoral artery associated with drug abuse.[4–15] In some urban institutions, these complications associated with injection of drugs of abuse have exceeded the incidence and complications caused by infected aneurysms in other anatomic locations.[10] In addition, recent reports[7–9] regarding the indications for revascularization under circumstances of grossly contaminated operative sites have stimulated some additional discussion. This chapter reviews the management of infected femoral false aneurysms caused primarily by injection of drugs of abuse and evaluates their selective management by arterial ligation or revascularization.

DIAGNOSIS AND PATHOPHYSIOLOGY

Infected femoral pseudoaneurysms (Fig. 25–1) among drug abusers generally present as tender groin masses, which are pulsatile in no more than one-half of cases.[9] Confirming the diagnostic uncertainties, Johnson and co-authors[4] reported an initial misdiagnosis of cellulitis or abscess alone in 17% of 52 cases. A draining puncture site may be visible over the area and other stigmata of chronic drug abuse, including evidence of contralateral groin injections, may be observed. Patients are frequently febrile with leukocytosis and commonly have a recent history of "missed" or "pink" (arterial)

TABLE 25–1. CLASSIFICATION OF SPONTANEOUS ARTERIAL INFECTION

Mycotic Aneurysm	
	Aneurysm occurring in a normal or atherosclerotic artery resulting from emboli of endocardial origin
Infected Aneurysm	
	Established aneurysm infected by bacteremia
Microbial Arteritis	
	Infection of normal or atherosclerotic artery by bacteremia, often resulting in rupture of the artery and pseudoaneurysm formation
Traumatic Infected Pseudoaneurysm	
	Aneurysm due to trauma (penetrating or blunt), iatrogenic injury, and injection sites in hemodialysis patients or narcotic addicts
Contiguous Arterial Infection	
	Arterial invasion from an adjacent septic focus
Septic Arterial Emboli	
	Infected peripheral emboli or infected pulmonary artery aneurysms
Spontaneous Aortoenteric Fistula	
	Duodenal or colonic

Modified with permission from Wilson SE, Van Wagenen P, Passaro E Jr. Arterial infection. *Curr Prob Surg.* 1978;15:5.

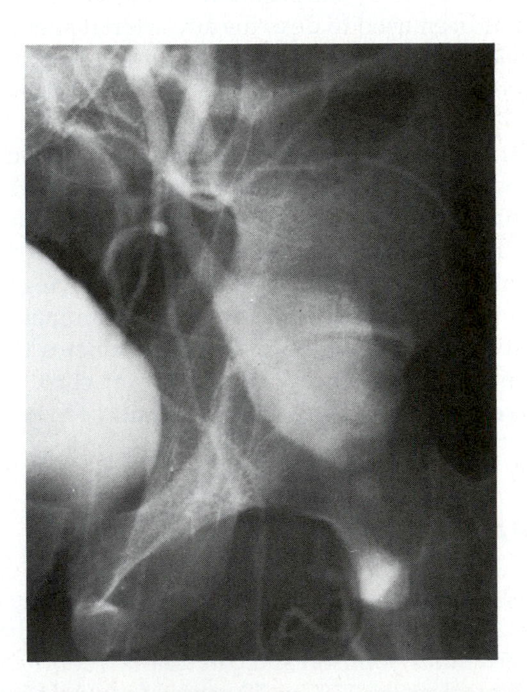

Figure 25–1. Arteriographic demonstration of a large common femoral infected pseudoaneurysm. *(Reprinted with permission from Padberg FT, Hobson RW II, Lee B, et al. Femoral pseudoaneurysm from drugs of abuse: ligation or reconstruction? J Vasc Surg.* 1992;15:642–648.)

injections. Distal septic emboli have been reported in 5% to 10% of patients, while rupture of pseudoaneurysms through necrotic overlying skin has been reported in 5% to 15%.[4,5,9] Infrequently, patients may present with evidence of distal ischemia at the time of admission. Furthermore, self-administration of antibiotics by members of the more experienced drug abuse group may mask the appearance of these lesions. Needle aspiration of suspected abscesses or pseudoaneurysms may yield serosanguinous fluid or may be misleading and delay the diagnosis. If the index of suspicion is not high enough for the diagnosis of pseudoaneurysm, the inexperienced surgeon may perform incision and drainage in an outpatient facility resulting in substantial hemorrhage.

Most surgeons have relied on arteriography, using intravenous or intra-arterial digital substraction techniques,[6] for the accurate diagnosis of these lesions as well as the determination of distal arterial run-off. Localization of the false aneurysm to the bifurcation of the common femoral artery carries with it a greater risk of limb ischemia should arterial ligation be performed in its for management. Conversely, involvement of the branches of the profunda or the superficial femoral arteries would be associated with a lesser risk of limb ischemia if ligation is performed initially. However, use of Doppler ultrasound for the detection of distal arterial flow signals and their quantitation by measurement of segmental Doppler pressures has enhanced the selective management of these patients by ligation or revascularization.[9]

Bacteriologically, the great majority of these infections are due to *Staphylococcus aureus*. However, *Pseudomonas aeruginosa* is common and other unusual organisms have also been cultured.[4,5,9] Other communicable infectious diseases, such as HIV, are common in these patients, and universal precautions in processing blood or tissue specimens becomes an essential feature of their clinical management.

Adjacent structures are commonly involved by the pseudoaneurysm that may have been present for several weeks. Extension of the abscess into the pelvis (Fig. 25–2) may require additional exploration above the inguinal ligament. Femoral nerve compression for example may result in substantial long-term disability. Furthermore, venous injections and local injury may result in femoral venous occlusion and chronic venous insufficiency.

SURGICAL MANAGEMENT: SELECTIVE MANAGEMENT WITH ARTERIAL LIGATION OR REVASCULARIZATION

Once an accurate diagnosis has been confirmed and board-spectrum intravenous antibiotics have been initiated, exploration and operative drainage and excision of the involved arterial segments should be performed in the operating room. Proximal control of the external iliac artery through a suprainguinal retroperitoneal approach is recommended in the more proximal common femoral and distal external iliac aneurysms. Arterial ligation and debridement to normal artery represents a straightforward plan of management, which will result in limb ischemia among a relatively small subset of patients. Reddy and colleagues[6] reported that no amputations were performed in the management of 26 aneurysms after ligation of isolated femoral arterial segments. However, involvement of the common femoral bifurcation in 28 cases resulted in triple ligation of the common profunda, and superficial femoral arteries resulted in six cases of limb ischemia requiring revascularization. These authors predicted an amputation rate of 33% in these late cases and reommended revascularization with autogenous saphenous vein reconstruction in these selected cases of limb ischemia. Similarly, Johnson et al.[4] reported severe limb-threatening ischemia in one-third of patients treated

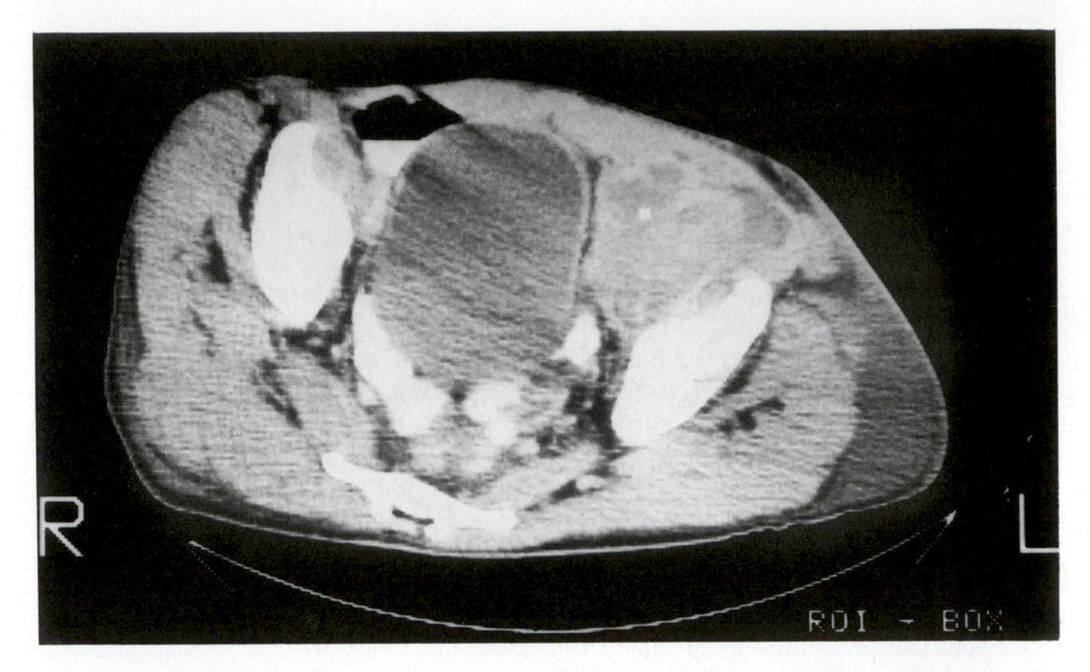

Figure 25–2. Computed tomographic image of an infected femoral pseudoaneurysm with extension of the abscess into the left pelvis. *(Reprinted with permission from Padberg FT. Infected femoral artery false aneurysm associated with drug abuse. In: Ernst C, Stanley J, eds. Current Therapy in Vascular Surgery. St. Louis, MO: Mosby–Year Book; 1995:319–321.)*

by excision of the femoral bifurcation resulting in a 21% amputation rate. Patients undergoing arterial ligation and selective revascularization generally fared better than those undergoing simultaneous reconstruction. Follow-up on patients undergoing simultaneous revascularization by our group[9,11] also has resulted in the identification of a substantial number of further complications requiring surgical intervention (Fig. 25–3). Although no mortalities were reported in our series of 18 femoral false aneurysms, 13 reoperations were performed in the reconstruction group with three amputations (25%), while two reoperations were performed in a group treated by ligation without incidence of amputation. Feldman and Berguer[5] reported a 22% incidence of graft infections and a 17% amputation rate among 23 patients treated by simultaneous revascularization. Excision, ligation, and selective delayed revascularization among 30 patients avoided graft infections, but the amputation rate remained at 17%.

Patel, Semel, and Clauss[7] have recommended routine revascularization in these cases using synthetic prosthetic bypass through the obturator foramen[14] or other extra-anatomical clean tissue planes. They argued that relief of limb-threatening ischemia, as well as subsequent symptoms of claudication, among 16 patients with infected pseudoaneurysms of the femoral artery had been accomplished with only one late failure and an amputation rate of 11%. However, it should be acknowledged that other authors using a selective approach to management also have reported equally low amputation rates.[8,9] Reddy,[8] furthermore, presents cogent arguments against routine revascularization, emphasizing the complexities associated with routine reconstruction, as well as the high recidivism among drug abusers, and the follow-up reconstructions that inevitably will be required in this group.

The presence of audible distal arterial Doppler signals after performance of proximal arterial ligation in trauma patients[16] has been associated with a prediction of limb

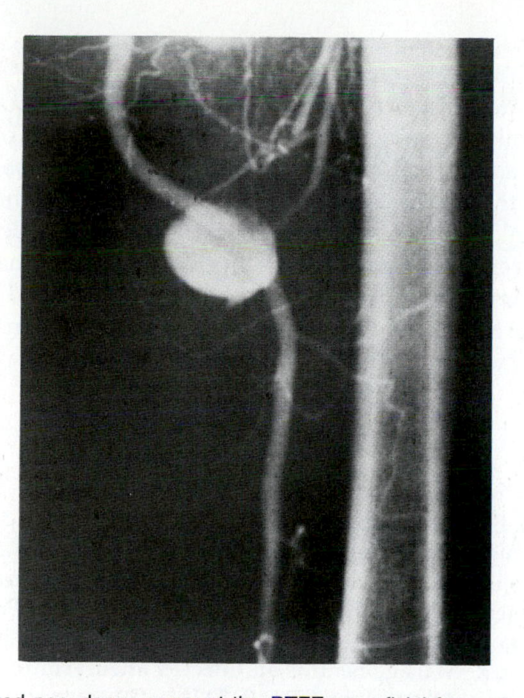

Figure 25–3. Infected pseudoaneurysm at the PTFE-superficial femoral arterial anastomosis following prior obturator foramen bypass. *(Reprinted with permission from Yeager RA, Hobson RW II, Wright CB. Vascular complications related to drug abuse. In: Veith FJ, Hobson RW, Williams RA, et al., eds. Vascular Surgery: Principles and Practice. 2nd ed. New York: McGraw-Hill; 1994:993–1005.)*

viability. Padberg and co-authors[9] have used this as a qualitative assessment after femoral arterial ligation, while we and others[13] have reported ankle-to-arm indices of greater than 0.3 to be associated with viable extremities even after triple ligation of the femoral arteries. Subsequent occurrence of chronic limb ischemia would result in follow-up arteriographic assessment and revascularization as indicated. Although Reddy and colleagues[6] recommended the use of autologous tissue bypasses, the availability of the saphenous vein is commonly restricted in these patients, making the immediate reconstruction with autologous tissue a less common option among our patients.[9]

Excision and drainage followed by arterial ligation and selective revascularization seems the most appropriate alternative. Extra-anatomic bypass through clean tissue planes has been recommended but requires use of prosthetic materials. If an adequate vein is available, the patient may benefit from a short bypass through an infected area, provided the proximal and distal anastomoses are located in areas not involved in the infection. In addition, coverage of these groin reconstructions with a mobilized sartorius muscle flap is also recommended.[6] However, prosthetic grafts should not be routed through areas of infection. The obturator foraman bypass is the preferred route for lower extremity revascularization in the presence of femoral infections,[14] but the acquisition of a clean tissue plane around a large false aneurysm in the groin can be difficult technically. Under these circumstances, subsequent development of an anastomotic false aneurysm may occur (Fig. 25–3) and require reoperation. While Patel and colleagues[7] have argued that absence of intermittent claudication through a program of immediate routine revascularization is meritorious, this complaint among the drug abuse population has been modest. Among this group, the risks associated with use of a prosthetic reconstruction outweigh the potential benefits of relieving claudication.[8,15]

CONCLUSION

Infected femoral pseudoaneurysm due to drugs of abuse infrequently require arterial reconstruction after initial management by arterial ligation. Consequently, defining clinical criteria for revascularization, which represents the unusual case, is most important. We have utilized the presence of audible Doppler signals at the ankle after proximal arterial ligation and ankle-to-arm indices above 0.3 as a reasonable method for selection of patients requiring revascularization. Absence of Doppler signals or lower ankle-to-arm indices indicate revascularization, preferentially performed with autologous bypass grafting procedures. However, it is recognized that extraanatomical bypass with prosthetic material inevitably will be required in most of these patients.

REFERENCES

1. Perler BA, Ernst CB. Infected aneurysms. In: Veith FJ, Hobson RW, Williams RA, et al., eds. *Vascular Surgery: Principles and Practice.* 2nd ed. New York: McGraw-Hill; 1994:589–608.
2. Osler W. The Gulstonian lectures on malignant endocarditis. *Br Med J.* 1885;1:467.
3. Wilson SE, Van Wagenen P, Passaro E Jr. Arterial infection. *Curr Prob Surg.* 1978;15:5.
4. Johnson JR, Ledgerwood AM, Lucas CE. Mycotic aneurysm. *Arch Surg.* 1983;118:577–582.
5. Feldman AJ, Berguer R. Management of an infected aneurysm of the groin secondary to drug abuse. *Surg Gynecol Obstet.* 1983;157:519–522.
6. Reddy DJ, Smith RF, Elliott JP, et al. Infected femoral artery false aneurysms in drug addicts: evolution of selective vascular reconstruction. *J Vasc Surg.* 1986;3:718–724.
7. Patel K, Semel L, Clauss RH. Routine revascularization with resection of infected femoral pseudoaneurysms from substance abuse. *J Vasc Surg.* 1988;8:321–328.
8. Reddy DJ. Treatment of drug-related infected false aneurysm of the femoral artery—is routine revascularization justified? *J Vasc Surg.* 1988;8:344–345.
9. Padberg FT, Hobson RW II, Lee B, et al. Femoral pseudoaneurysm from drugs of abuse: ligation or reconstruction? *J Vasc Surg.* 1992;15:642–648.
10. Brown SL, Busuttil RW, Baker JD, et al. Bacteriologic and surgical determinants of survival in patients with mycotic aneurysms. *J Vasc Surg.* 1984;10:635.
11. Yeager RA, Hobson RW II, Padberg FT, et al. Vascular complications related to drug abuse. *J Trauma.* 1987;27:305–308.
12. Yeager RA, Hobson RW II, Wright CB. Vascular complications related to drug abuse. In: Veith FJ, Hobson RW, Williams RA, et al, eds. *Vascular Surgery: Principles and Practice.* 2nd ed. New York: McGraw-Hill; 1994:993–1005.
13. Cheng SWK, Fox M, Wong J. Infected femoral pseudoaneurysm in intravenous drug abusers. *Br J Surg.* 1992;79:510–512.
14. Fromm SH, Lucas CE. Obturator bypass for mycotic aneurysm in the drug addict. *Arch Surg.* 1970;100:82–83.
15. Padberg FT. Infected femoral artery false aneurysm associated with drug abuse. In: Ernst C, Stanley J, eds. *Current Therapy in Vascular Surgery.* St. Louis, MO: Mosby–Year Book; 1995:319–321.
16. Lavenson GS, Rich NM, Strandness DE. Ultrasonic flow detector value in combat vascular injuries. *Arch Surg.* 1971;103:644–647.

26

Endovascular Grafts for the Treatment of Vascular Pathology

Michael L. Marin, MD, and Frank J. Veith, MD

Significant advances have occurred in the management of complex vascular diseases over the past 40 years, with treatment shifting from palliative measures to care for lethal or limb-threatening pathology to therapy focused on the precise diagnosis and open surgical correction of arterial disorders. In recent times, the operative mortality rate for elective repair of aortic aneurysms has markedly decreased, declining from 21% in surgical series carried out in the 1950s to under 5% reported in modern studies.[1–5] Multilevel lower extremity occlusive disease with gangrene that once mandated amputation can presently be treated with either interventional techniques or bypass surgery, resulting in favorable limb salvage rates.[6] Finally, despite advances in resuscitation, anesthesia, and intensive care, complex acute arterial injury from penetrating or blunt vascular trauma has remained a challenging problem with substantial morbidity and mortality, particularly when central vascular injuries occur in a setting with other severe injuries.[7–9] Despite important improvements in the management of all these vascular lesions, significant perioperative morbidity and mortality still occur, particularly in those patients with: (1) severe comorbid medical illnesses; (2) the need for operations in previous surgical sites; or (3) following multiorgan trauma.[10–16]

An increasing trend in surgery since the mid-1980s has been to develop less invasive procedures to accomplish treatment goals with reduced operative risks and complications, thus allowing therapy to be extended even to high-risk patients with severe comorbid medical illnesses. One such evolving technique for less invasive vascular surgery has involved the use of endovascular grafts, which are a blend of intravascular stent and prosthetic graft technologies.[17–38] These devices may be inserted through remote arterial access sites to treat vascular lesions without the need to directly expose the diseased artery through an extensive incision or dissection. To date, endovascular grafts have been successfully used to treat aortic and peripheral artery aneurysms, long segment arterial occlusive disease, and vascular trauma. Despite the potential advantages of these new techniques, the devices at present are primitive and will require further development before they are widely applied for the treatment of vascular disease. This report describes one center's initial experience over a 2½-year period with the use of 96 endovascular grafts for the treatment of arterial aneurysms, occlusions, and traumatic or iatrogenic vascular injuries.

ENDOVASCULAR STENTED GRAFT DEVICES

The endovascular stented graft devices used at the Montefiore Medical Center in New York were chosen according to the type of vascular lesion being treated (Table 26–1; Fig. 26–1). With the exception of the aortic devices, all endovascular grafts were composed of commercially available materials. Specific details regarding the balloon expandable aortic device and the Endovascular Technologies, Inc. (EVT) Endograft device are described elsewhere.[39,40]

TECHNIQUES FOR ENDOVASCULAR STENTED GRAFT INSERTION

The principles of endovascular stented graft insertion and deployment are similar for treating different vascular pathologies. Specific procedural modifications were made in accordance with the anatomic locations of the lesions as well as the presence or absence of arterial occlusive disease. Target lesions were generally approached through the largest available access vessel (i.e., common femoral or brachial). Following the insertion of a guide wire through the access vessel and the interpretation of preinsertion arteriograms, endovascular stented grafts, which were contained in delivery catheters, were advanced to the desired location by coaxial movement of the device over the guide wire under fluoroscopic control. In those instances in which stenotic or occluded arteries were treated, the diseased vessel was first diffusely balloon dilated, creating a widened tract prior to the insertion of the device (Fig. 26–2). Once proper positioning of the endovascular graft was confirmed, the delivery catheter was withdrawn, permitting deployment of the graft-to-artery attachment system (stent).[25,41] Each procedure was immediately followed by an intraoperative completion arteriogram and, in selected cases, intravascular ultrasound examination to evaluate the adequacy of the technique. All procedures were performed in the operating room using a portable C-arm fluoroscope.

TABLE 26–1. CHARACTERISTICS OF ENDOVASCULAR GRAFTS

Vascular Pathology	Graft Material	Attachment System	Introducer System
Aortic aneurysm			
Balloon expandable device	Thin walled knitted, crimped Dacron[a]	Balloon expandable stent[a]	Teflon, double sheath (24 Fr)[a]
EVT device	Woven Dacron[b]	Self-expanding, hooked, "Z" stent configuration[b]	Endovascular deployment assembly (26 Fr)[b]
Peripheral artery aneurysm	PTFE[c]	Palmaz balloon expandable stent[d]	Teflon, single sheath (12–14 Fr)
Chronic arterial occlusion	PTFE[c]	Palmaz balloon expandable stent[d]	Teflon, single sheath (14 Fr)
Arterial trauma	PTFE[c]	Palmaz balloon expandable stent[d]	Teflon, single sheath (12 Fr)

[a] Barone, Inc., Buenos Aires, Argentina.
[b] Endovascular Technologies Corporation, Menlo Park, CA.
[c] W.L. Gore and Associates, Flagstaff, AZ.
[d] Johnson and Johnson Interventional Systems, Warren, NJ.

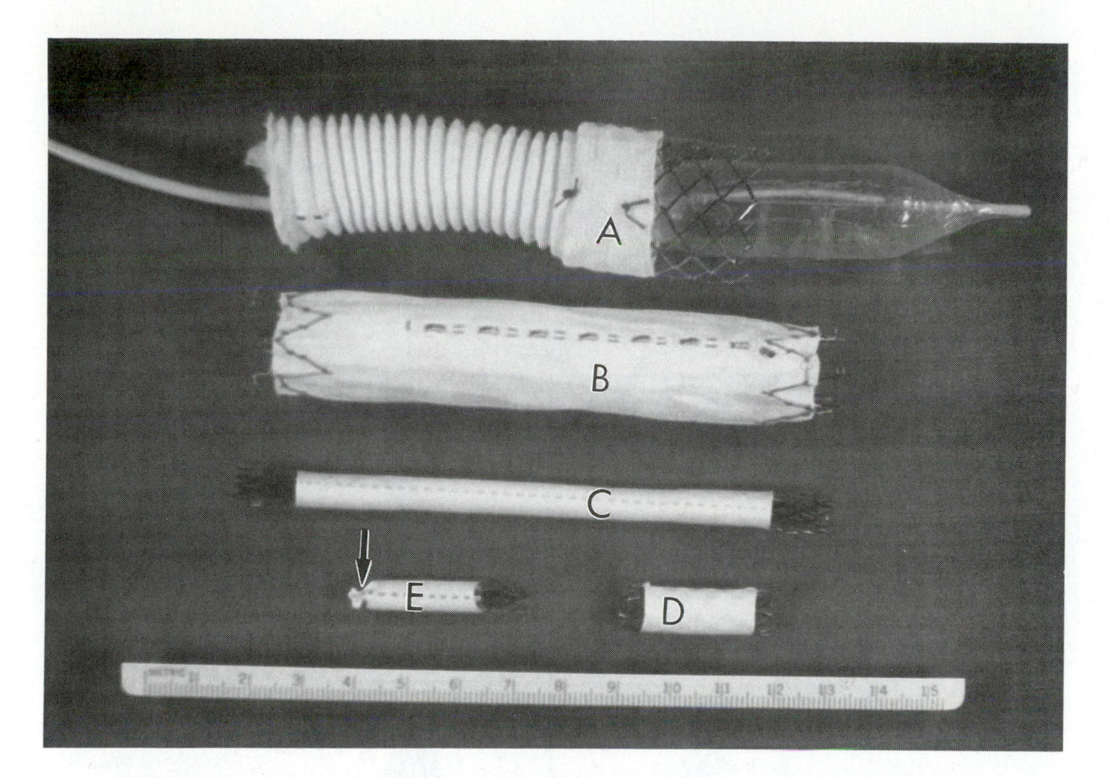

Figure 26–1. This is a photograph of the different endovascular grafts used for the repair of aortic and peripheral artery aneurysms, arterial occlusions, and traumatic vascular injuries. (**A**), A balloon expandable (Parodi) endovascular aortic device; (**B**), Endovascular Technologies' Endograft™; (**C**), a PTFE endovascular graft used for the treatment of peripheral artery aneurysms and arterial occlusive disease; (**D**), a PTFE-covered Palmaz balloon expandable stent used for the treatment of traumatic arterial injuries; and (**E**), an occluding PTFE covered Palmaz stent. One end of this device is closed with a purse-string suture (*arrow*). *(Reprinted with permission from Marin ML, Veith FJ, Cynamon J, et al. Initial experience with transluminally placed endovascular grafts for the treatment of complex vascular lesions. Ann Surg. 1995;222:449–469.)*

RESULTS

At Montefiore Medical Center in New York, the authors performed 96 endovascular stented graft procedures in 90 patients with 100 arterial lesions between November 1992 and April 1995 (Table 26–2). These grafts were used to treat 36 arterial aneurysms, 11 lesions secondary to penetrating vascular trauma, and 53 long segment arterial stenotic or occlusive lesions. Endovascular grafts were inserted under local (16 [17%]), epidural (42 [43%]), or general anesthesia (38 [40%]). The mean age of the patients with aneurysmal and occlusive lesions was 69 years compared with the relatively younger group of patients who were treated for penetrating traumatic vascular injuries (mean age, 38 years). Most of the patients in this study who were treated for aneurysmal or occlusive arterial disease also had significant comorbid medical illnesses or a major surgical contraindication to standard treatment.

Abdominal Aortic Aneurysms

Eighteen patients with abdominal aortic aneurysms (AAAs) were treated with two different endovascular graft devices. Four good-risk patients with suitable arterial anatomy had implantation of an EVT device (Figs. 26–3 and 26–4). Fourteen high-risk

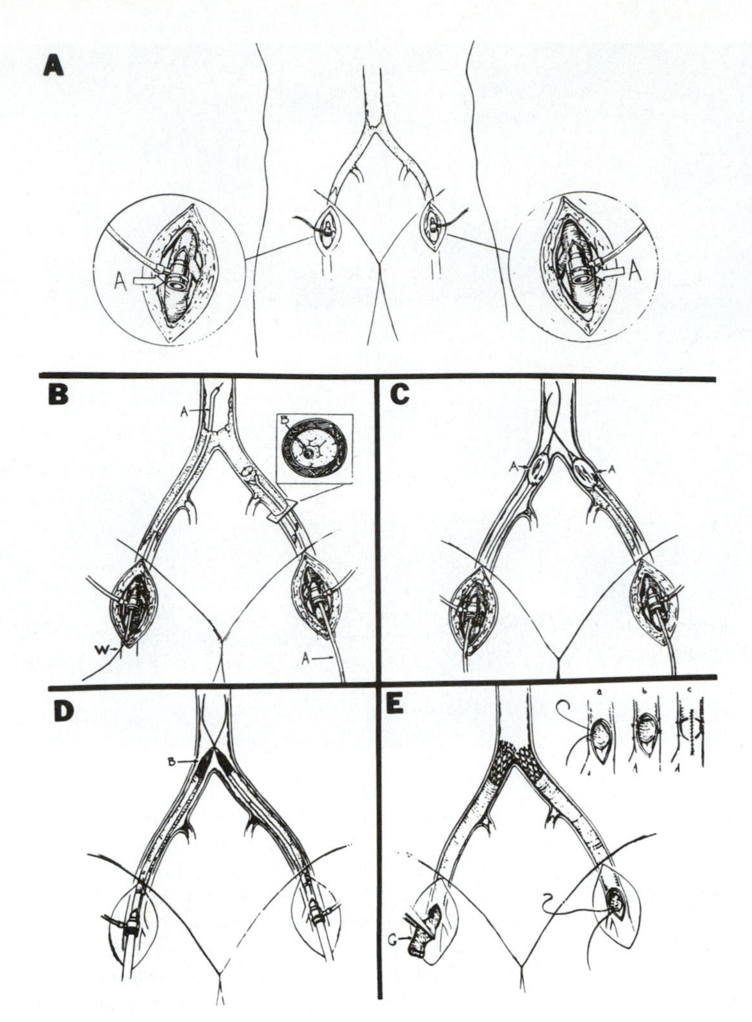

patients received balloon expandable endovascular grafts (Table 26–3; Fig. 26–5). All EVT procedures employed tubular, aorto-aortic grafts, while 6 of the 14 balloon expandable device procedures employed aortoiliofemoral reconstructions with the addition of femorofemoral bypasses and occlusion of the common iliac arteries contralateral to the main endovascular graft. There were no thromboses of the aortic grafts and no postimplantation structural device failures. One patient with a balloon expandable device demonstrated apparent cephalad migration of the distal stent seen on a CT scan at 13 months. During a mean follow-up period of 8 months, 2 of the 4 aneurysms treated with the EVT device decreased in size. Six of the 14 aneurysms repaired with the balloon expandable device decreased in size (1 to 3 mm), and 3 showed evidence of minimal enlargement (0.5 to 1 mm). No new aortic aneurysm ruptures occurred in this series after graft placement.

Three patients in this series had severe medical comorbidities in association with contained aortic ruptures. One patient had a ruptured 6-cm AAA and an acute anterior wall myocardial infarction; one patient with renal failure and severe congestive heart failure had complete anastomotic disruption (proximal and distal) of an infrarenal aortic graft with 2 contained pseudoaneurysms; and another patient with congestive heart failure and pulmonary insufficiency had a distal aortic disruption and a contained pseudoaneurysm that was secondary to the extension of a Pott's abscess of the lumbar spine to the wall of the infrarenal aorta (Fig. 26–6).

Peripheral Artery Aneurysms

Fifteen patients had aneurysms involving the popliteal, iliac, or subclavian arteries (Table 26–2; Figs. 26–7 and 26–8). Endovascular stented grafts were successfully placed in 11 patients who had a total of 14 iliac artery aneurysms, in 2 patients with popliteal artery aneurysms, and in 1 patient with a subclavian artery aneurysm. One endovascular graft that was inserted to treat a complex iliac artery aneurysm thrombosed at 9 months, and limb salvage was achieved with an axillofemoral bypass. One patient with a popliteal artery aneurysm underwent a standard vascular reconstruction when the endovascular graft device could not be successfully inserted. A second patient thrombosed a popliteal endovascular graft on the sixth postoperative day without apparent cause, and this endovascular graft procedure was successfully converted to a standard vascular reconstruction. A third patient with a popliteal artery aneurysm was treated with an endovascular stented graft that has maintained graft patency free of any hemodynamically significant lesions for 26 months.

A single patient with a subclavian artery aneurysm with distal embolization and a history of cervical rib resection for thoracic outlet syndrome 2 years previously had successful insertion of an endovascular graft. This graft abruptly thrombosed 6 weeks

←

Figure 26–2. This is a series of artist's drawings of the techniques for endoluminal aortoiliac bypass for occlusive disease. (**A**) Bilateral inguinal incisions are performed to expose the common femoral arteries. An introducer catheter, equipped with a hemostatic valve (A), is inserted in a retrograde fashion into the common femoral artery in each groin. It is through these introducer catheters that all subsequent catheter manipulations on the occluded or diseased arterial system are carried out. (**B**) A hydrophilic guide wire (W) is then inserted through each introducer catheter and guided through the occluded or stenotic segment of an artery by means of directional catheters (A). Inset: An effort is made to guide the recanalization process within the native lumen of diffusely stenotic arteries. In situations in which the entire vessel is chronically occluded, the recanalization process occurs in a relatively random fashion following the planes of least resistance within the subintimal plane (B). (**C**) After successful recanalization of an artery, long segment diffuse balloon dilatation is performed (A). Balloon catheters are inserted over the previously placed guide wires. Balloon dilatation creates a new tract within the diseased artery, which must communicate with the lumen of a patent proximal vessel. (**D**) An endovascular graft is inserted through an arteriotomy in the common femoral artery. Endovascular grafts, contained within introducer catheters, are advanced over the previously placed guide wires and into the patent proximal vessels. The delivery sheath is then withdrawn exposing the anchoring stent (B). (**E**) Following inflation of the coaxially loaded angioplasty balloon, the Palmaz balloon expandable stent expands, creating a friction seal between the stent, the attached graft and the underlying arterial wall. The introducer catheters on each side are then completely withdrawn, permitting the free end of the prosthetic endovascular graft (G) to be withdrawn from the common femoral arteriotomy and clamped. Vascular clamps are then positioned across the native proximal common femoral artery that will, in turn, compress its enclosed endovascular graft. An endoluminal anastomosis is then created between the endovascular graft and the internal surface of the common femoral artery with a series of interrupted "U" stitches (insets a–b). This anastomotic technique may be tailored to each individual vessel, depending on the extent of local disease. The endoluminal anastomosis may be completed with a running monofilament suture across the linear arteriotomy (inset c). Under some circumstances, a common femoral endarterectomy or a patch angioplasty of the arteriotomy site may be required to establish unobstructed flow through the endovascular graft and into the distal circulation. *(Reprinted with permission from Marin ML, Veith FJ, Cynamon J, et al. Initial experience with transluminally placed endovascular grafts for the treatment of complex vascular lesions. Ann Surg. 1995;222:449–469.)*

TABLE 26–2. DISTRIBUTION OF PATIENT CHARACTERISTICS AND LESIONS TREATED WITH ENDOVASCULAR GRAFTS

Vascular Pathology	No. of Patients	No. of Lesions	Sex Male/Female	Age Range (Mean)	Coexisting Coronary Artery Disease[a] No. (%)	Coexisting Chronic Obstructive Pulmonary Disease[b] No. (%)	Diabetes Mellitus No. (%)	Renal Insufficiency[c] No. (%)	Hostile Surgical Field[d] No. (%)
Abdominal aortic aneurysm	18	18	15 M; 3 F	66–88 (76)	17 (94)	11 (61)	5 (28)	6 (33)	3 (17)
Iliac artery aneurysm	11	14	11 M	58–89 (72)	11 (100)	5 (45)	5 (45)	3 (27)	5 (45)
Popliteal artery aneurysm	3	3	2 M; 1 F	63–84 (74)	2 (67)	1 (33)	1 (33)	0	0
Subclavian artery aneurysm	1	1	1 F	40	0	0	0	0	1 (100)
Traumatic arterial pseudoaneurysm	9	9	8 M; 1 F	18–78 (44)	1 (11)	1 (11)	1 (11)	0	0
Traumatic arteriovenous fistula	2	2	2 M	18–20 (19)	0	0	0	0	0
Aortoiliac occlusive disease	42	47	23 M; 19 F	43–86 (65)	36 (86)	9 (21)	22 (52)	7 (17)	13 (31)
Femoropopliteal occlusive disease	6	6	4 M; 2 F	62–82 (68)	6 (100)	5 (83)	4 (67)	1 (17)	0

[a] Ejection fraction less than 20% on echocardiography, thallium, or MUGA scans.
[b] FEV^1 <35% of predicted, room air PaO_2 <60 mmHg or $PaCO_2$ >50 mmHg.
[c] Creatinine ≥3.0.
[d] Hostile surgical field implies at least one previous dissection, scarring, or infection in the region of the vascular lesion treated by the endovascular graft.

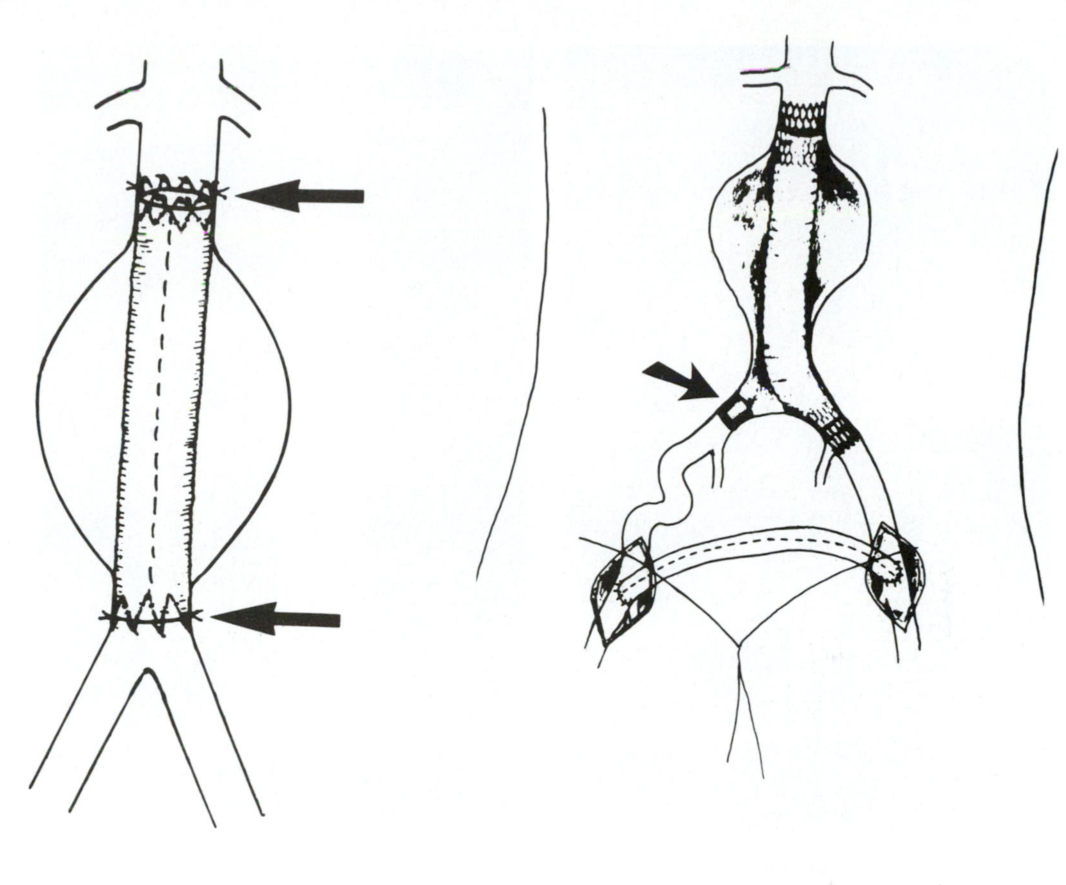

Figure 26–3. This is an artist's drawing of an aortic reconstruction following transfemoral, endoluminal repair of an abdominal aortic aneurysm. (**A**) Following transfemoral insertion of the Endovascular Technologies' Endograft™ self-expanding, hooked prosthesis, sealing of the graft to the underlying arterial wall is accomplished by movement of the self-expanding, hooked attachment system into the arterial wall (*arrows*). The current configuration of this device is useful only for those aneurysms that have a suitable segment of normal aorta both proximal and distal to the lesion. (**B**) For those aneurysms that extend to the aortic bifurcation, an aortoiliac reconstruction (after Parodi) may be performed. Flow through the contralateral common femoral artery is occluded by an endoluminal occlusion device (*arrow*) similar to that shown in Figure 26–1E. A femorofemoral extra-anatomic bypass is performed to restore arterial flow to the contralateral limb. Right hypogastric artery flow (not shown) was preserved.

after insertion without upper extremity limb-threatening consequences. No further interventions were performed in this patient.

Aortoiliac Occlusive Disease

Forty-two patients received 47 aortoiliofemoral endovascular grafts to treat 47 extremities at risk for limb loss (Table 26–4; Fig. 26–9). Most of these patients had significant comorbid medical illnesses or surgical conditions that precluded standard aortoiliac reconstructions, extra-anatomic bypasses, or treatment by balloon angioplasty and stent placement (Table 26–2). Technical success of graft insertion was achieved in 43 procedures (92%). Primary and secondary graft patency rates at 18 months were 77%

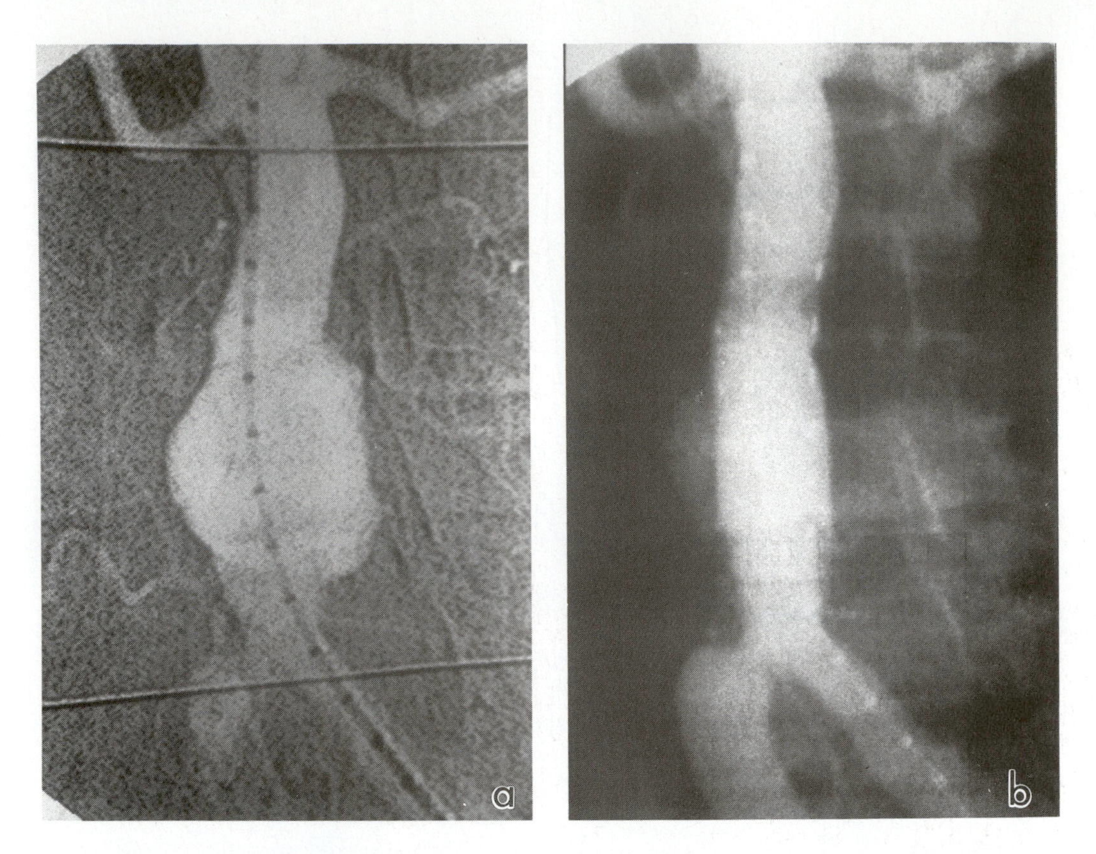

Figure 26–4. Transfemoral, endoluminal repair of an abdominal aortic aneurysm using the Endovascular Technologies' Endograft™. (**a**) Preoperative arteriogram demonstrates a suitable proximal and distal segment of normal aorta above and below the aneurysm. (**b**) Following transfemoral insertion of the Endograft™, the aneurysm lumen is excluded from the circulation. *(Reprinted with permission from Marin ML, Veith FJ, Cynamon J, et al. Initial experience with transluminally placed endovascular grafts for the treatment of complex vascular lesions. Ann Surg. 1995;222:449–469.)*

and 95%, respectively (Tables 26–5 and 26–6; Fig. 26–10). Limb salvage at 18 months was 98% (Table 26–7). There was a 7% major and a 17% minor complication rate associated with these procedures.

Femoropopliteal Occlusive Disease

Six patients with severe comorbid medical problems received endovascular femoropopliteal grafts to treat pedal gangrene. Two grafts were performed in association with an endovascular aortoiliofemoral graft. One endovascular femoropopliteal graft was performed in conjunction with an axillofemoral bypass after an unsuccessful attempt to perform an endovascular iliofemoral reconstruction. Three patients with patent grafts died from acute myocardial infarctions at 2, 7, and 15 months after their endovascular graft insertions. One graft to an isolated popliteal segment thrombosed at 1 week, and this patient maintained stable pedal gangrene until he died 2 months later of cardiac disease. Another endovascular femoropopliteal graft closed at 14 months following complete healing of a previously gangrenous foot. This limb has continued to remain healed with the graft closed. This patient has a patent endovascular aortofemoral graft

TABLE 26–3. ENDOVASCULAR GRAFTS FOR THE TREATMENT OF ABDOMINAL AORTIC ANEURYSMS

Endovascular Device	No. of Patients	Type of Anesthesia No. (%)			Successful Graft Insertion No. (%)	Hospital Stay[c] Days (Mean)	Perigraft Channel[d] No. (%)	Follow-up (in Months) (Mean)
		General	Epidural	Local				
EVT	4	4 (100)	0	0	4 (100)	2–7 (3.5)	2 (50)	4–22 (13.7)
Balloon expandable device[a]	11	1 (9)	8 (73)	2 (18)	9 (82)[e]	6–21 (12)	4 (36)	4–25 (13.3)
Balloon expandable device[b]	3	0	3 (100)	0	3 (100)	4–15 (9.5)	0	6–12 (9)

[a] Includes both aorto–aortic (8 patients) and aortoiliac with femorofemoral bypasses (3 patients).
[b] Endovascular graft for contained aortic rupture. All had aortoiliac grafts, contralateral iliac occlusion, and femorofemoral bypasses.
[c] Mean hospital length of stay is calculated exclusive of early postoperative deaths.
[d] Perigraft channel describes any contrast flow seen outside the lumen of the graft and into the aneurysmal sac on the initial follow-up CT with contrast.
[e] One procedure was converted to a standard repair, and one procedure was aborted without grafting.

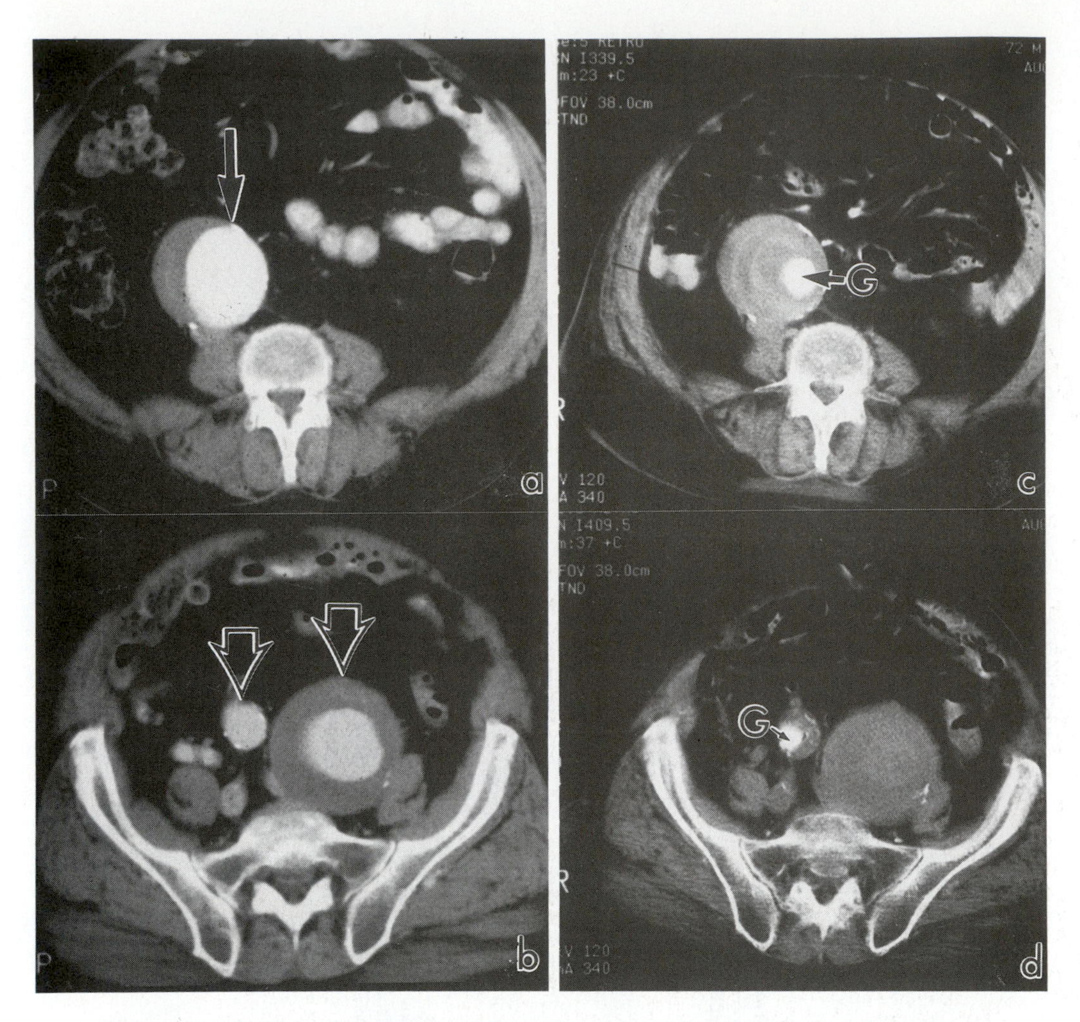

Figure 26–5. Transfemoral, endoluminal repair of a complex abdominal aortic aneurysm (**a,** *arrow*) and bilateral common iliac artery aneurysms (**b,** *open arrows*). (**c,d**) Following insertion of an endovascular graft (G), the aortic aneurysm and the bilateral common iliac artery aneurysms have thrombosed. *(Reprinted with permission from Marin ML, Veith FJ, Cynamon J, et al. Initial experience with transluminally placed endovascular grafts for the treatment of complex vascular lesions. Ann Surg. 1995;222:449–469.)*

with runoff only to the deep femoral artery. One endovascular femoropopliteal graft remains patent at 22 months.

Penetrating or Iatrogenic Arterial Trauma

Eleven patients sustained vascular trauma resulting in nine isolated pseudoaneurysms and two arteriovenous fistulas (Table 26–8; Fig. 26–11). Seven of these injuries were the result of gunshot wounds and two were secondary to iatrogenic needle injuries. Eight patients had sustained other injuries in conjunction with their vascular trauma. All penetrating and iatrogenic traumatic vascular injuries were repaired from 4 hours to 4 months after the primary injury. No endovascular grafts inserted for penetrating trauma have thrombosed during the follow-up period, which ranged from 2 to 28 months (mean, 15 months). Complications encountered with the use of endovascular

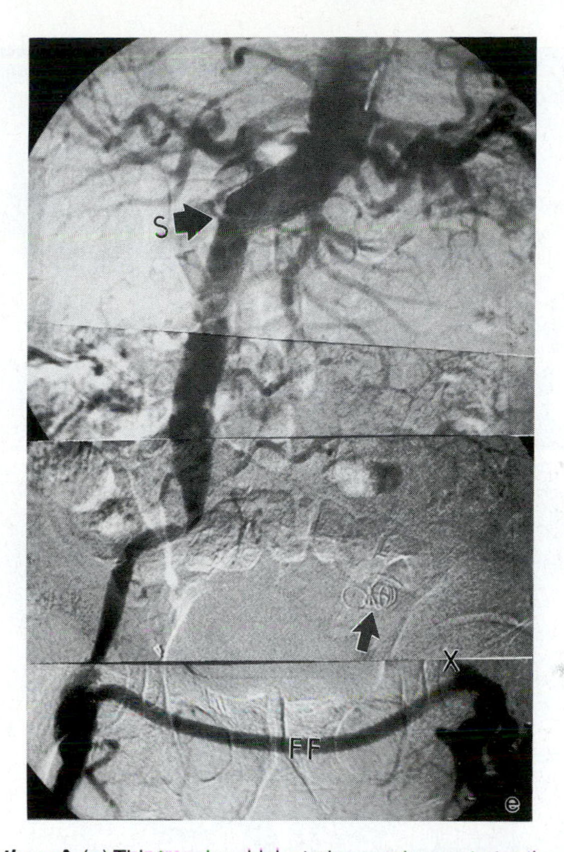

Figure 26–5 (*Continued*). (**e**) This transbrachial arteriogram demonstrates the completed reconstruction. Note the presence of embolization coils within the origin of the left hypogastric artery (*arrow*) that prevent backflow from this vessel into the left common iliac artery aneurysm. Ligation of the proximal left common femoral artery (x) followed by the creation of a femorofemoral bypass (FF) restores circulation to both lower extremities. (s = proximal stent fixation site) *(Reprinted with permission from Marin ML, Veith FJ, Cynamon J, et al. Initial experience with transluminally placed endovascular grafts for the treatment of complex vascular lesions. Ann Surg. 1995;222:449–469.)*

grafts for traumatic vascular injuries included one immediate insertion site stenosis that was successfully treated with a vein patch angioplasty. A single stent graft stenosis occurred at 8 months, which responded to percutaneous balloon angioplasty and remained patent for 23 months.

DISCUSSION

Transluminally placed endovascular grafting procedures are part of a growing trend to provide improved patient care in association with reduced cost by means of carefully planned, less invasive therapies. Such concepts have resulted in the successful development of important techniques such as transurethral prostatectomy, laparoscopic cholecystectomy, and a variety of other endoscopic procedures.

Less invasive endovascular therapies were conceptualized by Dotter, who first described catheter-based angioplasty and conceived of devices for intravascular stenting.[42,43] The use of balloon angioplasty procedures for the treatment of short segment arterial occlusive disease has become relatively well established in a variety of vascular

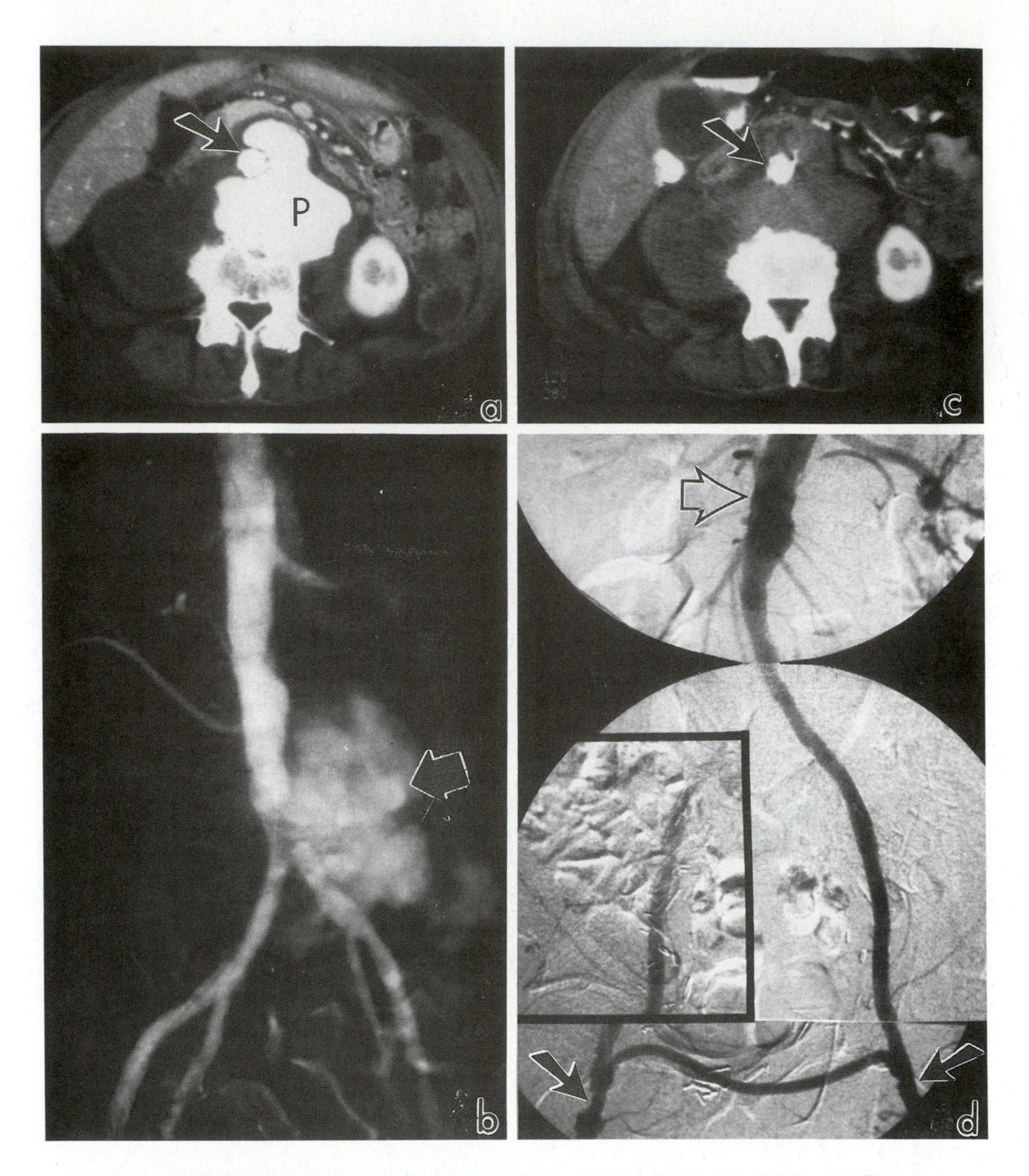

Figure 26–6. Transfemoral repair of a contained rupture of the distal aorta. (**a**) A spiral CT scan demonstrates extravasation of contrast material from the aorta (*arrow*) into a large, partially clot-filled pseudoaneurysm (P). (**b**) A transfemoral arteriogram confirms the presence of the large aortic pseudoaneurysm (*arrow*). (**c**) A spiral CT scan performed after transfemoral insertion of an endovascular graft demonstrates that the pseudoaneurysm is thrombosed, and vascular continuity within the lumen of the aorta (*arrow*) is preserved. (**d**) A postoperative transfemoral arteriogram at 1 week demonstrates vascular continuity between the aorta (*open arrow*) and the common femoral arteries (*arrows*). *(Reprinted with permission from Marin ML, Veith FJ, Cynamon J, et al. Initial experience with transluminally placed endovascular grafts for the treatment of complex vascular lesions. Ann Surg. 1995;222:449–469.)*

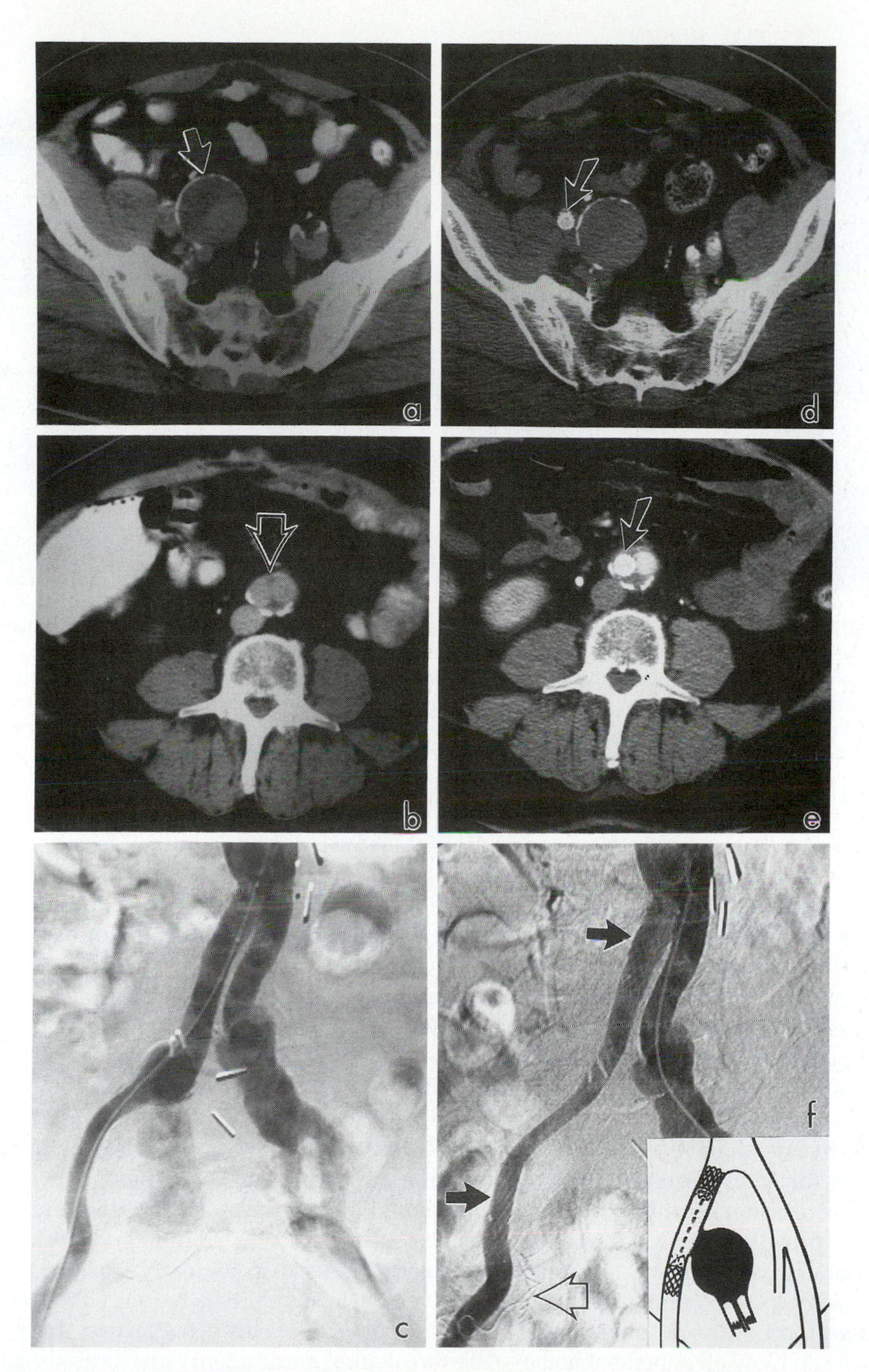

Figure 26–7. Transfemoral repair of a right internal iliac artery aneurysm 5 years after a bifurcated graft repair of aortic and common iliac artery aneurysms. (**a**) CT documents the presence of the right internal iliac artery aneurysm (*arrow*). (**b**) The two limbs of the bifurcated graft can be identified (*arrow*). (**c**) Transfemoral arteriography documents filling of the aneurysm prior to coil embolization of the anterior and posterior divisions of the vessel. (Note aneurysmal wall calcification [*small arrows*].) (**d**) Following endovascular graft repair, the aneurysm has thrombosed. Contrast can be identified within the endovascular graft (*arrow*). (**e**) This CT documents fixation of the proximal Palmaz stent (*arrow*) within the old bifurcated graft. (**f**) Postoperative digital arteriogram shows the anchoring stents (*arrows*) and coils in the posterior and anterior divisions of the right internal iliac artery to prevent retrograde flow (*open arrow*). Inset: Drawing of the completed repair. *(Reprinted with permission from Marin ML, Veith FJ, Cynamon J, et al. Initial experience with transluminally placed endovascular grafts for the treatment of complex vascular lesions. Ann Surg. 1995;222:449–469.)*

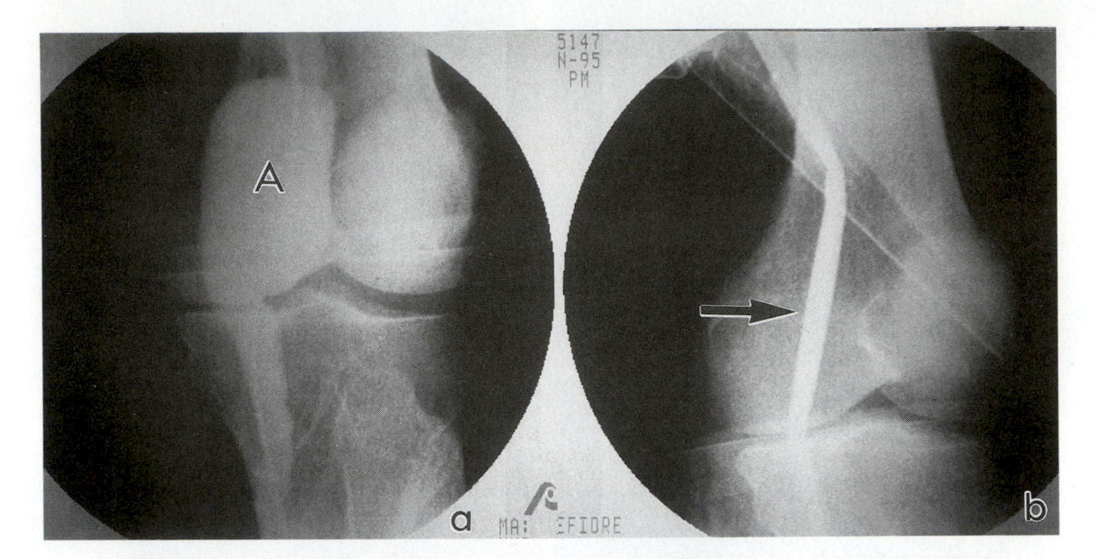

Figure 26–8. Transluminal repair of a popliteal artery aneurysm. (**a**) A transfemoral digital arteriogram demonstrates a large popliteal artery aneurysm (A). (**b**) Following insertion of an endovascular graft (*arrow*) that is fixed to the below-knee popliteal artery with a 1-cm Palmaz stent, the popliteal artery aneurysm is excluded. *(Reprinted with permission from Marin ML, Veith FJ, Cynamon J, et al. Initial experience with transluminally placed endovascular grafts for the treatment of complex vascular lesions. Ann Surg. 1995;222:449–469.)*

systems.[44–46] The supplemental use of arterial stents for more complex lesions has also proved beneficial.[47] The logical extension of transluminally placed endovascular grafting using covered stents and stent-fixed prosthetic conduits to treat more complex arterial lesions has followed a relatively ordered course with the development of new devices and animal models in which to test these devices.[48–54]

The earliest clinical experience using endovascular grafts is attributed to Volodos in Russia who described his experience with self-expanding endovascular grafts for the treatment of a thoracic aortic aneurysm and aortoiliac occlusive disease.[17,19] However, the true potential of this technology was only realized after Parodi, Palmaz, and Barone successfully treated a patient with an AAA in Argentina in 1990.[18] This and subsequent efforts by Parodi have sparked worldwide efforts to find new applications and improved devices for endovascular graft treatment of a variety of vascular lesions.[20–38,55–57]

The decision regarding which patients should initially be treated by this new technology has provoked controversy among vascular specialists.[18,25,28,58] Should good-risk patients without coexisting medical or surgical problems be used in the early trials of this new technology so as to permit rapid and safe conversion to standard techniques if the endovascular graft procedure is unsuccessful? Until such devices are proven effective, this philosophy would deny all patients who have life-threatening aortic aneurysms, limb-threatening ischemia, or central vascular injuries in the face of prohibitive cardiac, pulmonary, and other medical comorbidities possible benefit from receiving this treatment.

We have chosen the alternative approach of largely using these endovascular grafts in patients for whom standard surgical operations would be difficult or impossible to perform because of major medical or surgical comorbidities that precluded general or other major anesthesia and/or easy direct surgical access to the lesion. Although this approach offers the hope of great benefit to the patients if the new devices are effective, it largely denies them the possibility of a surgical "rescue" procedure should the device fail or have a complication. At the least, such a surgical "rescue" would be associated

TABLE 26–4. ENDOVASCULAR GRAFTS FOR THE TREATMENT OF OCCLUSIVE DISEASE

Disease Location	No. of Grafts	Indication for Surgery No. (%)	Proximal Graft Origin[a] No. (%)	Distal Graft Insertion[a] No. (%)	Graft Length cm (mean)	Associated Procedures No. (%)	Ankle/Brachial Indices (mean)	
							Pre	Post
Aortoiliac	47	Gangrene, 39 (83) Rest pain, 8 (17)	Aorta or CIA = 34 (72) EIA = 13 (28)	CFA = 29 (62) SFA = 4 (8.5) DFA = 11 (23) AKP = 3 (6)	15–46 (20)	35 (74)[b]	0.32	0.78
Femoropopliteal	6	Gangrene, 6 (100)	CFA = 3 (50) SFA = 3 (50)	AKP = 6 (100)	24–37 (29)	3 (50)[c]	0.30	0.71

[a] CIA = common iliac artery; EIA = external iliac artery; CFA = common femoral artery; SFA = superficial femoral artery; DFA = deep femoral artery; AKP = above-knee popliteal artery.
[b] Associated procedures include standard femoropopliteal, femoro-crural, femoro-femoral, and endoluminal femoropopliteal bypasses.
[c] Associated inflow procedure (axillofemoral or femorofemoral bypass or endoluminal aortoiliofemoral bypass).

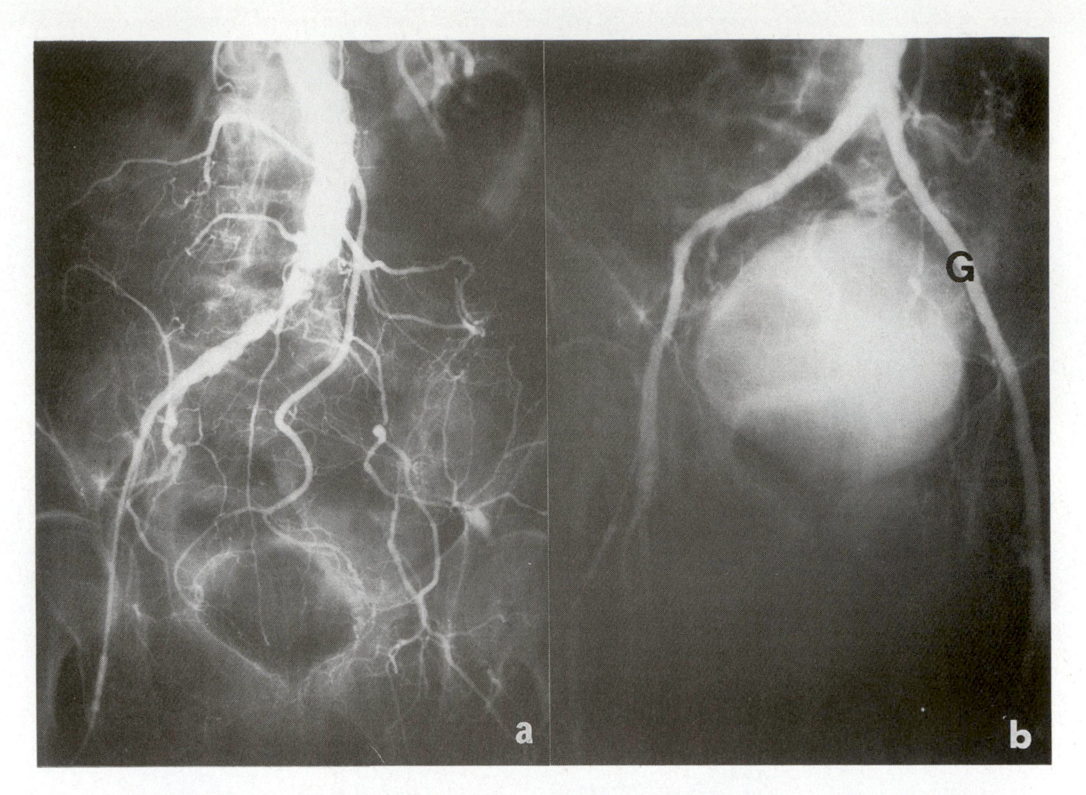

Figure 26–9. Transfemoral iliofemoral bypass for limb-threatening ischemia. (**a**) Prior to insertion of an endovascular graft, severe aortoiliac disease is demonstrated by this preoperative transfemoral arteriogram. Disease within the right common iliac artery system would preclude effective standard femorofemoral bypass to reestablish circulation to the left lower extremity in this 86-year-old woman. The left common and external iliac arteries are completely occluded. (**b**) Following long segment balloon dilatation of the left common and external iliac arteries and insertion of an endovascular graft (G), vascular continuity is established to the left lower extremity. A percutaneous balloon expandable stent has also been inserted into the right common iliac artery to treat the symptomatic high-grade common iliac artery stenosis and to protect the origin of the right common iliac artery during endovascular graft insertion. *(Reprinted with permission from Marin ML, Veith FJ, Cynamon J, et al. Initial experience with transluminally placed endovascular grafts for the treatment of complex vascular lesions. Ann Surg. 1995;222:449–469.)*

TABLE 26–5. PRIMARY PATENCY OF ENDOVASCULAR GRAFT PROCEDURES TO TREAT AORTOILIAC OCCLUSIVE DISEASE

Month	No. of Limbs at Risk	Closed	Dead	Duration	Interval Patency (%)	Cumulative Patency (%)	Standard Error
0–1	42	0	0	0	100	100	0
1–3	42	3	0	4	92.5	92.5	3.9
3–6	35	1	0	5	96.9	89.6	4.8
6–9	29	0	0	10	100	89.6	5.3
9–12	19	1	0	3	94.2	84.5	7.6
12–15	15	0	0	2	100	84.5	8.5
15–18	13	1	0	2	91.6	77.4	10.0

TABLE 26–6. SECONDARY PATENCY OF ENDOVASCULAR GRAFT PROCEDURES TO TREAT AORTOILIAC OCCLUSIVE DISEASE

Month	No. of Limbs at Risk	Closed	Dead	Duration	Interval Patency (%)	Cumulative Patency (%)	Standard Error
0–1	42	0	0	0	100	100	0
1–3	42	2	0	4	95	95	3.27
3–6	36	0	0	5	100	95	3.54
6–9	31	0	0	10	100	95	3.81
9–12	21	0	0	3	100	95	4.63
12–15	18	0	0	2	100	95	5.00
15–18	16	0	0	2	100	95	5.31

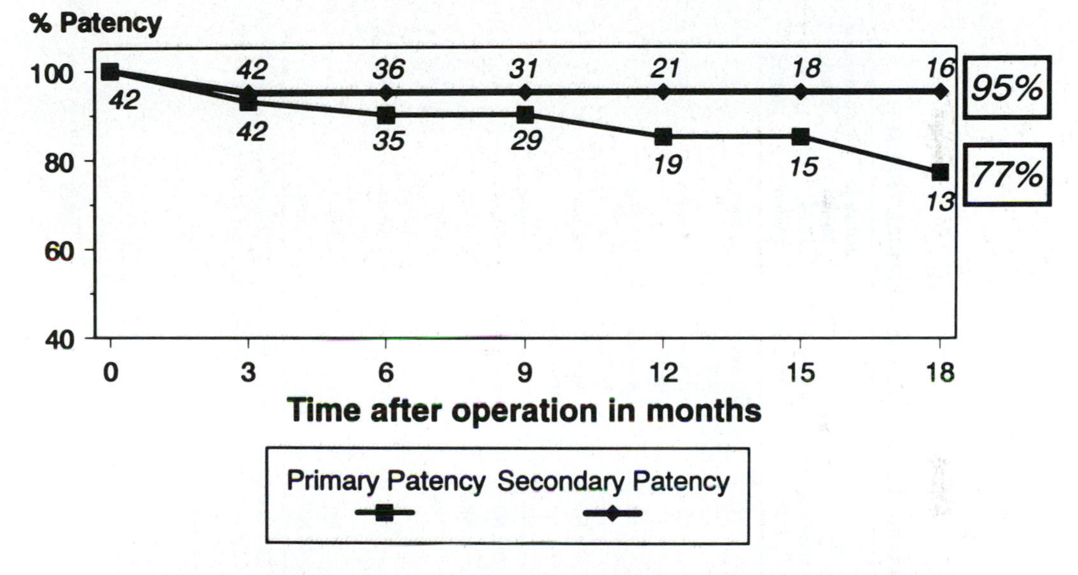

Figure 26–10. Cumulative 18-month primary and secondary patency rates for endovascular grafts. The numbers above or below each point indicate the number of grafts observed to be patent for that time period. *(Reprinted with permission from Marin ML, Veith FJ, Cynamon J, et al. Initial experience with transluminally placed endovascular grafts for the treatment of complex vascular lesions. Ann Surg. 1995;222:449–469.)*

TABLE 26–7. LIMB SALVAGE FOR PATIENTS WITH ENDOVASCULAR GRAFTS FOR THE TREATMENT OF AORTOILIAC OCCLUSIVE DISEASE

Month	No. of Limbs at Risk	Closed	Dead	Duration	Interval Patency (%)	Cumulative Patency (%)	Standard Error
0–1	42	0	0	0	100	100	0
1–3	42	1	0	4	97.5	97.5	2.3
3–6	37	0	0	5	100	97.5	2.5
6–9	32	0	0	10	100	97.5	2.7
9–12	22	0	0	3	100	97.5	3.2
12–15	19	0	0	2	100	97.5	3.5
15–18	17	0	0	2	100	97.5	3.7

TABLE 26–8. ENDOVASCULAR GRAFTS FOR PENETRATING OR IATROGENIC ARTERIAL TRAUMA

Sex/Age	Mechanism of Injury	Vessel(s) Involved[a]	Pseudoaneurysm	Arteriovenous Fistula	Associated Injuries	Injury to Repair Time Interval	Endovascular Graft Length (cm)	Access[a] Site	Hospital Stay (Days)	Patency
M/20	Bullet	LSFA LSFV	Yes	Yes	Soft tissue buttock	36 hours	3	LSFA percutaneous	5	28 months
M/28	Bullet	RSFA	Yes	No	Left open femur fracture	12 hours	3	RSFA arteriotomy	9	25 months
M/22	Bullet	LSFA	Yes	No	Soft tissue R. thigh, L. DVT	12 hours	3	LSFA arteriotomy	6	2 months[b]
M/24	Knife	LASA	Yes	No	Pneumothorax Hemothorax	4 hours	3	Left brachial arteriotomy	7	23 months
M/35	Bullet	RASA	Yes	No	Brachial plexus	3 weeks	3	Right brachial arteriotomy	4	19 months
F/78	Catheterization	RSA	Yes	No	Hemothorax	24 hours	3	Right brachial arteriotomy	56 weeks[c]	17 months
M/78	Catheterization	LCIA	Yes	No	None	4 months	2	LCFA arteriotomy	2	16 months
M/18	Bullet	RSA RSV	Yes	Yes	Rib fracture	1 week	3	LCFA arteriotomy	5	11 months
M/66	Iliac graft disruption	RCIA	Yes	No	None	2 weeks	12	LCFA arteriotomy	4	6 months
M/19	Bullet	RSA	Yes	No	Rib fracture	1 day	3	Right brachial arteriotomy	5	2 months
M/27	Bullet	RSA	Yes	No	None	4 hours	3	Right brachial arteriotomy	4	2 months

[a] LSFV = left superficial femoral vein; RSA = right subclavian artery; RSV = right subclavian vein; LCIA = left common iliac artery; RASA = right axillary-subclavian artery; LSFA = left superficial femoral artery; LASA = left axillary-subclavian artery; RSFA = right superficial femoral artery; RCA = right carotid artery; LCFA = left common femoral artery; RCIA = right common iliac artery.

[b] Died 2 months postprocedure (homicide).

[c] Hospitalized for multiple acute medical problems not directly related to the vascular trauma.

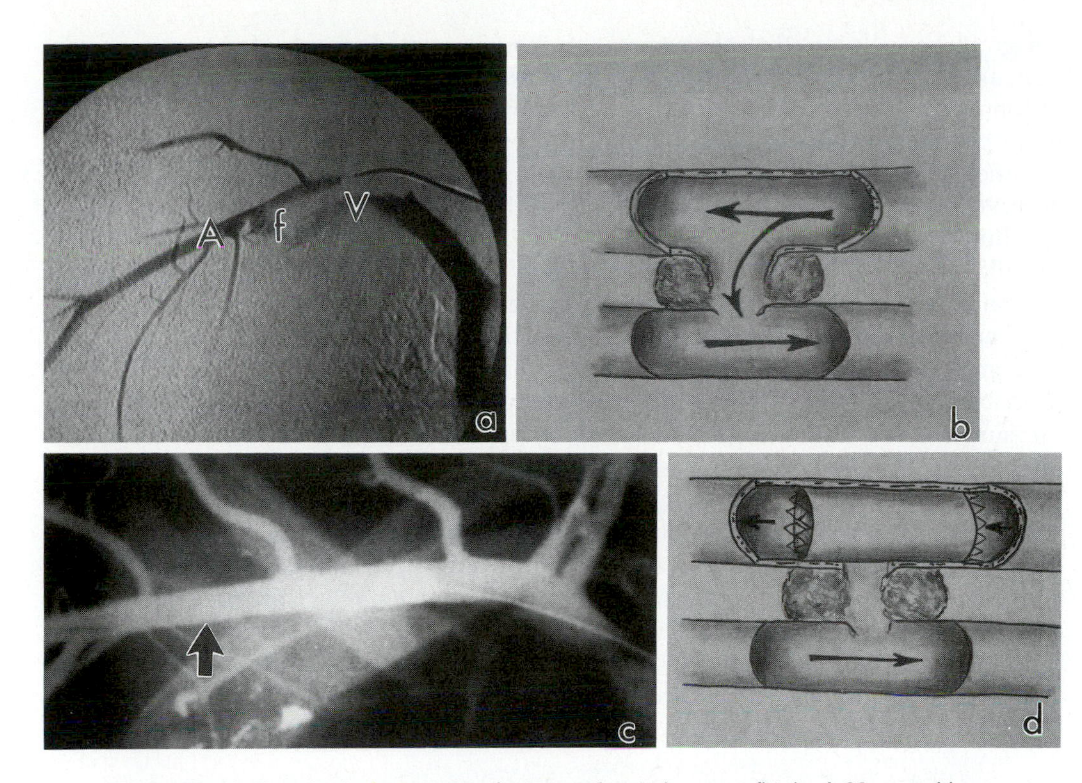

Figure 26–11. Transluminal treatment of a traumatic arteriovenous fistula. A 20-year-old man sustained a gunshot wound to the right upper chest. (**a**) A transfemoral arteriogram was performed that demonstrated a fistula between the distal subclavian artery and vein (f = fistula; v = vein; A = artery). (**b**) Schematic illustration of the fistula. (**c**) Under local anesthesia, an endovascular graft was inserted through a brachial artery cut-down. Following deployment of the device (*arrow*), a prograde arteriogram demonstrated occlusion of the arteriovenous fistula with preservation of the distal circulation. (**d**) Schematic drawing illustrating endovascular graft occlusion of a fistula. *(Reprinted with permission from Marin ML, Veith FJ, Cynamon J, et al. Initial experience with transluminally placed endovascular grafts for the treatment of complex vascular lesions. Ann Surg. 1995;222:449–469.)*

with a very high risk. These considerations have prompted us to treat with these endovascular graft devices those patients who were facing immediate loss of life or limb.

The advanced nature of the arterial pathology in most of our aneurysm and occlusive patients often made the endovascular grafting procedures lengthy and difficult and required that the endovascular graft be combined with some sort of relatively simple, open standard arterial surgical operation (e.g., a distal arterial reconstruction).[38] Even though these combined procedures were usually successful, they made it difficult to demonstrate that the endovascular approach reduced operating room usage or length of hospitalization. Such a demonstration was further hampered by the presence of advanced foot gangrene in many of our patients with occlusive disease. However, we believe the use of endovascular grafting techniques, when applied to lower-risk patients with less complex and advanced arterial pathology, will lead to a reduced requirement for hospitalization and lower costs. Suggestive evidence that this is so has already been documented with traumatic lesions and anatomically simple aortic aneurysms treated by endovascular grafts.[26,28]

Before endovascular grafts can be accepted for widespread use to treat aneurysms, they must be shown to effectively and permanently exclude the aneurysm from the arterial circulation and to prevent aneurysm expansion and rupture. The high rate of perigraft channels into the aneurysm sac and the associated reports of aneurysm expansion and rupture after endovascular graft treatment mandate caution before these techniques are used widely or without appropriately controlled studies.[59] Sealing of these channels by thrombosis may not prevent transmission of arterial pressure to the aneurysm wall. However, we are encouraged that aneurysm shrinkage has been observed in some of our cases and those of others.[32]

Endovascular stented grafts have a combined origin in the disciplines of both vascular surgery and interventional radiology. This and the fact that vascular surgeons and interventional radiologists have both been involved in the development and pioneering clinical use of these devices raises the question: Who should use them and who should control them? Both specialties have legitimate claims. The procedures described in this report have often been complex and difficult and have challenged the surgical and catheter guide wire skills of a combined group of surgeons and radiologists. Surgical and endovascular "rescue" techniques have often been required. It is, therefore, our belief that these devices should be used initially by a team of individuals who combine the highest levels of skill in vascular surgery and interventional radiology.[60,61] This has been effective in the developmental phase of these devices at our and other institutions. Ultimate development of a single, combined specialty or a group of specialists with dual skills working together will likely lead to the most rapid, effective advancement not only in the evolution of transluminally placed endovascular grafts but also in the treatment of vascular disease patients in general.

REFERENCES

1. Szilagyi DE, Smith RF, DeRusso FJ, et al. Contribution of abdominal aortic aneurysmectomy to prolongation of life. *Ann Surg.* 1966;164:678–679.
2. Crawford ES, Saleh SA, Babb JW III, et al. Infrarenal abdominal aortic aneurysm. Factors influencing survival after operation over a 25-year period. *Ann Surg.* 1981;193:699–709.
3. DeBakey ME, Crawford ES, Cooley DA, et al. Aneurysm of abdominal aorta: analysis of results of graft replacement therapy one to eleven years after operation. *Ann Surg.* 1964;160:622–639.
4. AbuRahma AF, Robinson PA, Boland JP, et al. Elective resection of 332 abdominal aortic aneurysms in a southern West Virginia community during a recent five-year period. *Surgery.* 1991;109:244–251.
5. Johnson KW, Scobie TK. Multicenter prospective study of nonruptured abdominal aortic aneurysms. I. Population and operative management. *J Vasc Surg.* 1988;7:69–81.
6. Veith FJ, Gupta SK, Wengerter KR, et al. Changing arteriosclerotic disease patterns and management strategies in lower-limb-threatening ischemia. *Ann Surg.* 1990;212:402–414.
7. Mattox KL, Feliciano DV, Burch J, et al. Five thousand seven hundred sixty cardiovascular injuries in 4459 patients. Epidemiologic evaluation 1958 to 1987. *Ann Surg.* 1989;209:698–707.
8. Lim RC Jr, Trunkey DD, Blaisdell FW. Acute abdominal aortic injury. An analysis of operative and postoperative management. *Arch Surg.* 1974;109:706–711.
9. Snyder WH III, Thal ER, Perry MO. Peripheral and abdominal vascular injuries. In: Rutherford RB, ed. *Vascular Surgery.* 2nd ed. Philadelphia: WB Saunders; 1984:460–500.
10. McCombs PR, Roberts B. Acute renal failure following resection of abdominal aortic aneurysm. *Surg Gyn Obstet.* 1979;148:175–178.
11. Gardner RJ, Gardner NL, Tarnay TJ, et al. The surgical experience and a one to sixteen year follow-up of 277 abdominal aortic aneurysms. *Am J Surg.* 1978;135:226–230.
12. Thompson JE, Hollier LH, Patman RD, et al. Surgical management of abdominal aortic aneurysms: factors influencing mortality and morbidity—a 20 year experience. *Ann Surg.* 1975;181:654–661.

13. Hollier LH, Reigel MM, Kazmier FJ, et al. Conventional repair of abdominal aortic aneurysm in the high-risk patient. A plea for abandonment of nonresective treatment. *J Vasc Surg.* 1986;3:712–717.
14. Sher MH. Principles in the management of arterial injuries associated with fracture/dislocations. *Ann Surg.* 1975;182:630–634.
15. Flint LM, Richardson JD. Arterial injuries with lower extremity fracture. *Surgery.* 1983;93:5–8.
16. Mattox KL, Whisennand HH, Espada R, et al. Management of acute combined injuries to the aorta and inferior vena cava. *Am J Surg.* 1975;130:720–724.
17. Volodos NL, Shekhanin VE, Karpovich IP, et al. Self-fixing synthetic prosthesis for endoprosthetics of the vessels. *Vestn Khir* 1986;137:123–125.
18. Parodi JC, Palmaz JC, Barone HD. Transfemoral intraluminal graft implantation for abdominal aortic aneurysms. *Ann Vasc Surg.* 1991;5:491–499.
19. Volodos NL, Karpovich IP, Troyan VI, et al. Clinical experience of the use of self-fixing synthetic prostheses for remote endoprosthetics of the thoracic and the abdominal aorta and iliac arteries through the femoral artery and as intraoperative endoprosthesis for aorta reconstruction. *Vasa Suppl.* 1991;33:93–95.
20. Marin ML, Veith FJ, Panetta TF, et al. Percutaneous transfemoral insertion of a stented graft to repair a traumatic femoral arteriovenous fistula. *J Vasc Surg.* 1993;18:299–302.
21. Cragg AH, Dake MD. Percutaneous femoropopliteal graft placement. *J Vasc Interv Radiol.* 1993;4:455–463.
22. May J, White G, Waugh R, et al. Transluminal placement of a prosthetic graft-stent device for treatment of subclavian artery aneurysm. *J Vasc Surg.* 1993;18:1056–1059.
23. Parodi JC, Barone HD. Transfemoral placement of aortic grafts in aortic aneurysms: clinical experience in patients. In: Yao JST, Pearce WH, eds. *Aneurysms: New Findings and Treatments.* Norwalk, CT: Appleton & Lange; 1994:341–349.
24. Marin ML, Veith FJ, Panetta TF, et al. Transfemoral endoluminal stented graft repair of a popliteal artery aneurysm. *J Vasc Surg.* 1994;19:754–757.
25. Marin ML, Veith FJ, Cynamon J, et al. Transfemoral endovascular stented graft treatment of aorto-iliac and femoropopliteal occlusive disease for limb salvage. *Am J Surg.* 1994;168:156–162.
26. Marin ML, Veith FJ, Panetta TF, et al. Transluminally placed endovascular stented graft repair for arterial trauma. *J Vasc Surg.* 1994;20:466–473.
27. Marin ML, Veith FJ. Transfemoral repair of abdominal aortic aneurysm. *N Engl J Med.* 1994;331:1751.
28. Moore WS, Vescera CL. Repair of abdominal aortic aneurysm by transfemoral endovascular graft placement. *Ann Surg.* 1994;220:331–341.
29. Dake MD, Miller DC, Semba CP, et al. Transluminal placement of endovascular stent-grafts for the treatment of descending thoracic aortic aneurysms. *N Engl J Med.* 1994;331:1729–1734.
30. May J, White G, Waugh R, et al. Treatment of complex abdominal aortic aneurysms by a combination of endoluminal and extraluminal aortofemoral grafts. *J Vasc Surg.* 1994;19:924–933.
31. May J, White GH, Yu W, et al. Endoluminal grafting of abdominal aortic aneurysms: causes of failure and their prevention. *J Endovasc Surg.* 1994;1:44–52.
32. Parodi JC. Endovascular repair of abdominal aortic aneurysms and other arterial lesions. *J Vasc Surg.* 1995;21:549–557.
33. Scott RAP, Chuter TAM. Clinical endovascular placement of bifurcated graft in abdominal aortic aneurysm without laparotomy. *Lancet.* 1994;343:413.
34. Yusuf SW, Baker DM, Chuter TAM, et al. Transfemoral endoluminal repair of abdominal aortic aneurysm with bifurcated graft. *Lancet.* 1994;344:350–351.
35. Mialhe C. Clinical experience with the Stentor bifurcated device for treatment of abdominal aortic aneurysmal disease. *International Congress VIII on Endovascular Interventions.* February 12–16, 1995; Scottsdale, AZ.
36. Marin ML, Veith FJ, Lyon RT, et al. Transfemoral endovascular repair of iliac artery aneurysms. *Am J Surg.* 1995;170:179–182.
37. Sanchez LA, Marin ML, Veith FJ, et al. Placement of endovascular stented grafts via remote access sites: a new approach to the treatment of failed aortoiliofemoral reconstructions. *Ann Vasc Surg.* 1995;9:1–8.

38. Marin ML, Veith FJ, Sanchez LA, et al. Endovascular aortoiliac grafts in combination with standard infrainguinal arterial bypasses in the management of limb-threatening ischemia: preliminary report. *J Vasc Surg.* 1995;22:316–325.
39. Parodi JC. Transfemoral intraluminal graft implantation for abdominal aortic aneurysm. In: Greenhalgh RM, ed. *Vascular and Endovascular Surgical Techniques.* 3rd ed. London: WB Saunders; 1994:71–77.
40. Moore WS. Transfemoral endovascular repair of abdominal aortic aneurysm using the endovascular graft system device. In: Greenhalgh RM, ed. *Vascular and Endovascular Surgical Techniques.* 3rd ed. London: WB Saunders; 1994:78–91.
41. Marin ML, Veith FJ. Endoluminal stented graft aorto-bifemoral reconstruction. In: Greenhalgh RM, ed. *Vascular and Endovascular Surgical Techniques.* 3rd ed. London: WB Saunders; 1994:100–104.
42. Dotter CT, Judkins MP. Transluminal treatment of arteriosclerotic obstruction. Description of a new technic and a preliminary report of its application. *Circulation.* 1964;30:654–670.
43. Dotter CT. Transluminally-placed coilspring endarterial tube grafts. Long-term patency in canine popliteal artery. *Invest Radiol.* 1969;4:329–332.
44. Johnston KW, Rae M, Hogg-Johnston SA, et al. 5-year results of a prospective study of percutaneous transluminal angioplasty. *Ann Surg.* 1987;206:403–413.
45. van Andel GJ, van Erp WFM, Krepel VM, et al. Percutaneous transluminal dilatation of the iliac artery: long-term results. *Radiology.* 1985;156:321–323.
46. King SB III, Schlumpf M. Ten-year completed follow-up of percutaneous transluminal coronary angioplasty: the early Zurich experience. *J Am Coll Cardiol.* 1993;22:353–360.
47. Palmaz JC, Laborde JC, Rivera FJ, et al. Stenting of the iliac arteries with the Palmaz stent: experience from a multicenter trial. *Cardiovasc Intervent Radiol.* 1992;15:291–297.
48. Dotter CT, Buschmann RW, McKinney MK. Transluminal expandable nitinol coil stent grafting: preliminary report. *Radiology.* 1983;147:259–260.
49. Cragg A, Lund G, Rysavy J, et al. Nonsurgical placement of arterial endoprostheses: a new technique using nitinol wire. *Radiology.* 1983;147:261–263.
50. Maass D, Kropf L, Egloff L, et al. Transluminal implantation of intravascular "double-helix" spiral prostheses: technical and biological considerations. *Eur Soc Artif Organs Proc.* 1982;9:252–256.
51. Balko A, Piasecki GJ, Shah DM, et al. Transfemoral placement of intraluminal polyurethane prosthesis for abdominal aortic aneurysm. *J Surg Res.* 1986;40:305–309.
52. Mirich D, Wright KC, Wallace S, et al. Percutaneously placed endovascular grafts for aortic aneurysms: feasibility study. *Radiology.* 1989;170:1033–1037.
53. Chuter TAM, Green RM, Ouriel K, et al. Transfemoral endovascular aortic graft placement. *J Vasc Surg.* 1993;18:185–197.
54. Laborde JC, Parodi JC, Clem MF, et al. Intraluminal bypass of abdominal aortic aneurysm: feasibility study. *Radiology.* 1992;184:185–190.
55. Chuter TAM, Wendt G, Hopkinson BR, et al. Early clinical experience with bifurcated endovascular grafts for abdominal aortic aneurysm repair. *International Congress VIII on Endovascular Interventions.* February 12–16, 1995; Scottsdale, AZ.
56. May J. Comparison of the Sydney and EVT prostheses for treatment of aneurysmal disease. *International Congress VIII on Endovascular Interventions.* February 12–16, 1995; Scottsdale, AZ.
57. Henry M, Amor M, Ethevenot G. Initial experience with the Cragg Endopro System 1 for intraluminal treatment of peripheral vascular disease: report of the first 64 cases. *International Congress VIII on Endovascular Interventions.* February 12–16, 1995; Scottsdale, AZ.
58. Veith FJ, Abbott WM, Yao JST, et al. Endovascular Graft Committee. Guidelines for development and use of transluminally placed endovascular prosthetic grafts in the arterial system. *J Vasc Surg.* 1995;21:670–685.
59. Lumsden AB, Allen RC, Chaikof EL, et al. Delayed rupture of aortic aneurysm following endovascular stent grafting. *Am J Surg.* 1995;170:174–178.
60. Veith FJ. Transluminally placed endovascular stented grafts and their impact on vascular surgery. *J Vasc Surg.* 1994;20:855–860.
61. Veith FJ, Marin ML. Endovascular surgery and its effect on the relationship between vascular surgery and radiology. *J Endovasc Surg.* 1995;2:1–7.

27

Wound Complications of the *In Situ* Saphenous Vein Technique

Jonathan B. Towne, MD

WOUND COMPLICATIONS OF THE *IN SITU* SAPHENOUS VEIN TECHNIQUE

The *in situ* saphenous vein bypass technique is an excellent way to revascularize the ischemic lower extremity when an adequate greater saphenous vein is available. The advantages of this technique include high patency rates, size matching of vein and artery at the anastomosis, decreased surgical trauma of the vein and its vaso vasorum, and the ability to use small diameter (<4 mm) veins successfully.[1] The technique's main disadvantage is its placement of the graft in the subcutaneous tissues, which leaves the bypass vulnerable to wound healing problems. Despite extensive use of this technique, wound healing problems are still common. This chapter describes the incidence and treatment of these problems.

SURGICAL TECHNIQUE

To understand our operative results, a familiarity with the technique used by the authors is necessary.[1] The entire saphenous vein as well as the distal and proximal arteries are exposed to a continuous incision beginning at the inflow artery and continuing below the knee. The saphenofemoral junction is completely dissected, and venous tributaries at the fossa ovalis are ligated and divided. After the administration of 5,000 units of heparin, the saphenous vein is divided at the saphenofemoral junction, and the common femoral vein is oversewn. The proximal two or three valves are incised. To bring the saphenous vein in juxtaposition with the common femoral artery for construction of a proximal anastomosis, an 8- to 10-cm length of proximal vein is mobilized and end-to-side anastomosis performed. Flow is restored down the vein to the next competent valve. All distal valves are incised with the Leather valvulotome. The distal saphenous vein is mobilized for approximately 15 cm and marked with methylene blue to prevent axial rotation. The posterior tibial and peroneal arteries are exposed through the incision used to expose the saphenous vein, and the anterior tibial artery is approached with an incision lateral to the tibia in the anterior compartment. The arteries are not circumferentially dissected, since a pneumatic tourniquet is used for distal vascular control for the construction of the distal anastomosis.

Following completion of the anastomosis, the tourniquet is released and the side branches of the saphenous vein are ligated. An intraoperative pulsed Doppler probe with real-time spectral analysis is used to find remaining vein side branches and to analyze the graft for incomplete valve incision and anastomotic technical defects. Operative arteriography is used to assure the ligation of arteriovenous fistulae and to document a technically satisfactory distal anastomosis. The skin is closed over the graft with either continuous or interrupted nylon mattress sutures, except in the groin where successive layers of absorbable suture are used to approximate the subcutaneous tissue prior to skin closure. Patients routinely receive perioperative Cefazolin (1 or 2 g) for 1 to 3 days and, if they are on antibiotics to treat an existing foot infection, these are continued in the postoperative period.

CLASSIFICATION OF WOUND INFECTION

A wound complication is defined as a problem with the incisional wound that consists of any or all of the following: (1) wound erythema or cellulitis for which antibiotics are prescribed; (2) skin edge or subcutaneous fat necrosis, or lymphatic leak that necessitates dressing changes and antibiotic therapy; and (3) infection.[2] The latter term is used for any wound that has signs and symptoms of infection with drainable purulence that on swab culture grew organisms.

Our wound treatment protocol consists of bed rest and dressing changes several times daily. All patients with wound problems received broad-spectrum parenteral antibiotics. Results of the wound cultures, or when not available, of recent pedal infections, are used to select antibiotic therapy. If no cultures are available, a broad-spectrum cephalosporin is empirically prescribed. Antibiotics were continued for 5 days or until the infection had subsided. If a deeper wound problem was suspected, patients were taken to the operating room for sharp debridement with inspection of the graft. If the graft was covered by viable tissue, bedside wound care was begun. If the graft was not incorporated, the surrounding necrotic or infected tissue was sharply debrided and the graft immediately covered with autogenous tissue.

Patients with wound complications were classified using the modification by Wengrovitz et al. of the Szialgyi system developed for grading wound complications after prosthetic arterial reconstruction.[3,4] These were: Class 1—wound edge skin necrosis or lymphatic leak treated with parenteral antibiotics; Class 2—wound infection or necrosis involving subcutaneous tissue; and Class 3—invasive wound infections to the depth of wound about the graft.

INCIDENCE OF GRAFT INFECTION

In order to determine the incidence of wound complication in our series, we reviewed 126 consecutive patients who underwent *in situ* bypasses, 45 (36%) of which were femoropopliteal, 75 (59%) were femorocrural, and 6 (5%) were popliteal-distal bypasses.[2] All but three operations were done for critical ischemia, and 55% of these patients had an ischemic ulcer, dry gangrene, or nonhealing toe amputation site as their operative indication. Of these patients, 46% were diabetic and 80% were smokers. Cefazolin was given in the perioperative period to 86% of the patients, with an average duration of coverage of 56 hours. The other patients received a variety of antibiotics on the basis of culture results of existing foot lesions.

Wound complications developed in 44% of the operative extremities. Twenty percent consisted solely of wound erythema, which resolved with parenteral antibiotic therapy. Thirty-five percent involved skin edge necrosis or lymphatic leaks with surrounding erythema and were considered Class 1 wounds. All these resolved with bed rest, protective dressings, and antibiotic therapy except for one, which required exploration and closure of a persistent lymph leak. Twenty-two percent of the patients developed Class 2 wound infections. Twenty-four percent of the wounds were Class 3.

RISK FACTORS THAT PREDISPOSE PATIENTS FOR INFECTION

Risk factor analysis was then performed to try to determine which factors showed a predisposition to cause infections. We found that age, race, diabetes, coronary artery disease, and smoking were not related to postoperative wound complications. Likewise, operative characteristics such as outflow vessel, duration of operation, preoperative antibiotic usage, preoperative gangrene or ulceration, and early reoperation also were not related to overall postoperative wound complications.

However, two predictors that influenced postoperative wound infections were found. If the patient had a graft revision within 4 days for a thrombosed graft, retained valve, large arterial venous fistula, or wound hematoma, these patients had a significantly higher risk of subsequent wound infection developing. More than one-half the patients with Class 3 wound infections in this series had early graft revision. The development of a postoperative lymph leak, a Class 1 wound complication, was also significantly related to subsequent wound infections. The presence of skin edge necrosis, however, did not reliably predate the onset of a wound infection.

Complete culture data were available from all the Class 3 wounds in this study. Wound infections were caused by a myriad of bacterial species, with 6 of 13 wounds having polymicrobial infections. Gram-positive cocci predominated in lower leg infections, with 7 of 13 cultures positive for *Staphylococcus aureus,* whereas gram-negative bacteria were involved in groin infections.

Patients with skin edge necrosis or lymphatic leaks, which are considered Class 1 wounds, were treated significantly earlier than patients with Class 2 or Class 3 wounds. Class 3 wounds tended to occur later than Class 2 wounds, although this did not reach statistical significance. Half of the patients with Class 2 wounds and 9 of the 13 with Class 3 wounds had already been discharged from the hospital and were found to have suppurating wounds at clinic follow-up, whereas all Class 1 wounds were detected during the patients' original admission. Of the 15 patients with Class 2 or Class 3 wounds that had been discharged before discovery of their problem, 8 had experienced either erythema, lymph leaks, skin edge necrosis, or blistered skin during their hospitalization that had resolved before discharge. The location of the wound problem also varied with the severity. Sixty-eight percent of Class 1 wounds occurred primarily in the groin, Class 2 wounds were evenly distributed down the leg, whereas 77% of Class 3 wounds were distally located.

All but one patient left the hospital with a patent graft and his or her wounds intact. That single patient required an above-knee amputation for persistent forefoot infection despite multiple debridements and a patent bypass graft. No deaths or limb loss occurred as a result of incisional wound problems. One patient who underwent femoroperoneal *in situ* bypass complicated by a Class 2 wound complication developed ipsilateral knee septic arthritis and subacute bacterial endocarditis over the ensuing 4 months. His wound, knee, and blood all grew the same staphylococcal organism. Another patient who had a femoroposterior tibial *in situ* bypass complicated by early postoperative wound erythema was admitted to an outside hospital 64 days later bleeding from a distal anastomotic disruption. The graft was ligated at the hospital as a life-saving measure, and the patient was immediately transferred. On arrival, his graft was still pulsatile and was therefore revised into a femoropopliteal bypass. Although his outflow at that level was diseased, the graft remained patent with subsequent limb salvage.

Wound complications are frequent with *in situ* bypass. In our series, 44% of the patients required additional treatment for wound problems. If wounds treated empirically with antibiotics for erythema are removed from analysis, then 35% of the limbs had open wound complications. This incidence is consistent with recent reports of *in situ* or subcutaneously placed vein grafts in which wound complication rates ranged from 17% to 33%, with one-third being major graft-threatening infections. Wengrovitz and associates[3] reported 17% incidence of wound complications following subcutaneous lower extremity bypass grafting. These included revised, nonrevised, and *in situ* grafts. They noted female gender, chronic steroid therapy, use of continuous incision, diabetes mellitus, ipsilateral limb ulcers, and pedal bypass as related to development of infection. On regression analysis, only diabetes, steroid therapy, ipsilateral ulcers, and pedal bypass predicted increased incidence of wound complication. Schwartz et al.[5] noted a 33% incidence of wound complications in a series of only *in situ* bypasses. These authors noted a significant relationship of a continuous incision and anterior tibial bypass. Regression analysis indicated that anterior tibial bypass and staple closure were the principle predisposing factors. Donaldson et al.[6] had an incidence of wound problems of only 7.2%, which is one of the best results in the literature.

TREATMENT ALTERNATIVES

The critical aspect in the treatment of Class 3 wounds is operative debridement and immediate coverage with autogenous tissue. Ouriel et al.[7] delayed coverage of exposed vein grafts until wounds were clean and granulating, and then coverage was obtained with split thickness skin grafts or musculocutaneous flaps. Despite these efforts graft rupture was a problem in 56%. With immediate coverage, we suffered no late failures. Although coverage of the grafts with muscle is preferable, expedient coverage with any autogenous tissue to avoid desiccation of the graft from exposure prevents subsequent rupture. In the groin, the sartorius muscle is easiest to use.[8] Since the blood supply originates from the profunda femoris artery, a patent profunda is required. Best results are obtained if the muscle is detached from its origin at the anterior superior iliac spine. The muscle is then rolled so that the lateral border becomes the medial border so as to not injure the blood supply as it enters the medial aspect of the muscle. The gracilis and rectus abdominus muscles can also be used. Their use requires additional incisions and are more involved. When distal grafts are exposed, adjacent muscle can often be mobilized to cover the conduit.

BACTERIOLOGY

The type of infecting organism has been implicated as a predictor of vein graft disruption. Although Ouriel et al.[7] had poor outcomes when exposed grafts were infected with gram-negative organisms, we did not find this to be the case. None of our patients, however, were infected with *Pseudomonas aeruginosa*, which can be particularly virulent. The only case of graft hemorrhage occurred in a wound from which *Staphylococcus aureus* was cultured.

PREVENTION

Because of the association with early graft revision and the development of Class 3 wounds, it is imperative to try as much as possible to prevent early reoperation. Meticulous hemostasis and the precise anastomosis are essential to minimize postoperative failures.

The wound problems in the groin and thigh are inherent to the area of the dissection. The groin lymphatics are traversed during dissection of the femoral vessels and proximal saphenous vein. To avoid postoperative lymph fistulas or lymphoceles, lymphatic channels should be ligated. Compounding this, in locating and exposing the saphenous vein, undermining of the skin with the creation of a skin flap is not unusual and may result in skin edge necrosis. Gentle surgical technique and accurately placed incisions will prevent many wound problems. Mapping of the saphenous vein before operation in the hope of eliminating wide skin flaps is recommended.

The etiology of Class 3 wounds, found mainly in the calf, were of a different etiology. These tended to occur at a mean time of 31.2 days, with most patients being readmitted with deep suppurating wounds. To control the infection and protect the graft, most of these patients need operative therapy. The cause of the delayed appearance and the etiology of these infections is undoubtedly multifactorial. Two of the Class 3 wounds were caused by infected hematomas. Ten had additional antibiotics for prophylaxis during secondary operations or to treat wound erythema. This may have suppressed any developing infection, allowing it to appear only after the antibiotics had been stopped. Postoperative edema, caused mainly by lymphatic disruption, may also contribute to delay wound healing and may promote infection.[9] Lastly, we believe that subcutaneous fat necrosis that becomes secondarily infected may be contributory. Fat necrosis is probably caused by surgical trauma and its poor inherent blood supply. Meticulous surgical technique cannot be stressed enough.

Recent improvements in angioscopy equipment now permit endoscopic visualization of the greater saphenous vein and its branches. This enables one to use smaller incisions when preparing the vein for bypass. Potentially, this can go a long way toward minimizing wound complications. Ultimately, perfecting surgical technique is the best measure of minimizing wound complications. This includes conducting the bypass procedure in a precise way, minimizing skin flap development, careful handling of all tissues, and meticulous wound closure.

REFERENCES

1. Bergamini TM, Towne JB, Bandyk DF, et al. Experience with *in situ* saphenous vein bypasses during 1981 to 1989: determinant factors of long-term patency. *J Vasc Surg*. 1991;13:137–147.
2. Reifsnyder T, Bandyk D, Seabrook GR, et al. Wound complications of the *in situ* saphenous vein bypass technique. *J Vasc Surg*. 1992;15:843–850.
3. Wengrovitz M, Atnip RG, Gifford RRM, et al. Wound complications of autogenous subcutaneous infrainguinal arterial bypass surgery: predisposing factors and management. *J Vasc Surg*. 1990;11:156–163.

4. Szilagyi DE, Smith RF, Elliot JP, et al. Infection in arterial reconstruction with synthetic grafts. *Ann Surg*. 1972;176:321–333.
5. Schwartz ME, Harrington EB, Schanzer H. Wound complications after *in situ* bypass. *J Vasc Surg*. 1988;7:802–807.
6. Donaldson MC, Whittemore AD, Mannick JA. Further experience with an all-autogenous tissue policy for infrainguinal reconstruction. *J Vasc Surg*. 1993;18:41–48.
7. Ouriel K, Geary KJ, Green RM, et al. Fate of the exposed saphenous vein graft. *Am J Surg*. 1990;160:148–150.
8. Mixter RC, Turnipseed WD, Smith DJ Jr, et al. Rotational muscle flap: a new technique for covering infected vascular grafts. *J Vasc Surg*. 1989;9:472–478.
9. Hunt TK, Rabkin J, Von Smitten K. Effects of edema and anemia on wound healing and infection. *Curr Stud Hematol Blood Trans*. 1986;53:101–111.

28

Aneurysms of the Gluteal and Persistent Sciatic Arteries

Eugene F. Bernstein, MD, PhD

Although extremely rare, aneurysms of the gluteal and sciatic arteries can be life-threatening if misdiagnosed and improperly treated. Therefore, a basic understanding of the most common presentations and the appropriate contemporary approaches to diagnosis and management are essential for those physicians who may be called on to identify and treat such pathology.

SURGICAL ANATOMY

All the visceral branches of the pelvis are derived from the internal iliac (hypogastric) artery.[1] The internal iliac runs medial to the psoas muscle, descends vertically into the pelvis, provides the iliolumbar and lateral sacral branches, and then divides into anterior and posterior divisions (Fig. 28–1A)*. The anterior division is the origin of the obturator, inferior gluteal, and internal pudendal branches, and is the main arterial supply to the pelvic viscera. The inferior gluteal artery leaves the pelvis through the infrapiriform space along with the sciatic nerve and proceeds to supply the gluteal musculature, as well as a small branch along the sciatic nerve—the sciatic artery. In cases of persistant sciatic artery, the inferior gluteal remains quite large as the sciatic artery (see "Embryology," later in this chapter). From the posterior approach, the inferior gluteal artery appears at the lower border of the pyriformis muscle and runs with the sciatic nerve to the interval between the greater trochanter and the tuberosity of the ischium (Fig. 28–1B)*. These vessels are covered by the thick gluteus maximus muscle layer.

The superior gluteal artery is the continuation of the posterior division of the internal iliac artery and is distributed to the gluteal muscles of the buttock after passing through the suprapiriform space (Fig. 28–1A)*. From a posterior approach, the superior gluteal artery enters the gluteal region through the greater sciatic foramen between the gluteus medius and pyriformis muscles, and then divides to provide the main arterial blood supply to the muscles of the buttock (Fig. 28–1C)*.

* Figure 28–1 is a color plate following page 138.

GLUTEAL ARTERY ANEURYSM

Historic Background

The earliest description of a successful surgical treatment of a traumatic gluteal aneurysm was published in the *British Medical Journal* in 1898 by William Henry Battle.[2] The patient was thrown from a horse, with his right buttock landing on a rock. Subsequently, a large swelling appeared in the gluteal region with expansile pulsation and pain down the back of the thigh and leg. There was no bruit, tenderness, or fever. The pulsating mass could be compressed by the examiners.

A diagnosis of aneurysm was made on these clinical grounds, with concern regarding the differential diagnosis of a pulsating sarcoma. Under ether anesthesia, an operation included a preliminary intraperitoneal incision for pressure control of the internal iliac artery. A right gluteal incision then permitted evacuation of blood and clot, exposure of the torn artery near the sciatic notch, and suture ligation of several bleeding sites. The patient survived.

The principles of diagnosis and treatment in this first reported surgical case are fundamental to understanding the current approaches to this entity, which has been reported in more than 100 cases.

Presentation

Gluteal artery aneurysm usually presents as a painful pulsating buttock mass with or without a bruit, murmur, thrill, or evidence of inflammation.[3-5] Pain, paresthesias, numbness, and paresis may be observed in the distribution of the sciatic nerve. A history of recent or distant penetrating injury, blunt trauma, and pelvic fracture should be sought. The superior gluteal artery is more commonly injured by penetrating trauma, while the inferior gluteal artery is more commonly injured in association with blunt trauma, and especially in association with pelvic fractures. Inferior gluteal artery injury is far more common than superior. Gluteal artery aneurysm is said to be more common on the left side, far more common in males than females, and most frequently observed in people between 20 and 40 years of age. Other important considerations include a history or evidence of prior endocarditis or other sources of systemic sepsis that might be associated with a septic embolus, evidence of a sciatic compartment syndrome, or a history consistent with polyarteritis nodosa or Type IV Ehlers-Danlos syndrome.[6-10] A summary of the presentations in reports since 1962 is found in Table 28–1.

TABLE 28–1. FREQUENCY OF PRESENTATION OF GLUTEAL ARTERY ANEURYSMS (STUDIES SINCE 1962)

Presentation	No. Reported	Incorrect Diagnosis	Mortality
Penetrating injury	12	7	2
Blunt trauma	3	3	0
Gluteal IM injection	2	0	0
Septic embolus	1	0	0
Polyarteritis nodosa	1	0	0
Ehlers-Danlos syndrome Type IV	1	0	0
Septic embolus	1	0	0

Diagnostic Considerations

With a history of recent trauma and the rapid development of a large pulsatile buttock mass, formal contrast angiography is the definitive initial diagnostic modality and will confirm the precise diagnosis, anatomic localization, and a method of treatment with endovascular techniques. Under less clearly defined and more chronic circumstances, however, preliminary CT or MRI scans are appropriate. Of these, the MRI appears to provide more precise soft-tissue information and can be coupled with an MR angiogram to define the vessels of origin, as well as the vascular nature of the primary lesion.[11]

Both true and false aneurysms of both the superior and inferior gluteal arteries have been described, but true aneurysms are very rare. The differential diagnosis must include abscess, chronic bursitis, sciatic hernia, lipoma, echinococcal cyst, and sarcoma. However, since gluteal artery aneurysm can be a life-threatening entity, swellings of the buttock should be considered gluteal aneurysms until an alternative diagnosis has been confirmed.

Treatment

Since Battle's initial report in 1898, the standard surgical approach has included a preliminary proximal arterial control procedure through either a retroperitoneal or transperitoneal approach, followed by a posterior approach to the aneurysm itself, with evacuation of the aneurysm contents and surrounding hematoma and endoaneurysmorrhaphy of the lesion by internal suture.[2,5] In those cases in which the diagnosis has been made preoperatively, surgical results have generally been excellent. However, serious problems have been reported when the aneurysm was unrecognized and an incision of a "pulsating abscess" was undertaken, frequently with massive, and occasionally fatal, hemorrhage. Ligation of the feeding arteries alone may not provide definitive control, with a return of pulsation from collateral sources several days later. Thus, opening the aneurysm and ligation of all vessels from within is considered essential for permanent resolution of the lesion.

Recently, endovascular approaches to the definitive control of gluteal aneurysms have been described, including balloon catheter occlusion of the aneurysm entrance, metal coil insertion, and superselective embolization. Each of these procedures has been successful with prolonged control of pulsation and expansion. However, the mass of blood and clot is not removed in these endovascular efforts and may be a nidus for subsequent infection or mass-induced pain. Late drainage of such residual masses has been reported.

PERSISTENT SCIATIC ARTERY ANEURYSM

Embryology

When the human embryo reaches 5 mm the lower limb bud appears, and at 6 mm the axial artery originates from the dorsal root of the umbilical artery, from which the external iliac and femoral arteries are subsequently derived[11,12] (Fig. 28–2A). During this period, the sciatic artery, a branch of the internal iliac, is the dominant blood supply to the lower limb through the 14-mm stage (Fig. 28–2B). As the femoral artery enlarges, the sciatic artery involutes, and its remnants participate in the formation of the inferior gluteal, profunda femoris, popliteal, peroneal, and pedal arterial systems (Fig. 28–2C).

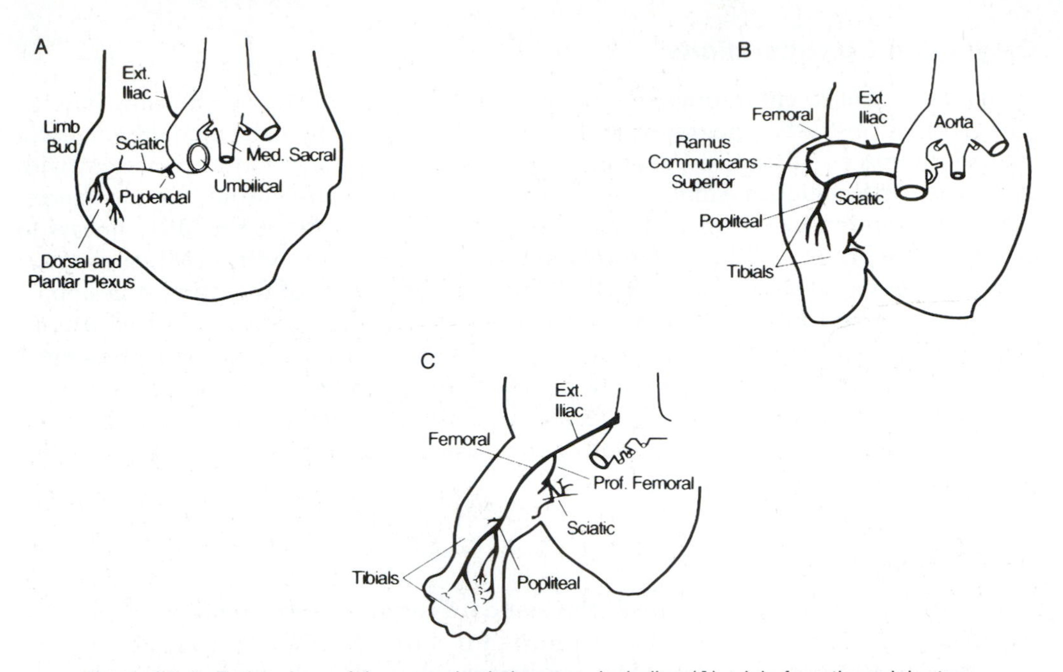

Figure 28–2. Embryology of the normal sciatic artery, including (**A**) origin from the axial artery, (**B**) parallel system of external iliac and sciatic arteries, and (**C**) involution of the sciatic artery. *(Adapted from Shutze WP, Garrett WV, Smith BL. Persistent sciatic artery: collective review and management. Ann Vasc Surg. 1993;7:303–310.)*

Pathology

If involution fails to occur, the axial system may persist as the dominant blood supply to the lower extremity in one of two forms: (1) the "complete" form of the anomaly in which the internal iliac artery extends through the persistent sciatic artery to continue as the popliteal artery with a hypoplastic or absent superficial femoral artery (Fig. 28–3A), and (2) the "incomplete" version of the anomaly (Fig. 28–3B), when the persistent sciatic artery either is broken in continuity or its connections to the internal iliac artery or popliteal artery are through smaller collaterals.[13–16] In a few cases, both the sciatic and the superficial femoral arteries exist and join at the level of the popliteal artery. In both versions of the anomaly, the profunda femoris is usually preserved and the superficial femoral artery is usually hypoplastic.

The persistent sciatic artery is usually associated with other vascular lesions, including hypertrophy or atrophy of the affected limb, venous varicosities or arteriovenous malformations, atherogenesis, and aneurysm formation, which appears to be the most common complication. Persistent sciatic arteries are frequently enlarged and tortuous, and aneurysmal degeneration has been described in 46% of the 167 reported cases. Most authors believe that repetitive trauma plays a role in the formation of aneurysms in the buttock region, with the abnormally enlarged artery more likely to degenerate with repeated exposure to intermittent pressure. In addition, 21% of the patients have provided a clear history of trauma at the site. Some of the aneurysms have been reported in the thigh. Acute rupture is rare, and some of the lesions are pseudoaneurysms. By 1914, Bryan had described 24 cases of aneurysm of this vessel, and 167 cases were described by 1994.[17–21] There is no clear predisposition regarding side or gender, and the ages of patients have varied from 6 months to 89 years. Bilateral aneurysms have

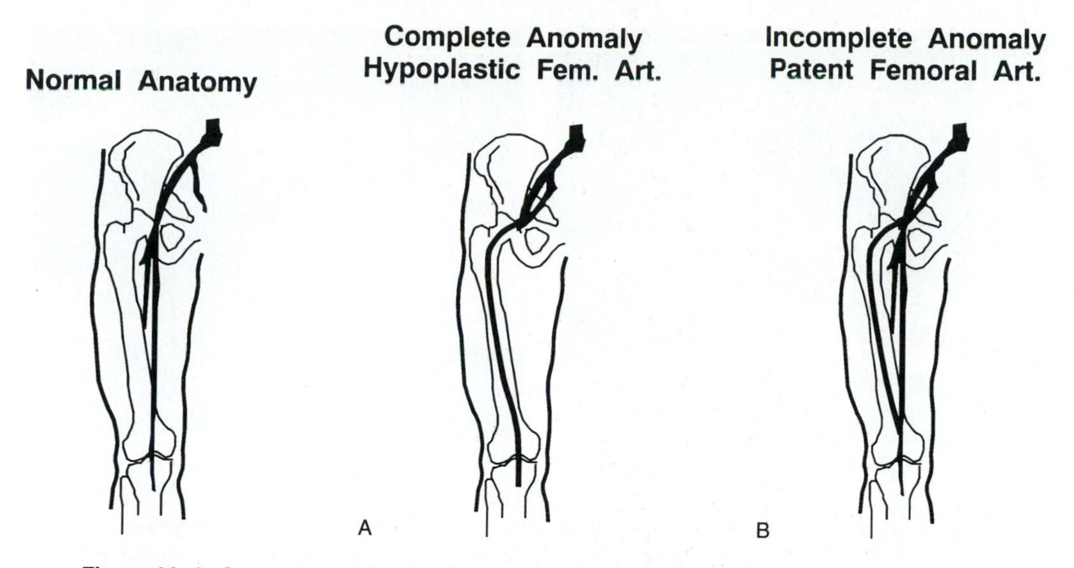

Figure 28–3. Comparison of (**A**) the "complete" form of the persistent sciatic artery with direct continuation to the popliteal artery with a bent superficial femoral artery, and (**B**) the "incomplete" form when the sciatic artery is not a continuous vessel, or its connections proximally or distally are not complete. *(Reprinted with permission from Wolf YG, Gibbs BF, Guzzetta VJ. Surgical treatment of aneurysm of the persistent sciatic artery. J Vasc Surg. 1993:17:218–221.)*

been described in 22%, and 69% of the reported cases were in persistent arteries of the complete type.

Historic Background

Persistent sciatic artery was initially described in 1832 by Green,[22] the first aneurysm of this artery was described by Fagge in 1864,[23] and the first surgical attempt at treatment was not reported until 1964 by Joffe,[24] who attempted proximal ligation of the vessel, with the subsequent complication of foot drop. Other early surgical procedures included exclusion or proximal ligation, with femoropopliteal bypass to reconstitute flow to the distal extremity.[25]

Presentation

The primary presenting complaints are buttock pain, sometimes associated with posterior thigh pain, presumably secondary to sciatic nerve compression.[25] Acute ischemia of the lower extremity, disabling claudication or toe gangrene are also common, usually associated with distal embolization or thrombosis. In three-fourths of the cases, a pulsatile mass is palpable. The pathognomonic physical sign of the arterial anomaly is an absent femoral pulse in the presence of a normal popliteal pulse.[26]

Diagnostic Considerations

The diagnosis of aneurysm of a persistent sciatic artery can be confirmed by ultrasound, CT, MRI (Fig. 28–4), or angiography[27,28] (Fig. 28–5). Ultrasound, particularly with real-time color and duplex capability, can provide a great deal of relevant information and

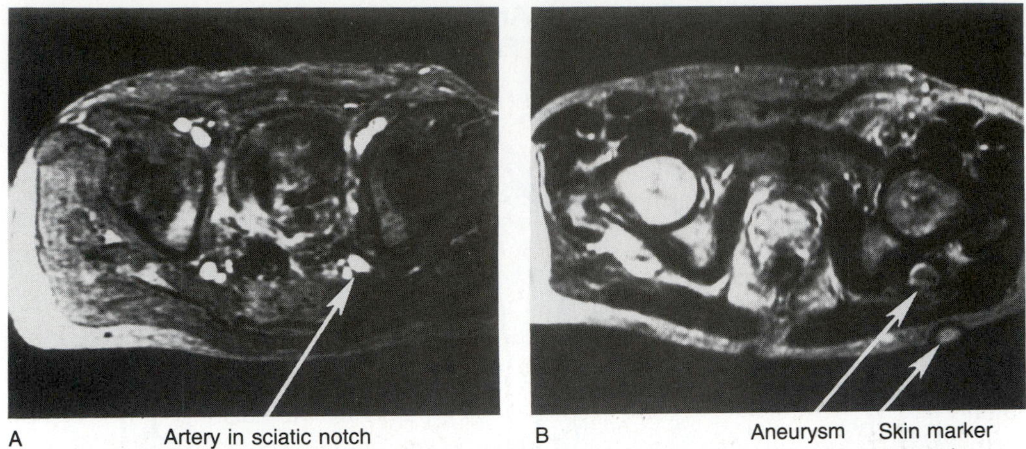

Figure 28–4. MRI scans documenting an aneurysm of the persistent sciatic artery with (**A**) normal vessel in the sciatic notch and pelvis, and (**B**) aneurysm just distal to the notch. *(Reprinted with permission from Wolf YG, Gibbs BF, Guzzetta VJ. Surgical treatment of aneurysm of the persistent sciatic artery. J Vasc Surg. 1993;17:218–221.)*

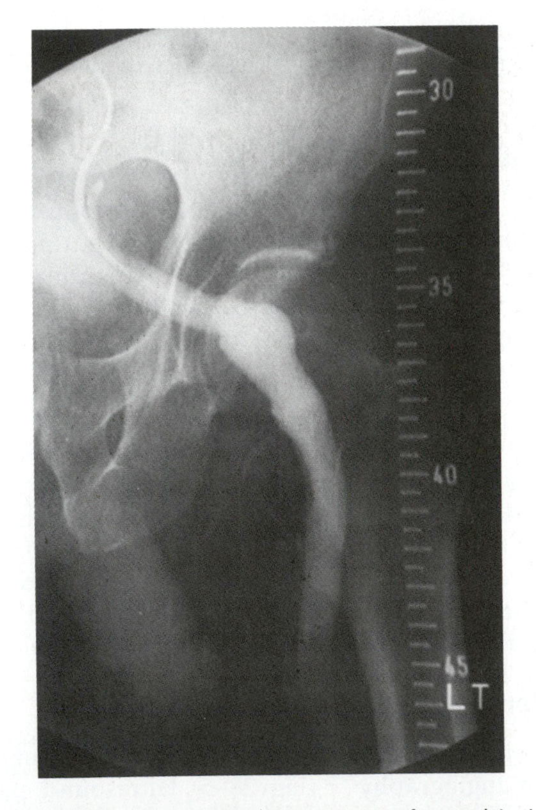

Figure 28–5. Angiogram demonstrating an aneurysm of a persistent sciatic artery.

probably should be the initial diagnostic modality, since it can rule out such other differential lesions as infection, hernia, and tumor, and characterize the lesion by pathology, size, arterial inflow source, and the pressure of a persistent sciatic artery. However, for detailed treatment plans, and to distinguish persistent sciatic from superior or inferior gluteal artery aneurysms, an angiogram with selective injections is usually necessary. CT and MRI scans are important when the lesion is large, and there is concern that the aneurysm protrudes proximally through the sciatic notch, which requires a dual pelvic and gluteal approach for surgical control and repair.

Treatment

The goals of treatment are the elimination of pain and the mass effect, cessation of distal embolism and prevention of future rupture. Thus, it is important that the aneurysm be excluded from the distal circulation, and that proximal arterial control be accompanied by relief of the aneurysmal mass. Current therapeutic approaches are both surgical and endovascular. Since 1964, 26 sciatic artery aneurysms have been repaired surgically and reported in the English literature.[14–25] Direct gluteal exposure with proximal ligation, endoaneurysmorrhaphy and distal reconstruction by femoropopliteal bypass is one satisfactory approach. Another successful surgical alternative involves posterior transgluteal dissection, excision of the aneurysm, and reconstruction with a local interposition graft. This plan obviates the need for a pelvic approach for proximal control and for a distal bypass. Some authors express concern regarding this direct approach to the aneurysm because of the possibility of injury to the sciatic nerve, which is immediately adjacent to it. However, concerns regarding the location of the reconstruction and potential injury due to frequent compression of the graft from sitting have not been borne out, and only one such graft occlusion has been reported. Some patients (approximately 25%) have required distal limb amputation because of severe ischemia at presentation.

A combined endovascular and surgical approach has also been successful, involving balloon catheter occlusion of the aneurysm (which required two angiographic efforts and eight pieces of Gel-foam), and a distal femoropopliteal bypass graft.[29,30] However, the same limitations of a residual mass effect as described under gluteal aneurysms pertain to aneurysms of the persistent sciatic artery, which are left *in situ*.

Additional endovascular maneuvers have included intra-arterial thrombolysis for an occluded aneurysm associated with distal ischemia, which then permitted direct surgical repair with interposition graft replacement and restoration of distal arterial flow.

COMMENTS

Both gluteal and persistent sciatic artery aneurysms are rare, but reports of their diagnosis and discovery are becoming more frequent. For example, in 1993, there were three reports regarding sciatic artery lesions, and four more in 1994! The vascular surgeon should be aware of these unusual conditions and have a clearly defined approach to the pathologic entities and their diagnosis and treatment. Most important, dissemination of information concerning these lesions will help alert other physicians to the deadly potential of approaching these treacherous aneurysms directly without adequate preliminary diagnostic information.

REFERENCES

1. Anson BJ, Maddock WG. *Callander's Surgical Anatomy*. Philadelphia: WB Saunders; 1952.
2. Battle WH. A case of traumatic gluteal aneurysm. *Br Med J*. 1898;2:1415–1416.
3. Gilroy D, Saadie R, Hide G, et al. Penetrating injury to the gluteal region. *J Trauma*. 1992;32:294–297.
4. Hultborn KA, Kjellman T. Gluteal aneurysm. Report of three cases and review of the literature. *Acta Chir Scand*. 1963;125:318–328.
5. Culliford ALT, Cukingham RA, Worth MH Jr. Aneurysms of the gluteal vessels: their etiology and management. *J Trauma*. 1974;14:77–81.
6. Williams W Jr, Jackson GF, Greene C. Superior gluteal artery aneurysm. *J Trauma*. 1977;17:477–479.
7. Gostigian J, Schlitt RJ. Aneurysm of the gluteal artery secondary to polyartritis nodosa. *Am J Surg*. 1963;105:267–268.
8. Schmalzried TP, Eckardt JJ. Spontaneous gluteal artery rupture resulting in compartment syndrome and sciatic neuropathy. *Clin Orthop*. 1992;275:253–257.
9. Demetriades D, Rabinowitz B, Sofianos C. Gluteal artery aneurysms. *Br J Surg*. 1988;75:494.
10. Benjamin JE, Lachman GS. A case of mycotic aneurysm of the gluteal artery. *JAMA*. 1924;82:1861–1862.
11. Zirinsky K, Markisz JA, Auh YH, et al. Computed tomography and magnetic resonance imaging of a superior gluteal artery pseudoaneurysm. *J Comput Tomogr*. 1988;12:75–78.
12. Vauthey JN, Maddern GH, Balsiger D, et al. Superselective embolization of superior gluteal artery pseudoaneurysms following intramuscular injection: a case report. *J Trauma*. 1991;31:1174–1175.
13. Arey LB. *Developmental Anatomy*. Philadelphia: WB Saunders; 1965.
14. Brantley SK, Rigdon EE, Raju S. Persistent sciatic artery: embryology, pathology and treatment. *J Vasc Surg*. 1993;18:242–248.
15. Izezawa T, Naiki K, Moriura S. Aneurysm of bilateral persistent sciatic arteries with ischemic complications: case report and review of world literature. *J Vasc Surg*. 1994;20:96–103.
16. Wolf YG, Gibbs BF, Guzzetta VJ. Surgical treatment of aneurysm of the persistent sciatic artery. *J Vasc Surg*. 1993;17:218–221.
17. Bryan RC. Aneurysm of the sciatic artery. *Ann Surg*. 1914;60:463–475.
18. Calleja F, Garcia Jimenez MA, Roman M. Operative management of the persistent sciatic artery aneurysm. *Cardiovasc Surg*. 1994;2:281–283.
19. Saey JP, Fastrez J. Acute ischemia of the lower limb and sciatic artery aneurysm. *Cardiovasc Surg*. 1994;2:271–274.
20. Valentine RJ. Optimal treatment of patients with complications of persistent sciatic artery. *Cardiovasc Surg*. 1994;2:270.
21. Ito H, Okadome K, Odashiro T. Persistent sciatic artery: two case reports and a review of the literature. *Cardiovasc Surg*. 1994;2:275–280.
22. Green PH. On a new variety of femoral artery. *Lancet*. 1832;1:730.
23. Fagge CH. Case of aneurysm, seated on an abnormal main artery of the lower limb. *Guy's Hosp Report*. 1864;10:151–159.
24. Joffe N. Aneurysm of persistent primitive sciatic artery. *Clin Radiol*. 1964;15:286–290.
25. Shutze WP, Garrett WV, Smith BL. Persistent sciatic artery: collective review and management. *Ann Vasc Surg*. 1993;7:303–310.
26. Cowie TN, McKellar NJ, McLean N. Unilateral congenital absence of the external iliac and femoral arteries. *Br J Radiol*. 1960;33:520–522.
27. Mandell VS, Jaques PF, Delany DJ, et al. Persistent sciatic artery: clinical, embryologic and angiographic features. *Am J Radiol*. 1985;144:245–249.
28. Wilms G, Storme L, Vandaele K, et al. CT demonstration of aneurysm of a persistent sciatic artery. *J Comput Assist Tomogr*. 1986;10:524–525.
29. Loh FK. Embolization of a sciatic artery aneurysm: an alternative to surgery: a case report. *Angiology*. 1985;36:472–476.
30. Becquemin JP, Gaston A, Coubret P, et al. Aneurysm of persistent sciatic artery: report of a case treated by endovascular occlusion and femoropopliteal bypass. *Surgery*. 1985;98:605–611.

29

Leg Inflow for Aortoiliac Occlusive Disease

Is Axillofemoral Bypass as Good as Aortofemoral Bypass?

Marc Passman, MD, Lloyd Taylor, Jr., MD, and John M. Porter, MD

The first extra-anatomic bypass was performed by Freeman and Leeds of San Francisco in 1952, when an endarterectomized superficial femoral artery was placed subcutaneously over the pubis as a femorofemoral conduit.[1] In 1959, Lewis of Perth, Australia, encountering an unworkable aorta during repair of a ruptured abdominal aortic aneurysm (AAA), placed a nylon graft to the left subclavian artery (SA) through a subcutaneous tunnel across the chest and into the abdomen and anastomosed to the proximal portion of a previously placed aortic homograft.[2] In 1963, Blaisdell and Hall[3] and Louw[4] independently reported the use of a bypass between the axillary and ipsilateral femoral arteries for unilateral lower extremity ischemia. In 1966, Sauvage and associates[5] added the femorofemoral extension to the axillofemoral graft, forming the first axillobifemoral procedure. Axillofemoral bypass was soon widely accepted as an alternative technique for lower extremity revascularization in clinical situations in which aortofemoral bypass was not feasible because of such contraindications as sepsis, advanced aortic calcification, and other examples of "hostile" abdomen. By the early 1970s, the indications for axillofemoral bypass had been expanded by some to include not only patients with a "hostile" abdomen, but also high-risk patients requiring revascularization for limb-threatening ischemia, as axillofemoral bypass was perceived as having less risk than aortofemoral reconstruction.[6–8]

As experience increased, it became clear that long-term results with axillofemoral grafting were remarkably variable (Table 29–1). Most investigators reported a high incidence of thrombosis for axillofemoral grafts, with intermediate-term patency distinctly inferior to aortofemoral bypass.[9–11] Moore et al.,[12] in a review of 52 axillofemoral bypasses performed over 8 years, including the original bypass performed by Blaisdell and Hall,[3] reported a primary patency of 60% at 1 year and 10% at 5 years. Similarily, Eugene et al.[13] reported a thrombosis rate of 50% at 2 years. Based on these and other

TABLE 29–1. CUMULATIVE PATENCY AND SURVIVAL RATES OF AXILLOFEMORAL BYPASS

Author	Year	*N*	Operative Mortality	Survival (%) 5 yr	Patency (%) 1 yr	Patency (%) 5 yr	Primary vs. Secondary
Mannick et al.[8]	1969	43	7.0	53	78	—[d]	Primary
Moore et al.[12]	1963–1970	44	9.0	29	60	10	Primary
Johnson et al.[21]	1965–1975	56	1.8	67	84	76	Primary
Eugene et al.[13]	1960–1975	59	8.0	26	60[a]/60[b]	30[a]/36[b]	Primary
LoGerfo et al.[17]	1966–1975	130	8.0	—	56[a]/87[b]	37[a]/74[b]	Secondary
Ray et al.[22]	1970–1979	54	3.7	65	75[a]/90[b]	67[a]/77[b]	Secondary
Burrell et al.[15]	1969–1979	106	8.0	50 (4 yr)	—	73 (4 yr)	Secondary
Ascer et al.[20]	1977–1982	56	5.3	43	95[a]/90[b]	71[a]/77[b]	Secondary
Donaldson et al.[16]	1970–1983	100	8.0	57	88	77	Secondary
Schultz et al.[24]	1978–1984	56	—	—	95	75[c]	Primary
Rutherford et al.[14]	1971–1985	42	13.0	—	—	37[a]/81[b]	Secondary
Kalman et al.[19]	1976–1985	90	8.8	50 (3 yr)	74[a]/90[b]	58[a]/77[b] (3 yr)	Primary
Harris et al.[26]	1983–1990	76	4.5	—	93	85[c]	Primary
Schneider et al.[43]	1985–1990	34	9.0	35 (3 yr)	92	76[c]	Secondary
El-Massry et al.[25]	1978–1990	79	5.1	23	97	79[c]	Secondary
Taylor et al.[27]	1984–1993	184	4.9	52	95	79[c]	Secondary

[a] Axillounifemoral graft configuration.
[b] Axillobifemoral graft configuration.
[c] Externally supported graft.
[d] —, no data.

reports, most vascular surgeons came to regard axillofemoral bypass as a "compromised" procedure with a limited clinical role. During this same period, however, other investigators experienced axillofemoral patency results comparable to aortofemoral bypass.[14–20] Johnson et al.,[21] in a review of their 10-year experience with aortofemoral and axillobifemoral bypass, reported operative mortalities of 5.5% and 1.8%, respectively, and an equivalent patency of 76% at 5 years for both. In 1979, Ray et al.[22] reported a 5-year primary patency of 91% for aortofemoral bypass compared to a secondary patency of 72% for axillofemoral bypass.

Since the mid-1980s, patency rates achieved with axillofemoral bypass have improved dramatically, probably due in large part to the introduction of the externally supported graft by Sauvage and associates in 1979.[23,24] Long-term follow-up of this series over a 12-year period demonstrated a primary patency of 78% at 5 years and 73% at 7 years with no change thereafter.[25] We began using externally supported polytetrafluoroethylene (PTFE) in the axillofemoral position at the Oregon Health Sciences University in Portland, Oregon in 1983, for axillofemoral bypass. Our experience with nonsupported prostheses in the axillofemoral position prior to 1983 was disappointing, with a 1-year primary patency of 51% (unpublished data), leading to placement of these grafts only when absolutely indicated.[26] Between 1984 and 1993, 184 axillofemoral bypasses with an externally supported prosthesis were performed in 164 patients for indications ranging from aortoiliac occlusive disease, aortic graft infection, aortoenteric fistula, and trauma. Life table 5-year primary patency, secondary patency, limb salvage, and survival of 71%, 79%, 92%, and 52%, respectively.

These contemporary patency results are noteworthy for both their superiority over previous axillofemoral series and for their striking similarity to the patency results from recently published aortofemoral series (Table 29–2). In the largest aortofemoral series, Szilagyi et al.[28] reported cumulative patency of 85%, 79%, 74%, and 70% at 5, 10, 15, and 20 years, respectively.

AORTOFEMORAL VERSUS AXILLOFEMORAL BYPASS

In our opinion, historic patency figures for aortofemoral bypass must be viewed in perspective. In the past, aortofemoral bypass was the standard treatment for all patients with symptomatic aortoiliac disease.[29–37] This included many patients with claudication, who today would be managed nonoperatively or with angioplasty. In all likelihood, inclusion of these minimal disease patients significantly improved historic aortofemoral patency results. In the series by Crawford et al.,[38] only 24% of 949 patients undergoing aortofemoral reconstruction had limb-threatening ischemia. Primary patency at 5 years was 84% and 71% for patients with claudication and limb-threatening ischemia, respectively, and survival was 76% and 66%, respectively. The improved functional outcome of aortofemoral reconstruction exclusively for claudication was further exemplified in the series by Sladen et al.[39] of 100 consecutive aortofemoral grafts performed for significant claudication secondary to aortoiliac occlusive disease. Primary patency was 84% and 78% at 5 and 10 years, respectively, whereas the secondary patency was a remarkable 97% and 93%. Long-term survival in these patients was 83% at 5 years and 56% at 10 years.

Another potential prejudice in historic series is that axillofemoral bypass was generally reserved for patients who had, in addition to limb-threatening ischemia, a prohibitive risk for intra-abdominal vascular reconstruction, thus clearly selecting the highest risk–worst outcome patient for axillofemoral bypass. Interestingly, there are no universally accepted criteria objectively defining the risk status of individual patients. In general, patients receiving axillofemoral bypass are a decade older than patients undergoing aortofemoral reconstruction and have an increased prevalence of coronary artery disease, hypertension, chronic pulmonary disease, cerebrovascular disease, and

TABLE 29–2. CUMULATIVE PATENCY AND SURVIVAL RATES OF AORTOFEMORAL BYPASS

Author	Year	*N*	Operative Mortality (%)	Survival (%) 5 yr	Patency (%) 1 yr	5 yr	10 yr	15 yr
Malone et al.[30,31]	1959–1974	282	2.5	80	96	85	66	—
Mulcare et al.[32]	1964–1975	114	0	—	98	95 (3yr)	—	—
Brewster et al.[33]	1963–1977	582	3.6	—	99	91	—	—
Jones et al.[36]	1974–1979	100	—[a]	—	96	89 (3yr)	—	—
van den Akker et al.[35]	1958–1980	518	3.0	69	90	82	69	59
Crawford et al.[38]	1955–1981	949	3.8	74	96	81	69	53
Szilagyi et al.[28]	1954–1983	1,748	5.0	63	92	85	79	74
Naylor et al.[37]	1975–1984	245	2.4	84	95	87	—	—
Sladen et al.[39]	1968–1986	100	0	83	97	84	78	—
Nevelsteen et al.[29]	1963–1987	869	4.5	70	92	82	74	70
Poulias et al.[40]	1966–1990	1,000	3.3	87	98	82	76	72

[a] —, no data.

diabetes mellitus (Table 29–3). Not surprisingly, increased comorbid risk factors have resulted in a higher operative mortality for axillofemoral bypass, ranging from 3.7% to 8.0% compared to the 2.5% to 5.1% for aortofemoral bypass, as well as a shorter life expectancy. In general, 5-year survival after axillofemoral bypass has ranged from 26% reported by Eugene et al.[13] to 65% reported by Ray et al.[22] In the latter study, the prevalence of comorbid factors was lower than most other axillofemoral series likely accounting for the improved long-term survival. In contrast, the 5-year survival for aortofemoral bypass has ranged from 59% reported by Szilagyi et al.[28] to 87% reported by Poulias et al.[40] Survival of patients requiring aortofemoral reconstruction has been estimated to be 10 years less than the "normal," nonatherosclerotic, age-adjusted male population,[41] and double that for patients requiring axillofemoral bypass.

Despite the numerous individual series on axillofemoral bypass and aortofemoral reconstruction for the treatment of aortoiliac occlusive disease, there have been only a few concurrent retrospective reports and no prospective, randomized series comparing both procedures (Table 29–4). While Johnson et al.[21] and Mason et al.[42] demonstrated excellent results with no significant difference in 5-year primary patency between axillofemoral and aortofemoral bypass, others have found inferior patency rates with axillofemoral bypass. Schneider et al.[43] reported a 3-year primary and secondary patency of 85% and 91% for aortofemoral bypass compared to 63% and 76% for axillofemoral bypass, respectively. Bunt[44] reported a life table primary patency of 94% at 2 years for aortofemoral bypass compared to 83% at 2 years for axillofemoral bypass. Aortofemoral procedures had a complication rate of 12% and operative mortality of 1.8% as opposed to a negligible degree of morbidity and mortality for axillofemoral bypass.

OREGON EXPERIENCE

We recently reviewed 139 aortofemoral and 117 axillofemoral grafts placed for aortoiliac occlusive disease and prospectively followed at our institution between 1988 and 1993, the largest concurrent series to date.[45] Patients undergoing axillofemoral bypass were on average a decade older and had a higher prevalence of associated medical conditions including heart disease, chronic renal failure, and prior intra-abdominal or aortic surgery than patients undergoing aortofemoral bypass (Table 29–5). Limb salvage defined as rest pain or ischemic ulcer/gangrene was also a more common indication in 80% of axillofemoral bypasses as compared to 42% of aortofemoral bypasses.

Despite these differences in the proportion of limb-threatening ischemia and associated medical problems, life table primary patency of 74% for the axillofemoral group was statistically no different from the 80% patency achieved for aortofemoral bypass by log-rank analysis. Primary patency was not influenced by surgical indication, superficial femoral artery patency, the need for deep femoral artery profundaplasty and/or endarterectomy, or the simultaneous placement of an infrainguinal bypass. Although there was no statistic difference in operative mortality (<1% for aortofemoral vs. 3.4% for axillofemoral), there was a significantly higher incidence of nonfatal major postoperative complications, most notably myocardial infarction, stroke, acute renal failure, and pulmonary failure after aortofemoral reconstruction (20.9% for aortofemoral vs. 10.3% for axillofemoral). Not surprisingly, long-term survival was significantly shorter after axillofemoral bypass with a 5-year survival of 45%, as compared to 72% for aortofemoral bypass. The most frequent cause of death, as in most series, was cardiac disease.

TABLE 29–3. COMPARISON OF OPERATIVE INDICATIONS AND RISK FACTORS

			Preoperative Risk Factors					Operative Indications		
Author	*N*	*Mean Age*	*Coronary Artery Disease (%)*	*Hypertension (%)*	*Chronic Pulmonary Disease (%)*	*Cerebral Vascular Disease (%)*	*Diabetes Mellitus (%)*	*Severe Claudication (%)*	*Limb Threatening Ischemia (%)*	*Other[a] (%)*
Axillofemoral										
Moore et al.[12]	44	—[b]	82	41	61	36	18	11	68	21
Eugene et al.[13]	59	66	76	41	61	31	19	12	65	23
LoGerfo et al.[17]	130	66	67	25	—	21	28	10	78	12
Ray et al.[22]	54	67	22	37	11	11	22	59	31	10
Burrell et al.[15]	106	66	91	52	45	20	22	34	69	7
Ascer et al.[20]	56	69	67	41	—	16	32	—	100	—
Donaldson et al.[16]	100	67	51	38	44	—	19	19	66	14
El-Massry et al.[25]	79	69	58	62	35	34	16	38	62	—
Taylor et al.[27]	184	67	80	—	13	—	25	14	69	17
Aortofemoral										
Malone et al.[30,31]	180	52	58	39	—	32	11	40	60	—
Nevelsteen et al.[29]	352	59	26	25	—	7	6	42	58	—
Crawford et al.[38]	949	59	36	—	—	—	12	76	24	—
Szilagyi et al.[28]	1748	59	46	35	—	19	18	66	44	—
Poulias et al.[40]	1000	55	24	19	—	—	16	71	29	—
van den Akker et al.[35]	518	55	25	31	13	4	7	77	23	—

[a] Aortic graft infection, aortoenteric fistula, trauma, or aortic aneurysm.
[b] —, no data.

TABLE 29–4. RETROSPECTIVE SERIES COMPARING AXILLOFEMORAL AND AORTOFEMORAL BYPASS

		Axillofemoral				Aortofemoral			
Author	**Year of Publication**	***N***	***Operative Mortality***	***Survival (%)(yr)***	***Patency (%)(yr)***	***N***	***Operative Mortality***	***Survival (%)(yr)***	***Patency (%)(yr)***
Johnson et al.[21]	1977	56	1.8	67 (5)	76 (5)	88	5.5	67 (5)	77 (5)
Ray et al.[22]	1979	54	3.7	65 (5)	72 (5)	105	—[b]	—	91 (5)
Bunt[44]	1986	33	—	—	83 (2)	55	1.8	—	94 (2)
Mason et al.[42]	1989	37	1.8	—	81 (3)	59	7.0	—	89 (3)
Schneider et al.[43]	1992	34	9.0	35 (3)	63/76[a] (3)	107	1.0	91 (3)	85/94[a] (3)

[a] Primary/secondary patency rates.
[b] —, no data.

In addition to the use of the externally supported prosthesis, our current success with axillofemoral bypass may be attributed in part to evolution of surgical technique. Our present operative approach for axillofemoral bypass is a variation of the technique originally described by Blaisdell and Hall[3] and uses a two-team approach. The axillary artery is approached by the first team through an infraclavicular incision, and the first portion between the chest wall and the medial border of the pectoralis minor is used for anastomosis because of its relatively fixed position and single collateral branch. Axillary anastomosis is performed in an end-to-side fashion to a longitudinal arteriotomy on the anterior surface, medial to the pectoralis minor and to the origin of the thoracoacromial artery. To prevent anastomotic disruption, the graft is routed parallel and adjacent to the axillary artery under the pectoralis minor and into the axilla before forming a gentle curve for its inferior course, thereby allowing for arm extension and distributing any potential tension across the curve of the graft rather than at the proximal anastomosis (Fig. 29–1).[46]

TABLE 29–5. ASSOCIATED MEDICAL CONDITIONS IN PATIENTS UNDERGOING AXILLOFEMORAL AND AORTOFEMORAL BYPASS AT OREGON HEALTH SCIENCES UNIVERSITY BETWEEN 1988 AND 1993

Condition	Axillofemoral Bypass (N = 108)	Aortofemoral Bypass (N = 139)
Age over 80	10 (9%)	0 (0)[a]
Tobacco abuse	93 (86%)	114 (82%)
Heart disease	91 (84%)	52 (38%)[a]
Chronic pulmonary disease	14 (13%)	17 (12%)
Diabetes mellitus	31 (29%)	27 (19%)
Chronic renal failure	12 (11%)	3 (2%)[a]
Prior intra-abdominal surgery	48 (44%)	42 (30%)[b]
Prior aortic surgery	17 (16%)	8 (6%)[b]

[a] $p < 0.001$ by chi square analysis.
[b] $p < 0.05$ by chi square analysis.

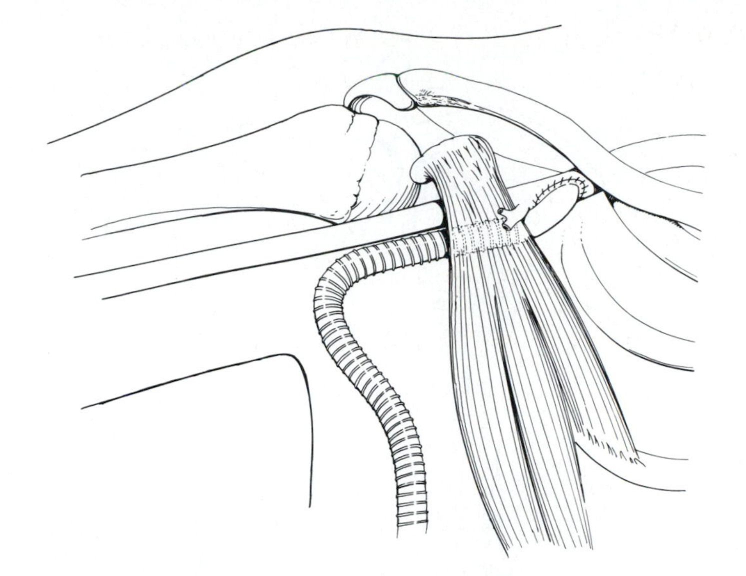

Figure 29–1. Axillofemoral proximal anastomosis. End-to-side anastomosis of the proximal graft to the first portion of the axillary artery. Note the parallel route of the graft adjacent to the axillary artery beneath the pectoralis minor for 8 to 10 cm before forming a gentle and redundant curve in the axilla prior to its inferior course. *(Reprinted with permission from Taylor LM Jr, Park TC, Edwards JM, et al. Acute disruption of polytetrafluoroethylene grafts. J Vasc Surg. 1994;20:520–528.)*

The femoral vessels are approached by the second team through vertical groin incisions, and a subcutaneous tunnel is formed between both femoral exposures. A second subcutaneous tunnel is formed using the Oregon tunneller, which allows passage of the graft without additional counterincisions, from the axilla, to the inferior border of the pectoralis major along the lateral aspect of the abdomen, curving medial to the anterior iliac spine, into the ipsilateral groin (Fig. 29–2). The common femoral artery at its bifurcation is preferred for the anatomosis; however, the profunda femoris artery can be used if there is significant atherosclerotic disease. The axillary anastomosis is performed first followed by anastomosis of the femorofemoral limbs to the respective femoral arteries. The distal end of the axillofemoral component is then anastomosed in an end-to-side fashion to the "cobra-head" of the ipsilateral femoral limb (Fig. 29–3). With use of multiple operative teams we are routinely able to perform an axillobifemoral bypass in less than 90 minutes.

Despite early disappointing results, primary patency of axillofemoral grafts in excess of 70% at 5 years has now been reported by a number of investigators, coinciding with the introduction of the externally supported prosthesis.[23-27] These results are not significantly different from those reported for aortofemoral reconstruction. Although aortofemoral bypass remains standard treatment for symptomatic aortoiliac occlusive disease, because of excellent long-term patency, consistently exceeding 80% at 5 years, these results must be viewed in perspective. Patients undergoing aortic revascularization today are characterized by advanced age and a higher prevalence of limb-threatening ischemia than patients undergoing aortofemoral bypass several decades ago. Although long-term results of aortofemoral bypass by modern reporting standards are largely unknown, it is logical to assume contemporary

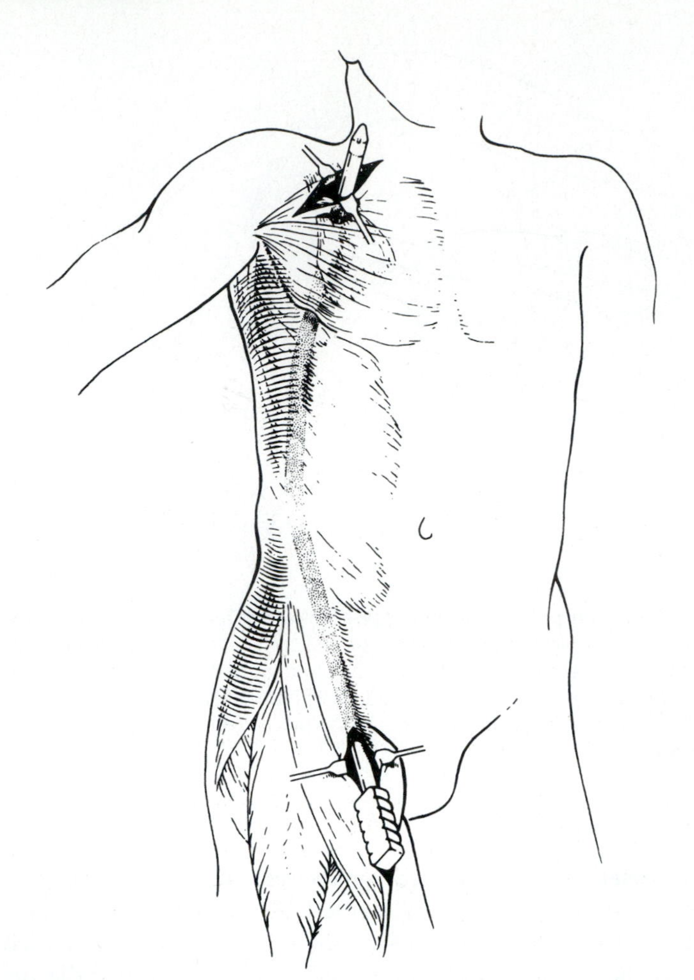

Figure 29–2. The use of the Oregon tunneller between axillary and femoral exposures. The graft is positioned in the subcutaneous position from the ipsilateral axilla, to the inferior border of the pectoralis major, medial to the anterior iliac spine to the femoral artery. *(Reprinted with permission from Taylor LM Jr, Moneta GL, McConnell DB, et al. Axillofemoral grafting with externally supported polytetrafluoroethylene. Arch Surg. 1994;129:588–595.)*

aortofemoral patency is less than that of 20 years ago, a finding certainly present in our series.

CONCLUSION

Modern vascular surgery is regularly called on to provide limb inflow in an increasing number of elderly, debilitated patients. In recent years we have come to rely increasingly on axillofemoral bypass in these patients. In order to assess the success of this procedure, we have reviewed our recent 5-year experience with axillofemoral and aortofemoral bypass performed concurrently and followed prospectively. On balance, axillofemoral patients had a slightly increased operative mortality, decreased operative complication rate, equal 5-year patency, and diminished 5-year survival. We conclude that axillofemoral bypass is a superior inflow procedure in elderly patients with associated comorbid risk factors, producing results at least as good as aortofemoral bypass.

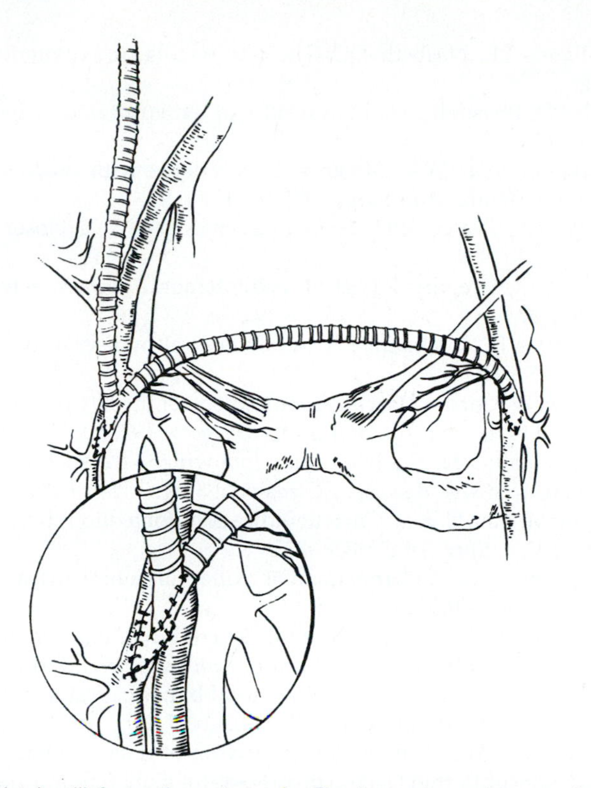

Figure 29–3. Distal axillofemoral anastomosis. The femorofemoral bypass is performed first, with the distal axillofemoral limb anastomosed to the "cobra head" of the ipsilateral femoral anastomosis (*insert*). *(Reprinted with permission from Taylor LM Jr, Moneta GL, McConnell DB, et al. Axillofemoral grafting with externally supported polytetrafluoroethylene. Arch Surg. 1994;129:588–595.)*

REFERENCES

1. Freeman NE, Leeds FH. Operations on large arteries: application of recent advances. *Calif Med*. 1952;77:229–233.
2. Lewis CD. A subclavian artery as the means of blood-supply to the lower half of the body. *Br J Surg*. 1961;574–575.
3. Blaisdell FW, Hall AD. Axillary-femoral artery bypass for lower extremity ischemia. *Surgery*. 1963;54:563–568.
4. Louw JH. Splenic-to-femoral and axillary-to-femoral bypass grafts in diffuse atherosclerotic occlusive disease. *Lancet*. 1963;29:1401–1402.
5. Sauvage LR, Wood SJ. Unilateral axillary bilateral femoral bifurcation graft: a procedure for the poor risk patient with aortoiliac disease. *Surgery*. 1966;60:573–577.
6. Alpert J, Brief DK, Parsonnet V. Vascular restoration for aortoiliac occlusion and an alternative approach to the poor risk patient. *J Newark Beth Israel Hosp*. 1967;18:4–7.
7. Pierangeli A, Guernelli N. The axillo-femoral bypass as a treatment of the aorto-iliac junction in the poor risk patient. *J Cardiovasc Surg*. 1967;8:353–360.
8. Mannick JA, Nasbeth DC. Axillofemoral bypass graft—a safe alternative to aortoiliac reconstruction. *N Engl J Med*. 1968;278:460–466.
9. Blaisdell FW, Hall AD, Lim RC, et al. Aorto-iliac arterial substitution utilizing subcutaneous grafts. *Ann Surg*. 1970;172:775–780.
10. Parsonnet V, Alpert J, Brief DK. Femorofemoral and axillofemoral grafts—compromise or preference. *Surgery*. 1970;67:26–33.

11. Mannick JA, Williams LE, Nasbeth DC. The late results of axillofemoral grafts. *Surgery.* 1970;68:1038–1043.
12. Moore WA, Hall AD, Blaisdell FW. Late results of axillary-femoral bypass grafting. *Am J Surg.* 1971;122:148–154.
13. Eugene J, Goldstone J, Moore WA. Fifteen year experience with subcutaneous bypass grafts for lower extremity ischemia. *Ann Surg.* 1977;186:177–183.
14. Rutherford RB, Patt A, Pearce WH. Extra-anatomic bypass: a closer view. *J Vasc Surg.* 1987;6:437–446.
15. Burrell MJ, Wheeler JR, Gregory RT, et al. Axillofemoral bypass: a ten-year review. *Ann Surg.* 1982;195:796–799.
16. Donaldson MC, Louras JC, Bucknam CA. Axillofemoral bypass: a tool with a limited role. *J Vasc Surg.* 1986;3:757–763.
17. LoGerfo FW, Johnson W, Corson D, et al. A comparison of the late patency rates of axillobilateral femoral and axillounilateral femoral grafts. *Surgery.* 1977;81:33–40.
18. Hepp W, de Jonge K, Pallua N. The late results following extra-anatomic bypass procedures for chronic aortoiliac occlusive disease. *J Cardiovasc Surg.* 1988;29:181–184.
19. Kalman PG, Hosang M, Cina C, et al. Current indications for axillounifemoral and axillobifemoral bypass grafts. *J Vasc Surg.* 1987;5:828–832.
20. Ascer E, Veith FJ, Gupta S, et al. Comparison of axillounifemoral and axillobifemoral bypass operations. *Surgery.* 1984;97:169–174.
21. Johnson WC, LoGerfo FW, Vollman RW, et al. Is axillo-bilateral femoral graft an effective substitute for aortic-bilateral iliac/femoral graft? *Ann Surg.* 1977;186:123–129.
22. Ray LI, O'Connor JB, Davis CC, et al. Axillofemoral bypass: a critical reappraisal of its role in the management of aortoiliac occlusive disease. *Am J Surg.* 1979;138:117–128.
23. Kenney DA, Sauvage LR, Wood SJ, et al. Comparison of noncrimped, externally supported (EXS) and crimped, nonsupported Dacron prostheses for axillofemoral and above-knee femoropopliteal bypass. *Surgery.* 1982;92:931–946.
24. Schultz GA, Sauvage LR, Mathisen SR, et al. A five- to seven-year experience with externally supported Dacron prostheses in axillofemoral and femoropopliteal bypass. *Ann Vasc Surg.* 1986;1:214–223.
25. El-Massry S, Saad E, Sauvage LR, et al. Axillofemoral bypass with externally supported, knitted Dacron grafts. A followup through twelve years. *J Vasc Surg.* 1993;17:107–115.
26. Harris EJ, Taylor LM Jr, McConnell DB, et al. Clinical results of axillobifemoral bypass using externally supported polytetrafluoroethylene. *J Vasc Surg.* 1990;12:416–421.
27. Taylor LM Jr, Moneta GL, McConnell DB, et al. Axillofemoral grafting with externally supported polytetrafluoroethylene. *Arch Surg.* 1994;129:588–595.
28. Szilagyi DE, Elliott JP Jr, Smith RF, et al. A thirty-year survey of the reconstructive surgical treatment of aortoiliac occlusive disease. *J Vasc Surg.* 1986;3:421–436.
29. Nevelsteen A, Suy R, Daenen W, et al. Aortofemoral grafting: factors influencing late results. *Surgery.* 1980;88:642–653.
30. Malone JM, Moore WS, Goldstone J. The natural history of bilateral aortofemoral bypass grafts for ischemia of the lower extremities. *Arch Surg.* 1975;110:1300–1306.
31. Malone JM, Goldstone J, Moore WS. Autogenous profundaplasty: the key to long-term patency in secondary repair of aortofemoral graft occlusion. *Ann Surg.* 1978;188:817–823.
32. Mulcare RJ, Royster TS, Lynn RA, et al. Long-term results of operative therapy for aortoiliac occlusive disease. *Arch Surg.* 1978;113:601–604.
33. Brewster DC, Darling RC. Optimal methods of aortoiliac reconstruction. *Surgery.* 1978;84:739–748.
34. Nevelsteen A, Wouters L, Suy R. Aortofemoral Dacron reconstruction for aorto-iliac occlusive disease: a 25-year survey. *Eur J Vasc Surg.* 1991;5:179–186.
35. van den Akker PJ, van Schelfgaarde R, Brand R, et al. Long-term success of aortoiliac surgery for arteriosclerotic obstructive disease. *SG&O.* 1992;174:485–496.
36. Jones AF, Kempczinski RF. Aortofemoral bypass grafting. A reappraisal. *Arch Surg.* 1981;116:301–305.
37. Naylor AR, Ah-See AK, Engeset J. Morbidity and mortality after aortofemoral grafting for peripheral limb ischaemia. *J R Coll Surg Edinb.* 1989;34:215–218.

38. Crawford ES, Bomberger RA, Glaeser DH, et al. Aortoiliac occlusive disease: factors influencing survival and function following reconstructive operation over a twenty-five year period. *Surgery.* 1981;90:1055–1067.
39. Sladen JG, Gilmour JL, Wong RW. Cumulative patency and actual palliation in patients with claudication after aortofemoral bypass—prospective long term follow-up of 100 patients. *Am J Surg.* 1986;152:190–195.
40. Poulias GE, Doundoulakis N, Prombonas E, et al. Aorto-femoral bypass and determinants of early success and late favourable outcome—experience with 1,000 consecutive cases. *J Cardiovasc Surg.* 1992;33:664–678.
41. Malone JM, Moore WS, Goldstone J. Life expectancy following aortofemoral arterial grafting. *Surgery.* 1977;81:551–555.
42. Mason RA, Smirnov VB, Newton B, et al. Alternative procedures to aortobifemoral grafting. *J Cardiovasc Surg.* 1989;30:192–197.
43. Schneider JR, McDaniel MD, Walsh DB, et al. Axillofemoral bypass: outcome and hemodynamic results in high risk patients. *J Vasc Surg.* 1992;15:952–963.
44. Bunt TJ. Aortic reconstruction vs. extraanatomic bypass and angioplasty. *Arch Surg.* 1986;121:1166–1170.
45. Passman MA, Taylor LM Jr, Moneta GL, et al. Comparison of axillofemoral bypass for aortoiliac occlusive disease. *J. Vasc Surg.* in press.
46. Taylor LM Jr, Park TC, Edwards JM, et al. Acute disruption of polytetrafluoroethylene grafts adjacent to axillary anastomoses: a complication of axillofemoral grafting. *J Vasc Surg.* 1994;20:520–528.

VI

Renal Artery Reconstruction

30

Magnetic Resonance Angiography of the Renal Arteries

Louis M. Messina, MD, James C. Stanley, MD, and Martin R. Prince, MD, PhD

As renovascular disease has become an important public health issue in our aging population, the need for a safe but accurate technique to diagnose renal artery stenosis has increased substantially. The significance of the problem of renovascular arterial occlusive disease is apparent if one considers that approximately 2% to 5% of people with hypertension have a renovascular etiology. If 20% to 30% of the U.S. population has hypertension, then between 2 to 4 million people have significant renal artery occlusive disease contributing to their hypertension.[1] It is important to recognize that the prevalence of renovascular hypertension varies significantly depending on race and ethnic make-up of the population under consideration. For instance, it has been estimated that of patients with accelerated or malignant hypertension, 43% of Caucasians have a renovascular etiology, whereas only 7% of African Americans have renovascular disease as an etiology for their hypertension.[2] In addition, it is estimated that 15% of all new cases of end-stage renal failure requiring dialysis are due to progressive renal artery occlusive disease.[1] Thus, there is good evidence that renovascular disease is underdiagnosed in current clinical practice in the United States.

Although traditional catheter-based, iodinated-contrast angiography provides accurate delineation of renal artery stenosis, the risks attendent to this technique have been a strong impetus for developing safer techniques of diagnosis.[3] In addition to other complications, the incidence of renal toxicity is an important consideration when undertaking conventional catheter-based renal angiography. The incidence of renal failure increases significantly as kidney function deteriorates. Renal insufficiency occurs in up to 10% of patients with mild to moderate renal insufficiency and in up to 90% of patients with diabetes and severe renal insufficiency. Newer generations of lower osmolar contrast media whether ionic or nonionic have not been shown conclusively to reduce the incidence of renal toxicity.[1] Of the newer techniques under development for the diagnosis of renal artery stenosis, perhaps none is more promising than magnetic resonance angiography. Magnetic resonance angiography can image the renal arteries without the nephrotoxic contrast agents or intra-arterial catheters. This chapter reviews the fundamentals of the technique of magnetic resonance imaging (MRI) and magnetic resonance angiography (MRA), including time of flight (TOF) and phase contrast (PC) modifications; reviews the studies that compare the accuracy of MRA to conventional angiography; and describes the promising early results of the new modification of MRA, breath-held 3D gadolinium MRA.

MAGNETIC RESONANCE IMAGING

Magnetic resonance imaging (MRI) is a technique based on the detection of radio-frequency waves emitted by protons as they precess within a strong magnetic field.[4–7] Protons in the form of hydrogen nuclei are abundant in human tissues.[4–5] When a strong static magnetic field is applied, protons tend to align in the direction of the applied static magnetic field. This is due to the fact that hydrogen atoms (protons) are charged nuclei that spin, thereby creating a magnetic dipole moment (MDM). It is this tiny MDM or spin that aligns with the externally applied static magnetic field. When a pulse of radio waves at the appropriate "resonant" frequency is applied to the tissue, it can exert force on the tiny proton dipoles. This force causes the protons to tip away from the axis of the original static magnetic field. After the pulse stops, the protons try to realign with the static magnetic field but fundamental laws of nature cause the protons to precess about the axis of the magnetic field like a spinning top or a gyroscope. While precessing, the protons emit radio waves that are detected by radio-frequency antennae. These antennae are often referred to as coils. The radio waves are the signal that eventually, after hundreds of pulses, is sufficient to create an image.

The magnitude of the signal depends primarily on two factors, referred to as T_1 and T_2 relaxation. These relaxation times vary among the different tissues of the body. T_1 relaxation represents the time required for the tissue to recover from a pulse so that it will be ready to generate signal from another pulse. T_2 relaxation indicates how long after a pulse that tissue will continue to emit a signal (radio waves). Tissues with a short T_1 recover rapidly from each pulse resulting in a brighter signal when the pulses are delivered in a rapid succession. Tissues with a short T_2 lose their signal rapidly after each pulse and thus tend to be dark if there is a delay between giving the pulse and listening for signal. Differences in relaxation times allow identification of different tissues.

It is the repetitive process of excitation and relaxation of the target tissues at regular short intervals (for MRI, 0.5 to 2.0 s; MRA, 10 to 50 ms) that ultimately produces an image. A typical MR pulse sequence is characterized by a time interval between pulses, known as the repetition time (TR), and a time interval between giving the pulse and listening for the signal known as the echo time (TE). When the TR is so short that the tissue does not have time to recover in between pulses, the tissue is said to be "saturated" and gives off very little signal. This is important in MRA where the recovery from each pulse depends on inflow of fresh "unsaturated" blood. If blood flow is too slow or in the image plane, it becomes saturated and has a reduced signal.

Cross-sectional MRI images are created by application of additional magnetic fields (referred to as gradients) that induce a change in frequency of precession of the protons depending on their location in relationship to the externally applied field. Sensing coils pass these changes onto computers where the signals undergo Fourier transformation to generate an image.[5]

MAGNETIC RESONANCE ANGIOGRAPHY

Magnetic resonance angiography is a noninvasive diagnostic technique that does not use ionizing radiation or nephrotoxic contrast media that can image blood vessels and measure blood flow based on the principles of MRI.[4–8] Magnetic resonance angiography utilizes many different reconstruction techniques all of which depend on selective imaging of moving blood within multiple thin cross-sectional slices in designated regions of the body. In so doing the signal from the moving blood is maximized and the signals from all of the other tissues is minimized. After different techniques of signal acquisition have been applied, reconstructions are accomplished using the *maximum intensity projection* (MIP) technique, which selects the maximum intensity of each pixel within a projection. Although there have been many rapid advances in the resolution of blood vessels achieved by MRA, imaging of the abdominal aorta and its branches has lagged behind other areas of the body due to the confounding problems of respiratory motion induced artifact, bowel motion, and relatively slow blood flow, which reduces signal and increases noise.

The principles and terminology associated with MRI and MRA are quite complex and can be confusing to the clinician. Nonetheless, one simplified functional classification of the different pulse sequences used during MRA is based on the velocity of blood necessary to achieve contrast.[6] One method, referred to as black blood imaging, utilizes a long TE, a long interval between giving the pulse and listening for signal, so that flowing blood has a chance to flow away and dephase. This yields images in which the vessel walls and surrounding organs are seen, while blood is dark, or black. This technique is useful for imaging large structures such as the aorta. A second method of MRA is phase contrast angiography (PCA), which is a map of proton velocity. Moving blood produces a bright signal, all other stationary tissues are dark. A third approach, TOF, detects protons moving into a designated area. Under these conditions, inflowing blood is fully relaxed and its large magnetic moment generates a bright signal. Stationary tissue is saturated and has a small magnetic moment. Finally, there is the intravenous injection of MR contrast agents such as gadolinium contrast, which is paramagnetic.[9,10] Gadolinium shortens the T_1 of blood, making it bright on heavily T_1 weighted images. Gadolinium has such a powerful magnetic effect that a small dose can brighten the entire blood pool. It has no nephrotoxicity and is routinely used in patients with renal insufficiency. It also has a low incidence of allergic reactions so that it can be used in patients with a history of severe reactions to iodinated contrast. These different techniques display different sensitivities to the detection of variant blood velocities. Gadolinium MRA is the most sensitive to low blood flow velocities because it does not require motion for its image.

Of the different techniques of MRA, TOF is used most commonly. The vascular signal on TOF is related to the amount of the blood flowing into the defined imaging area in between MR pulses. The intensity of this signal is related to the fraction of protons in their equilibrium state parallel to the static-applied magnetic field. If the pulse repetition rate is sufficiently rapid (short TR) that the protons do not have time to relax, they eventually lose their magnetization and generate minimal MR signal. The tissue is said to be "saturated." During MRA, the radio-frequency pulses are applied at 10 to 40 millisecond intervals; virtually all stationary tissues are saturated and produce little or no signal. In contrast, protons within the blood flowing into the region of interest are fully relaxed since they have not been exposed to the radio-frequency pulses. Such protons are fully magnetized in their equilibrium state and will rarely become saturated unless they remain within the region of interest for sufficient time to be subjected to several pulses. Thus, in TOF, moving blood has a bright white signal and the brightness or intensity of this signal is roughly proportional to the velocity of blood flow moving into the plane of imaging.

Time of flight images can be acquired either in two dimensions or three dimensions. Two-dimensional, time of flight (2D TOF) images are obtained from multiple continuous thin slices until an entire region of interest has been covered. Three-dimensional time of flight (3D TOF) acquires signal from a volume of tissue. Typically 6 to 15 minutes is required for 3D data acquisition. Three-dimensional TOF has good spatial resolution and is best suited to study rapid blood velocities. In contrast, 2D TOF is more sensitive to low blood flow velocities and thus able to distinguish between low flow and occlusion, but provides lower image resolution than does 3D TOF. For both techniques the flip angle used during data acquisition can be adjusted typically between 10° and 60° to maximize background tissue suppression and minimize image artifact due to the pulsatile nature of blood flow.[5] Repetition time is adjusted to maximize sensitivity to the anticipated blood flow velocity rates.

PHASE CONTRAST ANGIOGRAPHY

Phase contrast angiography reflects the relative direction or "phase" of a tissue magnetic moment. Phase contrast observes the phase shift signals rather than the absolute magnitude of the signals as in TOF sequences. Moving tissue such as blood and stationary tissue will have magnetic moments in different directions. Because this difference in phase is proportional to the velocity of moving blood, this technique can also be used to quantitate blood flow velocities. This technique overcomes the weakness of TOF whereby the radio-frequency pulses that are used to suppress the background tissue also to some extent suppress the blood signal. In the phase contrast method, two or more images are obtained at each slice. In one image, the phase of magnetization is changed in proportion to the blood flow velocity. In a second image, the direction is altered in an opposite manner. In stationary tissues, no change in the direction of magnetization or phase occurs. When the vectors of magnetization of the two acquisitions are subtracted, the moving tissues generate a brightness that is proportional to its velocity and background tissues are subtracted away. Thus, this phase contrast method is particularly sensitive to low flow velocities.[4–8]

GADOLINIUM-ENHANCED MAGNETIC RESONANCE ANGIOGRAPHY

Magnetic resonance angiography is particularly well suited to low-resistance vessels such as the internal carotid or renal arteries, which have continuous diastolic flow that is detected easily by TOF techniques. However, in certain circumstances, such as patients with vascular occlusive disease in which turbulent flow occurs, TOF images can be degraded. In addition, there can be loss of signal during low flow states in patients with low cardiac output. Finally, patients with tortuous vessels may have segments not oriented perpendicular to the point of imaging, causing loss of signal from in-plane saturation. All of these problems are exacerbated in the abdomen and pelvis where motion artifacts secondary to breathing and bowel motility induce further signal artifacts. In order to make MRA independent of blood flow rates or blood motion and thus avoid many of the problems of conventional TOF MRA, an intravenous paramagnetic contrast agent, gadolinium can be administered during 3D MRI. Administration of gadolinium shortens the T_1 of blood relative to that of fat, muscle, and other background tissues. Under such conditions one can image the arteries directly with excellent, high resolution in a 3D Fourier transform acquisition optimized for the shortened T_1 of the blood.

Infusion of gadolinium during the MR acquisition results in substantial arterial enhancement without confounding effects of excess venous or background tissue enhancement. Comparative studies applying angiographic and surgical correlation shows high sensitivity and specificity for the detection of arterial stenoses or occlusions and aneurysmal disease.[4,10,11]

Although gadolinium is a heavy metal, it can be chelated with a variety of compounds. The gadolinium chelates currently available for clinical use are safer than iodinated contrast. Gadolinium chelates have no nephrotoxicity and an extremely low incidence of allergic reactions. They are routinely administered in patients with renal insufficiency and in patients with a history of iodinated contrast allergy. These compounds include gadopentetate dimeglumine, gadoteridol, and gadodiamide.

COMPARISON OF MAGNETIC RESONANCE ANGIOGRAPHY TO OTHER RENAL ARTERY IMAGING MODALITIES

Due to the increasing importance of renal artery occlusive disease both as a mechanism of renal failure requiring chronic dialysis and for exacerbation of hypertension in the elderly, a number of centers have evaluated the role of MRA in the diagnosis of the renal artery occlusive disease.[11–27] In addition, since there are up to 9,000 renal transplants performed each year, MRI has been evaluated as an alternative to angiography to define renal artery anatomy prior to donor nephrectomy in living related donors. Of particular importance in the latter studies is the accurate identification of accessory renal arteries as well as branch renal artery disease. To date, the only diagnostic study that possesses sufficient resolution and accuracy is conventional catheter-based angiography. Both intravenous pyelography and radionuclide scintigraphy lack sufficient sensitivity in the detection of renal artery stenosis. Neither study is capable of identifying renal artery anatomy. Renal duplex scanning cannot reliably identify accessory renal arteries or branch artery disease. Finally intravenous digital subtraction angiography has not been proven to be sufficiently sensitive to be of clinical value as the study is nondiagnostic in approximately 10% of patients and both specificity and sensitivities are less than 90%.[20]

MRA is a noninvasive diagnostic modality that permits direct visualization of aortic and renal artery anatomy without the use of iodinated contrast agents. Preliminary work has shown that MRA can be used for a functional assessment of renal artery blood flow, glomerular filtration rates, and tissue perfusion. In addition, MRA can be used for serial renal size and volume measurements. Presently, its major disadvantages are that it is an expensive study in which any patient with a pacemaker, other electronic implants, or metal adjacent to a neurologic structure is excluded from study. In addition, the study requires substantial expertise to obtain the appropriate image acquisition and interpretation.

In the studies comparing the diagnostic accuracy, sensitivity, and specificity of MRA imaging of renal arteries relative to that obtained by conventional catheter-based arteriography shows sensitivities and specificities in the range of 70% to 100% to detect 50% or greater renal artery stenosis[12–24] (Table 30–1, Figs. 30–1 and 30–2). In one of the first studies examining reliability of MRI of renal arteries, Kent and associates at the Beth Israel Hospital in Boston used MRI to study 37 patients who had recently undergone renal angiography.[20] Fourteen patients had normal arteries. In 23 patients, the MRI results concurred with the angiographic reading in 70 of 77 arteries (91%). MRI predicted the presence of a greater than 50% stenosis of the proximal renal artery, with

TABLE 30–1. CORRELATION OF MRA AND CONVENTIONAL ANGIOGRAPHY FOR RENAL ARTERY OCCLUSIVE DISEASE

Study	No. of Patients	Technique	Sensitivity (%)	Specificity (%)
Kim et al. (1990)[19]	25	TOF	100	92
Kent et al. (1991)[20]	37	TOF	100	94
Debatin et al. (1991)[22]	25	PC, TOF	87	97
Yucel et al. (1993)[21]	16	TOF	100	93
Grist et al. (1993)[4]	35	PC, TOF	89	95
Servois et al. (1994)[23]	21	TOF	70	78
Hertz et al. (1994)[24]	16	TOF	91	94

PC = phase contrast; TOF = time of flight.

a sensitivity of 100% and a specificity of 94%. These MRA studies entailed 2D gradient echo acquisitions in the axial and coronal plane to form renal MRA images. Five-millimeter thick sections with 1 mm of overlap between consecutively acquired sections were obtained. Each of 15 overlapping sections required a single 8-second breath hold; therefore the total time of study was less than 30 minutes. The investigators indicated that most patients are able to cooperate fully with such a study. One potential concern was patients with severe chronic respiratory insufficiency. Another concern was that positional variations in the renal artery from one breath to the next could cover part of the renal artery to be missed even with 1 mm overlap.

Yucel and associates at Massachusetts General Hospital studied 16 patients with renal insufficiency using a combination of 2D and 3D TOF MRAs.[13] In comparison to results obtained by conventional catheter-based angiography, all renal arteries were identified correctly by MRA. Accuracy for determining the presence or absence of a moderately severe stenosis or an occluded artery was 91%. When the subset of patients were examined to determine the sensitivity to detect the presence or absence of a severe, 70% proximal stenosis, 100% were detected by MRA, with a specificity of 93%. As in other studies, these investigators could only evaluate the proximal renal arteries as saturation of the blood with loss of MR signal occurred in the mid and distal renal arteries. Nonetheless in this preliminary study the investigators demonstrate that the combination of 2D and 3D TOF MRAs was capable of identifying all renal arteries and diagnosing renal artery stenosis in patients with renal insufficiency.

Debatin and associates at Duke University examined 33 patients undergoing renal MRA consisting of axial 2D PC, coronal 2D PC, and coronal 2D TOF acquisitions, which were obtained within 48 hours of angiography.[22] In 25 patients, these studies were performed to evaluate the possibility of renovascular hypertension or as an aid in the preparation of patients for donor nephrectomy. The evaluation was limited to the proximal 35 mm of each renal artery. Renal artery visualization and detection of renovascular disease was more complete with coronal phase contrast (80% sensitivity, 91% specificity) than with TOF (53% sensitivity, 97% specificity) images. Combined axial and coronal phase contrast images allowed good resolution of the proximal renal arteries and detection of 13 of 15 stenosis. The investigators found that the phase contrast sequences had a higher sensitivity than that achieved by coronal breath-held TOF sequences. The investigators concluded that although the techniques are quite promising, further refinements, such as the implementation of surface coils, shorter TEs, use of gradient moment nulling, and modification of the velocity-encoding volume aid, would be necessary to reach a high degree of spatial resolution.

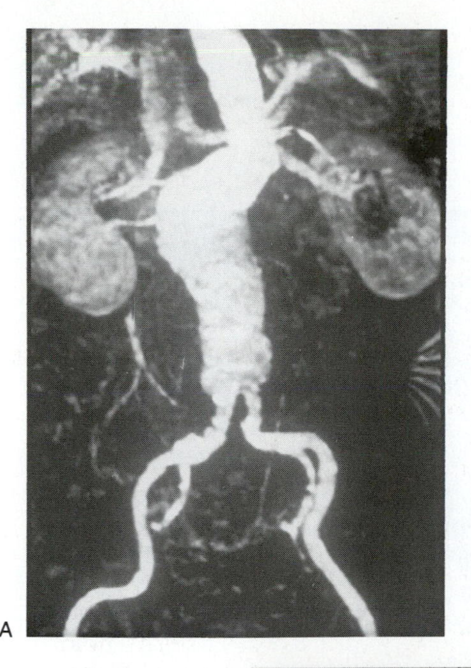

A

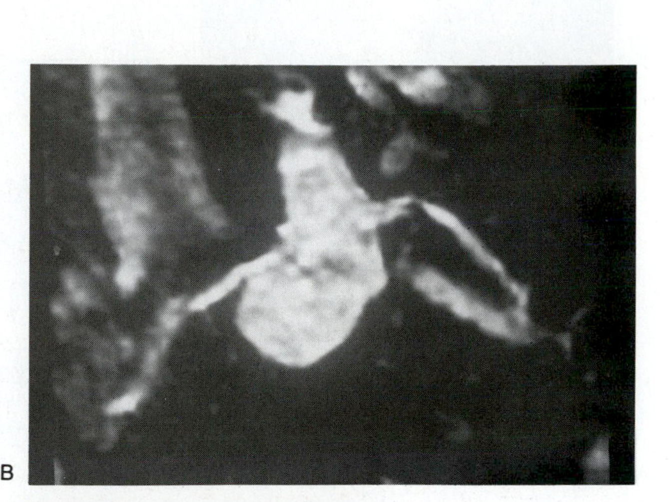

B

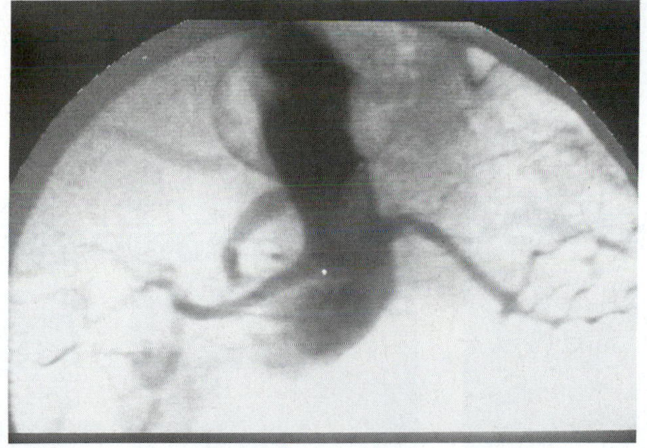

C

Figure 30–1. (**A**) Coronal MIP from a gadolinium-enhanced 3D MRA of an AAA showing that there is a proximal left renal artery stenosis. This left renal artery is better seen on an oblique reformation (**B**) and confirmed by digital subtraction arteriography (**C**). *(Reprinted with permission from Prince MR et al. J Vasc Surg. 21:256–269, 1995.)*

A recent study examined the role of 2D TOF MRA of renal arteries without maximum intensity projection in clinical decision making regarding renal artery stenosis.[23] Twenty-one patients underwent MRA and catheter angiography within a 3-day interval. Fifteen patients were suspected of having renovascular hypertension and six patients had multiple clinical manifestations of atherosclerotic occlusive disease including renal insufficiency. Conventional angiography showed 48 renal arteries. All main and three of six accessory arteries were identified correctly by MRA as well as 11 of 14 significant stenosis or occlusions. Overestimation of stenosis by MRA occurred in four circumstances. In two patients, the MRA provided a false-negative reading. The overall sensitivity and specificity for the detection of stenosis of the main renal arteries was 70% and 78%, respectively. The investigators concluded that 2D TOF MRA without 3D reconstruction is unable to substitute for traditional angiography mainly due to prob-

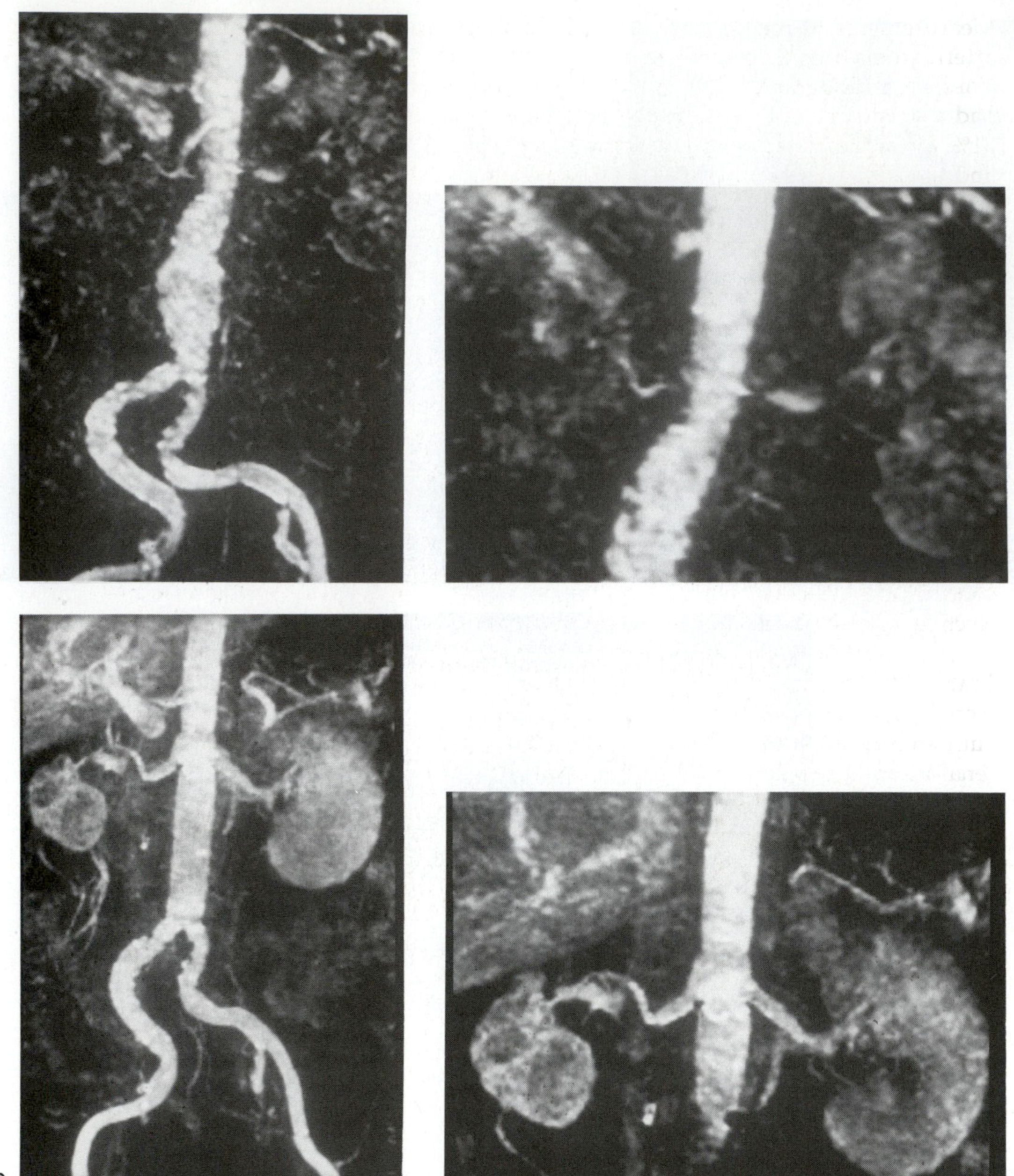

Figure 30–2. Coronary MIP (**A,B**) from a gadolinium-enhanced 3D MRA showing AAA and bilateral renal artery stenosis. After bilateral renal endarterectomy (**C,D**), there is improved visualization of the renal arteries and increased renal enhancement with the gadolinium. *(Reprinted with permission from Prince MR et al. J Vasc Surg. 21:256–269, 1995.)*

lems caused by anatomic variations and tortuosity of renal vessels. They concluded that in patients with nondiagnostic ultrasound exams, 2D TOF MRA was a useful screening tool prior to conventional angiography.

Hertz and colleagues at the University of Pennsylvania Hospital studied 16 adult patients who underwent 2D and 3D TOF MRA and conventional cut film angiography.[24]

Measurements of renal artery luminal diameter reduction were made from contrast arteriograms from three vascular radiologists blinded to the results of the other studies. Contrast arteriography revealed a 50% or greater stenosis in 11 of 32 patients. MRA had a sensitivity of 91%, negative predicted value of 94%, and an overall accuracy of 81%. Linear regression analysis demonstrated significant correlation between the MRA and the angiographic measurements ($r = 0.8$; $p < 0.001$). The false-negative study occurred due to a failure to detect a distal renal artery lesion in a patient with fibromuscular disease. As in other studies, resolution of the image of the orifice and proximal renal artery was far superior to that of the distal renal artery and its primary branches. Again, this loss of resolution in the distal artery was due to degradation of the MR signal by respiratory motion and in-plane saturation effects.[4]

Three studies have examined patients undergoing MRA and conventional catheter-based angiography in the evaluation of patients prior to elective kidney donation[25–27] (Table 30–2). Debatin and colleagues reported on 39 patients undergoing MRA using a 2D phase contrast technique in both coronal and axial planes.[25] In this patient group conventional arteriography showed 78 dominant and 13 accessory renal arteries. MRA identified the proximal 35 mm of all 78 dominant and of the 3 codominant renal arteries. Of the remaining 10 accessory arteries, only 4 were correctly identified with MRA. These investigators concluded that their high error rate (60%) indicated that phase contrast MRA was an inadequate diagnostic technique to evaluate patients prior to elective kidney donation.

Meyers and associates studied 17 patients who underwent post-processed 3D phase contrast MRA and conventional arteriography.[27] All 34 single or dominant renal arteries were identified correctly but only 8 of 10 accessory renal arteries were identified. These authors concluded that 3D MRA is a reliable technique of imaging single or dominant renal arteries but does not possess sufficient accuracy in the detection of accessory renal arteries in small arterial branches. Finally, Gedroyc and associates undertook a study of 50 renal transplant patients to determine the presence or absence of a significant renal artery stenosis in the transplanted kidney.[26] In this prospective study, of MRA and intra-arterial digital subtraction angiography, MRA had a sensitivity of 83% and a specificity of 97%, and when all images were graded respectively for severity of stenosis, the two techniques showed a significant correlation ($r = 0.74$; $p < 0.001$). These investigators concluded that 3D phase contrast MRA is both sensitive and specific for accurately imaging the renal transplant artery to determine the presence or absence of renal artery stenosis.

A consistent finding of all of these studies is that using a variety of imaging and reconstruction techniques, MRA is able in the majority of patients to accurately depict

TABLE 30–2. CORRELATION OF MRA AND CONVENTIONAL ANGIOGRAPHY FOR RENAL TRANSPLANTATION

Study	No. of Patients	Technique	Accuracy	Sensitivity (%)	Specificity (%)
Gedroyc et al. (1992)[25,a]	50	PC[c]	—[e]	83	97
Debatin et al. (1993)[26,b]	39	PC	60	—	—
Meyers et al. (1994)[27,b]	17	TOF[d]	80	—	—

[a] Transplant artery stenosis.
[b] Detection of all renal arteries.
[c] PC, phase contrast.
[d] TOF, time of flight.
[e] —, no data.

the location and the presence or absence of a stenosis in the dominant main proximal renal artery. All current techniques do not have sufficient resolution to diagnose distal or branch vessel renal artery disease or fibromuscular disease with sufficient accuracy. Other problems include overestimation of stenosis by MRA due to signal saturation caused by the presence of complex turbulent flow. Underestimation of renal artery stenosis is usually due to poor spatial resolution and poor signal-to-noise ratio. In this regard, 2D TOF is more sensitive to low flow rates and thus less apt to experience signal loss at high-grade stenosis or in patients with renal insufficiency. However, 2D TOF can be hampered by an underestimation of stenosis due to its relatively poor spatial resolution. Three-dimensional TOF achieves higher spatial resolution but suffers more from in-plant saturation. Blood is within the 3D imaging volume for such a long distance that by the time it reaches the mid-distal artery all the signal is gone and the artery image fades away.

Of these two shortcomings, overestimation of renal artery stenosis appears to be the greater hazard. Loss of signal in the area of a stenosis is due to "intravoxel dephasing."[4] It is caused by complex flow patterns that destroy the MR signal; MR signal is canceled due to the presence of multiple counteropposing phases within the smallest volume element or "voxel." Since the phase of the proton is proportional to the velocity of moving blood, the presence of a wide distribution of velocities in different direction results in a wide distribution of positive and negative proton phase resulting in cancellation of the overall signal.

The problem of saturation of the signal in renal arteries is amplified in patients with renal insufficiency and higher vascular resistance, which further reduces renal artery blood flow. One solution is to use an intravenous infusion of gadolinium-DPTA, which markedly reduces the T_1 relaxation time of blood making it bright on T_1 weighted images. This reduces the effect of spin saturation in the high resolution, heavily T_1 weighted 3D sequences. Image contrast with this approach is based on T_1 relaxation and less dependent on blood. It thus eliminates most of the flow and saturation artifacts that degrade the other techniques.

HIGH DOSE BREATH-HELD THREE-DIMENSIONAL GADOLINIUM

Although considerable progress has occurred in the development of MRA imaging of the renal arteries, loss of signal due to turbulent flow and poor resolution imaging of the distal renal artery continues to be an obstacle to a more widespread application of this technique. As stated earlier, the cost of the clinical consequences of renal artery occlusive disease, particularly those associated with the treatment of end-stage renal disease, has refocused our attention on the inadequacies of current alternatives to catheter-based, iodinated-contrast angiography. Both of the latter shortcomings of MRA, particularly blurring of the renal arteries due to respiratory motion, could potentially be remedied by a fast high dose 3D gadolinium MRA sequence performed during a breath-hold. We recently undertook a clinical study to examine this hypothesis more closely in which the resolution of breath-held shortened sequence images was compared to that of 3D gadolinium long, performed during quiet breathing as well as to conventional angiography. Whenever possible, the accuracy of these images was also substantiated by findings at surgery.

All patients were imaged with a 1.5 Tesla superconducting magnet (Signa, GE Medical Systems, Milwaukee, WI). The protocol for MRA renal artery imaging consisted of an initial sagittal T_1-weighted localizer sequence, coronal 2D TOF, a dynamic gadolinium-enhanced sequence, and a 3D phase contrast post-gadolinium images.

The 3D gadolinium-enhanced MRA image was acquired while the patients were holding their breath. It was possible to acquire a 12-slice volume in 29 s or a 28-slice volume in 58 s using a 16 kHz bandwidth.

Dynamic infusion of gadolinium during breath-holding produced a dramatic enhancement of the resolution of the aorta and renal artery images compared to those obtained prior to and immediately after gadolinium infusion. Reformation of the 3D data into axial, sagittal, and oblique planes provided perpendicular views of the renal arteries and lateral views of the celiac, proximal superior mesenteric, and inferior mesenteric arteries. In general, small arteries and renal artery stenosis were better visualized on individual raw data slices or on thin maximal intensity planes, while the aorta was better visualized on thicker maximal intensity planes. Analysis of the aorta, proximal, and distal renal arteries documented a higher signal-to-noise ratio and CNR with breath-holding compared to free breathing studies. The breath-held technique had superior resolution of the renal artery branches. Comparing breath-held examinations with the results obtained at conventional catheter-based angiography with surgical correlation, 22 arteries were graded as normal, 2 as mild stenosis, 1 as a moderate stenosis, and 3 as severe stenosis, as well as 1 occluded artery. This assessment by MR breath-held high-dose gadolinium imaging of the renal arteries correlated with the angiography in 27 arteries or at surgery in all but one patient. This patient had a complex clinical course after development of the Budd-Chiari syndrome and a severe left renal artery stenosis. At the time of angioplasty and subsequent to the MRA study, the renal artery was found to be occluded rather than to have a high-grade stenosis as the MRA suggested. However, the patient was taken off of Coumadin 5 days before the proposed angioplasty and progression from high-grade stenosis to total occlusion most likely occurred. When comparing studies in which the renal arteries were graded as moderate, severe, or occluded, the sensitivity and specificity for detecting renal artery stenosis were both 100%. A significantly worse correlation was found for MRA studies acquired during free breathing.

Of significance, the high-dose, breath-held gadolinium MRA studies demonstrated six accessory renal arteries, all of which were confirmed by angiography. In fact, one accessory renal artery was identified by MRA, that was not seen on the conventional catheter-based angiogram, but confirmed at the time of surgical exploration. In contrast, the free breathing technique identified only 71% of the accessory arteries in 30 patients in whom correlation was available.

A surprising outcome from this study was the lack of difficulty most patients had with a 58-second breath-hold. The procedure was well tolerated and although about half the patients began breathing in a shallow manner within the final 15 seconds of the 58-second breath-hold, they were able to suspend respiration throughout acquisition of the center of k-space. No contrast reactions occurred, and there was no evidence of nephrotoxicity from the gadolinium.

The accuracy and resolution of the high-dose, breath-held MRAs was clearly superior to those obtained during free breathing. However, this technique is more difficult to perform and requires the close attention of a radiologist throughout the procedure. These preliminary results suggest that these modifications of MRA may finally have elevated the resolution of the aorta and renal arteries to that of conventional angiography and thus allow this technique to be applied more widely in this very important high-risk group of patients. Breath-held gadolinium MRA used in combination with 3D phase contrast MRA (postgadolinium) and T_1-weighted images to evaluate renal size/mass and left ventricular hypertrophy will likely become the preferred approach to screening patients for renovascular hypertension.

REFERENCES

1. Rimmer JM, Gennari FJ. Atherosclerotic renovascular disease and progressive renal failure. *Ann Intern Med.* 1993;118:712–719.
2. Pickering TG. Functional significance of renal arterial occlusive disease. In: Ernst CB, Stanley JC, eds. *Current Therapy in Vascular Surgery.* St. Louis, MO: Mosby–Year Book; 1995:774.
3. Hansen KJ, Reavis SW, Dean RH. Duplex scanning for renal arterial occlusive disease. In: Ernst CB, Stanley JC, eds. *Current Therapy in Vascular Surgery.* St. Louis, MO: Mosby–Year Book; 1995:768.
4. Grist TM. Magnetic resonance angiography of renal artery stenosis. *Am J Kid Dis.* 1994;24:700–712.
5. Pearce WH, Salyapongse AN, Fitzgerald S. Computed tomography and magnetic resonance imaging in vascular disease. In: Rutherford RB, ed. *Vascular Surgery.* 4th ed. Philadelphia: WB Saunders; 1995:130.
6. Anderson CM. What is MRA? In: Anderson CM, Edelman RR, Tursi, eds. *Clinical Magnetic Resonance Angiography.* New York: Raven Press; 1993:1.
7. Anderson CM. Time-of-flight angiography. In: Anderson CM, Edelman RR, Tursi, eds. *Clinical Magnetic Resonance Angiography.* New York: Raven Press; 1993:11.
8. Anderson CM. Phase contrast angiography. In: Anderson CM, Edelman RR, Tursi, eds. *Clinical Magnetic Resonance Angiography.* New York: Raven Press; 1993:43.
9. Prince MR, Yucel EK, Kaufman JA, et al. Dynamic gadolinium-enhanced three-dimensional abdominal MR arteriography. *Radiology.* 1993;3:877–881.
10. Prince MR. Gadolinium-enhanced MR aortography. *Radiology.* 1994;191:155–164.
11. Belli AM. New approaches to the diagnosis and management of renal artery stenosis. *J Hum Hypertens.* 1994;8:593–594.
12. Lewin JS. Time-of-flight magnetic resonance angiography of the aorta and renal arteries. *Am J Neuroradiol.* 1994;15:1657–1664.
13. Yucel EK. Magnetic resonance angiography of the lower extremity and renal arteries. *Semin Ultrasound CT MR.* 1992;13:291–302.
14. Mukai J, Kershaw G, Hees PS. Application of magnetic resonance imaging to physiologic and morphologic characterization of renal artery stenosis before and after angioplasty. *Am J Physiol Imaging.* 1992;7:220–229.
15. Postma CT, Hartog O, Rosenbusch G, et al. Magnetic resonance angiography in the diagnosis of renal artery stenosis. *J Hypertens.* 1993;11:S204–S205.
16. Farrugia E, King BF, Larson TS. Magnetic resonance angiography and detection of renal artery stenosis in a patient with impaired renal function. *Mayo Clin Proc.* 1993;68:157–160.
17. Roditi GH, Smith FW, Redpath TW. Evaluation of tilted, optimized, nonsaturating excitation pulses in 3D magnetic resonance angiography of the abdominal aorta and major branches in volunteers. *Br J Radiol.* 1994;67:11–13.
18. Lundin B, Cooper TG, Meyer RA, et al. Measurement of total and unilateral renal blood flow by oblique-angle velocity-encoded 2D-cine magnetic resonance angiography. *Magn Reson Imaging.* 1993;11:51–59.
19. Kim D, Edelman RR, Kent KC, et al. Abdominal aortic and renal artery stenosis: evaluation with MR angiography. *Radiology.* 1990;174:727–731.
20. Kent KC, Edelman RR, Kim D, et al. Magnetic resonance imaging: a reliable test for the evaluation of proximal atherosclerotic renal arterial stenosis. *J Vasc Surg.* 1991;13:311–318.
21. Yucel EK, Kaufman JA, Prince M, et al. *Magn Reson Imaging.* 1993;11:925–930.
22. Debatin JF, Spritzer CE, Grist TM, et al. Imaging of the renal arteries: value of MR angiography. *Am J Roentgenol.* 1991;157:981–990.

23. Servois V, Laissy JP, Feger Ch, et al. Two-dimensional time-of-flight magnetic resonance angiography of renal arteries without maximum intensity projection: a prospective comparison with angiography in 21 patients screened for renovascular hypertension. *Cardiovasc Intervent Radiol.* 1994;17:138–142.
24. Hertz SM, Holland GA, Baum RA, et al. Evaluation of renal artery stenosis by magnetic resonance angiography. *Am J Surg.* 1994;168:140–143.
25. Debatin JF, Sostman HD, Knelson M, et al. Renal magnetic resonance angiography in the preoperative detection of supernumerary renal arteries in potential kidney donors. *Invest Radiol.* 1993;28:882–889.
26. Gedroyc WMW, Negus R, Al-Kutoubi A, et al. Magnetic resonance angiography of renal transplants. *Lancet.* 1992;339:789–791.
27. Meyers SP, Talagala SL, Totterman S, et al. Evaluation of the renal arteries in kidney donors: value of three-dimensional phase-contrast MR angiography with maximum-intensity-projection or surface rendering. *Am J Roentgenol.* 1995;164:117–121.

31

Combined Aortic and Renal Artery Surgery

Charles S. O'Mara, MD

Recent series[1-3] have documented a changing clinical profile for patients requiring operation for renal revascularization. These reports have shown a trend toward predominantly older patients with more diffuse atherosclerosis. Patients often have combined aortic and renal disease, and the renal occlusive lesions are frequently bilateral. These trends are reflected in the report of Hansen et al.[4] in which 64 of 157 patients (41%) treated for atherosclerotic renal artery disease required concomitant aortic replacement for correction of an aortic aneurysm or severe aortoiliac occlusive disease. Among these combined procedures, 32 patients (50%) had bilateral renal artery repair.

In the 1960s, DeBakey et al.[5] accumulated the first series of patients treated with combined aortic and renal artery reconstruction. Nevertheless, surgical management of these patients remains difficult. Furthermore, this aspect of vascular surgery encompasses many concepts and practices that are highly controversial. Such issues are exemplified by the following questions:

1. Is prophylactic repair of a renal artery stenosis (RAS) combined with aortic reconstruction justified in the absence of severe hypertension and renal insufficiency?
2. In current practice, is the risk of combined aortic and renal revascularization significantly higher than either aortic or renal reconstruction alone?
3. Should a severely diseased but asymptomatic aorta be replaced solely to provide optimal inflow to a renal artery graft?
4. Are nonaortic sources of inflow for renal revascularization durable enough to be used frequently when a severely diseased aorta precludes its use for inflow?
5. When combined with aortic replacement, which is the preferred operative technique for renal revascularization, bypass or endarterectomy?

These difficult questions, as well as other controversial aspects of this challenging problem, will be addressed in this chapter by considering results of studies in the recent literature along with personal experience.

PREVALENCE OF RENAL ARTERY STENOSIS IN PATIENTS WITH AORTIC DISEASE

Patients with aneurysmal and occlusive disease of the aorta have a substantial prevalence of moderate or severe RAS, even when renal artery occlusive disease is clinically unsuspected. A recent study by Olin et al.[6] from the Cleveland Clinic analyzed 395 consecutive patients undergoing arteriography without clinically suspected renal artery occlusive disease. RAS of greater than 50% was found in 38% of patients with an aortic aneurysm and 33% of patients with aortoiliac occlusive disease. A severely stenotic (75%–99%) or totally occluded renal artery was demonstrated in 18% of aneurysm patients and 15% of patients with aortoiliac occlusive disease.

As a result of this high prevalence of significant RAS among patients requiring aortic reconstruction, a decision often must be made about whether renal revascularization should be combined with aortic reconstruction. Although some of these patients have clinical findings that suggest functional renovascular disease, many patients with RAS exhibit neither severe hypertension nor renal insufficiency. Rational decisions regarding management of these uncomplicated renal artery lesions require a consideration of the long-term outcome of untreated RAS.

NATURAL HISTORY OF RENAL ARTERY OCCLUSIVE DISEASE

The natural history of atherosclerotic RAS has been evaluated by four retrospective studies[7–10] of patients undergoing serial arteriograms (Table 31–1). Incidence of progression of RAS in these reports ranged from 36% to 53%, while progression to total occlusion varied from 9% to 16%. In the study by Schreiber et al.[8], the risk of progression to occlusion was especially high (39%) in renal arteries with greater than 75% stenosis on the initial arteriogram. Moreover, the greater the degree of stenosis, the more quickly occlusion occurred. Tollefson and Ernst[9] found that the average RAS on the arteriogram immediately before occlusion was 80% (range, 61% to 94%). Among those renal arteries that developed progressive narrowing in their study, a predictable rate of about 5% per year was documented irrespective of the initial degree of stenosis.

The progressive nature of RAS was further documented in a recent prospective study by Zierler et al.[11] in which 80 patients with renal artery lesions were monitored with serial duplex ultrasonography for follow-up intervals extending to 26 months. The incidence of progression from less than 60% to 60% or greater RAS was approximately 20% per year. Alarmingly, the rate of occlusion among renal arteries with a previously documented 60% or greater stenosis was about 5% per year. All arteries

TABLE 31–1. STUDIES OF SERIAL RENAL ARTERIOGRAMS

Authors (Ref. No.)	Year Published	No. Patients	Follow-Up Interval	Progressive RAS (%)	Progression to OCC (%)
Meaney et al.[7]	1968	39	6 mo.–10 yr.	36[b]	10[b]
Wollenweber et al.[10]	1968	30	mean 28 mo.	50[a]	NG
Schreiber et al.[8]	1984	85	mean 52 mo.	44[b]	16[b]
Tollefson and Ernst[9]	1991	48	mean 54 mo.	53[a]	9[a]

[a] Percentages based on number of renal artery lesions.
[b] Percentages based on number of patients.
NG, not given; OCC, renal artery occlusion; RAS, renal artery stenosis.

that progressed to occlusion had 60% or greater stenosis at baseline assessment. Loss of renal mass was documented by a mean decrease in length of almost 2 cm among those kidneys associated with renal artery occlusion.

These studies clearly document the progressive nature of renal artery occlusive disease, especially when the degree of stenosis is severe. Progression to occlusion usually results in loss of renal mass and may complicate or preclude renal revascularization. Furthermore, reoperation for renal revascularization after aortic reconstruction may present technical problems that compromise safety as well as functional results.

INDICATIONS FOR ADJUNCTIVE RENAL ARTERY REVASCULARIZATION

Although no data in the literature proves that repair of asymptomatic RAS optimizes renal function or prolongs life, these natural history studies support concomitant renal revascularization for stenoses of 75% or greater, whether or not the patient has hypertension or renal insufficiency. Patients with stenosis of 60% to 74% should be individualized. Adjunctive renal artery repair should be done for patients with renovascular hypertension or vascular-related renal insufficiency and for selected patients with a reasonable life expectancy who have asymptomatic renal artery lesions, especially when such lesions are bilateral or involve a solitary kidney.

Excellent results without death or renal functional impairment after prophylactic renal revascularization combined with aortic reconstruction have been reported.[3,12] It is indeed imperative that individual centers monitor their morbidity and mortality results to verify that a low operative risk can be achieved to justify adjunctive renal artery repair. However, prophylactic renal revascularization is not recommended for patients with stenosis less than 60%.

RISK OF COMBINED AORTORENAL RECONSTRUCTION

Prior to the mid-1980s, numerous studies reported high operative mortality rates for synchronous aortic and renal revascularization. In 1975, the multicenter Cooperative Study of Renovascular Hypertension[13] reported an operative mortality rate of 25% for the combined operations. Four other series[14–17] published through 1984 reported operative mortality rates ranging from 12% to 27.4%. Such high figures for operative mortality should be considered in historic perspective, yet continued reference to them has led to the misperception that combined aortic and renal procedures still have an inordinately high risk.[18]

In contrast to these high mortality rates, seven reports[4,12,19–23] from different institutions published during the past decade involving a total of 410 patients have each documented an operative mortality for combined aortic and renal reconstruction of 3.2% or less (Table 31–2). The collective mortality rate for these series was 2.0%. These results demonstrate that combined aortorenal reconstruction can be performed currently with an operative mortality rate that is lower than previously reported and that even approaches the mortality rate of either aortic or renal revascularization done as a solitary procedure.

This comparable mortality rate is substantiated by the study of Branchereau et al.,[19] in which operative mortality for patients undergoing combined aortorenal reconstruction was 2% at their institution from 1980 to 1990. During the same interval,

TABLE 31–2. SIMULTANEOUS AORTIC AND RENAL RECONSTRUCTIONS

Authors (Ref. No.)	Year Published	No. Patients	Operative Mortality (%)
Stewart et al.[23]	1985	63	3.2
O'Mara et al.[22]	1988	32	3.2
Branchereau et al.[19]	1992	48	2.0
Hanson et al.[4]	1992	64	3.1
Chaikoff et al.[20]	1994	50	2.0
McNeil et al.[12]	1994	101	1.0
Dougherty et al.[21]	1995	52	0
Combined results		410	2.0

operative mortality was virtually the same for isolated aortic reconstruction for occlusive disease (2%), for isolated aortic aneurysm repair (2.8%), and for isolated renal artery revascularization (2.2%).

AORTIC REPLACEMENT SOLELY FOR INFLOW

When combined with renal revascularization, aortic reconstruction is usually required for correction of either an aneurysm or symptomatic aortoiliac occlusive disease. However, some patients have prominent aortic plaque formation angiographically with no hemodynamically significant aortoiliac stenosis and no lower extremity ischemic symptoms. In this circumstance, calcification and degenerative material within the plaque can render the native aorta unsuitable as a source of reliable inflow to a renal artery graft. Moreover, subsequent progression of aortic atherosclerosis may compromise long-term renal graft function.

Cambria et al.[24] emphasized the technical difficulties of originating a renal bypass graft from a diseased but asymptomatic aorta. They reported a 23.5% failure rate at 2 years for renal grafts originating from the native aorta. In contrast, their renal graft failure rate at 2 years was only about 5% when inflow was obtained from an aortic prosthetic graft.

Based on these considerations, our practice is to replace the aorta with a prosthetic graft in patients with severe aortorenal atherosclerosis, even in the absence of an aneurysm or symptomatic aortoiliac occlusive disease. This approach assures optimal long-term inflow to the renal graft and, in our experience, is technically easier and safer than alternatives such as localized aortic endarterectomy and patch aortoplasty.

NONAORTIC SOURCES OF INFLOW

Some authors[25–28] have advocated alternative techniques using nonaortic sources of inflow such as splenorenal, hepatorenal, and ileorenal bypass for patients who require renal revascularization and who also have an aorta unsuitable for use as an inflow source. However, the presence of occlusive disease in the celiac axis or the iliac arteries often precludes use of these remote sources. In addition, the potential for progression of atherosclerosis in these arteries raises concern about the durability of extra-anatomic grafting.

Although Cambria et al.[24] reported acceptable durability of various techniques for renal revascularization, analysis of their data suggests that late failures occurred almost twice as frequently with extra-anatomic grafts as with direct renal reconstructions.[29] As a result of these concerns, we limit use of extra-anatomic techniques to highly selected situations, such as when the retroperitoneum is densely scarred from previous aortic reconstruction or when inordinately high cardiopulmonary risk factors preclude aortic reconstruction.

MANAGEMENT OF BILATERAL RENAL ARTERY STENOSIS

Bilateral involvement is especially common in patients who have renal artery occlusive disease combined with severe aortic atherosclerosis. In the past, reports[18] have suggested a high operative risk for patients undergoing simultaneous bilateral renal revascularization. In the study of Tarazi et al.,[30] the operative mortality rate among patients having surgical treatment of bilateral renal artery occlusive disease was 15%, which was twice the mortality of their patients treated for unilateral disease. Concern about increased risk led some authors[31,32] to recommend a selective staged repair of bilateral lesions or correction of only the side with the more severe degree of stenosis or the higher renal vein renin value.

Recent studies, by contrast, have shown that simultaneous bilateral renal revascularization, even when combined with aortic reconstruction, can be accomplished with acceptable operative risk. O'Mara et al.[22] reported an operative mortality rate of 3.2% among 32 patients undergoing simultaneous aortic reconstruction and bilateral renal revascularization. In the study of Chaikof et al.[20] bilateral renal artery bypass was done in 21 of 50 patients (42%) undergoing combined aortorenal revascularization. The incidence of postoperative complications was similar for patients having bilateral renal artery bypass compared to those receiving unilateral repair. These results support the use of simultaneous bilateral renal revascularization when each renal artery warrants repair on its own merit.

PREOPERATIVE ASSESSMENT

Proper patient selection and careful preoperative evaluation with optimization of risk factors are paramount in achieving satisfactory outcome in patients undergoing these complex operations. RAS of 75% or more has been shown to be associated with a fourfold increase in the prevalence of clinically overt coronary artery disease.[33] This relationship emphasizes the importance of thorough cardiac assessment preoperatively. Cardiac function and valvular integrity are assessed by echocardiography, and dipyridamole-thallium radionuclide scanning is used to detect significant coronary artery occlusive disease. Coronary angiography is undertaken in patients with a history of progressive or unstable angina or with a reversibly ischemic area of myocardium demonstrated by dipyridamole-thallium scan.

These patients frequently have a significant cigarette smoking history with resultant chronic obstructive lung disease. Pulmonary status is evaluated using pulmonary function studies with bronchodilator responsiveness and baseline arterial blood gas determinations. Preoperative pulmonary preparation with bronchodilators and steroid therapy is important in selected patients with advanced lung disease.

Complete arteriographic evaluation with visualization of the entire abdominal aorta and its visceral branches is essential for planning the appropriate operation. When renal disease is the primary indication for evaluation, full arteriographic demonstration of the iliac and common femoral arteries is also important in determining the optimal inflow technique for renal revascularization. In patients evaluated primarily for aortic disease, RAS, when not readily apparent, should be suspected by the presence of a delayed nephrogram or by disparity in size of the kidneys. RAS in this circumstance can be detected by oblique views to define the renal artery origins. Restricting the volume of contrast material by the use of intra-arterial digital subtraction angiography and providing adequate intravenous hydration are important measures to minimize risk of contrast-induced nephrotoxicity.

PERIOPERATIVE MANAGEMENT

Advances in perioperative management are also essential in allowing these complex reconstructions to be accomplished with low operative mortality and morbidity. During operation patients now undergo monitoring of multiple physiologic parameters, including systemic arterial pressure, right atrial pressure, pulmonary arterial pressure, pulmonary capillary wedge pressure, pulmonary and systemic vascular resistance, cardiac output, and urinary output. Cardiac function is optimized by regulating intravascular volume and by the judicious use of vasopressor agents. Afterload reduction to minimize cardiac stress during aortic clamping is achieved with vasodilating agents.

Adjunctive epidural anesthesia provides excellent postoperative pain control and is especially helpful in facilitating satisfactory pulmonary toilet in patients with severe lung disease. Heparin is administered intravenously before vascular clamping, and protamine is given for heparin reversal after the reconstruction is completed. Shed blood is autotransfused routinely, and exogenous blood transfusion is infrequently needed.

Prior to renal artery repair, intravascular volume status is optimized and diuresis is initiated by administration of intravenous mannitol. Although renal revascularization can usually be accomplished with a renal clamp time of about 20 minutes, in our experience renal ischemic times up to 45 minutes are generally well tolerated, especially in patients with severely stenotic lesions. We have not utilized techniques either for cooling of the kidney or for direct renal artery perfusion.

OPERATIVE TECHNIQUES

Aortic reconstruction is accomplished by either aortofemoral or aortoiliac bypass or by infrarenal aortic replacement with a tube graft (Table 31–3). The three principal methods by which renal revascularization is done in conjunction with aortic reconstruction are transaortic renal endarterectomy, bypass from aortic graft to renal artery, and reimplantation of the renal artery into the aortic graft. Proximal renal artery exclusion and direct renal eversion endarterectomy are used in conjunction with both bypass and reimplantation.

Transaortic renal endarterectomy combined with aortic reconstruction can be done either transperitoneally[3] or via a left retroperitoneal approach.[34,35] This procedure is performed by initially clamping the aorta at or above the level of the superior mesenteric artery orifice. The aorta is transected just distal to the renal artery origins, and the plaque is separated circumferentially from the aortic wall. The endarterectomy is extended in

TABLE 31–3. OPERATIVE TECHNIQUES

Methods of Aortic Reconstruction
Aortofemoral bypass
Aortoiliac bypass
Infrarenal aortic replacement
Methods of Renal Artery Repair
Transaortic endarterectomy
Renal artery bypass/reimplantation
Proximal renal artery exclusion
Direct renal eversion endarterectomy

continuity into each involved renal artery. The renal endarterectomy is accomplished by exerting gentle traction on the aortic plaque and thereby prolapsing the renal artery into the aortic lumen (Fig. 31–1). Eversion of the renal artery for adequate plaque removal is facilitated by completely mobilizing the main renal artery prior to aortic clamping. With continued traction and teasing away of the renal artery wall, the plaque should separate with a smooth transition into normal distal intima.

After the renal lesion has been removed, the contiguous aortic plaque is transected proximal to and away from the renal artery orifice. The graft is then anastomosed to the aorta in end-to-end fashion. After vascular flushing, the aortic graft is clamped, renal perfusion is restored, and the aortic reconstruction is completed.

A longitudinal incision in the aorta from its transected end to a point alongside the superior mesenteric artery orifice may be necessary for adequate transluminal visualization of the renal orifice. This incision can subsequently be closed primarily, or a tongue of the graft can be fashioned for incorporation of this incision into the graft-aortic anastomosis.

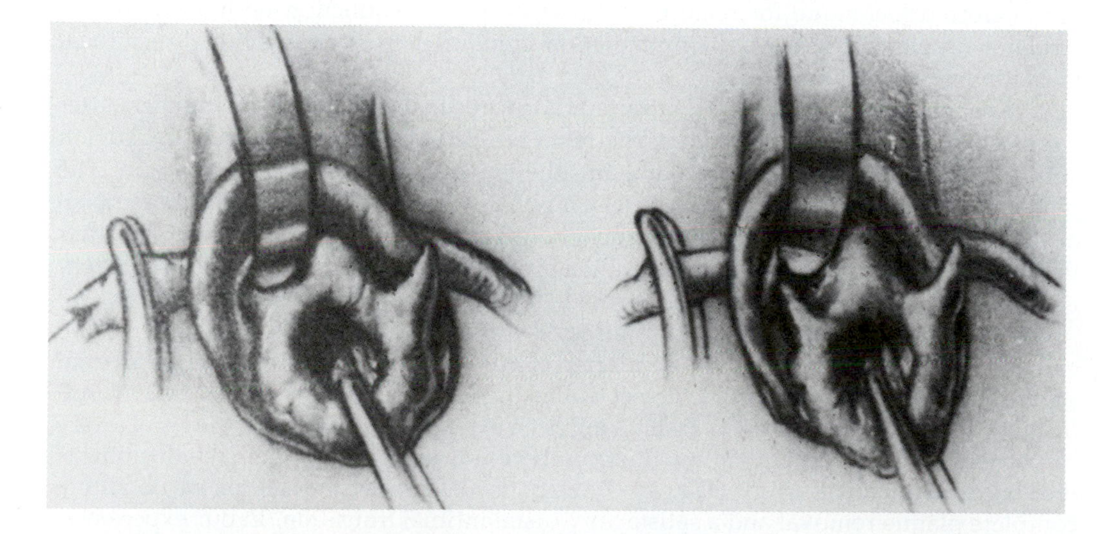

Figure 31–1. Drawings depict removal of plaque in continuity from the aorta and from each renal orifice using the technique of transaortic endarterectomy. *(Reprinted with permission from Stoney et al. Renal endarterectomy through the transected aorta: a new technique for combined aortorenal atherosclerosis—a preliminary report. J Vasc Surg. 1989;9:224–233.)*

Transaortic endarterectomy is well suited for lesions confined to the renal artery orifice, especially when multiple small stenotic renal arteries are present (Fig. 31–2). However, the technique should not be used when plaque extends into the distal renal artery. The principal advantage of this procedure is a relatively brief interruption of renal blood flow. A disadvantage is the obligatory interruption of blood flow to the contralateral kidney when only unilateral repair is required. In addition, satisfactory plaque removal may prove difficult because of limited exposure, poor visualization transluminally, or unanticipated extension of plaque into the distal renal artery. Indeed, precise determination of the distal extent of plaque is sometimes not possible by preoperative arteriography or even by findings at operation prior to undertaking the endarterectomy. Furthermore, the left retroperitoneal approach for transaortic endarterectomy of a right renal artery lesion should be used cautiously and only when definite poststenotic dilatation just beyond the renal artery orifice ensures proximal confinement of the plaque.

Despite these caveats, several reports[3,12] have documented good results with the technique of transaortic renal endarterectomy combined with aortic reconstruction. Dougherty et al.[21] recently reported the Mayo Clinic experience with transaortic renal endarterectomy in 26 patients and with renal artery bypass in another 26 patients during the same time period when either technique was combined with infrarenal aortic replacement. Patients in this study were not randomized, and no rigid criteria were used for choice of technique. Bypass patients generally had more advanced cardiovascular and renal disease, while endarterectomy patients required more intraoperative technical revisions (12% vs. 4%) than bypass patients. However, both groups experienced no operative mortality, had similar cardiopulmonary morbidity, and achieved equal improvement in hypertension.

These results suggest that both transaortic endarterectomy and renal artery bypass can be used effectively in conjunction with aortic surgery. We use transaortic endarterectomy for orificeal lesions in multiple or small renal arteries, especially when such lesions are conducive to being approached through the obliquely transected aorta to permit satisfactory transluminal visualization of the renal orifice (Fig. 31–2). However, our preferred technique for renal revascularization in conjunction with aortic reconstruction is either bypass or reimplantation combined frequently with direct renal eversion endarterectomy.

With this approach, standard infrarenal aortic reconstruction is done initially. After completion of aortic reconstruction, the renal artery is ligated with a silk transfixion suture secured to the adventitia adjoining the aorta and the renal artery origin. The renal artery, which has been completely mobilized from aorta to the primary renal artery branches prior to aortic reconstruction, is transected just beyond its origin. After the renal revascularization is completed, the proximal transected end of the renal artery is oversewn with vascular suture to provide a secure renal artery stump closure.

If plaque is present in the distal transected end of the artery, a direct renal eversion endarterectomy is performed. This endarterectomy is accomplished by circumferential separation of the plaque from the vessel wall using fine instruments and optical magnification. Unattached to the aorta and having been extensively mobilized, the renal artery can be everted upon itself to allow unencumbered direct transluminal visualization of the entire main renal artery (Fig. 31–3). Such visualization is essential in obtaining complete plaque removal and a satisfactory distal intimal transition. In our experience, this method of endarterectomy has been superior in most situations to transaortic renal endarterectomy, which sometimes provides only a momentary, partially obscured view of the transition from plaque to normal intima and leaves doubt about achieving complete plaque removal.

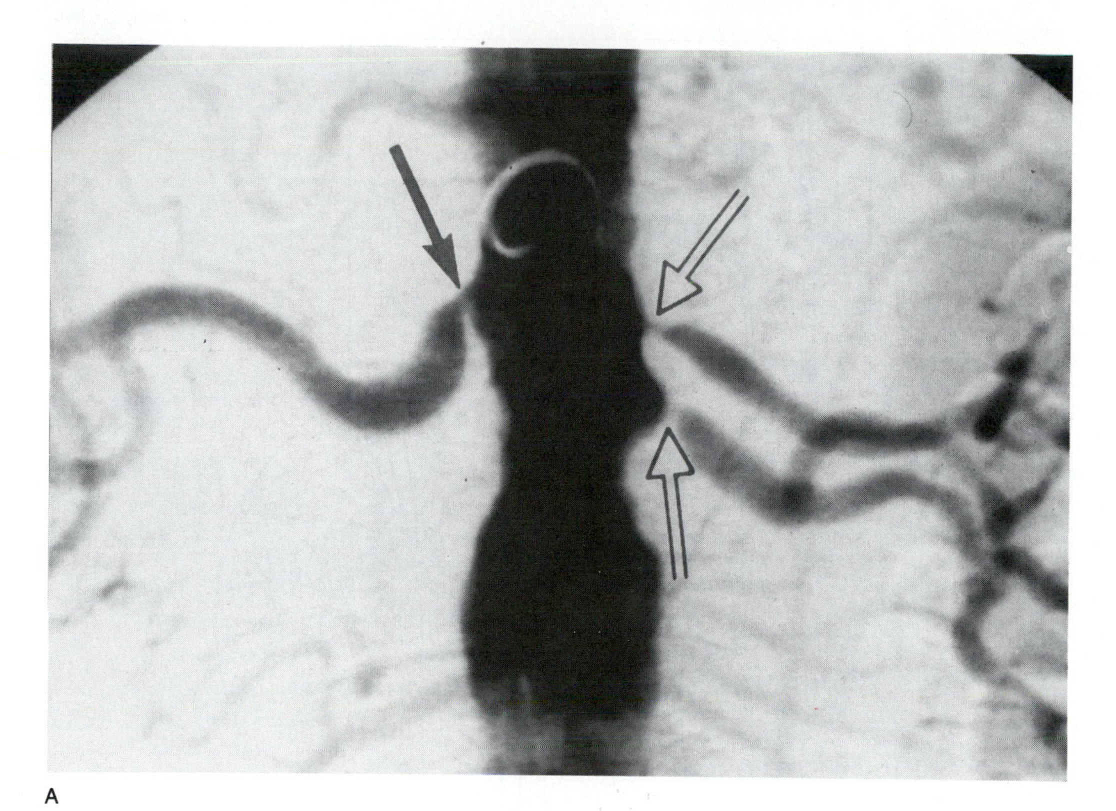
A

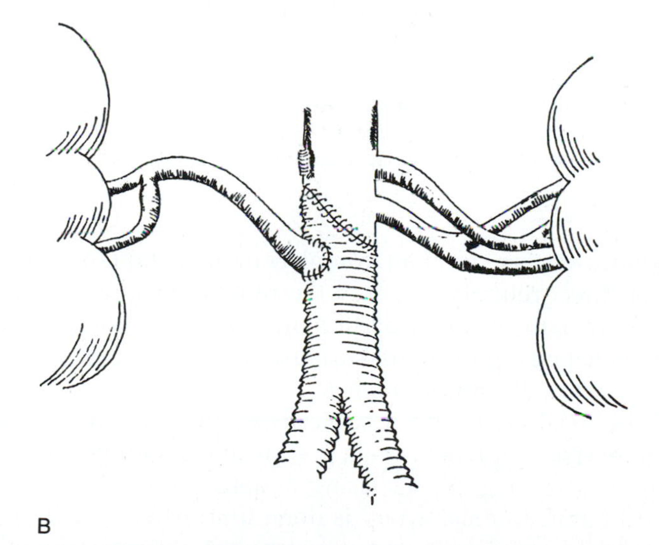
B

Figure 31–2. (**A**) Aortogram demonstrating stenosis of the right renal artery (*solid arrow*) and stenosis of two left renal arteries (*open arrows*). This patient also had a large abdominal aortic aneurysm. (**B**) Repair was accomplished by transaortic endarterectomy of the two left renal arteries through the obliquely transected aorta, aortoiliac bypass, and direct eversion endarterectomy of the right renal artery. Redundancy of the right renal artery allowed its reimplantation into the prosthetic graft without need for an intervening graft.

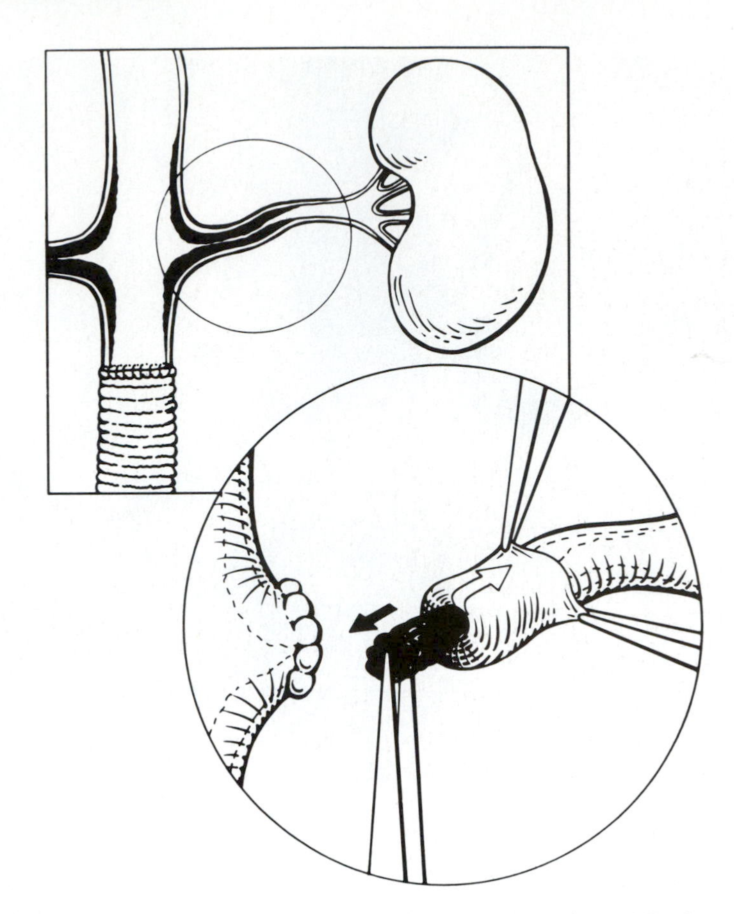

Figure 31–3. Direct renal eversion endarterectomy is done following full mobilization and proximal transection of the renal artery. The vessel can then be everted upon itself to permit complete plaque removal with direct transluminal visualization throughout its entire length.

When the renal artery is redundant, complete mobilization of the vessel may permit enough length for direct reimplantation of the renal artery into the side of the aortic graft (Fig. 31–2). Vascular control for performance of this anastomosis can be obtained either with a tangential clamp for partial occlusion or by clamping both the infrarenal aorta and the graft below the anastomotic site.

If length of the renal artery is not sufficient to permit direct reimplantation into the aortic graft, a reversed saphenous vein graft is interposed between the renal artery and the aortic prosthesis (Fig. 31–4). Using a spatulated end-to-end technique, the anastomosis of vein graft to renal artery is done first. After this distal anastomosis is completed, appropriate graft length and curvature are determined while gently instilling heparinized saline from a syringe attached to the proximal end of the vein graft. The proximal end of the graft is anastomosed to a window cut in the side of the aortic graft using a tangential clamp for partial occlusion. The same procedure is then done for the contralateral renal artery if bilateral lesions warrant repair.

An end-to-end technique for the distal anastomosis of a renal artery bypass has several advantages over end-to-side anastomosis. The principal benefit is that transection of the proximal renal artery just beyond its origin combined with mobilization distally permits the transected end of the artery to be easily elevated out of the depths of the retroperitoneum to afford optimal exposure for a technically precise anastomosis.

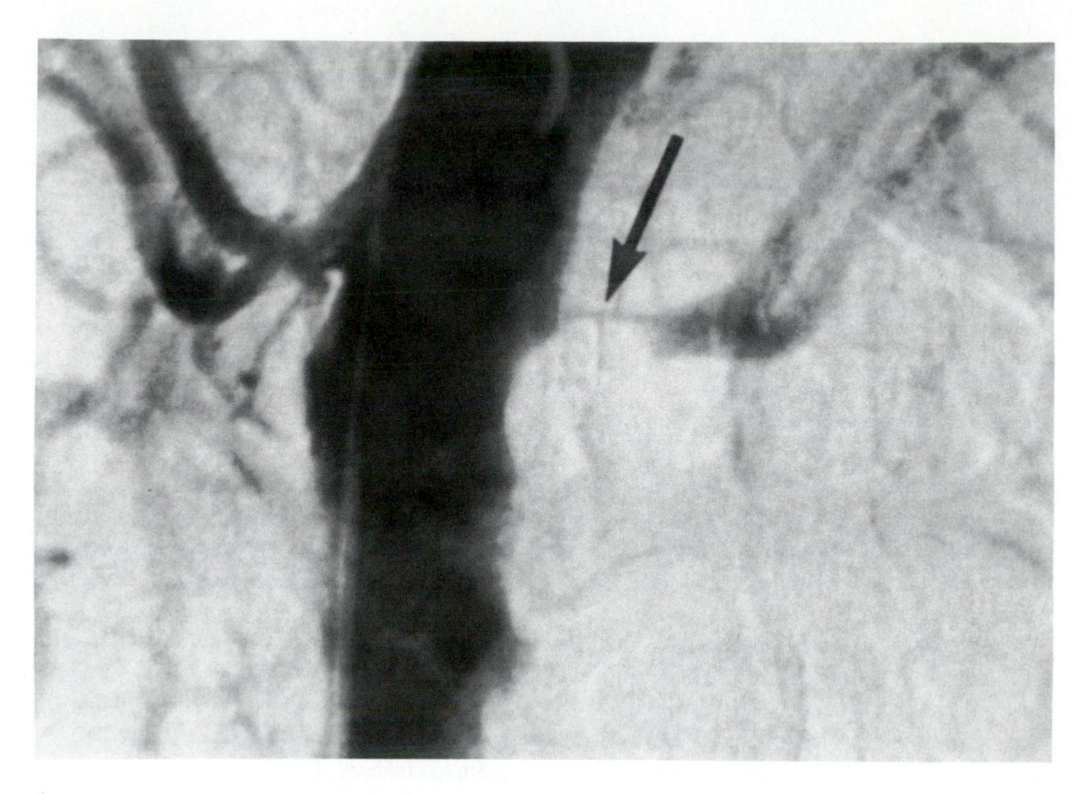

A

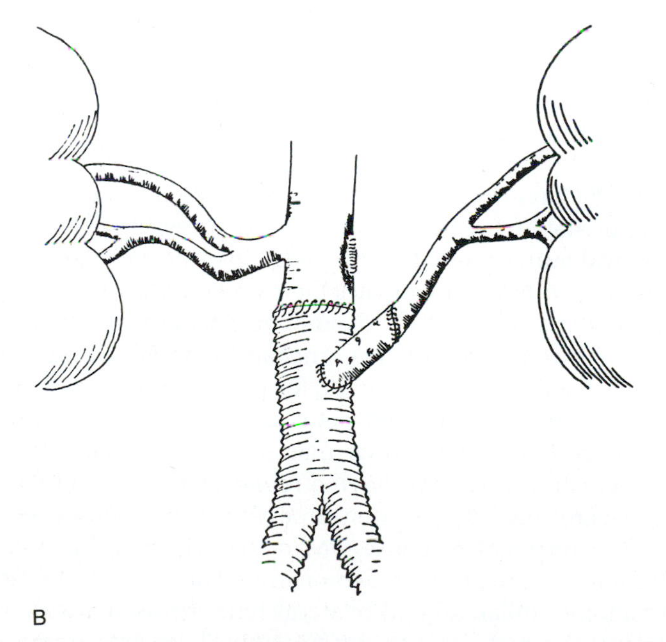

B

Figure 31–4. (**A**) Aortogram showing high-grade left RAS (*arrow*). The study also documented right common iliac artery occlusion. (**B**) This patient underwent aortofemoral bypass for lower extremity revascularization and direct left renal eversion endarterectomy along with placement of an interposition saphenous vein graft between the renal artery and the aortic prosthesis for renal revascularization.

Also, end-to-end anastomosis eliminates the potential for competing flow through the native renal artery. Finally, plaque extending into the distal renal artery can be completely removed by direct renal eversion endarterectomy prior to performing the renal artery anastomosis.

Intraoperative duplex ultrasonography has been shown to be effective in assessment of the technical result of renal revascularization. Significant problems such as a distal intimal flap or an anastomotic narrowing were recognized in about 11% of patients in each of two series.[4,36] Most of these defects were immediately correctable without adverse outcome.

BLOOD PRESSURE RESPONSE

The effectiveness of isolated renal revascularization in treating hypertension is well established. Several authors[2,37] have reported a beneficial blood pressure response in 90% of carefully selected patients. Long-term improvement in hypertension after combined aortic and renal artery reconstruction is achieved in comparable series at rates that range from 60% to 75%.[3,21,38,39]

This less beneficial blood pressure response for combined operation compared to isolated renal revascularization is probably related principally to differences in diagnostic evaluation. Methods currently used for establishing the diagnosis of renovascular hypertension have recognized limitations, especially in the presence of bilateral RAS, which is common in patients with aortorenal atherosclerosis. Furthermore, these diagnostic methods have not been widely applied in patients undergoing operation for combined aortic and renal artery disease, even when only unilateral RAS exists.

RENAL FUNCTIONAL RESPONSE

Numerous reports[37,40,41] have documented the importance of isolated renal revascularization in improving or stabilizing renal function and preserving renal tissue in selected patients. Studies evaluating patients with renal insufficiency undergoing combined aortorenal reconstruction have shown variable results in the extent and clinical setting of this functional benefit. Chaikof et al.[20] documented that renal function early postoperatively was improved in 42% of patients, unchanged in 54%, and worse in only 4%. In contrast, other authors[12,21] have found that, for patients with preexisting renal insufficiency, mean serum creatinine level did not change significantly from preoperatively to discharge. Some reports have shown that improvement in renal function early postoperatively is greatest in patients having repair of significant bilateral RAS[23,42] and in patients with severe renal dysfunction preoperatively.[22] However, Chaikof et al.[20] reported that early functional response was not predictable by preoperative serum creatinine level. Moreover, their study demonstrated similar renal functional response for patients undergoing unilateral and bilateral renal revascularization.

Although transient elevations in serum creatinine level are common early postoperatively, need for dialysis during this period is unusual.[22] However, during late follow-up 17% to 20% of patients undergoing combined aortorenal reconstruction primarily for renal insufficiency eventually require chronic dialysis despite high long-term patency rates for the renal reconstructions.[20,21,38] The likelihood of requiring late dialysis is greatest among those patients with low preoperative renal functional reserve (serum creatinine ≥3 mg/dL).[20] These findings indicate that, despite revascularization, renal preservation may not be sustainable in patients with markedly compromised preoperative function. Conversely, intervention before the occurrence of profound functional decline may offer the best option for minimizing the risk of eventual dialysis.

LATE SURVIVAL

The benefits of combined aortic and renal artery surgery must be weighed against the advanced age and associated medical problems that are characteristic of these patients and that inherently limit their life expectancy. The actuarial survival rate at 5 years after combined aortorenal reconstruction is between 62% and 72%.[19,20,30] This range, which is perhaps better than anticipated in a population afflicted with such advanced atherosclerosis, is similar to survival rates after isolated repair of either an AAA or aortoiliac occlusive disease.[43,44]

Like late survival after other atherosclerotic vascular procedures, clinically overt coronary artery disease is the strongest indicator of limited longevity. Myocardial infarction accounts for more than one-half of late deaths.[24] Other factors associated with limited survival are advanced age (older than 70 years), poorly controlled hypertension, and extreme preoperative renal insufficiency, especially when such impaired renal function does not improve after operation and progresses to dependence on dialysis.[4]

CONCLUSION

Recent studies have enhanced our understanding of the management of patients with combined aortic and renal atherosclerosis. Such information helps to resolve some of the controversial aspects of this topic exemplified by questions listed in the beginning of this chapter. However, addressing these issues only leads to further questions. For instance, can the formulation of specific morphologic and physiologic criteria permit better patient selection for operative intervention? Does adjunctive repair of an asymptomatic RAS optimize renal function and prolong life? Can further refinements in operative technique make combined revascularization even safer and more effective? Attempting to answer such questions begs for prospective randomized trials, which would give additional insight into treating patients with this challenging disease.

REFERENCES

1. Bredenberg CE, Sampson LN, Ray FS, et al. Changing patterns in surgery for chronic renal artery occlusive disease. *J Vasc Surg.* 1992;15:1018–1024.
2. Novick AC, Ziegelbaum M, Vidt DG, et al. Trends in surgical revascularization for renal artery disease: ten years' experience. *JAMA.* 1987;257:498–501.
3. Stoney RJ, Messina LM, Goldstone J, et al. Renal endarterectomy through the transected aorta: a new technique for combined aortorenal atherosclerosis—a preliminary report. *J Vasc Surg.* 1989;9:224–233.
4. Hanson KJ, Starr SM, Sands RE, et al. Contemporary surgical management of renovascular disease. *J Vasc Surg.* 1992;16:319–331.
5. DeBakey ME, Morris GC Jr, Morgen RO, et al. Lesions of the renal artery: surgical technique and results. *Am J Surg.* 1964;107:84–96.

6. Olin JW, Melia M, Young JR, et al. Prevalence of atherosclerotic renal artery stenosis in patients with atherosclerosis elsewhere. *Am J Med.* 1990;88:46–51.
7. Meaney TF, Dustan HP, McCormack LJ. Natural history of renal arterial disease. *Radiology.* 1968;91:881–887.
8. Schreiber MJ, Pohl MA, Novick AC. The natural history of atherosclerotic and fibrous renal artery disease. *Urol Clin North Am.* 1984;11:383–392.
9. Tollefson DFJ, Ernst CB. Natural history of atherosclerotic renal artery stenosis associated with aortic disease. *J Vasc Surg.* 1991;14:327–331.
10. Wollenweber J, Sheps SG, David GD. Clinical course of atherosclerotic renovascular disease. *Am J Cardiol.* 1968;21:60–71.
11. Zierler RE, Bergelin RO, Isaacson JA, et al. Natural history of atherosclerotic renal artery stenosis: a prospective study with duplex ultrasonography. *J Vasc Surg.* 1994;19:250–258.
12. McNeil JW, String ST, Pfeiffer RB Jr. Concomitant renal endarterectomy and aortic reconstruction. *J Vasc Surg.* 1994;20:331–337.
13. Franklin SS, Young JD, Maxwell MH, et al. Operative morbidity and mortality in renovascular disease. *JAMA.* 1975;231:1148–1153.
14. Dean RH, Keyser JE III, Dupont WD, et al. Aortic and renal vascular disease: factors affecting the value of combined procedures. *Ann Surg.* 1984;200:336–344.
15. Diehl JT, Cali RF, Hertzer NR, et al. Complications of abdominal aortic reconstruction: an analysis of perioperative risk factors in 557 patients. *Ann Surg.* 1983;197:49–56.
16. Libertino JA, Selman FJ. Alternatives to aortorenal revascularization. *J Cardiovasc Surg.* 1982;23:18–22.
17. Shahian DM, Najafi H, Javid H, et al. Simultaneous aortic and renal artery reconstruction. *Arch Surg.* 1980;115:1491–1497.
18. Novick AC. Management of renovascular disease: a surgical perspective. *Circulation.* 1991;83(suppl 1):I–167–71.
19. Branchereau A, Espinoza H, Magnan PE, et al. Simultaneous reconstruction of infrarenal abdominal aorta and renal arteries. *Ann Surg.* 1992;3:232–238.
20. Chaikof EL, Smith RB, Salam AA, et al. Ischemic nephropathy and concomitant aortic disease: a ten-year experience. *J Vasc Surg.* 1994;19:135–148.
21. Dougherty MJ, Hallett JW Jr, Naessens J, et al. Renal endarterectomy vs. bypass for combined aortic and renal reconstruction: is there a difference in clinical outcome? *Ann Vasc Surg.* 1995;9:87–94.
22. O'Mara CS, Maples MD, Kilgore TL, et al. Simultaneous aortic reconstruction and bilateral renal revascularization. *J Vasc Surg.* 1988;8:357–366.
23. Stewart MT, Smith RB III, Fulenwider JT, et al. Concomitant renal revascularization in patients undergoing aortic surgery. *J Vasc Surg.* 1985;2:400–405.
24. Cambria RP, Brewster DC, L'Italien GL, et al. The durability of different techniques for atherosclerotic renal artery disease. *J Vasc Surg.* 1994;20:76–87.
25. Fichelle JM, Colacchio G, Farkas JC, et al. Renal revascularization in high-risk patients: the role of iliac renal bypass. *Ann Vasc Surg.* 1992;6:403–407.
26. Khauli RB, Novick AC, Ziegelbaum M. Splenorenal bypass in the treatment of renal artery stenosis: experience with sixty-nine cases. *J Vasc Surg.* 1985;2:547–551.
27. Moncure AC, Brewster DC, Darling RC, et al. Use of the splenic and hepatic arteries for renal revascularization. *J Vasc Surg.* 1986;3:196–203.
28. Reilly JM, Rubin BG, Thompson RW, et al. Long-term effectiveness of extraanatomic renal artery revascularization. *Surgery.* 1994;116:784–791.
29. Dean RH. In: Cambria RP, Brewster DC, L'Italien GL, et al. The durability of different techniques for atherosclerotic renal artery disease. *J Vasc Surg.* 1994;20:76–87.
30. Tarazi RY, Hertzer NR, Beven EG, et al. Simultaneous aortic reconstruction and renal revascularization: risk factors and late results in 89 patients. *J Vasc Surg.* 1987;5:707–714.
31. Dean RH, Oates JA, Wilson JP, et al. Bilateral renal artery stenosis and renovascular hypertension. *Surgery.* 1977;81:53–62.
32. Straffon R, Siegel DF. Saphenous vein bypass graft in the treatment of renovascular hypertension. *Urol Clin North Am.* 1975;2:337–350.

33. Valentine RJ, Clagett GP, Miller GL, et al. The coronary risk of unsuspected renal artery stenosis. *J Vasc Surg.* 1993;18:433–440.
34. O'Mara CS, Williams GM. Extended retroperitoneal approach for abdominal aortic aneurysm repair. In: Bergan JJ, Yao JST, eds. *Aneurysms: Diagnosis and Treatment.* New York: Grune and Stratton; 1982:327–343.
35. Williams GM, Ricotta JJ, Zinner M, et al. The extended retroperitoneal approach for treatment of extensive atherosclerosis of the aorta and renal vessels. *Surgery.* 1980;88:846–855.
36. Dougherty MJ, Hallett JW Jr, Naessens J, et al. Optimizing technical success of renal revascularization: the impact of intraoperative color-flow duplex ultrasonography. *J Vasc Surg.* 1993;17:849–857.
37. Dean RH, Lawson JD, Hollifield JW, et al. Revascularization of the poorly functioning kidney. *Surgery.* 1979;85:44–52.
38. Atnip RG, Neumyer MM, Healy DA, et al. Combined aortic and visceral arterial reconstruction: risks and results. *J Vasc Surg.* 1990;12:705–715.
39. Piquet P, Ocana J, Verdon E, et al. Atherosclerotic lesions of the aorta and renal arteries: results of simultaneous surgical treatment. *Ann Vasc Surg.* 1988;2:319–325.
40. Hallett JW Jr, Fowl R, O'Brien PC, et al. Renovascular operations in patients with chronic renal insufficiency: do the benefits justify the risks? *J Vasc Surg.* 1987;5:622–627.
41. Novick AC, Pohl MA, Schreiber M, et al. Revascularization for preservation of renal function in patients with atherosclerotic renovascular disease. *J Urol.* 1983;129:907–912.
42. Sterpetti AV, Schultz RD, Feldhaus RJ, et al. Aortic and renal atherosclerotic disease. *Surg Gynecol Obstet.* 1986;163:54–59.
43. Crawford ES, Bomberger RA, Glaeser DH, et al. Aortoiliac occlusive disease: factors influencing survival and function following reconstructive operation over a twenty-five-year period. *Surgery.* 1981;90:1055–1064.
44. Hollier LH, Plate G, O'Brien PC, et al. Late survival after abdominal aortic aneurysm repair: influence of coronary artery disease. *J Vasc Surg.* 1984;1:290–299.

32

Surgical Treatment of Aneurysms of the Renal Artery and Its Branches

James C. Stanley, MD

Renal artery aneurysms are infrequently encountered by most physicians and surgeons. Furthermore, the clinical significance of these lesions appears to have been overstated in the existing literature, which for the most part, describes surgical experiences where complicated lesions are common.[1–5] Nevertheless, a better understanding of true renal artery aneurysms is important since they are being recognized more frequently with increasing arteriographic studies, computed tomography (CT) scans, and magnetic resonance imaging (MRI) studies for other illnesses.[6–9] It is important to differentiate true renal artery aneurysms from limited mural dilatations accompanying fibrodysplastic disease, arteritis-related microaneurysms, and renal artery dissections. This chapter addresses the diagnosis and surgical treatment of true renal artery aneurysms.

INCIDENCE

The frequency of true renal artery aneurysms in the adult population is approximately 0.1%, as determined by the findings in more than 8,500 patients undergoing arteriography for nonrenal disease.[6] By contrast, select retrospective studies have documented nearly a 7-fold increase of these aneurysms among hypertensive patients and more than a 90-fold increase in patients exhibiting renal artery fibrodysplasia.[6] In fact, aneurysms associated with dysplastic renal artery disease undoubtedly account for the slightly greater overall occurrence of these lesions in women, and the more frequent involvement of the right renal artery, which is known to be more likely than the left to exhibit medial fibrodysplasia.[10]

Most renal artery aneurysms are saccular and 90% occur in extrarenal vessels, with the remaining 10% occurring within the renal parenchyma. More than 75% of all renal artery aneurysms arise at branchings of the main renal artery or its first-order branches (Fig. 32–1). The 1.3-cm mean diameter of renal artery aneurysms described in an earlier University of Michigan experience with 94 of these lesions is typical of incidentally diagnosed aneurysms.[6]

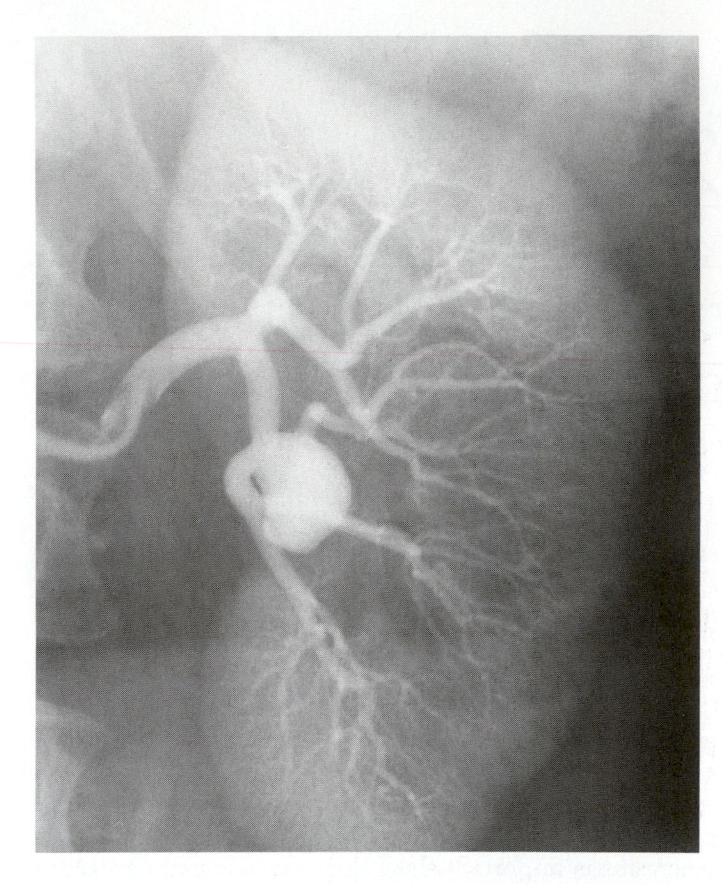

Figure 32–1. Renal artery aneurysm at a second-order branch of an adult, presenting as a saccular lesion. *(Reprinted with permission from Stanley JC, Whitehouse WM Jr. Renal artery macroaneurysms. In: Bergan JJ, Yao JST, eds. Aneurysms. New York: Grune & Stratton; 1982:417–431.)*

PATHOGENESIS

The cause of renal artery aneurysm formation, like that of aneurysms affecting other similar-sized muscular arteries, appears related to loss of medial smooth muscle and an accompanying congenital or acquired deficiency of the internal elastic lamina. Vessel dilation in these circumstances may become accentuated in the presence of arterial fibrodysplasia or blood pressure elevations. Hypertension affects nearly 80% of patients with renal artery aneurysms and may be considered a dominant risk factor for the development of medial degeneration. Aneurysms affecting pediatric-age patients often appear due to other factors and frequently occur as a consequence of post-stenotic dilations resulting in amorphous globular lesions (Fig. 32–2).

Most large renal artery aneurysms are composed of acellular fibrous tissue. The latter may contain areas of complicated arteriosclerotic plaque with deposition of cholesterol crystals, mural necrosis, and calcification. The arteriosclerotic process in most of these aneurysms is a secondary event rather than a primary etiologic process. This is evident by the presence of calcific arteriosclerosis in some but not all aneurysms of certain patients having multiple aneurysms.[6] However, the arteriosclerotic process in these instances may contribute to further dilation of the aneurysm.

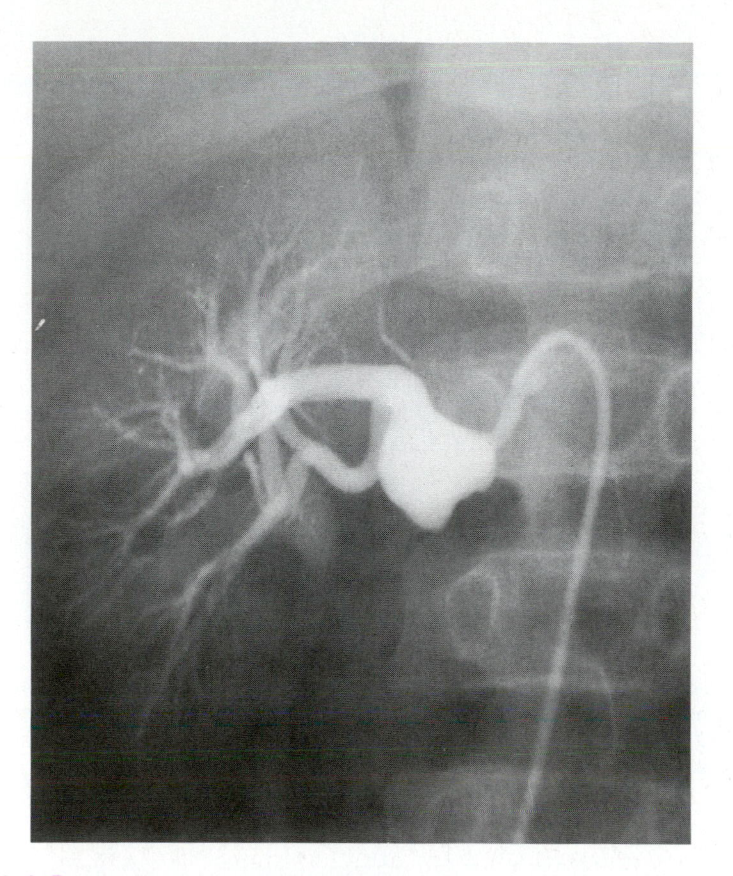

Figure 32–2. Renal artery aneurysm in a child, presenting as a globular, post-stenotic lesion. *(Reprinted with permission from Stanley JC, Whitehouse WM Jr. Renal artery macroaneurysms. In: Bergan JJ, Yao JST, eds. Aneurysms. New York: Grune & Stratton; 1982:417–431.)*

MANIFESTATIONS

Most true renal artery aneurysms are asymptomatic, with serious clinical complications of these lesions being uncommon.[7–9] Nevertheless, approximately 2% of reported patients with these lesions exhibit occluded cortical vessels within the kidney, due to dislodgment and peripheral embolization of aneurysmal thrombus[6] (Fig. 32–3). In many of these cases, simple segmental renal infarction may occur, but often the renal parenchyma surrounding the infarcted tissue remains viable, hypoperfused, and the source of considerable renin secretion that results in secondary hypertension (Fig. 32–4). Aneurysmal compression or torsion of adjacent renal arteries may also occur in occasional cases, with attendant reductions in renal blood flow, renal ischemia, and secondary renovascular hypertension. This latter cause of blood pressure elevations in patients with renal artery aneurysms is often controversial. Hypertension is more likely to be due to intrinsic renal artery occlusive disease, such as medial fibrodysplasia, than effects of the aneurysm on neighboring arteries[6,11–13] (Fig. 32–5).

Rupture of renal artery aneurysms represents the most serious complication of these lesions and has been reported in up to 3% of cases.[6] However, rupture is probably less common because of the select populations included in most published reports.

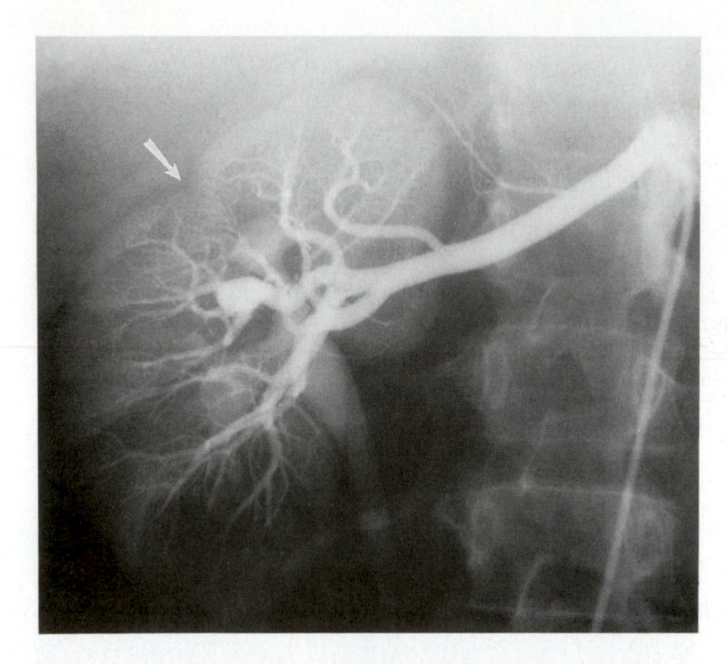

Figure 32–3. Small nonatherosclerotic intraparenchymal aneurysm associated with segmental thromboembolic renal ischemia and cortical infarct (*arrow*). *(Reprinted with permission from Stanley JC, Whitehouse WM Jr. Renal artery macroaneurysms. In: Bergan JJ, Yao JST, eds. Aneurysms. New York: Grune & Stratton; 1982:417–431.)*

Rupture, when it does occur, may be covert into an adjacent vein, or overt with initial bleeding into the extraperitoneal tissues (Figs. 32–6 and 32–7). These two forms of rupture appear to occur with near equal frequencies. Covert rupture may be asymptomatic, although hematuria and hypertension have frequently accompanied this complication.

Overt renal artery rupture is usually manifest by severe abdominal or flank pain. Initial bleeding may be contained within the perirenal retroperitoneum before life-threatening free rupture occurs into the peritoneal cavity. Approximately 10% of patients with reported ruptured renal artery aneurysms succumb from such an event, usually because of delays in operative intervention. Loss of the kidney in survivors of aneurysm rupture is considered inevitable in all but the rarest case.[6,14,15] Anecdotal statements that renal artery aneurysms do not rupture when they are less than 1.5 cm in diameter, are calcified, or are present in normotensive patients is refuted by contemporary experience.

Renal artery aneurysms in women who become pregnant are difficult management problems.[16–18] Among those renal artery aneurysms reported during pregnancy, rupture has occurred in all but a few, causing maternal and fetal death in 55% to 85% of these cases, respectively.[17] There appears to be no obvious relation of repeated pregnancies to the evolution of renal artery aneurysms, as has been the case with splenic artery aneurysms. However, many of these lesions undoubtedly evolved in young women who have previously completed gestational activities without major complications. Although most published figures regarding rupture and mortality during pregnancy are likely to be overstated, renal artery aneurysms must be considered a serious and life-threatening entity in young women who are pregnant or apt to conceive.

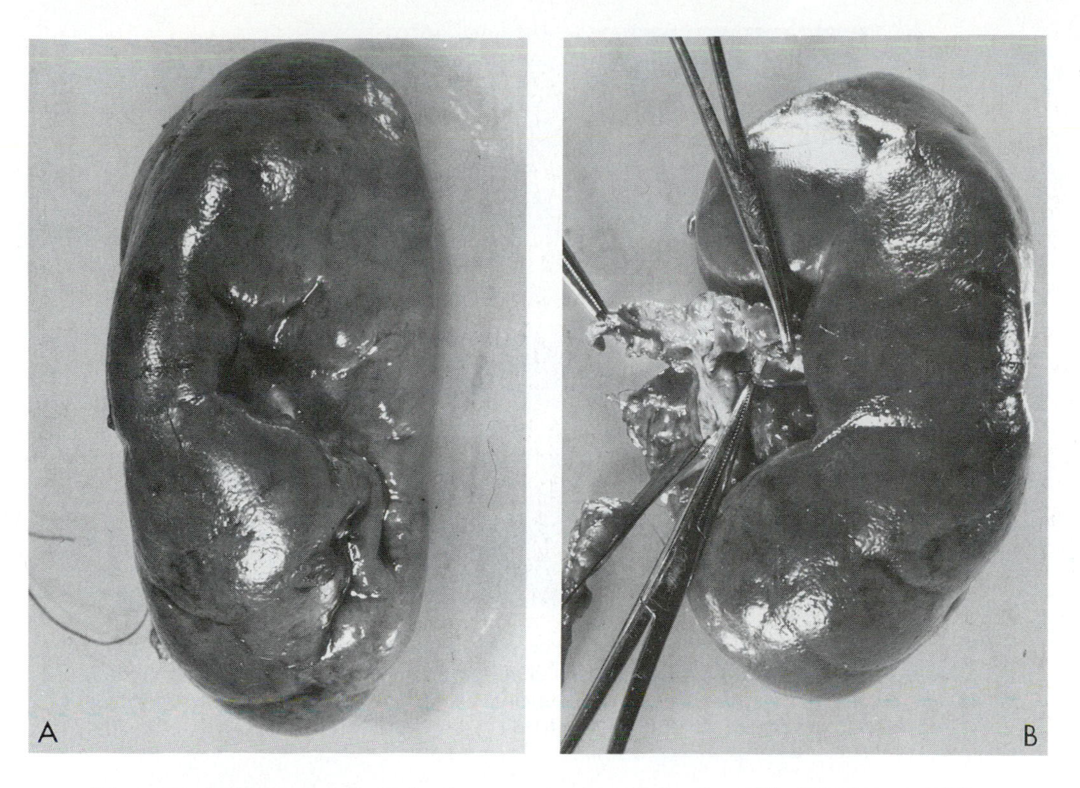

Figure 32–4. (**A**) Renal cortical infarction secondary to embolism from (**B**) a thrombus containing renal artery aneurysm. *(Reprinted with permission from Stanley JC, Whitehouse WM Jr. Renal artery macroaneurysms. In: Bergan JJ, Yao JST, eds. Aneurysms. New York: Grune & Stratton; 1982:417–431.)*

SURGICAL MANAGEMENT

Operations for renal artery aneurysms are recommended in: (1) all patients with symptomatic aneurysms, (2) patients with coexistent renovascular hypertension due to stenotic vessels or embolization of thrombus from the aneurysm itself, (3) women of childbearing age who are likely to conceive, and (4) bland aneurysms greater than 1.5 cm in diameter. The latter indication should only be exercised by those experienced in renal artery reconstructive surgery, because of the relative risk of nephrectomy that accompanies operative treatment of these lesions. Bland aneurysms smaller than 1.5 cm in diameter are perhaps best not subjected to operation. In such circumstances, serial ultrasonography, CT, or MRI can provide documentation of the aneurysm's stability. Arteriographic assessments should be pursued in patients who develop pain suggestive of aneurysmal expansion, exhibit hematuria, or become hypertensive.

Operations for renal artery aneurysms are often complex.[6,19–22] In most circumstances, transverse abdominal incisions are favored, extending from the contralateral anterior axillary line to the ipsilateral posterior axillary line. Subsequent medial visceral reflection of the colon and foregut structures to the opposite side provides for a generous extraperitoneal exposure of the renal artery. This affords visualization of the renal artery from the aorta to the kidney substance itself, and facilitates performance of arterial reconstructive procedures *in situ*.

Most moderate-sized aneurysms cause elongation and displacement of adjacent veins. This makes exposure of the aneurysm and the arteries about it much easier than

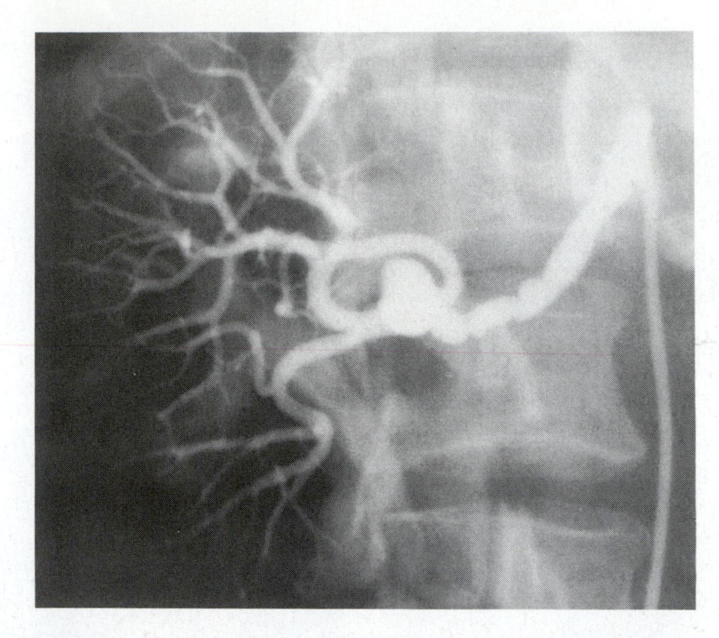

Figure 32–5. Saccular renal artery aneurysm occurring at the primary bifurcation of renal artery exhibiting medial fibroplasia. *(Reprinted with permission from Ernst CB, Stanley JC, Fry WJ. Multiple primary and segmental renal artery revascularization utilizing autogenous saphenous vein. Surg Gynecol Obstet. 1973;137:1023–1026.)*

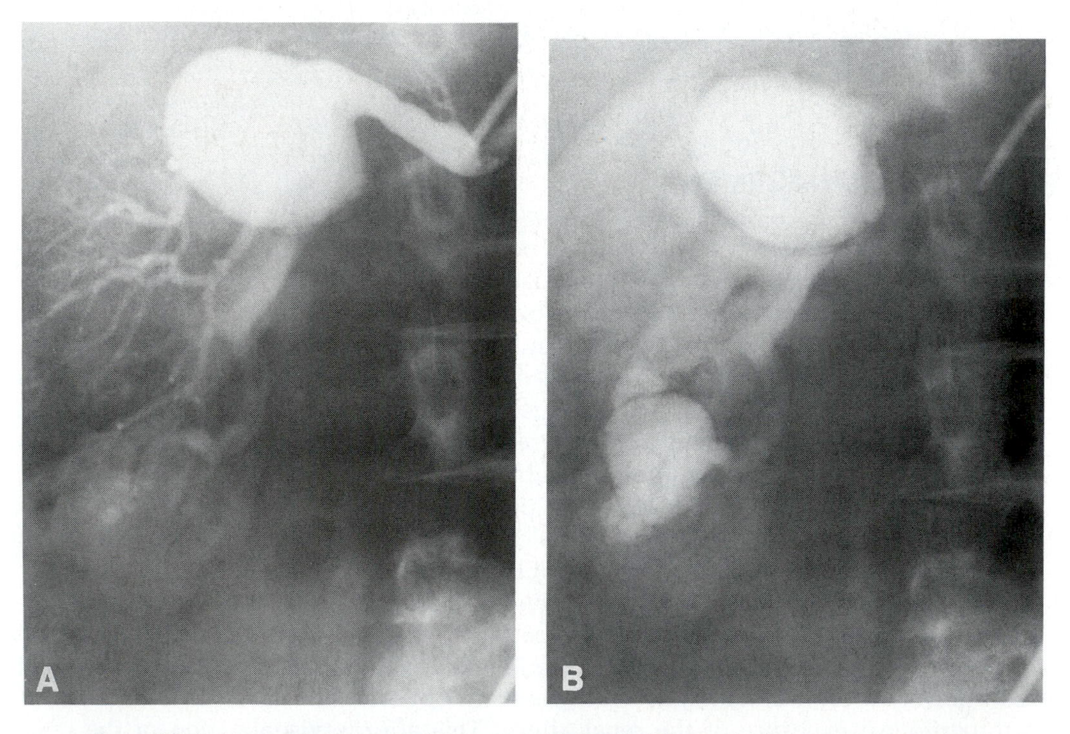

Figure 32–6. Large arteriovenous fistula associated with (**A**) covert inferior pole renal artery aneurysm rupture, (**B**) into a dilated vein. Superior pole aneurysm is intact. *(Reprinted with permission from Stanley JC, Whitehouse WM Jr. Renal artery macroaneurysms. In: Bergan JJ, Yao JST, eds. Aneurysms. New York: Grune & Stratton; 1982:417–431.)*

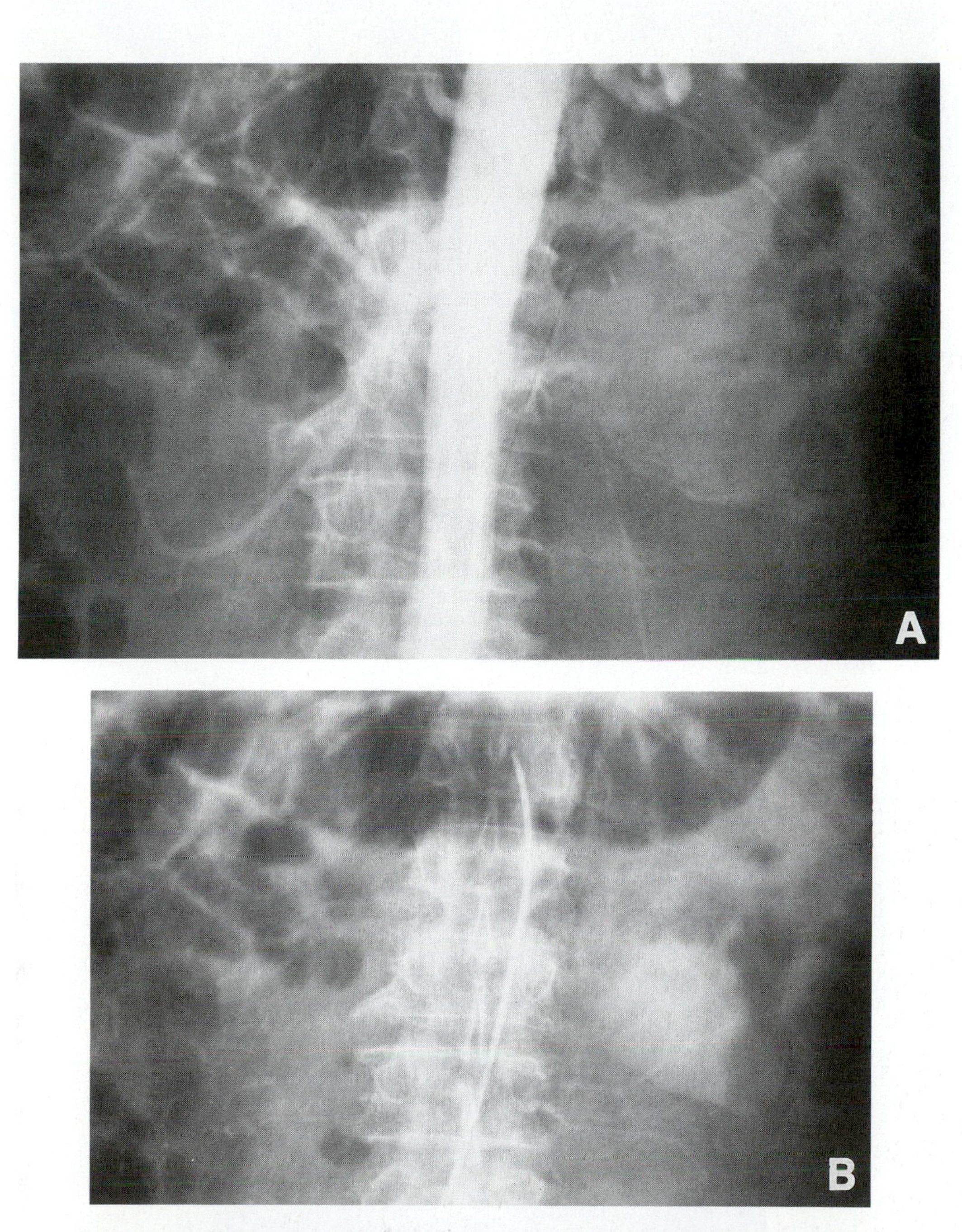

Figure 32–7. Aortographic demonstration of renal artery aneurysm rupture with no evidence of (**A**) distal parenchymal vessels and (**B**) latter peripelvic collection of contrast media. *(Reprinted with permission from Stanley JC, Whitehouse WM Jr. Renal artery macroaneurysms. In: Bergan JJ, Yao JST, eds. Aneurysms. New York: Grune & Stratton; 1982:417–431.)*

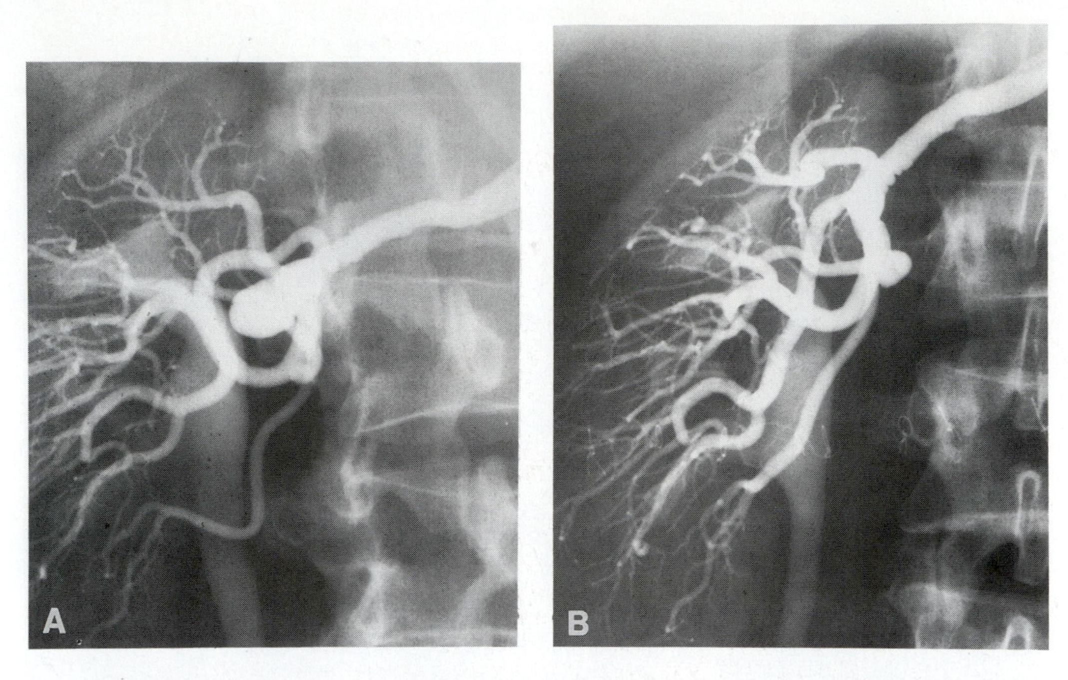

Figure 32–8. Renal artery aneurysm located at bifurcation of main renal artery (**A**). Surgical treatment included aneurysmectomy with vein patch graft closure of the artery (**B**). *(Reprinted with permission from Stanley JC. Renal artery aneurysms and dissections. In: Veith FJ, ed. Current Critical Problems in Vascular Surgery. St. Louis, MO: Quality Medical Publishing; 1991;3:311–319.)*

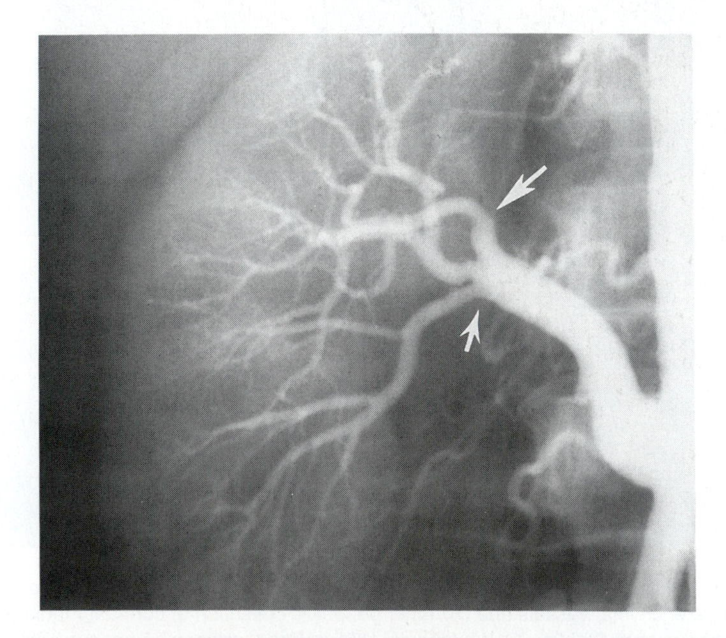

Figure 32–9. Aortorenal bypass with reversed autogenous saphenous vein, following excision of an aneurysm in a fibrodysplastic vessel (same patient as Fig. 32–5), with end-to-end anastomosis to one first-order segmental branch (*large arrow*) and end-to-side implanation of the other first-order segmental branch (*small arrow*). *(Reprinted with permission from Ernst CB, Stanley JC, Fry WJ. Multiple primary and segmental renal artery revascularization utilizing autogenous saphenous vein. Surg Gynecol Obstet. 1973;137:1023–1026.)*

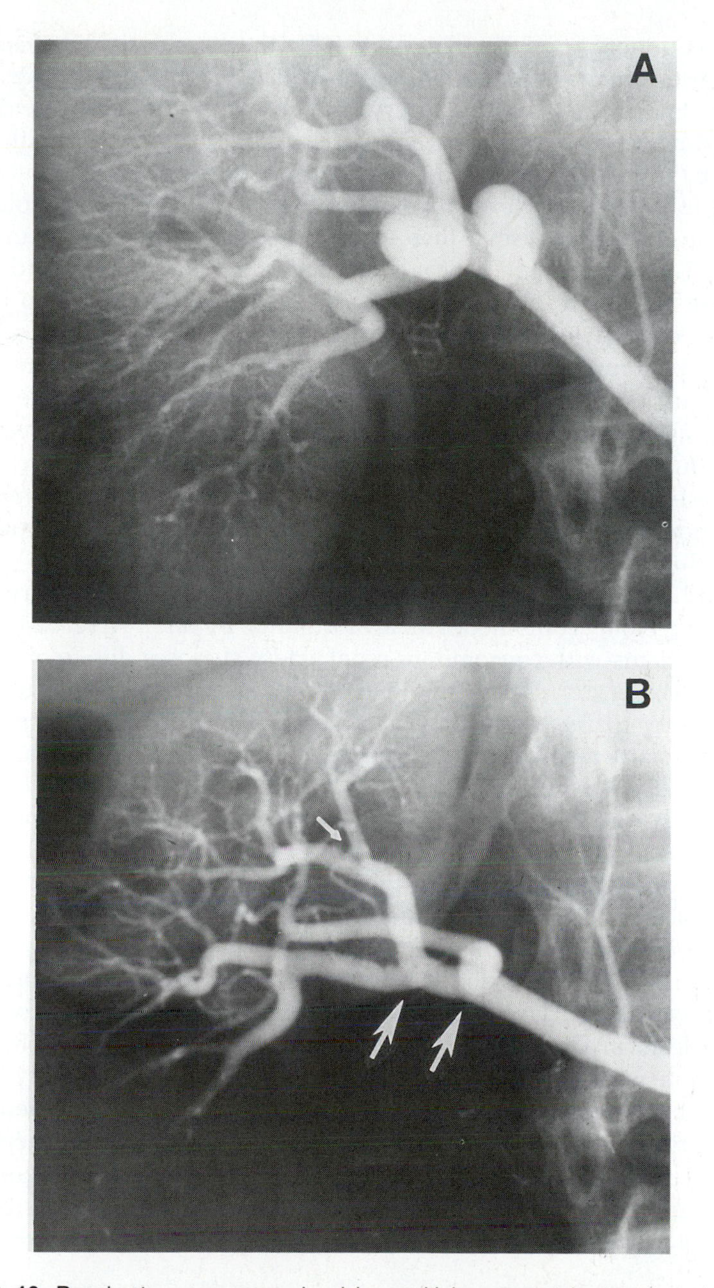

Figure 32–10. Renal artery aneurysms involving multiple segmental artery branchings (**A**). Surgical treatment included aneurysmectomy and end-to-side reimplantation (*large arrows*) of segmental vessels into adjacent artery, and (*small arrow*) closed aneurysmorrhaphy (**B**). *(Reprinted with permission from Stanley JC. Renal artery aneurysms and dissections. In: Veith FJ, ed. Current Critical Problems in Vascular Surgery. St. Louis, MO: Quality Medical Publishing; 1991;3:311–319.)*

dissections for comparable occlusive disease. Certain aneurysms that are difficult and hazardous to dissect anteriorly may be best approached posteriorly. This is accomplished by elevating the kidney from its bed and reflecting it medially, similar to the exposure of the aorta in performing a thoracoabdominal aneurysmectomy.

The most commonly performed operation for these lesions is an aneurysmectomy and primary arterioplasty, with or without a vein patch closure[6,21] (Fig. 32–8). Once the aneurysm, its proximal entering artery, and all exiting branches are dissected free from surrounding veins and tissues, the patient is anticoagulated with intravenous heparin (150 u/kg). A diuresis is established and intravenous Mannitol (12.5 g) is administered, following which microvascular clamps are applied to isolate the aneurysm. The dome of the aneurysm is then excised, leaving a border of aneurysmal tissue, approximately 1.5 mm in width. If the reconstruction is to be complex, and if preexisting stenotic disease has not resulted in a sufficient collateral circulation to the kidney, a cold hypertonic electrolyte solution may be infused into the distal renal artery in order to lessen ischemic injury to the kidney. If the site of aneurysm excision can be closed primarily without compromising the renal artery lumen, such is done. If it appears that a primary closure is impossible, then a small segment of saphenous vein is used as a patch closure. The latter is particularly needed when complete excision of the aneurysm is necessary in arteries less than 2 or 3 mm in diameter. Use of lupe magnification and fine monofilament cardiovascular suture with exacting technique allows most of these procedures to be completed *in situ* without difficulty.

The second most common means of managing renal artery aneurysms involves simple aneurysmectomy combined with an aortorenal bypass[6,21] (Fig. 32–9). This occurs most often in patients with concomitant renal artery stenoses due to arterial fibrodysplasia. In some centers, *ex vivo* repairs and bypass procedures, often using branched internal iliac artery grafts, are routinely undertaken in treating these patients.[23,24] All surgeons treating patients with renal artery aneurysms should be prepared to perform *ex vivo* reconstructions if necessary.

Recently, aneurysmectomy with reimplantation of the involved vessel or vessels into a normal adjacent or proximal renal artery has been advocated[5,21] (Fig. 32–10). It is important to spatulate the artery to be implanted, so as to not narrow the reimplantation anastomosis. These procedures are usually accomplished *in situ*, although some surgeons prefer *ex vivo* reconstructions in this setting. Lastly, renal artery aneurysms in the range of 2 to 3 mm may be plicated, by way of a closed aneurysmorrhaphy, using a fine running cardiovascular suture. Very small aneurysm, often encountered when treating larger lesions, are usually managed in this manner by the author.

The aforenoted operative techniques should allow aneurysmectomy to be successfully performed with kidney preservation in greater than 95% of patients. However, treatment of certain intraparenchymal aneurysms may entail partial nephrectomy. In exceptional circumstances intraparenchymal aneurysms may be embolized using a percutaneous transcatheter technique, after the distal cortical tissue has been infarcted with infusion of an agent such as absolute alcohol.

REFERENCES

1. DeBakey ME, Lefrak EA, Garcia-Rinaldi R, et al. Aneurysm of the renal artery: a vascular reconstructive approach. *Arch Surg*. 1973;106:438–443.
2. Hageman JH, Smith RF, Szilagyi DE, et al. Aneurysms of the renal artery: problems of prognosis and surgical management. *Surgery*. 1978;84:563–572.
3. Hubert JP Jr, Pairolero PC, Kazmier FJ. Solitary renal artery aneurysm. *Surgery*. 1980;88:557–565.
4. Martin RS III, Meacham PW, Ditesheim JA, et al. Renal artery aneurysm: selective treatment for hypertension and prevention of rupture. *J Vasc Surg*. 1989;9:26–34.

5. Stanley JC. Renal artery aneurysms. In: Ernst CB, Stanley JC, eds. *Current Therapy in Vascular Surgery*. 3rd ed. St. Louis, MO: Mosby–Year Book; 1995:813–817.
6. Stanley JC, Rhodes EL, Gewertz BL, et al. Renal artery aneurysms: significance of macroaneurysms exclusive of dissections and fibrodysplastic mural dilations. *Arch Surg*. 1975;110:1327–1333.
7. Henriksson C, Bjorkerud S, Nilson AE, et al. Natural history of renal artery aneurysm elucidated by repeated angiography and pathoanatomical studies. *Eur Urol*. 1985;11:244–248.
8. Henriksson C, Lukes P, Nilson AE, et al. Angiographically discovered, nonoperated renal artery aneurysms. *Scand J Urol Nephrol*. 1984;18:59–62.
9. Tham G, Ekelund L, Herrlin K, et al. Renal artery aneurysms. Natural history and prognosis. *Ann Surg*. 1983;197:438–452.
10. Stanley JC, Gewertz BL, Bove EL, et al. Arterial fibrodysplasia: histopathologic character and current etiologic concepts. *Arch Surg*. 1975;110:561–566.
11. Cummings KB, Lecky JW, Kaufman JJ. Renal artery aneurysms and hypertension. *J Urol*. 1973;109:144–148.
12. Ruberti U, Miani S, Scorza R, et al. Aneurysms of the renal artery. *Int Angiol*. 1987;6:407–414.
13. Soussou ID, Starr DS, Lawrie GM, et al. Renal artery aneurysm: long-term relief of renovascular hypertension by *in situ* operative correction. *Arch Surg*. 1979;114:1410–1415.
14. Poutasse EF. Renal artery aneurysms: their natural history and surgery. *J Urol*. 1966;95:297–306.
15. Vaughan TJ, Barry WF, Jeffords DL, et al. Renal artery aneurysms and hypertension. *Radiology*. 1971;99:287–293.
16. Burt RL, Johnson FF, Silverthorne RG, et al. Ruptured renal artery aneurysm in pregnancy: report of a case with survival. *Obstet Gynecol*. 1956;7:229–233.
17. Cohen JR, Shamash FS. Ruptured renal artery aneurysms during pregnancy. *J Vasc Surg*. 1987;6:51–59.
18. Cohen SG, Cashdan A, Burger R. Spontaneous rupture of a renal artery aneurysm during pregnancy. *Obstet Gynecol*. 1972;39:897–902.
19. Mercier C, Piquet P, Piligian F, et al. Aneurysms of the renal artery and its branches. *Ann Vasc Surg*. 1986;1:321–327.
20. Ortenberg J, Novick AC, Straffon RA, et al. Surgical treatment of renal artery aneurysms. *Br J Urol*. 1983;55:341–346.
21. Stanley JC, Messina LM, Wakefield TW, et al. Renal artery reconstruction. In: Bergan JJ, Yao JST, eds. *Techniques in Arterial Surgery*. Philadelphia: WB Saunders; 1990:247–263.
22. Stanley JC, Messina LM, Zelenock GB. Splanchnic and renal artery aneurysms. In: Moore WS, ed. *Vascular Surgery: A Comprehensive Review*. 3rd ed. Philadelphia: WB Saunders; 1991:335–349.
23. Bugge-Asperheim B, Sdal G, Flatmark A. Renal artery aneurysm. *Ex vivo* repair and autotransplantation. *Scand J Urol Nephrol*. 1984;18:63–66.
24. Dubernard JM, Martin X, Gelet A, et al. Aneurysms of the renal artery: surgical management with special reference to extracorporeal surgery and autotransplantation. *Eur Urol*. 1985;11:26–30.

33

Reoperative Surgery for Renal Artery Stenosis

Richard H. Dean, MD, and Stanley B. Fuller, MD

Occlusive lesions of the renal arteries occur from a variety of congenital and acquired causes. They may present at any age and can be located at any site from the ostium of the main renal artery to the intraparenchymal branches. Although each lesion type and location has its own unique natural history of progression or stability, the development of new lesions at new sites during even decades of observation is rare. For this reason, recurrent ischemia in a previously revascularized kidney most commonly is secondary to the presence of a stenosing lesion in the anastomotic sites, in the body of the graft or related to the site of endarterectomy. Two classes of recurrent lesions can be seen. Lesions occurring in the early postoperative period are usually technical. Recurrent lesions occurring during later follow-up usually relate to progressive stenosing lesions at a site of injury to either the vessel or the graft at the initial procedure. Therefore, this discussion of recurrent renal artery stenosis is divided into considerations of early and late reoperations for recurrent occlusive lesions.

EARLY REOPERATION

The vast majority of cases of early recurrent renal ischemia necessitating reoperation represent errors either in operative technique or judgment committed at the initial operation and that were avoidable. Therefore, a brief description of common pitfalls is appropriate. Acute angulation, kinking, and twisting of the graft can occur when graft length is inappropriate or axial orientation is not obtained. Similarly, inappropriately deep placement of sutures in the heel area of the graft will create a band-like constriction across the suture line. Further, the aortic anastomosis can be made stenotic unless a large button of aorta is excised when end-stage atherosclerosis is present. Such aortas have minimal capacity to alter their configuration and unless a large orifice for the graft is created by excision, the graft may have a stenotic origin. Suture line stenoses also can result from a "purse string" when using a continuous suture line. To avert this problem, a spatulated anastomosis is always used in which the smaller of the two vessels being connected is opened to at least three times its cross-sectional diameter.

In each of these instances, the technical error can and should be recognized at the time of operation and, when present, should prompt the surgeon to "redo" the anastomosis.

Peculiar to renal artery endarterectomy, residual intimal plaque, and unrecognized intimal flap creation usually are produced by blind renal artery endarterectomy performed through the transaortic route. For this reason, we routinely perform intraoperative duplex sonography on all renal artery reconstructions prior to closure of the abdomen.[1,2] Although residual lesions or internal flaps are most commonly found after transaortic endarterectomy, anastomotic errors and unrecognized lesions in the bypass graft itself can be observed in any reconstruction and should be excluded or corrected prior to completion of the initial operation. Through employment of appropriate microvascular technique and intraoperative completion duplex sonography we have experienced early renal revascularization failure in only 3 (0.5%) of a recent consecutive 541 renal artery reconstructions. Interestingly, all of these were in patients undergoing *ex vivo* reconstruction and led to the need for nephrectomy in each case.

Clinical characteristics suggesting the presence of acute graft thrombosis include onset of accelerated hypertension in the early postoperative period or deterioration in renal function. Neither of these characteristics is accurate, however, for either can be present in spite of a functioning graft and be absent in the presence of graft thrombosis. In the instance of an end-to-side distal graft anastomosis, the graft anastomosis can function as a patch and result in improved perfusion even when the graft itself is thrombosed (Fig. 33–1).

Although graft thrombosis can lead to clot propagation into the distal renal artery branches and lead to the necessity of nephrectomy, renal revascularization is frequently

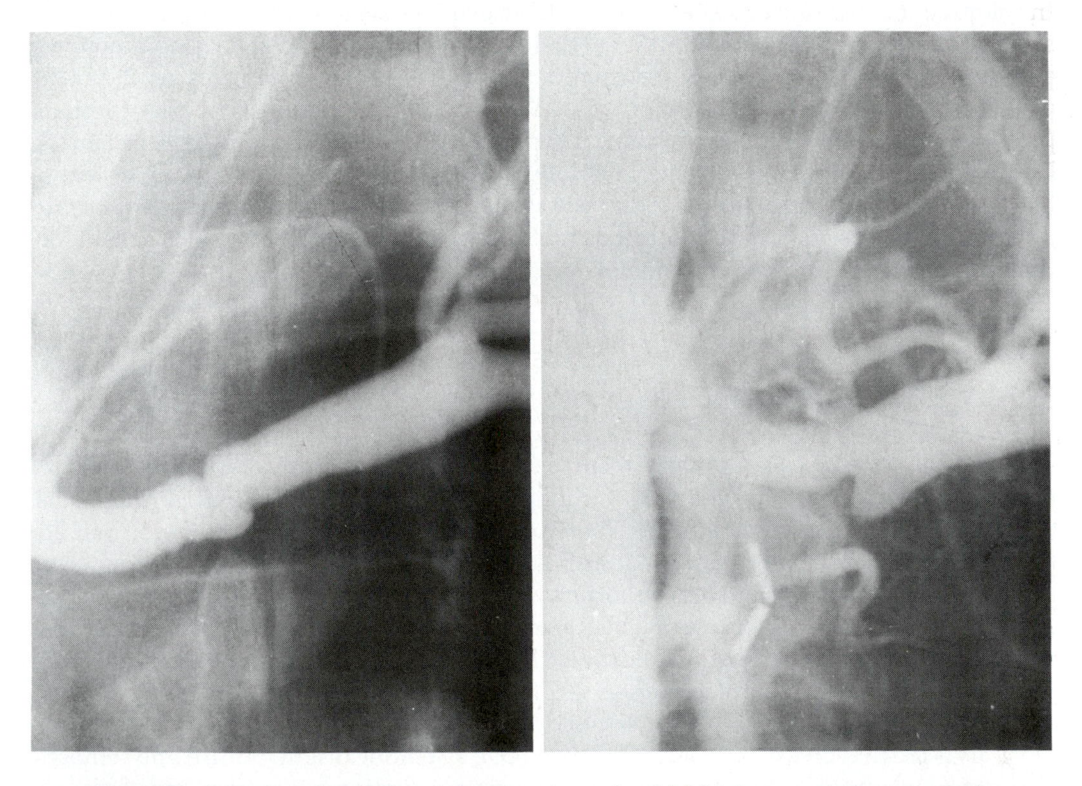

Figure 33–1. Preoperative (*left*) and 2-year postoperative (*right*) follow-up arteriogram empirically obtained in a patient cured by hypertension. Note the thrombosed graft but patient renal artery.

possible at reoperation. Since the original occlusion usually has prompted the development of significant collateral pathways for renal perfusion, the kidney, although ischemic, may have retained perfusion and patent distal vessels through these collateral networks (Fig. 33–2).

LATE REOPERATION

Lesions producing a need for late reoperation after an initially successful operation are relatively uncommon and have been found in less than 10% of renal artery reconstructions followed angiographically from 1 to 23 years after a successful operation in our center.[3] Causes of recurrent lesions include fibrotic stenosis of venous valves in saphenous vein grafts, tubular subendothelial fibroblastic proliferation, anastomotic lesions, and the development of new stenosing lesions beyond the initial graft.

Valves in the reversed saphenous vein do not lie against the vein wall but instead assume a nonobstructing neutral position. If such valves become fibrotic in that position and undergo contracture, a web-like stenosis of the vein graft is created (Fig. 33–3). Although we have rarely identified such lesions in our follow-up studies, it suggests that a valveless segment of vein should be used if possible. Percutaneous transluminal angioplasty has been used successfully in one of these patients to relieve the hemodynamic significance of the lesion. Most such lesions, however, are managed by longitudinal venotomy, excision of the fibrotic valve, and patch angioplasty (Fig. 33–4).

Subendothelial fibroblastic proliferation of saphenous vein aortorenal grafts (Fig. 33–5) also have been identified in follow-up angiographic studies in our center. In each instance, the grafts were in *ex vivo* reconstructions or the second side of bilateral simultaneous reconstructions. In these circumstances, the veins were subjected to a prolonged ischemia time without the benefit of any specific measure designed to provide protection against intimal damage. Whether use of cold, heparinized blood or other preservative solutions would have prevented late tubular stenosis in these patients, however, is conjectural.

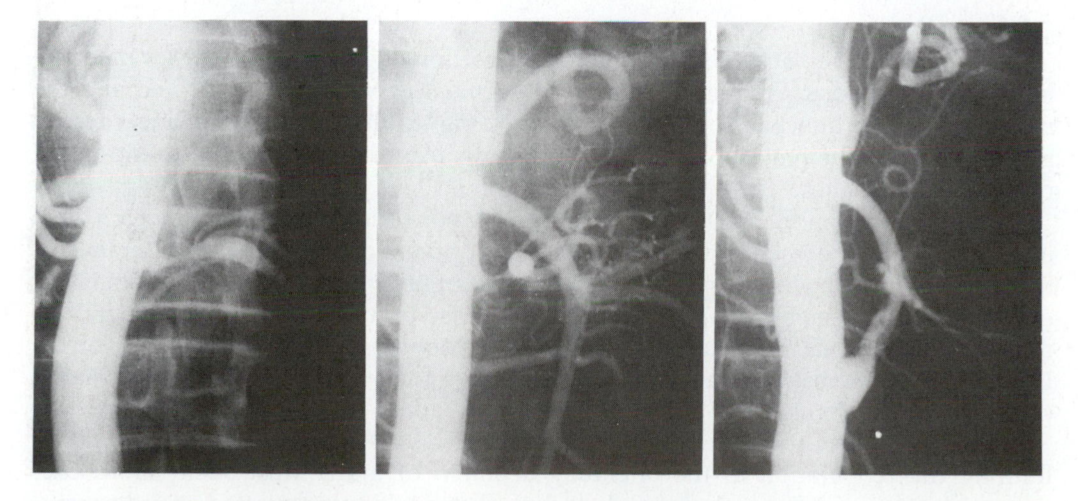

Figure 33–2. Serial arteriograms showing severe left renal artery stenosis (*left*). Although early occlusion of an end-to-end saphenous vein graft (*middle*) occurred, continued perfusion of the distal renal artery through collaterals allowed successful repeat bypass (*right*).

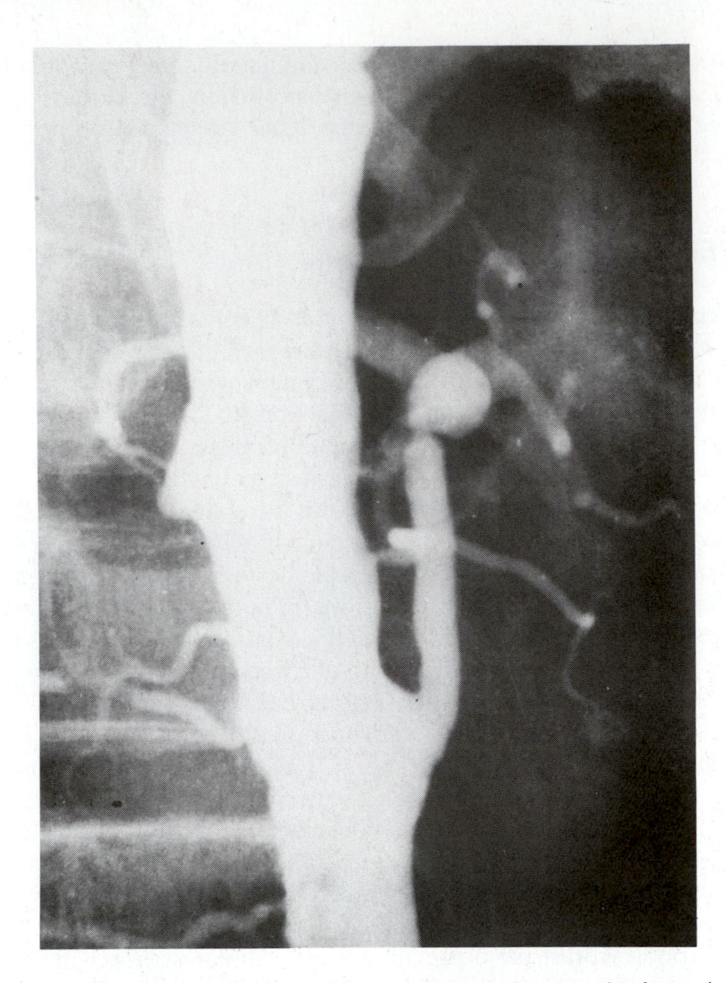

Figure 33–3. Angiographic appearance of the web-like valvular stenosis of a saphenous vein graft that was identified 1 year after operation.

In any event, replacement of the involved portion of graft is required for management of such lesions. Frequently, the distal segment of vein is not involved and the new graft can be attached to the old graft proximal to the distal suture line, thereby not requiring definitive mobilization of the previously dissected and scar-entrapped renal artery branches.

Finally, anastomotic stenoses may represent suture line "purse string," which went unrecognized at the initial operation or the development of neointimal proliferation at the anastomotic site when a synthetic graft had been used initially (Fig. 33–6). In either circumstance, repeat bypass may be limited to insertion of an interposition graft to replace the proximal or distal anastomotic site. Mobilization and transection of the Dacron graft with reattachment to a larger new aortotomy was possible in one instance of a stenotic proximal anastomotic site.

Total occlusion of a previously placed aortorenal graft removes the possibility of limiting the reoperation to the offending segment of graft. Most such thromboses represent progressive sequelae of early technical errors left uncorrected or progressive stenoses that were unrecognized before total thrombosis. In our experience, the development of late graft occlusion has occurred in 2% of our patients followed by sequential postoperative angiography.

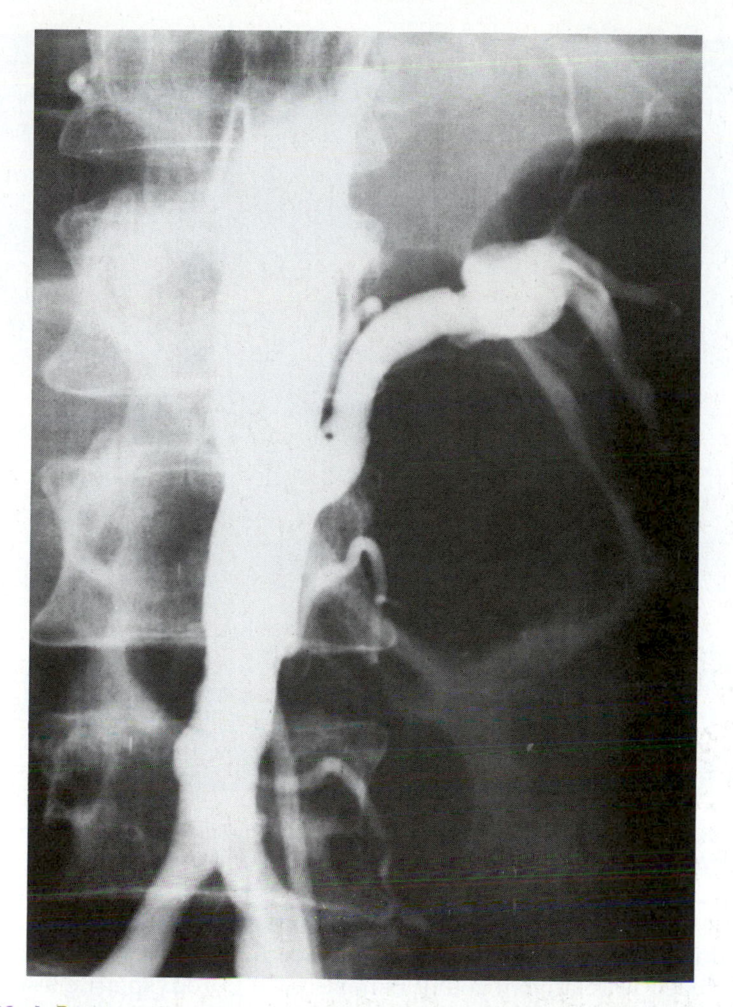

Figure 33–4. Postoperative arteriogram of lesion shown in Figure 33–3 showing the valvular stenosis corrected by vein patch angioplasty.

Development of new lesions in the renal artery beyond a patent graft is exceedingly rare in our experience and has only been seen twice in the management of more than 700 patients with renovascular hypertension. Both instances occurred in young patients. The first child, age 7 years, developed progressive branch stenoses to the lower pole of the kidney 2 years after a proximal branch repair (Fig. 33–7). A new segment of saphenous vein placed from the old patent graft to the distal branches beyond the stenoses restored renal perfusion and relieved recurrent hypertension. The second child developed a severe stenosis of the distal renal artery at the site of distal vessel cross-clamping early in our experience, which probably represented fibrotic healing of a vessel wall injury from the occluding clamp. This child underwent nephrectomy at another hospital without benefit of attempted repeat revascularization.

Two additional problems not producing recurrent renovascular hypertension merit comment as reasons for reoperation. These are aneurysmal degeneration of vein grafts and anastomotic false aneurysms.

Aneurysmal degeneration has been a widely publicized complication of the use of autogenous saphenous vein for aortorenal bypass (Fig. 33–8). Its development, however, is predictable and is primarily limited to its use in young patients. Although

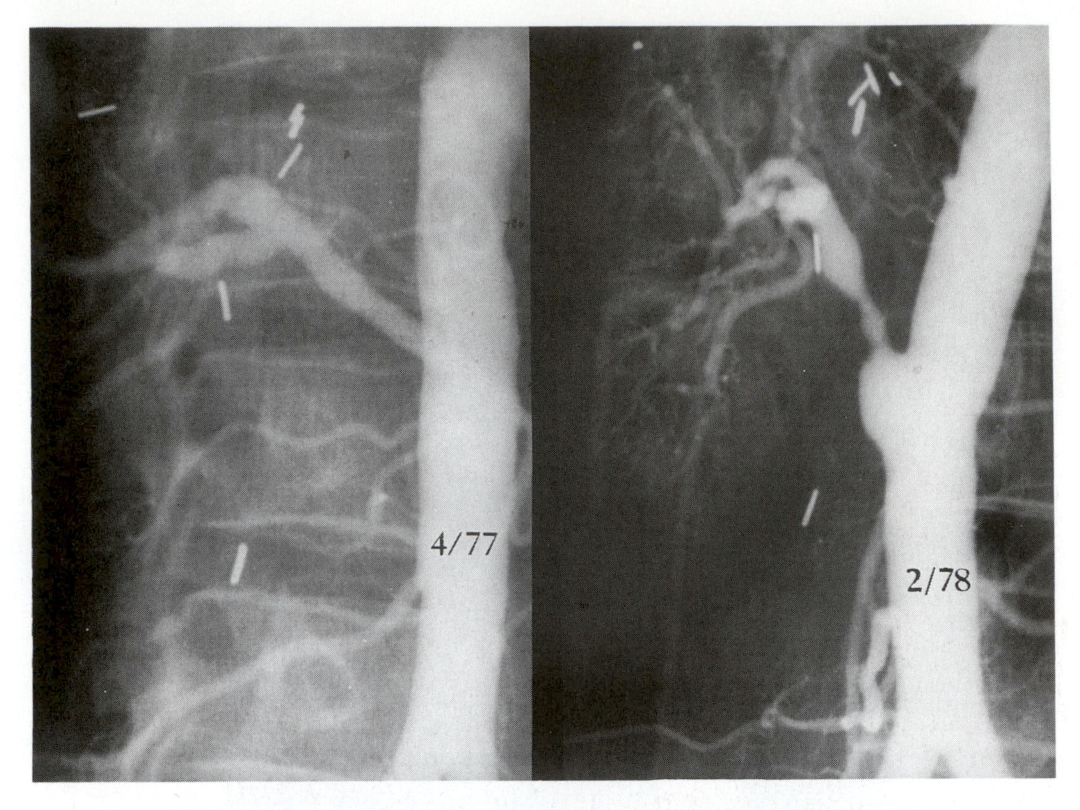

Figure 33–5. Angiographic appearance of tubular subendothelial fibroblastic proliferation in a saphenous vein graft that developed during the first year after insertion.

it has occurred in only 4% of saphenous veins used in all age groups in our center, all these have occurred in relatively young patients with fibrodysplastic lesions in whom the saphenous vein was used to provide total flow to the normal kidney. The fact that all of these aneurysmal grafts occurred in such patients who were also cured of hypertension by surgery suggests an interesting hypothesis. Specifically, when the vessel and kidney beyond the stenosis are normal, cure of hypertension and relatively higher flow rates should be expected. In this situation and in children whose saphenous vein is structurally less mature, flow through the graft is disproportionately higher and aneurysmal degeneration more likely. Circumstantial support for this hypothesis is drawn from the fact that we have not seen aneurysmal degeneration of saphenous vein aortorenal grafts placed in patients with atherosclerotic lesions. Since most of these patients have some intrarenal arteriolar nephrosclerosis that results in lower graft flow rates, this group would be at reduced risk for aneurysmal degeneration of the graft. Finally, although we have replaced one aneurysmally dilated aortorenal bypass, most such dilated grafts stabilize in size and can be followed without replacement.

Although uncommonly identified, false aneurysm formation at the anastomotic suture lines can occur with aortorenal grafting (Fig. 33–9). In all instances, these were noted at late follow-up angiography and occurred in patients having synthetic graft insertion (Dacron). Since the structural integrity of synthetic to artery anastomoses is permanently dependent on suture line integrity, this complication is probably peculiar to nonautogenous grafts. Their demonstration in a patient 20 years after insertion, however, suggests that such synthetic grafts should be empirically evaluated at a point in late follow-up to exclude the presence of silent false aneurysms.

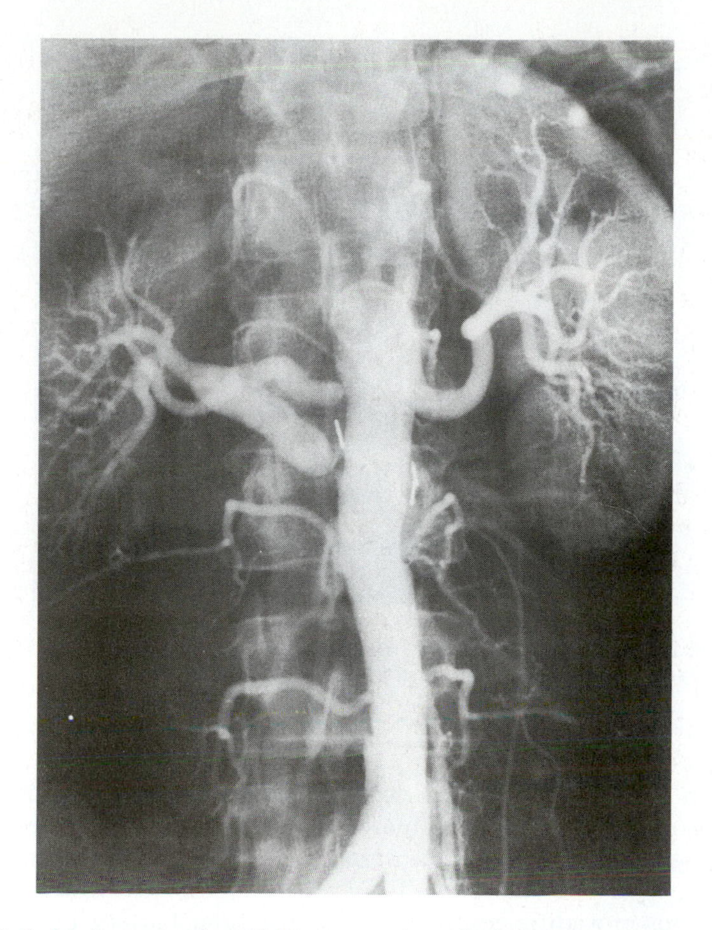

Figure 33–6. Arteriogram performed 11 years postoperatively that demonstrates stenosis of the aortic anastomosis of a Dacron aortorenal graft. By mobilization of the graft and elliptical excision anastomotic site, the revascularization was achieved by graft anastomosis to the larger aortotomy.

TECHNICAL CONSIDERATIONS AT REOPERATION

Finally, a few technical points are peculiar to operations on previously dissected renal arteries. These points apply both to our experience with reoperation after failed prior operative reconstructions[4] as well as failed prior percutaneous transluminal angioplasty.[5] Reoperation for proximal anastomotic suture line stenoses or valvular stenoses of saphenous vein grafts may be relatively simple without significantly increased technical difficulties. Mobilization of the previously dissected distal renal artery is particularly hazardous and must be performed by tedious, precise dissection. Since the renal vein is intimately associated with the renal artery, it is frequently densely adherent and easily entered in the process of its separation from the distal artery. To obtain the best topography of the respective vessels in the previously directed area, attention is first directed to the renal hilum at the edge of the kidney. By identifying each of the renal artery branches at this previously unmolested site, the surgeon can minimize inadvertent trauma to the branch points that are usually arising within the dissected scarred area of the more proximal branching sites. To carry this technical point to its logical conclusion, we will usually approach the kidney and renal vasculature

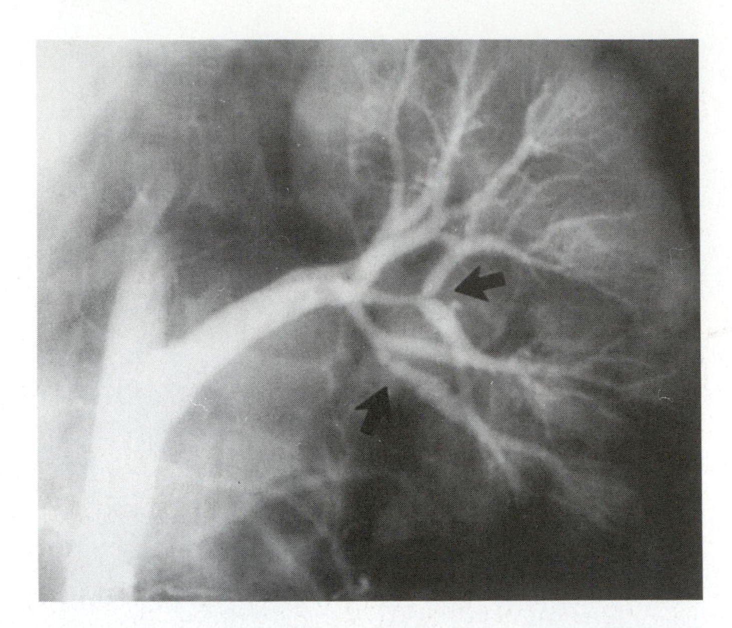

Figure 33–7. Postoperative arteriogram 2 years after insertion of a hypogastric artery graft that demonstrates the development of severe branch renal artery stenoses.

from an entirely new route. For instance, if the left renal artery has previously been approached through the base of the mesentery we will expose the renal hilar area by reflecting the left colon medially and approach the renal vasculature from this lateral direction.

If the previous procedure has involved the distal renal artery and a branch repair is anticipated, preparations for an *ex vivo* repair are always made[6] and held in "standby." Such preparations are frequently made even when branch repair is not anticipated, for removal of the kidney, *ex vivo* perfusion and preservation, and subsequent dissection of the fused renal arterial and venous system in this controlled manner may be the only means by which precise correction, without unacceptable venous bleeding and potential irretrievable renal arterial trauma, can be obtained.

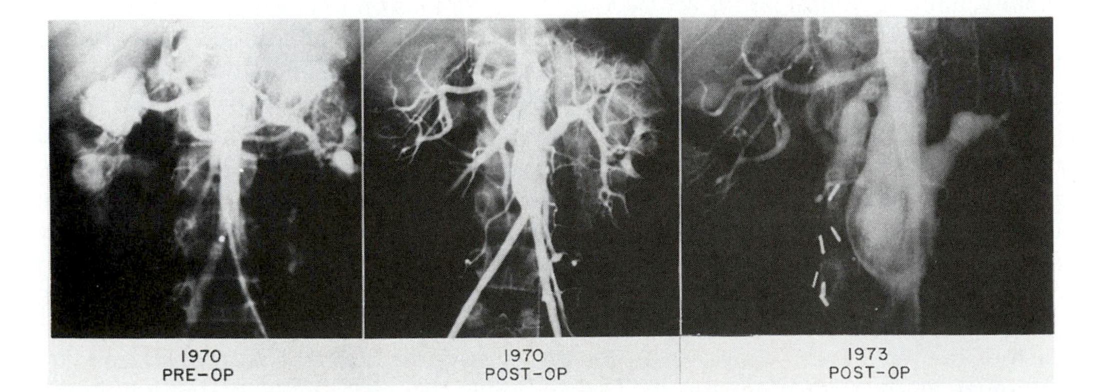

Figure 33–8. Sequential postoperative arteriograms that demonstrate progressive aneurysmal dilation of a hypogastric artery aortorenal bypass and a vein graft used for aortomesenteric grafting.

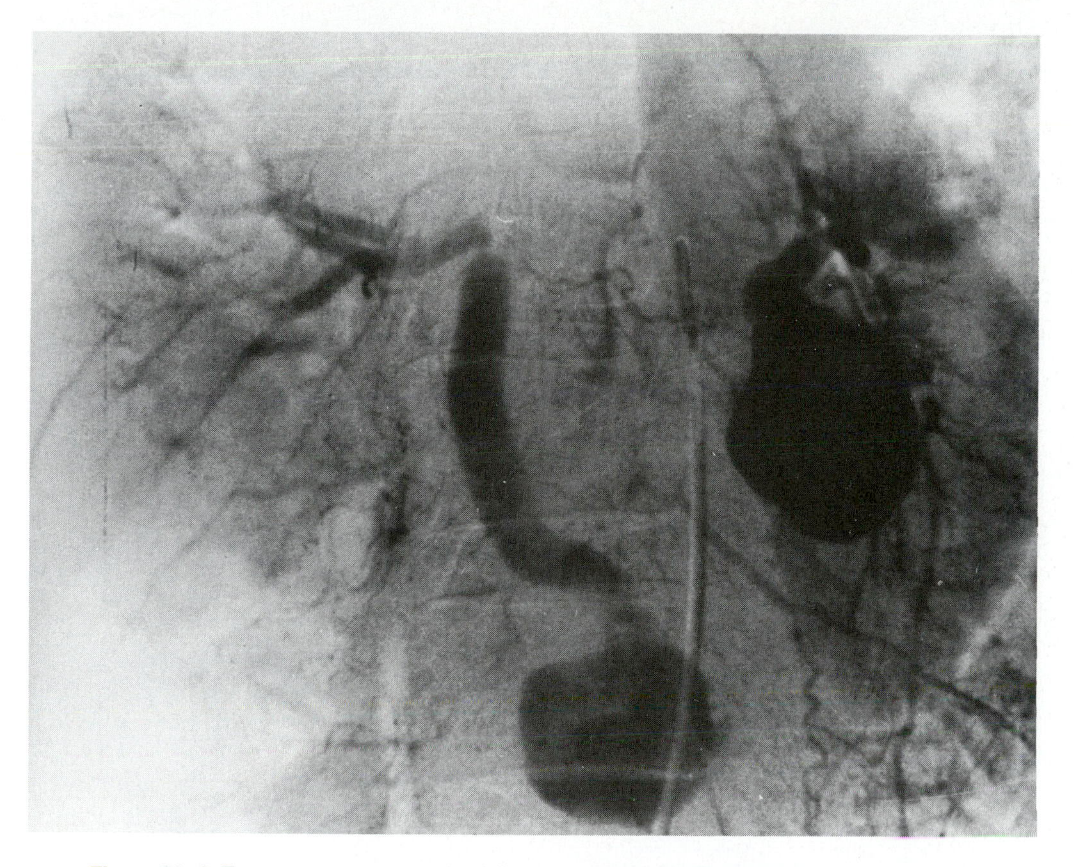

Figure 33–9. Twenty-year postoperative follow-up arteriogram demonstrating large false aneurysms at the aortic suture lines of bilateral Dacron aortorenal bypasses.

REFERENCES

1. Hansen KJ, O'Neil EA, Reavis SW, et al. Intraoperative duplex sonography during renal artery reconstruction. *J Vasc Surg*. 1991;14:364–374.
2. Hansen KJ, Starr SM, Sands RE, et al. Contemporary surgical management of renovascular disease. *J Vasc Surg*. 1992;16:319–331.
3. Dean RH, Krueger TC, Whiteneck JM, et al. Operative management of renovascular hypertension: results after follow-up of fifteen of twenty-three year. *J Vasc Surg*. 1984;1:234–242.
4. Dean RH, Hansen KJ. Renal revascularization: how to make a difficult operation easier. In: Veith FJ, ed. *Current Critical Problems in Vascular Surgery*. St. Louis MO: Quality Medical Publishing, Inc; 1989:306–308.
5. Dean RH, Callis JT, Smith BM, et al. Failed percutaneous transluminal renal angioplasty: experience with lesions requiring operative intervention. *J Vasc Surg*. 1987;6:301–307.
6. Dean RH, Meacham PW, Weaver FA. *Ex vivo* renal artery reconstructions: indications and techniques. *J Vasc Surg*. 1986;4:546–552.

34

Surgical Treatment of Acute and Chronic Renal Artery Occlusion

Andrew C. Novick, MD

Renal arterial occlusion resulting in a poorly functioning or nonfunctioning kidney can be either an acute or chronic process. In 1940, Hoxie and Coggins reviewed 1,411 consecutive autopsies and found renal infarction in 205 patients, for an incidence of 1.4%[1] A greater incidence of renal infarction, 3.2%, was reported by Schoenbaum and associates in 1971, following a review of the results of 17,300 autopsies.[2] These studies highlight that renal arterial occlusion is a relatively common postmortem finding. In clinical practice, such cases are being identified with increasing frequency, particularly in older patients with generalized atherosclerosis. This chapter reviews the most common causes of acute and chronic renal arterial occlusion along with available forms of management in such cases.

ACUTE RENAL ARTERY OCCLUSION

Renal artery embolism is a relatively rare entity that may result in acute occlusion of the renal artery or its branches.[3,4] The vast majority (>90%) are cardiac in origin and approximately 30% will involve both kidneys. Renal artery embolism should be suspected when there are features of acute renal ischemia in the presence of atrial fibrillation, myocardial ischemia, heart failure, a history of rheumatic heart disease, cardiomyopathy, or a prosthetic heart valve. In many cases, the embolic occlusion is only partial, allowing some renal perfusion to be maintained and affording the opportunity for renal salvage with prompt treatment.

Acute renal artery thrombosis with or without intramural dissection may occur in a variety of settings. Dissection of the renal artery is most commonly secondary to an aortic dissection, and isolated renal artery dissections are rare.[5,6] These dissections occur when the intima is disrupted to create a subintimal false lumen. Enlargement of the false lumen may compromise the true arterial lumen with a resulting decrease in renal blood flow, renal ischemia, hypertension and, in some cases, vascular occlusion with renal infarction. The causes of isolated renal artery dissection and thrombosis include blunt trauma, selective renal arteriography, percutaneous transluminal renal angioplasty, and underlying primary renal artery diseases, such as atherosclerosis, fibrous dysplasia, and arteritis.

Blunt abdominal trauma, especially that seen in acceleration–deceleration injuries, may result in artery dissection and thrombosis if sufficient force is exerted on the relatively inelastic intima to cause its disruption.[7] The typical clinical presentation is in a multiply injured patient with flank pain, tenderness, and hematuria. Hypertension may also be present. The possibility of this injury should be suspected in any recently traumatized patient with delayed visualization of the kidney upon an intravenous pyelogram or CT scan with contrast medium.

Acute renal artery thrombosis may be a consequence of percutaneous transluminal renal angioplasty (PTRA), which is now widely used in the treatment of both fibrous and atherosclerotic renal artery stenosis.[8,9] This can occur due to trauma from the guide wire or from overstretching of the arterial wall with disruption of the intima with resulting dissection and thrombosis. The risk of this occurrence is particularly significant in patients with abdominal aortic atherosclerosis and associated ostial renal artery stenosis. To ensure prompt detection and management of this problem, PTRA should always be done with the availability of a vascular surgeon, and an immediate postangioplasty angiogram should be obtained routinely. Rarely, renal artery dissection may also occur as a complication of selective renal arteriography alone.

Acute renal artery occlusion in the absence of trauma or angiographic intervention may occur as a complicating event in the natural history of primary underlying renal artery disease. Those disorders with the greatest potential for acute occlusion are atherosclerosis, intimal fibroplasia, and perimedial fibroplasia.[10] The latter two conditions are particularly worrisome since they generally occur in younger patients and may involve both kidneys. Rarely, acute renal artery thrombosis may be associated with other disorders such as arteritis, polycythemia vera, and tumors.

Acute renal artery occlusion in children occurs mainly in neonates with aortic thrombosis secondary to placement of an umbilical arterial catheter for intensive care monitoring.[11,12] The clinical picture is one of aortic thrombosis of variable extent usually compromising the visceral aorta with extension to the renal arterial circulation. Associated hypertension may be managed medically; however, when oligoanuria and renal failure are present, immediate intervention to restore renal arterial blood flow is necessary.

CHRONIC OCCLUSION OF THE RENAL ARTERY

Normally, the kidney can remain viable for 1 to 2 hours after complete interruption of its arterial supply, beyond which renal infarction occurs. However, in some patients with gradual renal artery occlusion, although renal function may be impaired severely, renal viability can be maintained by the development of collateral arterial supply from ureteral, lumbar, adrenal, or capsular vessels.[13] Early experimental studies demonstrated that canine kidneys exposed to low arterial pressures that were inadequate to ensure renal function would survive and have good function when normal pressure was resumed several days later. From a clinical standpoint, this circumstance is most often encountered in patients with existing atherosclerotic renal artery stenosis that progresses to complete occlusion.

Therefore, in some patients who have complete atherosclerotic renal artery occlusion, revascularization can yield significant recovery of renal function. This presents the clinical problem of differentiating the salvable kidney maintained by collateral blood flow one that has sustained irreversible ischemic damage. Currently, there are several clinical assessments that allow this distinction to be made with a high degree of accuracy prior to attempted revascularization.

With an abundant collateral arterial supply, retrograde filling of the distal renal arterial tree may be observed on angiography and is an excellent prognostic sign favoring renal viability. This also is manifested intraoperatively by the presence of significant backbleeding from the kidney when the renal artery is transected beyond the point of obstruction. Urographic or isotopic function of the involved kidney is another favorable sign that often, unfortunately, is absent in such cases. Several authors have referred to a critical renal size below which revascularization is ill advised. It is generally accepted that total arterial occlusion leads to a decrease in renal size, but this may be attributed to several factors, ranging from simple reduction in renal blood flow to irreversible ischemic atrophy or progressive cellular damage and fibrosis. This is the likely explanation for discrepant reports of a critical renal size (from 7 to 9 cm) for predicting renal salvage with total arterial occlusion. It would appear that therapeutic decisions in such patients should not be used on renal size alone.

Perhaps the most useful predictive criterion is histologic evidence of intact viable glomeruli upon intraoperative renal biopsy.[13] Extensive tubular atrophy, interstitial fibrosis, and arteriolar sclerosis do not appear to be of major prognostic importance. However, the finding of widespread glomerular hyalinization reflects irreversible ischemic renal injury and should preclude attempted vascular reconstruction.

In patients with advanced atherosclerotic renovascular disease and azotemia, the finding of complete arterial occlusion is important because it suggests that genuine recovery of renal function may be possible. Occasional patients with end-stage renal failure have been encountered in whom renal function has been salvable with revascularization.[14,15] The basis for this has been the presence of chronic bilateral total renal arterial occlusion where, fortuitously, the viability of one or both kidneys has been maintained through collateral vascular supply. In such cases, revascularization can yield dramatic recovery of renal function. Unfortunately, this clinical presentation is rare and a less favorable outcome of bilateral arterial occlusion or renal viability is far more common.

FIBRINOLYTIC THERAPY

Fibrinolytic therapy has several theoretic advantages over traditional treatment methods such as systemic anticoagulation, thrombectomy, embolectomy, and surgical renovascular reconstruction. Systemic anticoagulation simply limits extension of thrombus formation facilitating fibrinolysis by endogenous plasminogen activators. This process is slow and may take weeks to achieve complete lysis of a major clot. Fibrinolytic therapy avoids general anesthesia and theoretically entails less risk to the patient than a major vascular operation. Fibrinolytic therapy also enables clearance of thromboembolic material from distal renal vessels that may not be amenable to surgical treatment. Contraindications to fibrinolytic therapy include patients at particular risk for hemorrhage such as those with a history of recent bleeding, a recent stroke, a coagulation disorder, major trauma, recent surgery, a knitted vascular prosthesis, or active peptic ulcer disease.

Three fibrinolytic agents are currently available for direct intra-arterial renal infusion in cases of acute thrombosis or embolism.[11,12,16,17] These include streptokinase, urokinase, and recombinant tissue plasminogen activator. It is appropriate to consider fibrinolytic therapy in patients with unilateral renal arterial thromboembolism and a normal functioning contralateral kidney. In patients with bilateral complete renal arterial occlusion or where a solitary functioning kidney is affected, emergency surgical intervention is indicated to effect immediate restoration of renal blood flow.

In patients with acute unilateral renal artery thrombosis or embolism, with early diagnosis and a possible salvable kidney, immediate heparinization should be administered. The patient should then be taken promptly to the angiography suite for selective catheterization of the renal artery and local infusion of a fibrinolytic agent. Approximately 30 cases of acute renal artery embolism treated by intra-arterial fibrinolysis have been reported and most were treated with streptokinase or urokinase. Technically successful clot lysis was achieved in most cases but good long-term renal function was achieved in less than half. Partial or segmental renal arterial occlusion and the finding of a good collateral circulation have been associated with a favorable outcome. There are fewer reported cases of successful fibrinolytic therapy for acute renal artery thrombosis; however, as PTRA and endovascular stenting are increasingly performed, there may be a wider role for this approach to treat iatrogenic renal arterial thromboses.

SURGICAL MANAGEMENT OF RENAL ARTERY OCCLUSION

A variety of operative approaches are available to treat patients with acute and chronic renal artery occlusion. Advances in surgical renal vascular reconstruction have limited the role of total or partial nephrectomy in such cases. The latter operations are occasionally indicated in patients with frank renal infarction, noncorrectable intrarenal branch arterial disease, or an elderly poor surgical risk patient with a normal contralateral kidney.

In patients undergoing surgical treatment for renal artery embolism, a transabdominal approach is used to expose one or both renal arteries.[18,19] A transverse arteriotomy is made in the main renal artery and an embolectomy catheter is inserted, inflated and withdrawn, taking care to avoid intimal trauma. The artery may be closed primarily with fine vascular sutures, or alternatively, a vein patch may be applied. Occasionally, if both renal arteries are involved, embolectomy is performed through a longitudinal aortotomy following temporary occlusion of the proximal and distal aorta.

In patients with renal artery occlusion from acute thrombosis or dissection, surgical revascularization may be rendered more difficult by perivascular scarring of the diseased arterial segments, which is a particularly common associated finding in cases of intramural dissection.[5] When vascular disease is limited to the main renal artery, aortorenal bypass with a free graft of autogenous hypogastric artery or saphenous vein remains a useful approach for patients with a nondisease abdominal aorta.[20,21] In older patients, with severe atherosclerosis of the abdominal aorta, alternate extra-anatomic bypass techniques are preferable. These include hepatorenal bypass,[22] splenorenal bypass,[23] iliorenal bypass, and supraceliac or thoracic aortorenal bypass.[24] In some patients, intramural dissection and thrombosis may extend into the branches of the renal artery. Some of these patients will require management with extracorporeal microvascular branch arterial reconstruction and autotransplantation.[25] The indications and efficacy of these various reconstructive renal vascular operations are described in detail elsewhere.

REFERENCES

1. Hoxie HJ, Coggins CB. Renal infarction: statistical study in 205 cases. *Arch Intern Med.* 1940;65:587.

2. Schoenbaum SG, Goldman MA, Seigelman SS. Renal arterial embolization. *Angiology.* 1971;22:332.
3. Gasparini M, Hofmann R, Stoller M. Renal artery embolism: clinical features and therapeutic options. *J Urol.* 1992;147:567–572.
4. Lessman RK, Johnson SF, Coburn JW, et al. Renal artery embolism: clinical features and long-term follow-up of 17 cases. *Ann Intern Med.* 1978;89:477–482.
5. Slavis S, Hodge E, Novick AC, et al. Surgical treatment for isolated dissection of the renal artery. *J Urol.* 1990;144:233.
6. Smith BM, Holcomb GW III, Richie RE, et al. Renal artery dissection. *Ann Surg.* 1984;200:134–146.
7. Clark DE, Georgitis JW, Ray FS. Renal arterial injuries caused by blunt trauma. *Surgery.* 1981;90:87–96.
8. Dean RH, Callis JT, Smith BM, et al. Failed percutaneous transluminal renal angioplasty: experience with lesions requiring operative intervention. *J Vasc Surg.* 1987;6:301.
9. Martinez AG, Novick AC, Hayes JM. Surgical treatment of renal artery stenosis after failed percutaneous transluminal angioplasty. *J Urol.* 1990;144:1094–1096.
10. Schreiber MJ, Pohl MA, Novick AC. The natural history of atherosclerotic and fibrous renal artery disease. *Urol Clin North Am.* 1984;11:383–392.
11. Molteni KH, George J, Messersmith R, et al. Intrathrombic urokinase reverses neonatal renal artery thrombosis. *Pediat Nephrol.* 1993;7:413–415.
12. Berger C, Fancoise M, Durand C, et al. Treatment of neonatal aortic thrombosis with recombinant tissue plasminogen activator (tPA). *Arch Pediatr.* 1994;1:1014–1018.
13. Schefft P, Novick AC, Stewart BH, et al. Renal revascularization in patients with total occlusion of the renal artery. *J Urol.* 1980;124:184–186.
14. Wasser WG, Krakoff LR, Haimov M, et al. Restoration of renal function after bilateral renal artery occlusion. *Arch Intern Med.* 1981;141:1647–1651.
15. Kaylor W, Novick AC, Ziegelbaum M, et al. Reversal of end-stage renal failure with surgical revascularization in patients with atherosclerotic renal artery occlusion. *J Urol.* 1989;141:486–488.
16. Blum V, Billman P, Krause T, et al. Effect of local low-dose thrombolysis on clinical outcome in acute embolic renal artery occlusion. *Radiology.* 1993;189:549–554.
17. Salam TA, Lumsden AB, Martin LG. Local infusion of fibrinolytic agents for acute renal artery thromboembolism: report of ten cases. *Ann Vasc Surg.* 1993;7:21–26.
18. Lacombe M. Surgical versus medical treatment of renal artery embolism. *J Cardiovasc Surg.* 1977;18:281–290.
19. Bouttier S, Valverde JP, Lacombe M, et al. Renal artery emboli: the role of surgical treatment. *Ann Vasc Surg.* 1988;2:161–168.
20. Ernst CB, Stanley JC, Marshall FF, et al. Autogenous saphenous vein aortorenal autografts: a ten-year experience. *Arch Surg.* 1972;105:855–864.
21. Stoney RJ, Olofsson PA. Aortorenal arterial autografts: the last two decades. *Ann Vasc Surg.* 1988;2:169–173.
22. Chibaro EA, Libertino JA, Novick AC. Use of hepatic circulation for renal revascularization. *Ann Surg.* 1984;199:406–411.
23. Khauli R, Novick AC, Ziegelbaum W. Splenorenal bypass in the treatment of renal artery stenosis: experience with 69 cases. *J Vasc Surg.* 1985;2:547–551.
24. Novick AC, Stewart R, Hodge E, et al. Use of the thoracic aorta for renal arterial reconstruction. *J Vasc Surg.* 1994;19:605–609.
25. Novick AC, Jackson CL, Straffon RA. The role of renal autotransplantation in complex urological reconstruction. *J Urol.* 1990;143:452.

35

Management of Patients with Advanced Hypertension and Renal Failure

John W. Hallett, Jr., MD

Advanced aortic atherosclerosis tends to narrow or occlude the ostia of the renal arteries (Fig. 35–1). With time, bilateral renal arterial occlusive disease can precipitate a variety of difficult clinical syndromes, including malignant hypertension, "flash" pulmonary edema, and atheroembolism. In addition, some patients have aortoiliac arterial occlusive disease or large aneurysms that need urgent treatment.

All these challenging clinical presentations occur in the setting of significant medical comorbidity,[1-8] the most common of which is coronary heart disease. Physicians and surgeons appreciate that these medical factors increase operative risk, and current controversy revolves around whether the benefits justify the risks of renal revascularization. Furthermore, surgeons realize that operations for such patients can be technically challenging. The challenge is usually due to associated aortic disease and to the need for bilateral renal revascularization or nephrectomy in some patients.

THE CONTROVERSIAL ISSUES

The management of patients with advanced hypertension and renal insufficiency is surrounded by several controversial questions.[1-10] This chapter focuses on the most controversial issues: Who are these patients and which of them can be helped by either surgery or angioplasty? How does the physician determine which intervention to use? Should the intervention be surgery or angioplasty? If surgery appears to be the better choice, which operation should be performed? What are the surgical risks? And, finally, what are the expected outcomes?

METHODS OF ANSWERING THE DIFFICULT QUESTIONS

Most of the recent data on the management of patients with advanced hypertension and renal failure are based on retrospective studies from specialized surgical centers.[1-10]

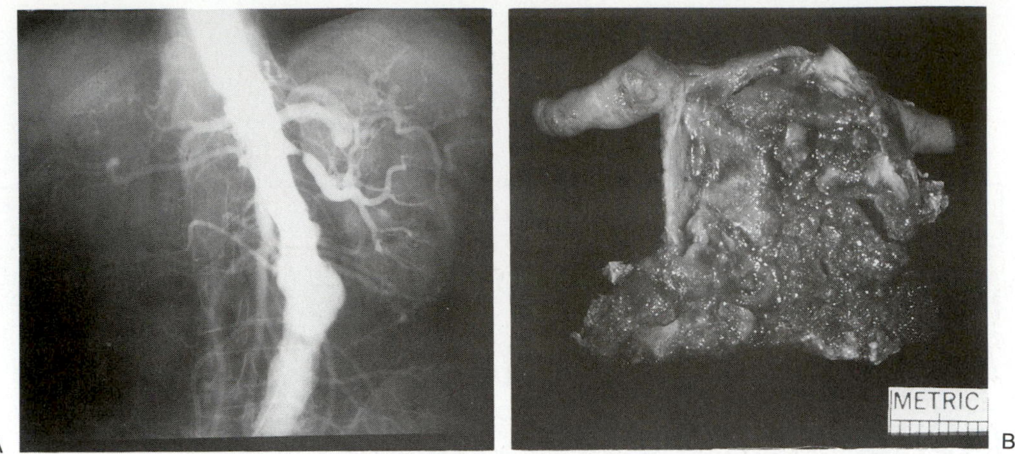

Figure 35–1. (**A**) Aortogram of advanced aortic atherosclerosis with bilateral renal artery disease causing uncontrolled hypertension and renal insufficiency. (**B**) Operative specimen following bilateral transaortic renal endarterectomy and infrarenal aortic grafting.

Although a few randomized clinical trials are being planned or are under way, only one randomized comparison of renal angioplasty versus surgical reconstruction appears in the recent literature.[11,12]

This chapter is based on a retrospective analysis of 1,643 patients who underwent renovascular surgery between 1970 and 1993 at the Mayo Clinic.[13] Advanced renal insufficiency is defined as a serum creatinine of more than 2 mg/dL. This level of renal failure was present in 402 patients. Comparative analysis was made between 1970 and 1980 and 1980 and 1993. The second time period was selected because balloon angioplasty became another alternative in our practice in 1980. Consequently, 1,315 total interventions for renovascular hypertension were performed between 1980 and 1993 (Fig. 35–2). A surgical procedure was performed in 74.6% (n = 991) and balloon angioplasty in 25.4% (n = 324). Thirty-one percent (n = 304) of the surgical patients had chronic renal insufficiency, while only 13.6% (n = 44) of the angioplasty patients had a creatinine of more than 2 mg/dL (Fig. 35–3).

WHAT ARE THE CLINICAL CHARACTERISTICS OF THESE PATIENTS?

The most recent 304 azotemic surgical patients (1980–1993) included 218 men and 86 women, with a median age of 68 years (range, 33–85 years). The gender distribution

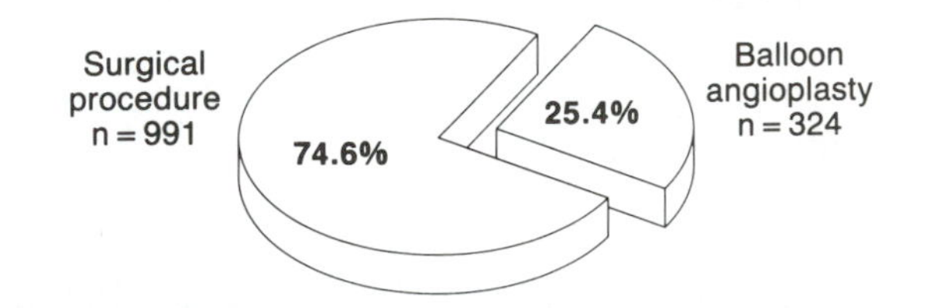

Figure 35–2. Relative use of a surgical procedure versus percutaneous balloon angioplasty to treat renal arterial occlusive disease (n = 1,315 interventions) at the Mayo Clinic between 1980 and 1993.

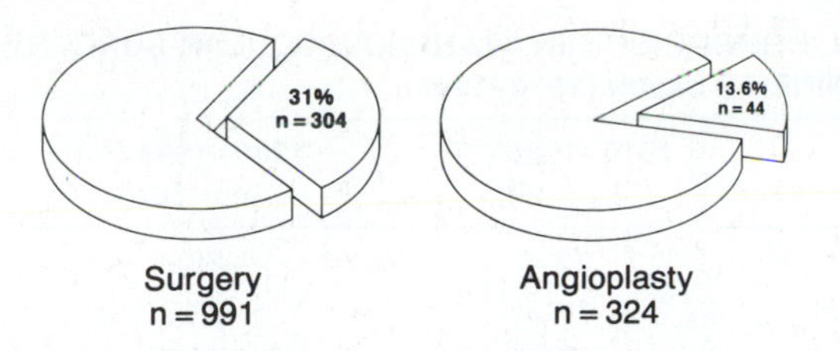

Figure 35–3. Percentage of patients with chronic renal insufficiency (serum creatinine >2 mg/dL) undergoing renal artery surgery or angioplasty, 1980–1990.

did not change between 1970 and 1993. In contrast, the mean age increased significantly from 63.5 years in the 1970s to 68 years in the 1980s ($P < .05$).

The primary indication for renal revascularization was progressive renal insufficiency (controlled hypertension) in 51% of the patients and both progressive azotemia and uncontrolled hypertension) in 49%. Mean preoperative serum creatinine was 3.29 mg/dL (range, 2.0–9.6 mg/dL) (Fig. 35–4). Median systolic blood pressure was 180 mm Hg (range, 124–270 mm Hg), with a diastolic pressure of 90 mm Hg (range, 60–150 mm Hg). The median number of antihypertensive medications was three, with a maximum number of six.

Several serious medical risk factors increased in prevalence between the two time periods (1970–1980 vs. 1980–1993) (Table 35–1). Fifty-two percent of the patients had clinical evidence of coronary heart disease. Twenty percent of the patients in the past 10 years were hospitalized preoperatively with malignant hypertension, pulmonary edema, and renal insufficiency.

Previous cardiovascular interventions were also common after 1980. For example, the most frequent vascular procedures were coronary artery bypass grafting (16.4%), carotid endarterectomy (15.5%), prior renal artery surgery (14.2%), prior percutaneous transluminal renal angioplasty (5.3%), and percutaneous transluminal coronary

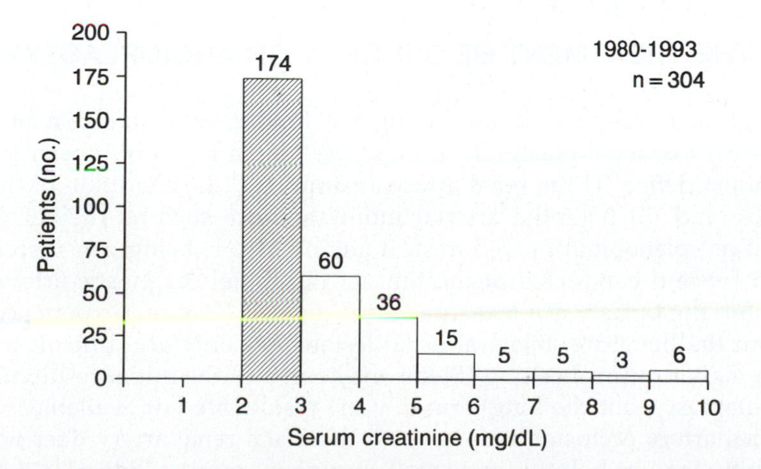

Figure 35–4. Preoperative serum creatinine in 304 azotemic patients undergoing surgical renal artery reconstruction at the Mayo Clinic, 1980–1993. *(From Hallett JW Jr, Textor SC, Kos PB, et al. Advanced renovascular hypertension and renal insufficiency: trends in medical comorbidity and surgical approach from 1970 to 1993. J Vasc Surg. 1995;21:753.)*

TABLE 35–1. MEDICAL COMORBIDITY IN 402 RENOVASCULAR SURGERY PATIENTS WITH SERUM CREATININE ≥2 mg/dL (1970–1993)

Risk Factor	1970–1980 (%) (*n* = 98)	1980–1993 (%) (*n* = 304)	*P* Value
Angina pectoris	21.4	29.9	.12
Past myocardial infarction	16.3	27.0	.04
Congestive heart failure	12.2	23.7	.02
Cerebrovascular disease	11.2	24.8	.01
Diabetes mellitus	7.1	18.1	.01
Claudication	35.7	56.4	.001

(From Hallett JW Jr, Textor SC, Kos PB, et al. Advanced renovascular hypertension and renal insufficiency: trends in medical comorbidity and surgical approach from 1970 to 1993. *J Vasc Surg.* 1995;21:753.)

angioplasty (1.3%). Thus, 19.5% of the patients underwent previous attempts to revascularize renal blood flow prior to referral for the current operation.

WHO CAN BE HELPED?

The question of which patients can be helped remains one of the most perplexing in the management of patients with advanced hypertension and renal failure. In general, we look for *three favorable features* indicating that revascularization will benefit the patient: (1) a high-grade proximal renal artery stenosis or focal occlusion; (2) a patent distal renal artery; and (3) a reasonable renal size (e.g., >8–9 cm). Although renal duplex ultrasonography, magnetic resonance renal angiography, and renal scans may assist in identifying these favorable features, standard arteriography remains essential to defining the anatomy. Further deterioration in renal function can be minimized by preangiographic hydration and limited contrast loads. Intra-arterial digital subtraction techniques can enhance the acquisition of high-quality films without excessive contrast nephrotoxicity.

SHOULD THE TREATMENT BE SURGERY OR ANGIOPLASTY?

The arteriogram is essential to answering the fundamental question of whether to perform surgery or angioplasty and should be a biplane study (posteroanterior and lateral). It must define (1) the renal artery anatomy; (2) the condition of the aorta and iliac arteries; and (3) potential arterial inflow sources such as the celiac axis (e.g., hepatorenal or splenorenal procedures). If angioplasty is being considered, it should be planned for and conducted at the time of the initial diagnostic arteriogram. The best lesion for angioplasty is a focal, midrenal stenosis.[9,11] In our experience and in the reports from the literature, bilateral ostial lesions not only are difficult to dilate, but also have a higher recurrence rate.[9] Stents may enhance the initial result of ostial renal balloon angioplasty, but the long-term (5-year) results are not available.[12]

If a renal artery occlusion is found and the distal renal artery does not visualize, a nephrectomy may be helpful for a small, shrunken, pressor kidney (<8 cm). In such cases, we often obtain vena cava and bilateral renal vein renins. If the shrunken kidney is clearly a renin-producing source, a nephrectomy is often performed at the time of the contralateral renal revascularization.

IF SURGERY IS THE BEST OPTION, WHICH OPERATION SHOULD BE PERFORMED?

For most patients in our series (87%), surgical renal reconstruction appeared to be the best choice in managing advanced renovascular hypertension and renal insufficiency. Several surgical series have documented the durability of this procedure.[1–8,14,15] A surgical approach also allows simultaneous treatment of (1) both renal arteries and (2) an aorta that has significant occlusive or aneurysmal change.

Although surgeons have personal biases about techniques,[14–27] the operation must be tailored to the patient (Table 35–2). In general, the basic options include endarterectomy, aortorenal bypass, and one of the extra-anatomic approaches (e.g., hepatorenal, splenorenal, or iliorenal bypass). One of the most significant trends in our experience was a shift toward bilateral simultaneous transaortic endarterectomy (18% in 1980–1985 vs. 53% in 1986–1993; $P < .01$). This procedure simplified and achieved complete renal revascularization, especially in patients having multiple renal artery stenoses and those needing aortic grafting for occlusive or aneurysmal disease (56% in 1970–1980 vs. 75% in 1980–1993).

Surgical results are also maximized currently by intraoperative color-flow duplex ultrasonographic assessment of the technical outcome.[28] In approximately 8% to 10% of our patients, a technical problem (intimal flap, residual stenosis, or occlusion) was identified and corrected. Patients who had correctable intraoperative technical problems demonstrated long-term outcomes similar to those of patients who had no technical problems.[29] In addition, we are currently studying the predictive value of the resistive index measured in the renal artery after revascularization. The resistive index is an indication of the amount of intraparenchymal renal disease. A higher index, indicating less diastolic flow, has been correlated with patients who have an eventual serum creatinine that remains above 1.5 mg/dL after surgical revascularization.

WHAT ARE THE SURGICAL RISKS?

The perioperative morbidity and mortality depend on three primary factors: (1) medical comorbidity, particularly clinically evident coronary heart disease; (2) the patient's age; and (3) the extent of the procedure, particularly the necessity for aortic replacement.

The three clinical characteristics with the strongest trends in predicting 30-day mortality are clinically evident coronary heart disease, a serum creatinine greater than 3 mg/dL, and age older than 70 years. Patients with low risk (0 or 1 of these comorbid

TABLE 35–2. OPERATIVE COMBINATIONS FOR 402 PATIENTS WITH RENOVASCULAR HYPERTENSION AND CHRONIC RENAL INSUFFICIENCY

Operation	1970–1980 (%) (n = 98)	1980–1993 (%) (n = 304)
Unilateral revascularization	38	36
Unilateral revascularization plus contralateral nephrectomy	25	14
Bilateral renal revascularization	26	50
Nephrectomy alone	11	0
Combined aortic grafting	55	75

(From Hallett JW Jr, Textor SC, Kos PB, et al. Advanced renovascular hypertension and renal insufficiency: trends in medical comorbidity and surgical approach from 1970 to 1993. *J Vasc Surg.* 1995;21:753.)

TABLE 35–3. EFFECT OF MULTIPLE MAJOR COMORBIDITIES ON 30-DAY OPERATIVE MORTALITY IN AZOTEMIC PATIENTS (*n* = 304)

Patients (%)	No. of Major Risk Factors[a]	30-Day Mortality (%)	*P* Value
60[b]	Low-risk group: 0 to 1	5.6	.016
40[c]	High-risk group: 2 to 3	15.5	

[a] The three major risk factors were age older than 70 years, clinically evident coronary heart disease (angina pectoris, past myocardial infarction, or congestive heart failure), and serum creatinine of more than 3 mg/dL.
[b] None of these risks was present in 18.6% of all patients, while 41.4% had one major comorbidity.
[c] Two major risk factors were present in 28.1% of all patients, and 11.9% had all three major comorbidities.
(From Hallett JW Jr, Textor SC, Kos PB, et al. Advanced renovascular hypertension and renal insufficiency: trends in medical comorbidity and surgical approach from 1970 to 1993. *J Vasc Surg.* 1995;21:755.)

factors) have a mortality of 5.6%, whereas patients with high risk (2 or 3 risk factors) have a mortality of 15.5% (P = .016) (Table 35–3). Age reflects the stage of the lifelong battle with systemic atherosclerosis (Table 35–4).

The type and the extent of the surgical procedure also affect 30-day mortality. Concomitant aortic grafting is associated with an increased mortality (12%) compared with that of renal revascularization without aortic replacement (3.6%) (P = .07). In addition, the 30-day mortality for patients undergoing renal endarterectomy (4.3%) appeared lower than that for those undergoing renal bypass grafting (12.2%) (P = .07).

WHAT ARE THE OUTCOMES?

The outcomes for blood pressure and renal function can be defined by various criteria. Because of the diverse array of antihypertensives used after operation, the simple

TABLE 35–4. DESCRIPTIVE STATISTICS OF 304 AZOTEMIC PATIENTS UNDERGOING RENOVASCULAR OPERATIONS, BY AGE GROUP (1980–1993)

	Age Group (yr)[a]			
Factor	*50–65 (n = 101)*	*65–70 (n = 86)*	*70–75 (n = 75)*	*>75 (n = 37)*
Gender				
Male (%)	67.3	69.8	76.0	81.1
Female (%)	32.7	30.2	24.0	18.9
30-Day mortality (%)	7.9	8.1	12.0	18.9
90-Day mortality (%)	7.9	12.8	16.0	24.3
Prior congestive heart failure (%)	21.1	19.6	20.8	42.3
Angina pectoris (%)	22.5	32.1	37.7	26.9
Past myocardial infarction (%)	21.1	26.8	32.1	26.9
Cerebrovascular disease (%)	22.5	26.8	24.5	19.2
Diabetes mellitus (%)	17.1	16.1	22.6	11.5
Preoperative creatinine (mg/dL) (median)	3.12 ± 0.13 (2.6)	3.16 ± 0.16 (2.2)	3.47 ± 0.18 (2.8)	3.75 ± 0.35 (2.6)

[a] Five patients younger than 50 years were excluded.
(From Hallett JW Jr, Textor SC, Kos PB, et al. Advanced renovascular hypertension and renal insufficiency: trends in medical comorbidity and surgical approach from 1970 to 1993. *J Vasc Surg.* 1995;21:756.)

classification of postoperative or postangioplasty blood pressure may not reflect quality of life. Quality of life is often affected negatively by side effects from various medications. Consequently, we focus not only on improvement in blood pressure and creatinine, but also on the number of medications necessary to attain these levels. In addition, we use relatively strict criteria to identify stabilization, improvement, or worsening of renal function (change in serum creatinine of 1 mg/dL).

Balloon angioplasty was technically successful for only a limited number of our patients with chronic renal insufficiency. Specifically, balloon angioplasty was used for only 13.6% of all patients undergoing treatment. Serum creatinine improved in 21% ($n = 9$), stayed the same in 52% ($n = 23$), and worsened in 27% ($n = 12$). In a total group of 44 patients, long-term mean serum creatinine was not changed significantly by balloon angioplasty.

Conversely, most patients with advanced renovascular hypertension and renal insufficiency benefited from surgical revascularization (Table 35–5). The median postoperative systolic blood pressure was 150 mm Hg (preoperative, 180 mm Hg), with a diastolic pressure of 80 mm Hg (preoperative, 90 mm Hg). These blood pressure levels

TABLE 35–5. POSTOPERATIVE OUTCOMES FOR 304 PATIENTS WITH RENOVASCULAR HYPERTENSION AND CHRONIC RENAL INSUFFICIENCY

	BLOOD PRESSURE (BP) CONTROL[a]	
	Systolic BP (mm Hg)	*Diastolic BP (mm Hg)*
Preoperative	180 (range, 124–270)	90 (range, 60–150)
Hospital discharge	150 (range, 96–190)	80 (range, 50–104)
Follow-up	146 (range, 96–236)	80 (range, 46–112)
	NO. OF ANTIHYPERTENSIVE MEDICATIONS	
	No.	***Range***
Preoperative	3	0–6
Hospital discharge	2	0–5
Follow-up	2	0–5
	RENAL FUNCTION	
	Serum Creatinine (Median, mg/dL)	
	Preoperative	2.7
	Hospital discharge	2.2
	Later follow-up[c]	2.3
	Change in Serum Creatine (% of Patients)[b]	
	Increase (≥1 mg/dL)	27.3
	Same (<1 mg/dL)	52.6
	Decrease (≥1 mg/dL)	20.1
	Stable or improved	72.7
	Chronic Dialysis (% of Patients)	
	<21 Days postoperatively	4.6
	>21 Days postoperatively[c]	13.5

[a] Blood pressure, median values.
[b] Postoperative: hospital discharge.
[c] Mean follow-up, 17.5 months.
(From Hallett JW Jr, Textor SC, Kos PB, et al. Advanced renovascular hypertension and renal insufficiency: trends in medical comorbidity and surgical approach from 1970 to 1993. *J Vasc Surg.* 1994;21:757–758.)

were maintained at later follow-up. Furthermore, this control was achieved with fewer antihypertensive drugs (preoperative median, three vs. postoperative median, two). Although only 44% of our patients took fewer than three antihypertensive drugs preoperatively, 70% improved and required fewer than three drugs to control high blood pressure after operation ($P = .0005$). An additional 10.9% of the patients were cured (i.e., no antihypertensive medications and a diastolic blood pressure ≤90 mm Hg).

In addition, the majority of patients (73%) had stabilized or improved renal function. Twenty percent experienced a postoperative fall in creatinine of at least 1 mg/dL, while in 53% the creatinine remained unchanged. In contrast, 27% of the patients had an increase in creatinine of more than 1 mg/dL.

One of the most important long-term outcomes was the relatively small need for chronic dialysis, which was necessary within 30 days for only 4.6% of all 304 azotemic patients. Subsequently, another 13.5% progressed to chronic dialysis at a mean follow-up of 17.5 months. During this time period, the need for dialysis remained low (9%) for patients with a preoperative creatinine of 2.0 to 2.9 mg/dL, compared with the need of those with a creatinine of greater than 3 mg/dL (35%) ($P < .01$).

Survival in these patients was impaired compared with that of matched controls without atherosclerosis, but reasonably good compared to similar patients undergoing other major cardiovascular procedures. Five-year survival was 65%, compared with 83% for an age-matched control group (Fig. 35–5). This survival, however, is similar to that of patients undergoing coronary artery bypass grafting, carotid endarterectomy, and abdominal aortic aneurysm repair. Survival has clearly been better for patients who have an initial serum creatinine of less than 3 mg/dL.

CONCLUSION

Medical comorbidity and age have increased in patients presenting with advanced renovascular hypertension and renal insufficiency. The most important predictors

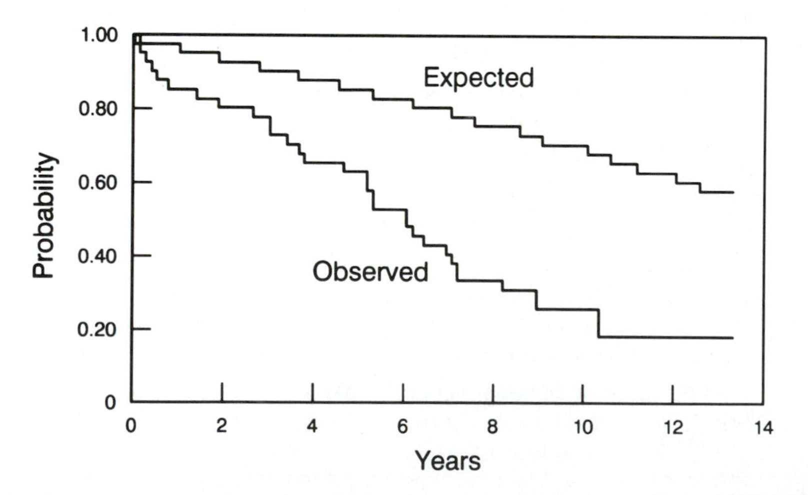

Figure 35–5. Five-year survival after renal artery revascularization for advanced hypertension and/or renal insufficiency ($n = 98$, 1970–1980, Mayo Clinic. *(Reproduced with permission from Hallett WJ Jr, Fowl R, O'Brien PC, et al. Renovascular operations in patients with chronic renal insufficiency: do the benefits justify the risks? J Vasc Surg. 1987;5:622–627.)*

of higher operative mortality are age older than 70 years, a creatinine of more than 3 mg/dL, and the need for simultaneous aortic grafting. Low-risk patients have an operative mortality of 5.6%, compared with a 15.5% mortality for high-risk patients.

RECOMMENDATIONS

Transaortic renal endarterectomy simplifies and expedites renal revascularization in patients with ostial renal atherosclerosis. Bilateral transaortic endarterectomy plus aortic grafting provides complete renal revascularization and aortic reconstruction at a reasonable mortality (4.6%). The best surgical outcomes for patients with advanced renovascular hypertension and renal insufficiency are achieved when such patients undergo renal revascularization before the serum creatinine exceeds 3 mg/dL.

Acknowledgments
The author acknowledges the following individuals who have participated in the care and study of the patients whose cases are discussed in this chapter: Stephen C. Textor, M.D.; Paul B. Kos, B.S.; Gregory Nicpon, B.A.; Thomas C. Bower, M.D.; Kenneth J. Cherry, Jr., M.D.; Peter Gloviczki, M.D.; and Peter C. Pairolero, M.D. The author also gratefully acknowledges the editorial assistance of Mrs. Renee Brandt.

REFERENCES

1. Novick AC, Pohl MA, Schreiber M, et al. Revascularization for preservation of renal function in patients with atherosclerotic renovascular disease. *J Urol.* 1983;129:907–912.
2. Ying CY, Tifft CP, Gavras H, et al. Renal revascularization in the azotemic hypertensive patient resistant to therapy. *N Engl J Med.* 1984;311:1070–1075.
3. Hallett WJ Jr, Fowl R, O'Brien PC, et al. Renovascular operations in patients with chronic renal insufficiency: do the benefits justify the risks? *J Vasc Surg.* 1987;5:622–627.
4. Mercier C, Piquet P, Alimi Y, et al. Occlusive disease of the renal arteries and chronic renal failure: the limits of reconstructive surgery. *Ann Vasc Surg.* 1990;4:166–170.
5. Elmore JR, Ray FS, Dillihunt RC, et al. Renal failure and advanced atherosclerotic lesions. *Arch Surg.* 1988;123:610–613.
6. Messina LM, Zelenock GB, Yao KA, et al. Renal revascularization for recurrent pulmonary edema in patients with poorly controlled hypertension and renal insufficiency: a distinct subgroup of patients with arteriosclerotic renal artery occlusive disease. *J Vasc Surg.* 1992;15:73–82.
7. Hansen KJ, Starr SM, Sands RE, et al. Contemporary surgical management of renovascular disease. *J Vasc Surg.* 1992;16:319–331.
8. Chaikof EL, Smith RB, Salam AA, et al. Ischemic nephropathy and concomitant aortic disease: a ten-year experience. *J Vasc Surg.* 1994;19:135–148.
9. Sos TA. Angioplasty for the treatment of azotemia and renovascular hypertension in atherosclerotic renal artery disease. *Circulation.* 1991;83(suppl I):I-162–I-166.
10. Textor SC. Renovascular hypertension. *Endocrinol Metab Clin North Am.* 1994;23:235–253.
11. Weibull H, Bergqvist D, Bergentz S-E, et al. Percutaneous transluminal renal angioplasty versus surgical reconstruction of atherosclerotic renal artery stenosis: a prospective randomized study. *J Vasc Surg.* 1993;18:841–852.
12. Bacharach JM, Graor RA, Olin JW, et al. Utility of stenting for ostial renal artery stenosis. *J Vasc Surg.* (Presented at the International Society for Cardiovascular Surgery, June 6, 1994.)
13. Hallett JW Jr, Textor SC, Kos PB, et al. Advanced renovascular hypertension and renal insufficiency: trends in medical comorbidity and surgical approach from 1970 to 1993. *J Vasc Surg.* 1995;21:750–760.

14. Cambria RP, Brewster DC, L'Italien GJ, et al. The durability of different reconstructive techniques for atherosclerotic renal artery disease. *J Vasc Surg.* 1994;20:76–87.
15. Lawrie GM, Morris GG Jr, Soussou ID, et al. Late results of reconstructive surgery for renovascular disease. *Ann Surg.* 1980;191:528–533.
16. Dean RH, Keyser JE III, Dupont WD, et al. Aortic and renal vascular disease. *Ann Surg.* 1984;200:336–344.
17. Stewart MT, Smith RB, Fulenwider JT, et al. Concomitant renal revascularization in patients undergoing aortic surgery. *J Vasc Surg.* 1985;2:400–405.
18. Tarazi RY, Hertzer NR, Beven EG, et al. Simultaneous aortic reconstruction and renal revascularization: risk factors and late results in eighty-nine patients. *J Vasc Surg.* 1987;5:707–714.
19. Branchereau A, Espinoza H, Magnan P-E, et al. Simultaneous reconstruction of infrarenal abdominal aorta and renal arteries. *Ann Vasc Surg.* 1992;6:232–238.
20. Katz DJ, Stanley JC, Zelenock GB. Operative mortality rates for intact and ruptured abdominal aortic aneurysms in Michigan: an eleven-year statewide experience. *J Vasc Surg.* 1994;19:804–817.
21. Novick AC, Straffon RA, Stewart BH, et al. Diminished operative morbidity and mortality in renal revascularization. *JAMA.* 1981;246:749–753.
22. Kannel WB, Castelli WP, McNamara PM, et al. Role of blood pressure in the development of congestive heart failure. *N. Engl J Med.* 1987;287:781–788.
23. Dean RH, Kieffer RW, Smith BM, et al. Renovascular hypertension. *Arch Surg.* 1981;116:1408–1415.
24. Novick AC, Ziegelbaum M, Vidt DG, et al. Trends in surgical revascularization for renal artery disease. *JAMA.* 1987;257:498–501.
25. Stanley JC. The evolution of surgery for renovascular occlusive disease. *Cardiovasc Surg.* 1994;2:195–202.
26. Stoney RJ, Skioldebrand CG, Qvarfordt PG, et al. Juxtarenal aortic atherosclerosis. *Ann Surg.* 1984;200:345–354.
27. Moncure AC, Brewster DC, Darling RC, et al. Use of the splenic and hepatic arteries for renal revascularization. *J Vasc Surg.* 1986;3:196–203.
28. Fichelle J-M, Colacchio G, Farkas J-C, et al. Renal revascularization in high-risk patients: the role of iliac renal bypass. *Ann Vasc Surg.* 1992;6:403–407.
29. Dougherty MJ, Hallett JW Jr, Naessens JM, et al. Optimizing technical success of renal revascularization: the impact of intraoperative color-flow duplex ultrasonography. *J Vasc Surg.* 1993;17:849–857.

36

Visceral Artery Aneurysms

Sandra C. Carr, MD, Robert L. Vogelzang, MD, and James S. T. Yao, MD, PhD

Aneurysms of the visceral arteries are an uncommon but important form of vascular disease. The natural history of most of these aneurysms appears to be expansion and eventual rupture, producing life-threatening hemorrhage. The most commonly involved vessels, in order of decreasing frequency, include the splenic, hepatic, superior mesenteric, celiac, gastric–gastroepiploic, jejunal–ileal–colic, pancreatoduodenal–pancreatic–gastroduodenal, and inferior mesenteric arteries.

The earliest report of a visceral artery aneurysm was in 1770 by Beaussier,[1] who discovered a splenic artery aneurysm (SAA) while injecting the aorta and femoral veins of a 60-year-old female cadaver for anatomic demonstration. A hepatic artery aneurysm (HAA) was first described in 1809 by Wilson.[2] In 1834, Jackson first published a report of a case of hemobilia caused by an HAA with intrabiliary rupture.[3] In 1871, Quincke described the classic triad of abdominal pain, hemobilia, and obstructive jaundice due to HAA.[3] An important event in American history was in 1881 when President James A. Garfield died from a ruptured SAA 2 months after being shot in the abdomen by an assassin.[4] The first successful surgical therapy was reported in 1903 by Kehr, who successfully treated a common HAA with ligation.[3] In 1932, the first preoperative diagnosis of an SAA followed by a successful operation was made by Lindboe.[5] The first maternal survivor following SAA rupture in pregnancy was not described until 1940 by Macleod.[1] In 1967, Nassalotti and Schaller reported the first case of both fetal and maternal survival after an SAA rupture.[5]

In the past, visceral artery aneurysms were primarily mycotic, syphilitic, or traumatic in origin. Currently, most true aneurysms are due to atherosclerosis or to medial degenerative diseases, while false aneurysms are usually due to trauma. Until recently, most visceral artery aneurysms were discovered at autopsy, with rupture the cause of death. Today, with the increasing use of computed tomography (CT) and angiography, many aneurysms are being discovered in the asymptomatic state. Still, nearly 22% of all reported visceral artery aneurysms present as clinical emergencies, including 8.5% that result in death.[6]

Although the various types of visceral artery aneurysms have many features in common, the etiology, presentation, and natural history of the disease differ. Thus, splenic, hepatic, superior mesenteric, celiac, gastric–gastroepiploic, jejunal–ileal–colic, pancreatoduodenal–pancreatic–gastroduodenal, and inferior mesenteric artery aneurysms are discussed separately.

SPLENIC ARTERY ANEURYSMS

Splenic artery aneurysms are the most common of the visceral artery aneurysms and account for more than 60% of these lesions. Splenic artery aneurysms are usually saccular, occur commonly at bifurcations, and are multiple in 20% of the patients. These aneurysms occur far more frequently in women, with a female-to-male ratio of 4:1 (Fig. 36–1). Forty-five percent of all female patients with SAAs have had six or more pregnancies, 88% have had two or more pregnancies, and 98% have had at least one pregnancy.[4] About 70% of all SAAs are solitary, and most of the multiple aneurysms are small and saccular.[2] Approximately 80% are located in the distal part of the artery.[2]

In addition to pregnancy, other conditions that are sometimes associated with the SAA include portal hypertension, fibromuscular dysplasia, and pancreatitis. In the patient with portal hypertension, the development of an SAA is thought to be a consequence of a hyperkinetic state in the spleen.[7] The pathogenesis of SAAs in pregnant women is thought to depend on hemodynamic and hormonal factors. It is possible that estrogen or the hormone relaxin, which is secreted during the last trimester of pregnancy, has some effect on the elastic support of the arteries.[8] Fibromuscular dysplasia is the cause in 13% of all cases of SAAs. Aneurysms of the splenic artery may occur in association with fibromuscular dysplasia of the renal arteries; 4% of all patients with renal artery fibromuscular dysplasia have a concomitant SAA. In the patient with pancreatitis, an aneurysm may form as a result of the inflammatory process, which erodes into the adjacent vessel wall. Many of these aneurysms show evidence of atherosclerosis; this usually represents secondary changes resulting from increased turbulence, not a primary process.[9]

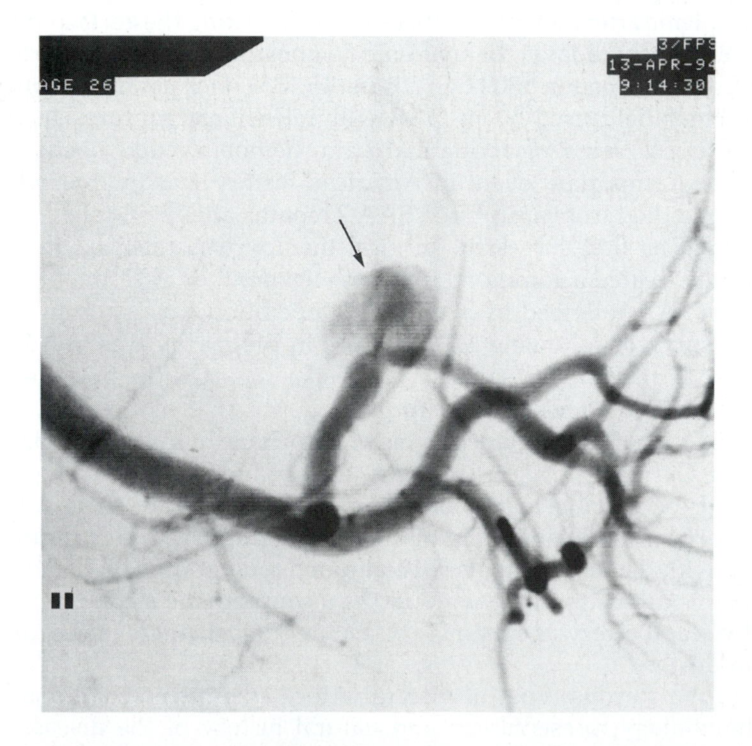

Figure 36–1. Splenic artery aneurysm (*arrow*) in a 26-year-old woman.

Most patients with SAAs (80%) are asymptomatic, but some may have symptoms of vague left upper quadrant or epigastric pain, sometimes with radiation to the left subscapular region. A few patients, 11%, have an audible abdominal bruit.[5] The abdominal pain worsens with acute expansion or rupture and may be accompanied by hypotension, diaphragmatic irritation, and diaphoresis. Aneurysm rupture often presents with hemorrhage initially confined to the lesser sac. Exsanguinating hemorrhage follows as blood escapes through the foramen of Winslow into the peritoneal cavity.[10] This *double-rupture phenomenon* was first described by Brockman in 1930.[5] In patients with pancreatitis, the aneurysm may present with gastrointestinal hemorrhage after rupture into the gastrointestinal tract, pancreatic duct, or splenic vein.[11] Less commonly, the aneurysm may rupture into the retroperitoneum (16%), stomach (11%), colon (8%), or pancreas (6%).[11]

Fortunately, rupture of an SAA is rare, occurring in only 2% of all cases not associated with pregnancy. However, more than 98% of the aneurysms reported during pregnancy present with rupture, the majority during the last trimester. Rupture during pregnancy is accompanied by a maternal mortality rate of 70% and a fetal death rate of 95%.[6] Twenty percent to 50% of all SAA ruptures occur during pregnancy, and another 20% occur in patients with portal hypertension.[5] Treatment of an SAA is therefore indicated for pregnant patients or for women of childbearing age who might become pregnant. Treatment is also indicated for patients with symptomatic or enlarging lesions. Aneurysm size greater than 2.5 cm is also considered a relative indication for therapy.[6]

HEPATIC ARTERY ANEURYSMS

Hepatic artery aneurysms are the second most common of the visceral artery aneurysms and account for 20% of these lesions. Approximately 80% of all HAAs are extrahepatic and 20% are intrahepatic. Sixty-three percent of the aneurysms are in the common hepatic artery, 28% in the right hepatic artery, 5% in the left hepatic artery, and 7% in both the right and left hepatic arteries.

Although in the past, infection was the most common cause of HAAs, the current causes are atherosclerosis in 32% of the cases, medial degeneration in 24%, trauma in 22%, and infection associated with illicit drug use in 10%.[6,10] Aneurysms of traumatic origin may be caused by a major crush injury, a penetrating wound, or surgery.[2] An increasingly common source of these aneurysms is the percutaneous placement of a transhepatic biliary drainage catheter for relief of benign or malignant biliary obstruction. Periarteritis nodosa, cystic medial necrosis, and other arteriopathies also cause HAAs. Men are affected twice as often as women. Except for aneurysms secondary to trauma, most of these lesions occur in patients in the sixth decade of life.

As with SAA patients, most patients with HAAs are asymptomatic. Patients may have right upper quadrant or epigastric pain that may mimic symptoms of pancreatitis. The pain may radiate to the back or to the right shoulder and is unrelated to meals. Rarely, a large aneurysm can obstruct the biliary tract, and this obstruction leads to jaundice.[6] Usually, HAAs do not produce physical signs such as a bruit or a palpable abdominal mass. The classic triad of pain, hemobilia, and obstructive jaundice is seen in only one-third of the patients. Unfortunately, in as many as 80% of all patients with HAAs, rupture of the aneurysm is the reason for first medical consultation.[2,3] Of these patients, 70% present with pain and 62% with gastrointestinal hemorrhage.[2]

Hepatic artery aneurysms that rupture into the peritoneal cavity and those that rupture into the biliary tract occur with equal frequency. Rupture may also occur into the duodenum, gallbladder, portal vein, or stomach.[2] The frequency of HAA rupture is thought to be less than 20%. The mortality rate with rupture, however, approaches 35%.[6] Because the natural history of the HAA appears to be progression to rupture, most of these aneurysms should be treated aggressively. In contrast to abdominal aortic aneurysms, the size at which HAAs are likely to become symptomatic is not well defined.

SUPERIOR MESENTERIC ARTERY ANEURYSMS

Aneurysms of the superior mesenteric artery (SMA) are rare, comprising between 5% and 8% of all visceral artery aneurysms.[12] In autopsy series, the reported incidence is 1 in 12,000. Most of these aneurysms occur in the proximal 5 cm of the vessel. Men and women are affected equally.[10]

The majority of SMA aneurysms (60%) are mycotic, usually due to septic emboli from endocarditis. More than any other muscular artery, the SMA is involved with mycotic aneurysm from left-sided bacterial endocarditis due to nonhemolytic streptococci (Fig. 36–2). Superior mesenteric artery aneurysms in patients less than 50 years of age are usually mycotic, whereas those in older patients are most frequently noninfectious. Noninfectious causes of an SMA aneurysm include medial degeneration, athero-

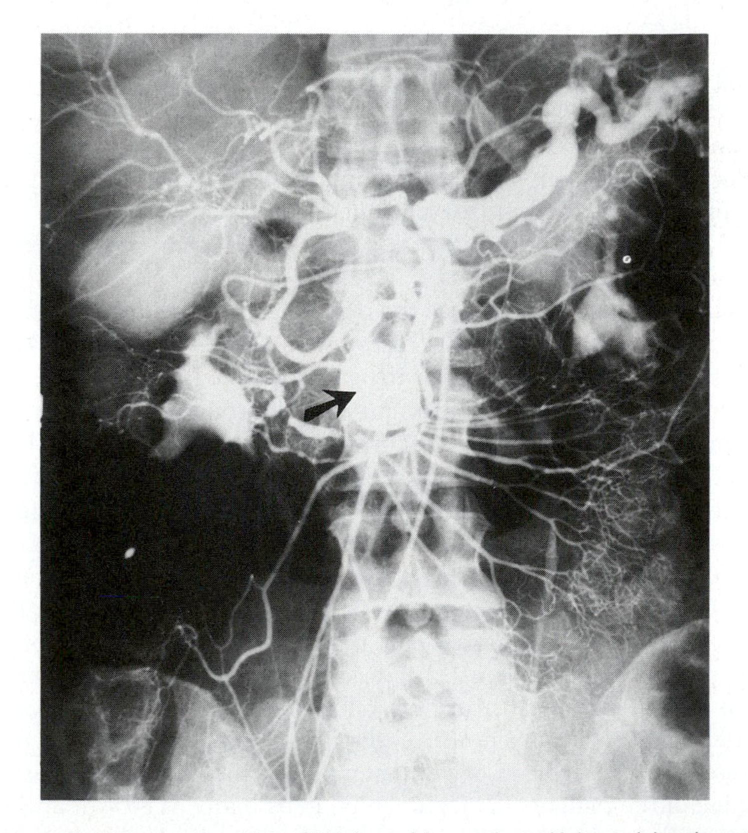

Figure 36–2. Mycotic aneurysm of the SMA (*arrow*) in a patient with bacterial endocarditis. The aneurysm was treated with ligation.

sclerosis, polyarteritis nodosa, and trauma.[6,12] Atherosclerosis is seen in 20% of these aneurysms but may be a secondary process.

Many patients with SMA aneurysms manifest with intermittent upper abdominal or epigastric pain. Some present with symptoms suggestive of mesenteric ischemia. Although physical findings are uncommon, some patients present with a tender, mobile, pulsatile abdominal mass.

The incidence of rupture of untreated SMA aneurysms appears to be high, up to 50%.[2,12] Expansion of the aneurysm accompanied by dissection or propagation of an intraluminal thrombus may occlude collateral flow, leading to intestinal ischemia. Because complications from this disease can lead to mesenteric infarction and because the natural history of these lesions appears to be progressive expansion and rupture, intervention is indicated for essentially all lesions, even if asymptomatic.

CELIAC ARTERY ANEURYSMS

Celiac artery aneurysms (CAAs) represent only 4% of all visceral artery aneurysms. The mean patient age is 52 years, and the male-to-female ratio is 1 : 1.[10] Most CAAs are due to atherosclerosis or to medial degeneration. Other causes of CAAs include post-stenotic dilation, trauma, re-entry from aortic dissection, and infection. Associated diseases include hypertension in 20% of the patients, abdominal aortic aneurysms in 20%, and other visceral artery aneurysms in 40%.

Approximately two-thirds of all patients with CAAs are symptomatic. More than 60% of the patients complain of abdominal pain, which is often an epigastric discomfort radiating to the back. Others describe vague abdominal pain that is associated with nausea and vomiting. The pain may increase with meals, mimicking intestinal angina. Nearly 30% of the patients have a palpable abdominal mass and 37% have an abdominal bruit on physical examination. Involvement of adjacent organs may result in gastrointestinal bleeding or obstructive jaundice.[2] Most CAAs in asymptomatic patients are discovered on arteriograms or CT scans obtained for another disease process.

The natural history of the CAA appears to be expansion and rupture. Current series report the rupture rate of CAAs to be 12.5%. Rupture can be complicated by intestinal infarction, with a mortality rate of 50%. These aneurysms usually do not rupture into the gastrointestinal tract, but they may result in hemoperitoneum. Currently, operative treatment is indicated for all symptomatic aneurysms. Treatment is also recommended for the asymptomatic CAA discovered as an incidental finding, except in the very high risk patient.

GASTRIC AND GASTROEPIPLOIC ARTERY ANEURYSMS

Gastric artery (GA) and gastroepiploic artery (GEA) aneurysms account for only 4% of all visceral artery aneurysms. Gastric artery aneurysms are 10 times more frequent than the GEA type, and most patients are in the sixth or seventh decade of life. The male-to-female ratio is 3 : 1. The cause of these lesions is medial degeneration, periarterial inflammation, or atherosclerosis. Atherosclerosis is often thought to represent a secondary process rather than a primary cause. Most GA and GEA aneurysms are solitary.[6]

Although a few GA and GEA aneurysms are discovered during angiography for other diseases, 90% of the patients present emergently with rupture. About two-thirds of the ruptured aneurysms cause upper gastrointestinal bleeding, while the remainder rupture into the peritoneal cavity. Hemobilia can result from rupture of left GA aneurysms.[2] Rupture of GA and GEA aneurysms is often accompanied by exsanguinating hemorrhage, with a 70% mortality rate. Of the patients who present emergently, 70% have gastrointestinal bleeding and 30% have life-threatening intraperitoneal hemorrhage. Because of the serious complications associated with aneurysm rupture, operative therapy is recommended for nearly all GA and GEA aneurysms.

JEJUNAL, ILEAL, AND COLIC ARTERY ANEURYSMS

Aneurysms of the jejunal, ileal, and colic arteries represent only 3% of all visceral artery aneurysms. These lesions are seen in the seventh decade of life, and men and women are affected equally. Medial defects are the cause in most cases. Other causes include trauma and arteritis from septic emboli. As with the other visceral artery aneurysms, arteriosclerosis is usually a secondary process, occurring in 20% of the cases. Except for lesions associated with connective tissue disorders, most jejunal, ileal, and colic artery aneurysms are solitary.

Seventy percent of all patients with these aneurysms present with abdominal pain, bleeding, or a tender abdominal mass. Most jejunal, ileal, and colic artery aneurysms are discovered during exploratory celiotomy for gastrointestinal or intraperitoneal bleeding. Although the risk of rupture is thought to be low, the mortality rate, 20%, supports an aggressive therapeutic approach to these aneurysms.[6]

PANCREATODUODENAL, PANCREATIC, AND GASTRODUODENAL ARTERY ANEURYSMS

Aneurysms of the pancreatic artery (PA) and the pancreatoduodenal artery (PDA) represent only 2% of all visceral artery aneurysms. Gastroduodenal artery (GDA) aneurysms account for an additional 1.5% These three types of aneurysms occur most commonly in the sixth decade of life, with men affected four times as frequently as women (Fig. 36–3). Many of these lesions are associated with pancreatitis, which leads to periarterial inflammation or vessel erosion from an adjacent pseudocyst. Approximately 60% of all GDA aneurysms and 30% of all PDA aneurysms are related to pancreatitis.

Because of this relationship to pancreatitis, most patients with these aneurysms have symptoms of abdominal pain and discomfort; few patients are asymptomatic. Pancreatic artery, PDA, and GDA aneurysms rupture into the gastrointestinal tract, or, less commonly, into the biliary or pancreatic ductal system. Seventy-five percent of the inflammatory lesions and 50% of the noninflammatory lesions are associated with rupture into the gastrointestinal tract. The mortality rate accompanying rupture is high, nearly 50%. Thus, an aggressive therapeutic approach is indicated and usually involves operative treatment of the associated pancreatitis or pseudocyst.[6]

INFERIOR MESENTERIC ARTERY ANEURYSMS

Aneurysms of the inferior mesenteric artery (IMA) are the most rare of all visceral artery aneurysms. Discussions of their clinical presentation and therapy are almost anecdotal. The sources of IMA aneurysms vary but include medial dissection, atherosclerosis, and mycotic causes. Younger patients tend to have mycotic aneurysms.

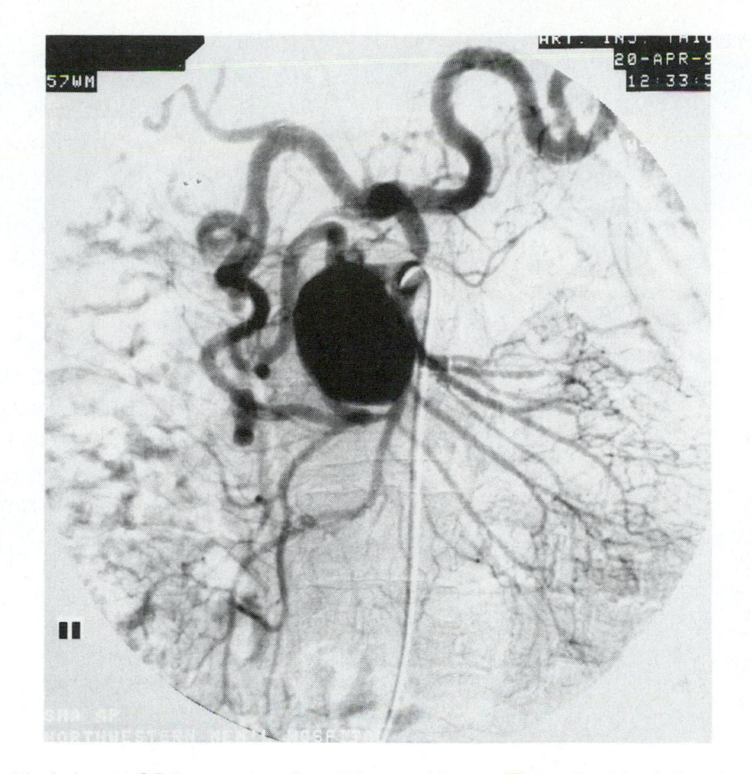

Figure 36–3. Large GDA aneurysm in a 57-year-old man. The patient had chronic occlusion of the proximal celiac artery with the development of an aneurysm in an enlarged collateral vessel. The patient was treated surgically with a saphenous vein graft bypass to the celiac artery and ligation of the vessels feeding the aneurysm.

The natural history of IMA aneurysms is undefined. It has been suggested that all mycotic lesions and large IMA aneurysms be treated.[13]

DIAGNOSIS

In many cases, the diagnosis of a visceral artery aneurysm can be suspected from the abdominal plain film. As many of these aneurysms have secondary atherosclerosis and calcification, a characteristic curvilinear "eggshell" pattern may be seen in the epigastrium, in the right of left upper quadrant. About two-thirds of all SAAs have this feature, which is localized to the left upper quadrant.[2]

Computed tomography has become a useful diagnostic modality for these lesions (Fig. 36–4). Not only are intact aneurysms well demonstrated, but ruptured aneurysms also produce characteristic findings. A contained hematoma within the lesser sac is often found with ruptured SAAs, before the blood escapes through the foramen of Winslow into the peritoneal cavity.[14] On dynamic contrast CT scans, a visceral artery aneurysm may appear as a brightly enhancing lesion with a variable amount of luminal thrombus.[15]

Many visceral artery aneurysms are discovered incidentally during routine abdominal ultrasonography or CT scanning for unrelated symptoms. The lesion appears as an isolated hypoechogenic nodule or an anechoic cystic mass. The connection of the mass with the feeding artery and the presence of parietal linear calcifications can help

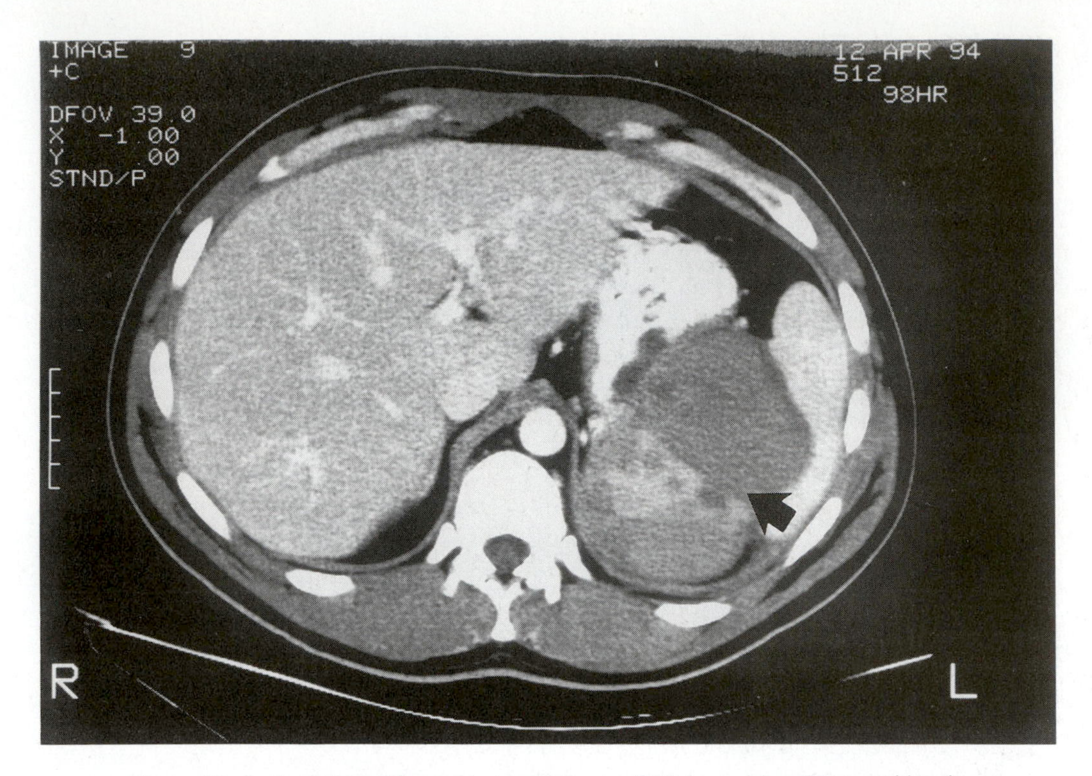

Figure 36–4. Abdominal CT scan demonstrating an SAA (*arrow*) in a 26-year-old male.

to make the diagnosis. However, the finding of an abdominal cystic mass on CT scans is not specific for a visceral artery aneurysm and is commonly due to some other pathology. Color-flow Doppler ultrasound can be used in adjunct to determine the nature of the lesion by demonstrating arterial flow.[15,16]

Recently, magnetic resonance imaging (MRI) has been used to diagnose visceral artery aneurysms. The presence of a central flow void and thrombus are characteristic (Fig. 36–5). However, with MRI it is often difficult to distinguish between arterial and venous flow.[15]

Although plain films, ultrasound, CT, and MRI can often detect a visceral artery aneurysm, angiography is usually necessary to confirm the diagnosis. Arteriography is the method of choice for diagnosis and is recommended for all elective cases. Biplanar angiography with selective injection is needed to define the extent of the aneurysm, to visualize collaterals, to define the distal vasculature, and to exclude the presence of associated aneurysms (splenic artery aneurysms, for example, are multiple in 20% of all cases). Such high definition is especially important in the visceral arteries, as there is much anatomic variation. Angiography is also important with HAAs because the hepatic artery and its branches can arise from either the celiac axis or the SMA.

SURGICAL TREATMENT

The main methods of therapy for visceral artery aneurysms are surgery and transcatheter occlusion of the aneurysm. Surgical options differ somewhat for each type of visceral artery aneurysm.

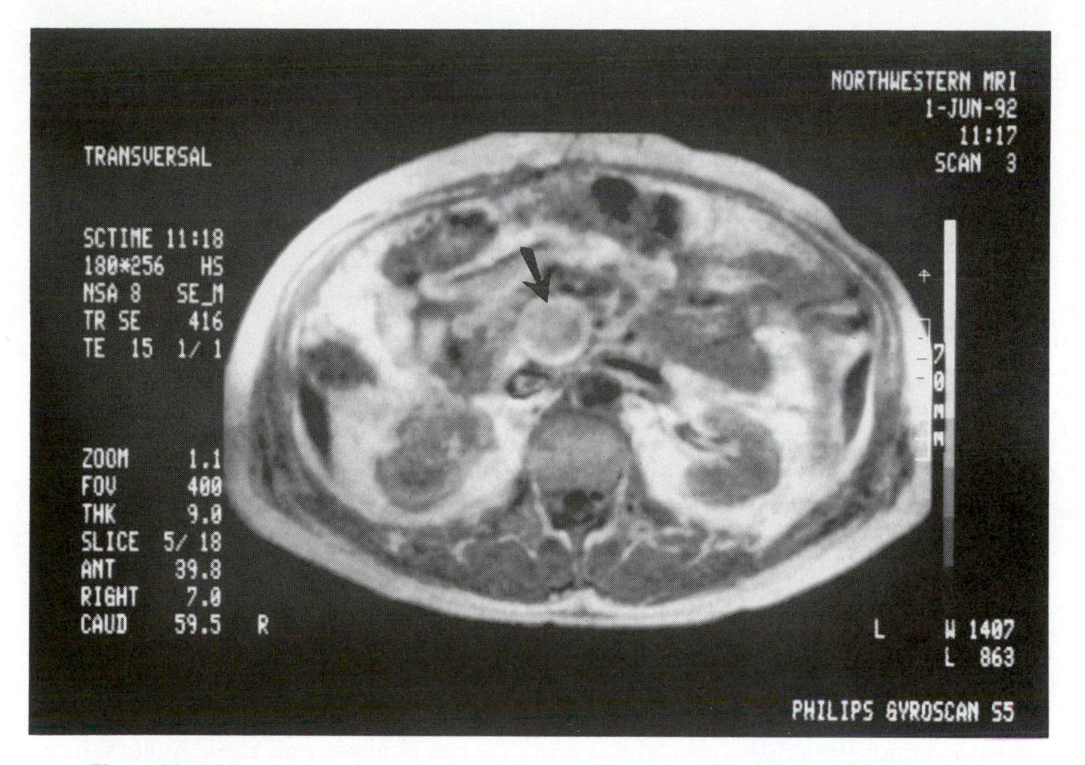

Figure 36–5. Magnetic resonance imaging study demonstrating an aneurysm of the GDA (*arrow*) in a 57-year-old male.

Splenic Artery Aneurysms

For SAAs, surgical therapy usually consists of splenectomy and removal of the portion of the splenic artery containing the aneurysm. Proximal SAAs may be treated with aneurysmectomy with proximal and distal ligation, without splenectomy. Because of excellent collateral flow, it is usually not necessary to revascularize the spleen. The extensive blood supply from the stomach through the short gastric arteries usually prevents infarction in these cases. In cases where extensive dissection of the pancreas or adjacent structures is required, aneurysm exclusion with ligation of contributing vessels is appropriate. Arterial ligation from within the aneurysm may be necessary if the lesion is located in the midportion of the splenic artery or is embedded in the pancreas.[6] Laparoscopic ligation has also been described for SAAs, with good results.[17,18] It is important to examine the artery for multiple aneurysms, especially in emergent cases, when preoperative angiograms are not obtained.

No procedural guidelines exist for an SAA that is identified during pregnancy. Options include elective surgery during the second trimester and elective cesarean section with operative treatment of the aneurysm at the same time.[5] Because of the high risk of rupture during the third trimester, observation of SAAs in obstetric patients is not recommended.

Hepatic Artery Aneurysms

Aneurysms of the proximal hepatic artery can be treated by excision or by exclusion without reconstruction. There is usually sufficient collateral circulation through the SMA to the GDA. In distal lesions or in those involving the GDA, revascularization may be necessary. A transient 5-minute intraoperative occlusion of the hepatic artery can help the surgeon assess the need for revascularization.[19] When revascularization is necessary, autogenous saphenous vein is the conduit of choice for most visceral artery aneurysms, although prosthetic grafts have been used. Reconstruction may take the form of an aortohepatic artery bypass, splenohepatic anastomosis, or interposition grafting with GDA reimplantation. For intra–hepatic artery aneurysms, surgical correction may require hepatic resection of the area involving the aneurysm or simple ligation of the involved artery before it enters the liver parenchyma.[3,19,20]

Superior Mesenteric Artery Aneurysms

Superior mesenteric artery aneurysms are usually treated operatively through a transmesenteric or retroperitoneal approach. Simple ligation of vessels entering and exiting the aneurysm has been successful in 30% of the reported cases.[2,6,12] Aneurysmectomy with reconstruction is sometimes necessary if there is doubt about sufficient collateral circulation. With proximal SMA lesions, proximal anastomosis to the aorta is accomplished with techniques similar to those used for mesenteric occlusive disease. Endoaneurysmorrhaphy is an alternative, especially for saccular aneurysms.[10]

Celiac Artery Aneurysms

For CAAs, aneurysmectomy with arterial reconstruction is the preferred treatment. Although celiac artery ligation can be done if adequate collateral circulation to the foregut is demonstrated, this procedure carries the risk of hepatic necrosis. Aneurysmorrhaphy may be used for discrete saccular lesions.[6] Most CAAs can be approached through the abdomen with vascular control of the aorta obtained after division of the crus of the diaphragm.[10]

Gastric–Gastroepiploic and Pancreatoduodenal–Pancreatic–Gastroduodenal Artery Aneurysms

With GA and GEA aneurysms that occur in an extragastric location, ligation of the aneurysm vessels with or without aneurysm excision is appropriate. Intramural lesions are best excised with the involved portion of the stomach.[6] With PDA, PA, and GDA aneurysms, simple ligation is often difficult because of multiple communicating vessels. The aneurysm may be opened, and suture ligation of entering and exiting vessels can be accomplished from within the aneurysm.[6,10]

Mesenteric Branch Artery Aneurysms

Aneurysms of the mesenteric branch vessels are usually treated with arterial ligation, aneurysmectomy, and resection of ischemic bowel segments. As with other visceral artery aneurysms, a search for multiple branch vessel aneurysms is appropriate. Inferior mesenteric artery aneurysms can be treated with ligation with or without revascularization, depending on the status of the intestinal circulation.

TRANSCATHETER EMBOLIZATION

Angiographic embolization has been used for several years in patients with visceral artery aneurysms who are poor surgical risks. Greater experience with the techniques of transcatheter embolization has made this procedure an option for primary treatment of these aneurysms. The process involves selective catheterization of the involved vessel, followed by injection of Gelfoam particles or steel coils. Detachable balloons may be used as an alternative.

Transcatheter embolization may be used for SAAs.[20–22] Treatment of SAAs involves occlusion of the splenic artery or direct embolization of the aneurysm. Multiple coils placed into the neck of the aneurysm cause occlusion of the aneurysm and the more proximal splenic artery, but modern coaxial microcatheter techniques make it possible to fill the aneurysm with coils and maintain flow in the main splenic artery. It is important to occlude the neck or origin of the aneurysm. Otherwise, collateral circulation will result in filling of the aneurysm and recurrence. With modern catheterization techniques, it is possible to occlude the main splenic artery at the level of the aneurysm or to primarily occlude only the aneurysm with preservation of the spleen.[21]

Embolization is especially useful for intra–hepatic artery aneurysms. A percutaneous transhepatic route allows better access to distally located aneurysms, especially in patients with tortuous proximal vessels. It is important to thrombose the vessel as distally as possible, as embolization of a more proximal vessel that is feeding the aneurysm may result in recurrence (Fig. 36–6).

The availability of wires and catheters for superselective catheterization permits precise localization and treatment of aneurysms of the mesenteric artery branches. Several centers use these techniques to treat large aneurysms by filling the aneurysm or by occluding only the neck of the lesion, thus avoiding bowel ischemia (Fig. 36–7).[23] Submucosal aneurysms and small aneurysms that are difficult to reach surgically are also good candidates for transcatheter embolization.

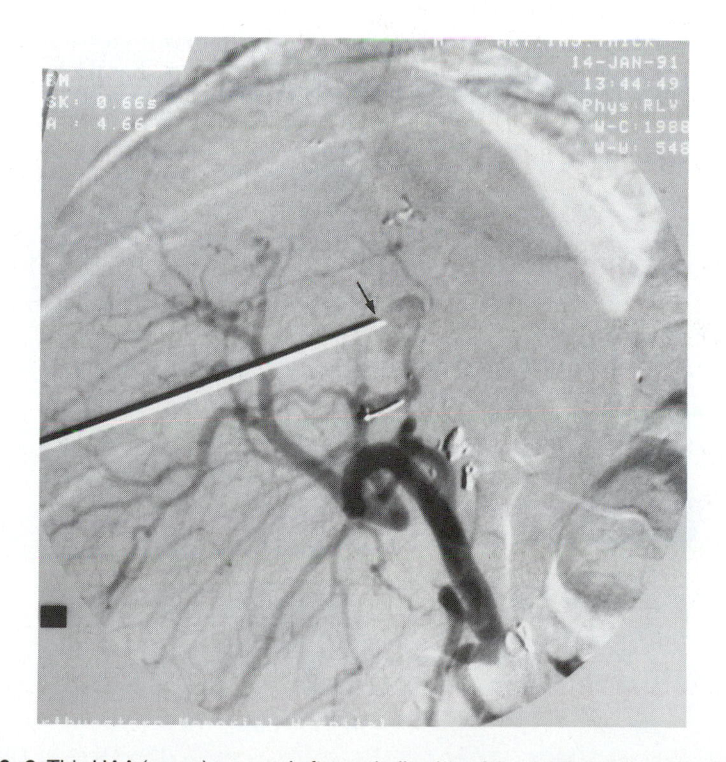

Figure 36–6. This HAA (*arrow*) recurred after embolization of the right hepatic artery. Successful thrombosis was obtained after a combined percutaneous transhepatic and transarterial approach was taken. Note the needle approaching the aneurysm for direct occlusion.

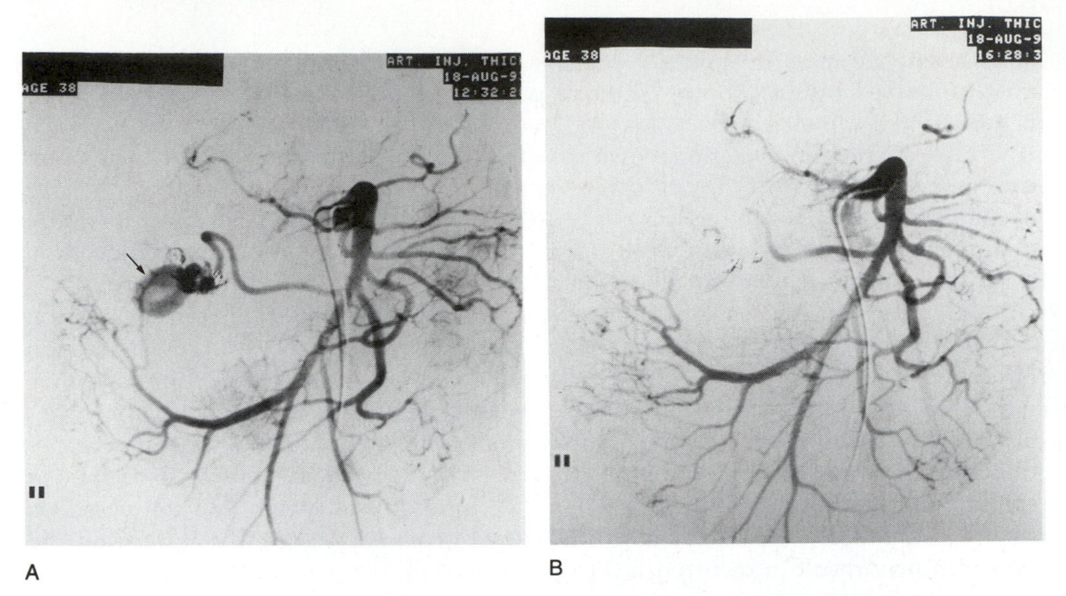

Figure 36–7. An aneurysm of a branch of the SMA was successfully occluded by using transcatheter embolization. (**A**) The aneurysm originated from a branch of the SMA (*arrow*). (**B**) Successful thrombosis was achieved with coils.

Recently, a few centers used a combined percutaneous and transarterial approach to treat visceral artery aneurysms. Percutaneous puncture of the aneurysm can provide direct access to the aneurysm and can be used to achieve complete thrombosis in aneurysms with tortuous feeding vessels (Fig. 36–8). Transcatheter treatment can also be used for patients who are not good surgical candidates (e.g., have a hostile abdomen) or who failed surgical treatment.

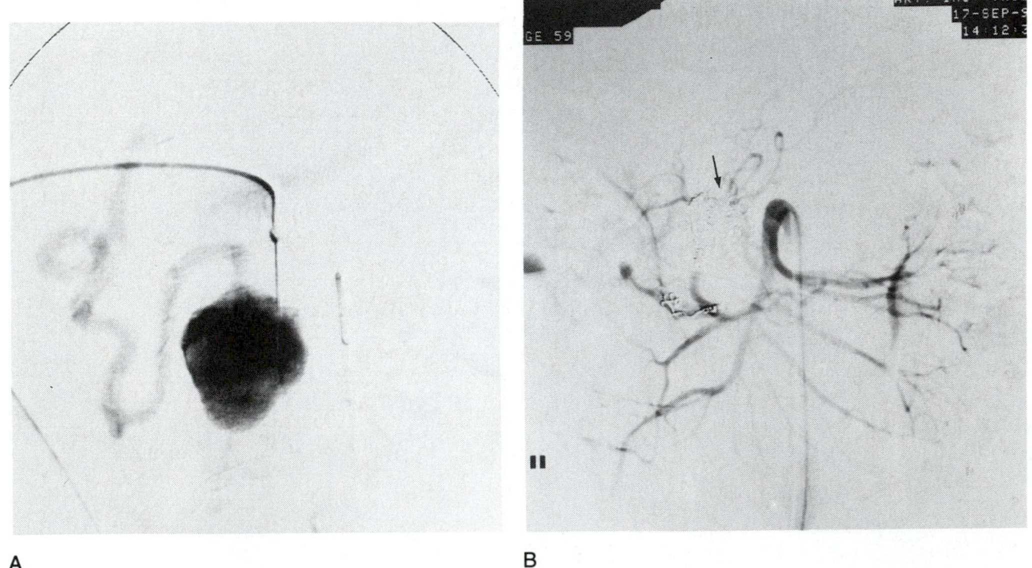

Figure 36–8. A large GDA aneurysm was treated by combined percutaneous and transarterial embolization. (**A**) Direct percutaneous puncture of the aneurysm. (**B**) Follow-up SMA angiogram obtained after occlusion.

Transcatheter embolization may be the treatment of choice for many visceral artery aneurysms, as it offers several advantages. This is particularly true with the widespread use of microcatheterization techniques for aneurysm exclusion or primary aneurysm thrombosis. Advantages include precise localization of the aneurysm, assessment of collateral flow, lower risk for patients who are not good operative candidates, and easier approach to aneurysms for which surgical exposure would be difficult.[24] Transcatheter occlusion may also be a less risky option for some patients with connective tissue disorders, such as Ehlers-Danlos syndrome.[25]

NORTHWESTERN MEMORIAL HOSPITAL EXPERIENCE

Since 1980, 29 patients at Northwestern Memorial Hospital in Chicago, Illinois, were diagnosed with visceral artery aneurysms. The majority of aneurysms, 19, were in the splenic artery. There were 8 hepatic, 4 superior mesenteric, 2 celiac, 2 left gastric, 1 jejunal, 1 gastroduodenal, and 1 inferior mesenteric artery aneurysm (Table 36–1). Four patients had multiple visceral artery aneurysms, usually due to septic emboli. Three patients had aneurysms secondary to trauma, two secondary to blunt wounds and one secondary to a gunshot wound. Other causes included pancreatitis, portal hypertension, and atherosclerosis. The treatment of each of these aneurysm types is summarized in Table 36–2.

At our institution, SAAs accounted for 50% of all visceral artery aneurysms discovered since 1980. The average age of these patients was 59 years, and 74% were female. None of the patients treated at this hospital were pregnant. Four patients (21%) presented with acute rupture of the aneurysm and underwent emergent celiotomy. Ten aneurysms were found incidentally during evaluation for concomitant disease. Associated conditions included portal hypertension, hypersplenism, pancreatitis, and atherosclerosis. Seven of the 19 patients with SAAs were treated with splenectomy. Many of these splenectomies were performed emergently for ruptured aneurysms. Three patients were treated with ligation of the aneurysm, and one aneurysm was successfully thrombosed by using transcatheter embolization.

In our series, eight patients had HAAs. Three lesions were secondary to trauma; one of these was related to percutaneous biliary drainage. Other causes were infection and atherosclerosis, and one aneurysm was associated with pancreatitis. The three patients with aneurysms that were due to trauma presented with abdominal pain and hemobilia. Other aneurysms were discovered during ultrasonography for suspected cholelithiasis. Three of the eight patients with HAAs underwent surgical correction.

TABLE 36–1. VISCERAL ARTERY ANEURYSMS AT NORTHWESTERN MEMORIAL HOSPITAL

Artery	No.	Percent
Splenic	19	50.0
Hepatic	8	21.1
Superior mesenteric	4	10.5
Celiac	2	5.3
Gastric	2	5.3
Jejunal	1	2.6
Gastroduodenal	1	2.6
Inferior mesenteric	1	2.6

TABLE 36–2. TREATMENT OF VISCERAL ARTERY ANEURYSMS

Aneurysm[a]	Intervention (No.)
Splenic artery	Splenectomy (7) Ligation (3) Embolization (1)
Hepatic artery	Excision with bypass (2) Ligation (1) Embolization (4)
SMA	Excision with bypass (1) Ligation of feeding vessels (1) Embolization (1)
Celiac artery	Excision with bypass (2)
GA	Ligation (1)
Jejunal artery	Ligation (1)
GDA	Ligation of feeding vessels (1) (Embolization of recurrent aneurysm)
IMA	Embolization (1)

[a] SMA = superior mesenteric artery; GA = gastric artery; GDA = gastroduodenal artery; IMA = inferior mesenteric artery.

One patient had ligation of the aneurysm, and two patients underwent excision with a saphenous vein bypass to the distal vessel. Four of our patients with HAAs, three resulting from trauma and one secondary to pancreatitis, were treated with transcatheter embolization. One of the patients suffered recurrence of an HAA 2 months after embolization of a proximal hepatic artery branch. Successful occlusion of the lesion was obtained by using combined percutaneous and transarterial routes for embolization.

Four of our patients, two males and two females, had aneurysms of the SMA. Three of the aneurysms were mycotic due to septic emboli, and the cause of one was thought to be atherosclerosis. None of these aneurysms ruptured. Of the two patients in our series that underwent operation for SMA aneurysms, one was treated by ligation of the vessels feeding the aneurysm and one was treated with aneurysm resection and a saphenous vein bypass. We also successfully treated one patient with an SMA aneurysm by using transcatheter embolization to occlude the small vessels feeding the aneurysm.

Two of our patients had aneurysms of the celiac artery. One aneurysm was mycotic, and one was atherosclerotic and associated with an abdominal aortic aneurysm. Both patients with CAAs had other, associated visceral artery aneurysms. None of these patients presented with aneurysm rupture or intestinal ischemia. The two patients with CAAs who were treated at our institution underwent operative repair with resection of the aneurysm and saphenous vein revascularization.

Since 1980, we have seen only two patients with GA aneurysms, both in the left GA. These lesions were due to septic emboli and were accompanied by multiple other visceral artery aneurysms. Neither aneurysm ruptured, but the patients presented with symptoms of chronic abdominal pain. The aneurysms were discovered during angiography done to evaluate other visceral aneurysms.

Only one patient had an aneurysm of a jejunal artery branch, and one had an aneurysm of the IMA. These aneurysms were thought to result from septic emboli and were associated with multiple aneurysms in each patient. The jejunal artery aneurysm was treated surgically with ligation. The IMA aneurysm was treated with transcatheter embolization of the small vessels feeding the aneurysm.

One of our patients at Northwestern had an aneurysm of the GDA. This 57-year-old male had chronic occlusion of the proximal celiac artery with the development of an aneurysm in the enlarged collateral vessel. This patient presented with complaints of abdominal pain but no evidence of aneurysm rupture. He was treated with bypass of a chronically occluded celiac artery and ligation of the vessels feeding the large GDA aneurysm. Postoperatively, the GDA aneurysm recurred. The patient was then treated with a combined percutaneous and transarterial embolization procedure that resulted in successful thrombosis of the aneurysm.

CONCLUSION

Visceral artery aneurysms are rare but clinically important lesions. Most of these aneurysms are associated with atherosclerosis or medial degenerative disease, although trauma and infection are still common causes. With the increasing use of CT and MRI, many aneurysms are being discovered prior to rupture or thrombosis. Improvements in ultrasound, CT, and MRI technology have led to the detection of more visceral artery aneurysms in patients who are being evaluated for abdominal pain or other intra-abdominal disease. At this time, however, angiography remains the method of choice to determine the extent of an aneurysm and to define the anatomy of the collateral circulation.

Most visceral artery aneurysms, even if asymptomatic, require some form of therapy to prevent the complications of rupture or end-organ ischemia. Surgical options include splenectomy with removal of the aneurysm, aneurysm exclusion with ligation, excision with or without vascular reconstruction, and ligation of the vessels entering and exiting the aneurysm. As laparoscopic technology continues to improve, more aneurysms may be amenable to laparoscopic ligation or repair. Transcatheter embolization is a newer form of therapy that has been employed to treat visceral artery aneurysms. As new technology becomes available and as more experience with interventional techniques is obtained, our methods of diagnosing and treating these rare aneurysms will continue to evolve.

REFERENCES

1. Beaussier M. Sur un aneurisme de l'artère splenique dont les parois se sont ossifiees. *J Med Toulous.* 1770;32:157.
2. Jorgensen BA. Visceral artery aneurysms. *Dan Med Bull.* 1985;32:237–242.
3. Psathakis D, Muller G, Noah M, et al. Present management of hepatic artery aneurysms. *Vasa.* 1992;21(2):210–215.
4. McGinnis HD, Deluca SA. Splenic artery aneurysms. *Am Fam Physician.* 1993;47(5):1119–1202.
5. Holdsworth RJ, Gunn A. Ruptured splenic artery in pregnancy. A review. *Br J Obstet Gynaecol.* 1992;99:595–597.
6. Stanley JC, Wakefield TW, Graham LM, et al. Clinical importance and management of splanchnic artery aneurysms. *J Vasc Surg.* 1986;3(5):836–840.
7. Ohta M, Hashizume M, Tanoue K, et al. Splenic hyperkinetic state and splenic artery aneurysms in portal hypertension. *Hepatogastroenterology.* 1992;39:529–532.
8. Martinez E, Menendez AR, Ablanedo P. Splenic artery aneurysms. *Int Surg.* 1986;71:95–99.
9. Graham LM, Mesh CL. Celiac, hepatic, and splenic artery aneurysms. In: Ernst CB, Stanley JC, eds. *Current Theory in Vascular Surgery.* St. Louis, MO: Mosby-Yearbook; 1995:714–718.

10. Graham LM, Rubin JR. Visceral artery aneurysms. In: Strandness DE, Breda A, eds. *Vascular Diseases: Surgical and Interventional Therapy.* New York, NY: Churchill Livingstone; 1994:811–821.
11. Wagner WH, Cossman DV, Treiman RL, et al. Hemosuccus pancreaticus from intraductal rupture of a primary splenic artery aneurysm. *J Vasc Surg.* 1994;19:158–164.
12. Lindberg CG, Stridbeck H. Aneurysms of the superior mesenteric artery and its branches. *Gastrointest Radiol.* 1992;17:132–134.
13. Graham LM, Hay MR, Cho KJ, et al. Inferior mesenteric artery aneurysms. *Surgery.* 1985;97(2):158–162.
14. Brunet WG, Greenberg HM. CT demonstration of a ruptured splenic artery aneurysm. *J Comput Assist Tomogr.* 1991;15(1):177–178.
15. Warshauer DM, Keefe B, Mauro MA. Intrahepatic hepatic artery aneurysm: computed tomography and color-flow Doppler ultrasound findings. *Gastrointest Radiol.* 1991;16:175–177.
16. Bret PM, Bretagnolle M, Enoch G, et al. Ultrasonic features of aneurysms of splanchnic arteries. *Assoc Radiol J.* 1985;36:226–229.
17. Hashizume M, Ohta M, Ueno K, et al. Laparoscopic ligation of splenic artery aneurysms. *Surgery.* 1993;113(3):352–354.
18. Saw EK, Ku W, Ramachandra S. Laparoscopic resection of a splenic artery aneurysm. *J Laparoendosc Surg.* 1993;3(2):167–171.
19. Salo JA, Aarnio PT, Jarvinen AA, et al. Aneurysms of the hepatic arteries. *Am Surg.* 1989;55(12):705–709.
20. Blue JM, Burney DP. Current trends in the diagnosis and treatment of hepatic artery aneurysms. *South Med J.* 1990;83(8):966–969.
21. Reidy JF, Rowe PN, Ellis FG. Technical report: splenic artery aneurysm embolization—the preferred technique to surgery. *Clin Radiol.* 1990;41(4):281–282.
22. Tarazov PG, Polysalov VN, Ryzhkov VK. Transcatheter treatment of splenic artery aneurysms: report of two cases. *J Cardiovasc Surg (Torino).* 1991;32:128–131.
23. Ku A, Kadir S. Embolization of a mesenteric artery aneurysm: case report. *Cardiovasc Intervent Radiol.* 1990;13:91–92.
24. Baker KS, Tisnado J, Cho SR, et al. Splanchnic artery aneurysms and pseudoaneurysms: transcatheter embolization. *Radiology.* 1987;163:135–139.
25. Nosher JL, Trooskin SZ, Amorosa JK. Occlusion of a hepatic arterial aneurysm with Gianturco coils in a patient with the Ehlers-Danlos syndrome. *Am J Surg.* 1986;152:326–328.

37

Mesenteric Venous Thrombosis

Peter Gloviczki, MD, Robert Y. Rhee, MD,
Linda G. Canton, RN, BSN, and
C. Michael Johnson, MD

Mesenteric venous thrombosis is a rare but lethal disease. First reported by Elliot[1] in 1895, this form of acute intestinal ischemia was described in detail in 1935 by Warren and Eberhard.[2] These authors reported a 34% mortality rate following intestinal resection for venous thrombosis. Because of the insidious presentation with nonspecific signs and symptoms, delay in diagnosis of acute mesenteric venous thrombosis is still frequent, and mortality remains substantial. Progress has been made, however, in recognizing the most important risk factors of this disease, by identifying and treating rare, previously unknown abnormalities of coagulation, and by the increased awareness of this lethal condition. The more frequent use of abdominal imaging modalities, such as ultrasonography, computed tomography (CT), and magnetic resonance imaging (MRI), helped to improve detection of mesenteric venous thrombi. It also helped us to recognize a separate, small group of patients with a more benign, chronic form of mesenteric venous thrombosis.

INCIDENCE

Mesenteric venous thrombosis is an infrequent form of intestinal ischemia. A review of the literature until 1984 revealed only 372 published cases. Ottinger and Austen[3] found that mesenteric venous thrombosis comprised only 0.006% of hospital admissions and less than 2% of autopsy cases. Kazmers[4] estimated that intestinal infarction due to mesenteric venous thrombosis is encountered in fewer than 1 in 1,000 laparotomies for acute abdominal disease. Rhee et al[5] found that only 72 (6.2%) of 1,167 patients treated for mesenteric ischemia at the Mayo Clinic had mesenteric venous thrombosis.

ETIOLOGY

Patients with no known cause of the disease are classified as having spontaneous, idiopathic, or *primary* mesenteric venous thrombosis. The number of patients in this group has decreased substantially since the 1980s because of improvement in diagnosis and recognition of previously unknown, natural, circulating anticoagulants. The number of patients with *secondary* venous thrombosis is, therefore, increasing. Of the hematologic disorders, protein C and S deficiency, antithrombin III deficiency, dysfibrinogenemia, abnormal plasminogen, polycythemia vera, thrombocytosis, and sickle-cell disease are diagnosed in patients with mesenteric venous thrombosis. Tumor, portal hypertension, and previous abdominal surgery are also frequent causes of mechanical venous occlusion. Localized mesenteric venous thrombosis caused by volvulus, intussusception, or strangulation of the bowel is not discussed in this chapter since other factors, primarily mechanical bowel obstruction and arterial occlusion, are the important clinical features.

Penetrating or blunt abdominal trauma, iatrogenic injury to the mesenteric vessels, and endoscopic sclerotherapy may also lead to mesenteric venous thrombosis. Abdominal infections, pancreatitis, and congestive heart failure are additional causes described in the literature.[4] In our material, previous abdominal surgical procedures, hematologic abnormalities, and previous mesenteric venous thrombosis were the most frequent etiologic factors identified (Table 37–1).

CLINICAL CLASSIFICATION

Patients with symptoms of less than 4 weeks' duration are classified as having *acute mesenteric venous thrombosis.* Patients with symptoms beyond 4 weeks but without evidence of bowel infarction, or asymptomatic patients in whom mesenteric venous thrombosis is discovered during evaluation of other abdominal pathology, are classified as having *chronic mesenteric venous thrombosis.* Patients with symptoms of portal hypertension, such as gastrointestinal bleeding, and with documented mesenteric venous thrombosis also belong to this chronic group. Boley et al[6] distinguished a subgroup of patients with chronic disease: The term *subacute mesenteric venous thrombosis* can be used for these patients, who have symptoms of abdominal pain of only several weeks' or months' duration.

ACUTE MESENTERIC VENOUS THROMBOSIS

Clinical Presentation

The patient with acute mesenteric venous thrombosis may present with typical signs and symptoms of acute bowel ischemia, characterized by pain out of proportion to physical findings, nausea, vomiting, and constipation, with or without bloody diarrhea. Such an acute presentation, however, is rare. Much more frequent is a diffuse, increasing, sometimes intermittent abdominal pain of several days' or even weeks' duration. In the Mayo Clinic material,[5] which included 30 males and 23 females with acute mesenteric venous thrombosis and a mean age of 56.6 years (range, 23–81 years), only 4 (8%) presented with symptoms of less than 24 hours' duration. However, 75% of the patients had symptoms for more than 48 hours at diagnosis of the disease. Abdominal pain was the most frequent symptom, and it was documented in 83% of the cases. Fifty-three percent of the patients had anorexia and 43% had diarrhea (Table 37–2). Only one-fourth of the patients had evidence of lower gastrointestinal bleeding and only 13% had constipation. The abdominal pain was diffuse and nonspecific in 57%

TABLE 37–1. CONDITIONS ASSOCIATED WITH MESENTERIC VENOUS THROMBOSIS IN 72 PATIENTS TREATED AT THE MAYO CLINIC BETWEEN 1972 AND 1993

Condition	No. of Patients (%)
Previous abdominal surgical procedure	37 (51)
Hypercoagulable state	30 (42)
Previous mesenteric venous thrombosis	25 (35)
Smoker	23 (32)
Previous deep venous thrombosis	20 (28)
Alcohol abuse	15 (21)
Malignant tumor	13 (18)
Cirrhosis	13 (18)
Oral contraceptive use	4 (6)

of the patients. If it was localized, it occurred in the right lower quadrant in three of four patients.

Abdominal distension was the most frequent sign, and it occurred in half the patients (Table 37–3). Peritonitis was present in 36% of the patients, and 21% had tachycardia. Leukocytosis was found in 51%, but the lactates were above 1.65 mmol/L in only 28% of the patients.

Diagnostic Tests

Plain abdominal films show a pattern of ileus in only two-thirds of the cases. Marked abdominal wall thickening is seen most frequently. Air in the portal system or in the abdominal cavity is a rare finding of advanced disease.

If mesenteric venous thrombosis is suspected but peritonitis is absent, CT is our first test of choice. Twenty of our patients were studied with CT, and thrombus in the superior mesenteric vein was demonstrated in 11 (55%) (Fig. 37–1). Portal venous thrombosis and splenic venous thrombosis were documented equally, each in 35% of the patients. Other findings of bowel ischemia included a thickened bowel wall, pneumatosis, and streaky mesentery (Fig. 37–2). Computed tomography was 100% sensitive to show abdominal findings suggesting mesenteric venous thrombosis or ischemic bowel. Similar good diagnostic accuracy was reported by other investigators as well. Vogelzang et al[7] correctly diagnosed meseneric venous thrombosis in 14 patients studied, and Harward et al[8] diagnosed mesenteric venous thrombosis in 9 of 10 patients imaged with CT.

TABLE 37–2. SYMPTOMS OF ACUTE MESENTERIC VENOUS THROMBOSIS IN 53 PATIENTS TREATED AT THE MAYO CLINIC BETWEEN 1972 AND 1993

Symptom	No. of Patients (%)
Abdominal pain	44 (83)
Anorexia	28 (53)
Diarrhea	23 (43)
Nausea and vomiting	22 (42)
Upper gastrointestinal bleeding	15 (28)
Lower gastrointestinal bleeding	12 (23)
Constipation	7 (13)

TABLE 37–3. SIGNS OF ACUTE MESENTERIC VENOUS THROMBOSIS IN 53 PATIENTS TREATED AT THE MAYO CLINIC BETWEEN 1972 AND 1993

Signs	No. of Patients (%)
Abdominal distension	27 (51)
Blood on rectal examination	17 (32)
Peritonitis	19 (36)
Ascites	5 (9)
Hypotension (<90 mm Hg)	3 (6)
Tachycardia (>110 beats/min)	11 (21)
Fever (>38°C)	13 (24)
Leukocytosis (10×10^9L)	27 (51)
Lactate (>1.65 mmol/L)	15 (28)
Amylase (>115 U/L)	10 (19)
Creatinine kinase (>350 U/L)	4 (8)

If CT is nondiagnostic or equivocal, or if mesenteric arterial occlusion cannot be excluded, mesenteric arteriography with venous phase has to be performed. We studied seven patients and identified thrombus or nonfilling of the mesenteric vein in five (71%).

Abdominal ultrasonography was also sensitive in our experience. It confirmed thrombus in the superior mesenteric vein in 8 (80%) of 10 patients studied. Miller and

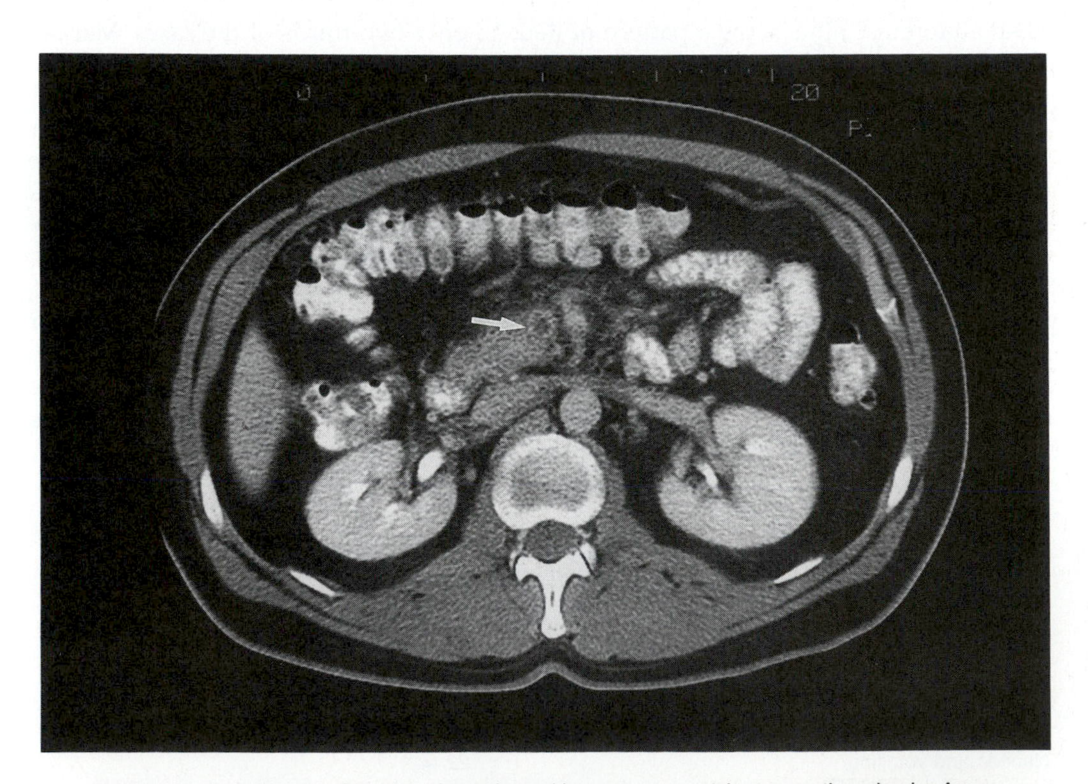

Figure 37–1. Abdominal CT scan of a patient with acute mesenteric venous thrombosis. *Arrow* shows the thrombus in the superior mesenteric vein. *(From Rhee RY, Gloviczki P, Mendonca CT, et al. Mesenteric venous thrombosis: still a lethal disease in the 1990s. J Vasc Surg. 1994;20:688–697.)*

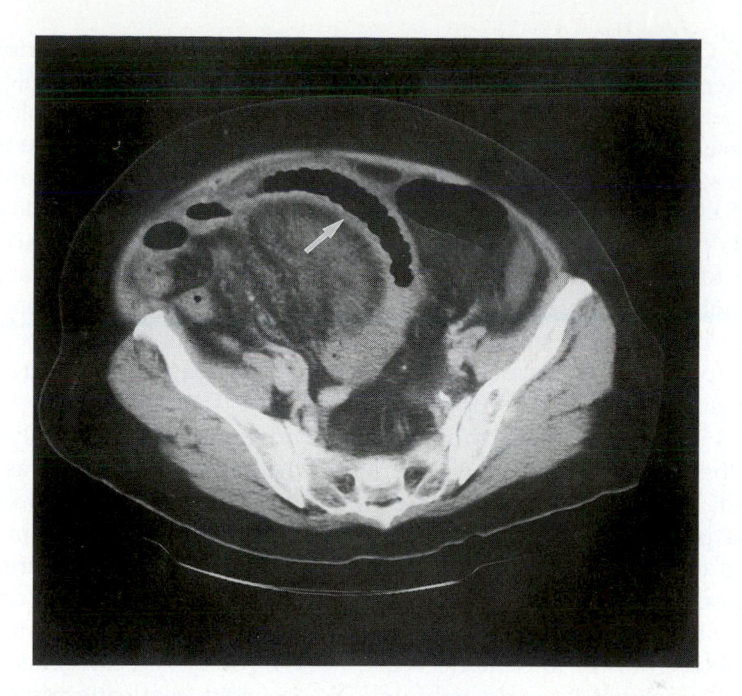

Figure 37–2. Abdominal CT scan of a patient with acute mesenteric venous thrombosis. The small bowel is distended, its walls are thickened, and the mesentery shows streaking and edema. *Arrow* shows the thickened bowel wall. *(From Rhee RY, Gloviczki P, Mendonca CT, et al. Mesenteric venous thrombosis: still a lethal disease in the 1990s. J Vasc Surg. 1994;20:688–697.)*

Berland[9] found that abdominal duplex scanning was as useful as CT for diagnosing mesenteric venous thrombosis.

Magnetic resonance imaging is being used with increasing frequency to diagnose abdominal pathology. Using MRI, Gehl et al[10] identified an abdominal venous obstruction in each of 15 patients. They found the results of MRI similar to those obtained with CT.

Despite advancement in imaging techniques, mesenteric venous thrombosis is still frequently diagnosed only at the time of operation.[5] In our material, in 16 (30%) of 53 patients the diagnosis of acute mesenteric venous thrombosis was established only at the time of operation. The median delay in diagnosis was 48 hours (mean, 83 ± 17 hours). The delay in diagnosis did not change significantly during the two decades of our study.

Treatment

Patients with acute mesenteric venous thrombosis need rapid fluid resuscitation to increase the intravascular volume. Broad-spectrum antibiotics are started immediately, with coverage of anaerobes as well, in every patient with signs of peritonitis. Once the diagnosis is established, heparin anticoagulation is instituted.

Surgical Management

Abdominal exploration is necessary in every patient who has signs of peritonitis. In our review of 53 patients with acute mesenteric venous thrombosis, 34 (64%) underwent abdominal exploration.[5] Intraoperative assessment of the bowel and mesentery is important since venous thrombus may not extend into the proximal superior mesenteric vein. The arterial supply is almost always intact, with pulsatile flow palpable in the superior mesenteric artery. Edema of the mesentery and cyanotic discoloration of the involved bowel are characteristic of mesenteric venous thrombosis. Once the diagnosis of mesenteric venous thrombosis is confirmed, and if the patient was not anticoagulated previously, 5,000 units of heparin are given and a heparin infusion is started at a rate of 1,000 units per hour, with continuous monitoring of the activated partial thromboplastin time to keep it above 80 seconds. This is the only type of acute mesenteric ischemia for which we fully heparinize the patient intraoperatively and maintain continuous heparin perfusion, even in the early perioperative period. Although the risk of bleeding complications is increased, perioperative anticoagulation decreases the risk of rethrombosis and improves survival.

Intestinal infarction caused by mesenteric venous thrombosis usually involves the jejunum or the distal ileum. In our experience, the ascending colon was involved in only 13.5% of the cases, and the duodenum in 8.1% (Fig. 37–3). Transmural bowel necrosis was present in 85% of our patients, with bowel perforation in 21%. Bowel resection had to be performed in 30 patients (88%) during the first operation.

Single case reports have been published of successful thrombectomy of the superior mesenteric vein by using a Fogarty balloon catheter together with manual expression of the thrombus from the mesenteric veins.[4,11,12] We performed thrombectomy in only one patient. Unfortunately, early rethrombosis occurred, requiring resection of additional bowel during a "second-look" procedure. Although an occasional patient with early thrombosis could be treated with thrombectomy, most patients present with diffuse venous thrombosis, frequently following previous thrombotic episodes, with distal extension of thrombus into the mesentery. These patients have a poor chance of successful treatment with venous thrombectomy.

A second-look operation should be decided, as in the instance of a patient with acute mesenteric arterial occlusion, at the time of the first operation. Indeed, during 14 second-look operations that we performed, additional bowel was resected in all.

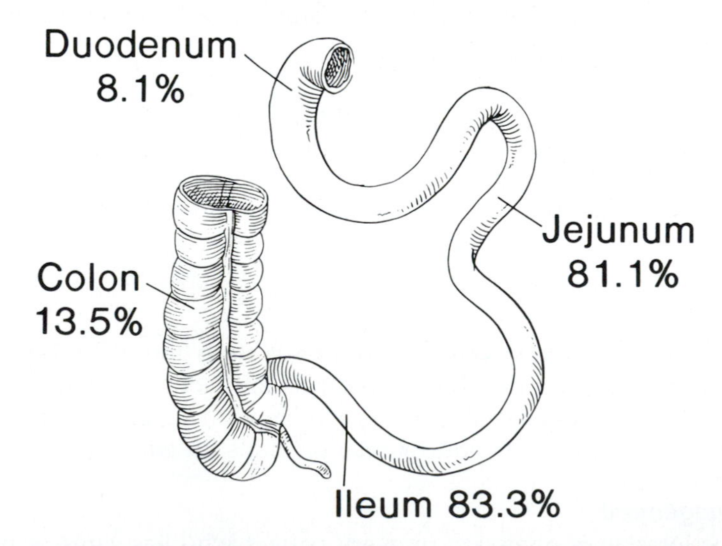

Figure 37–3. Intraoperative findings of the distribution of infarcted bowel secondary to acute mesenteric venous thrombosis. *(From Rhee RY, Gloviczki P, Mendonca CT, et al. Mesenteric venous thrombosis: still a lethal disease in the 1990s. J Vasc Surg. 1994;20:688–697.)*

Nonoperative management

Patients without peritonitis who have documented acute mesenteric venous thrombosis can be observed and managed nonoperatively with fluid resuscitation and heparin anticoagulation. The use of fibrinolytic treatment involving urokinase, streptokinase, or tissue-type plasminogen activator[13,14] is controversial at present. The increased risk of hemorrhagic complications from an infarcted bowel makes these types of treatment less attractive. Most patients need long-term anticoagulation with Coumadin, unless bleeding complications due to portal venous hypertension clearly contraindicate its use.

Clinical Outcome

Most patients who present with peritonitis and have infarcted bowel requiring resection have multiple complications and prolonged hospitalization. The mean hospital stay for patients with acute venous thrombosis, in our experience, was beyond 22 days, ranging from 1 to 98 days. Complications occurred in 55% of our patients; the most frequent complications were short-bowel syndrome, wound infection, and sepsis (Table 37–4). Five patients suffered pulmonary embolism, but in our retrospective study we noted that only one of the five was anticoagulated at the time of the event.

The 30-day mortality continues to be significant. For our patients, it was 27%. Although there was a decrease from 32% in the first decade of the study to 24% in the last decade, this difference was statistically insignificant. Early mortality in other published series was similar, ranging from 13% to 50%.[15–21] The use of anticoagulation significantly increased early survival in our study (Fig. 37–4).

Late survival of patients with acute mesenteric venous thrombosis is poor; in our patients, it was 36% at 3 years (Fig. 37–5). The cause of death in 38% of these patients was the mesenteric venous thrombosis.

Current Management

Figure 37–6 depicts the management algorithm that we follow for patients who are suspected of having acute mesenteric venous thrombosis. Patients with localized or diffuse peritonitis require abdominal exploration. Preparation for surgery includes fluid resuscitation and broad-spectrum antibiotics. Once the diagnosis of acute mesenteric venous thrombosis is confirmed, the patient is heparinized. During operation, we perform bowel resection if necessary and evaluate the possibility of venous thrombectomy. We inject two ampullae of fluorescein intravenously and observe the bowel under Wood's lamp to confirm adequate perfusion. If any question exists about the viability of the remaining bowel, a second-look laparotomy is decided at the time of

TABLE 37–4. COMPLICATIONS IN 53 PATIENTS WITH ACUTE MESENTERIC VENOUS THROMBOSIS

Complication	No. of Patients (%)
Short-bowel syndrome	12 (23)
Wound infection	11 (21)
Sepsis	9 (17)
Pneumonia	7 (13)
Pulmonary embolus	5 (9)
Renal failure	5 (9)
Gastrointestinal bleeding	3 (6)

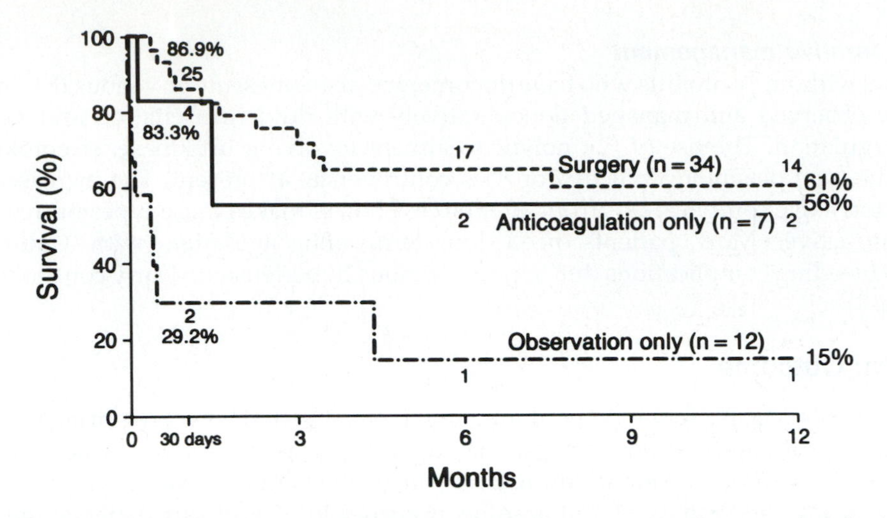

Figure 37–4. Short-term (Kaplan-Meier) survival curves of acute mesenteric venous thrombosis treated with surgery and anticoagulation, anticoagulation alone, and observation. *(From Rhee RY, Gloviczki P, Mendonca CT, et al. Mesenteric venous thrombosis: still a lethal disease in the 1990s. J Vasc Surg. 1994;20:688–697.)*

the operation. Postoperatively, the patients are anticoagulated with heparin and if no surgical exploration is planned and the patient's overall condition improves, we switch to Coumadin. For patients who do not present with peritonitis, the diagnosis is confirmed by CT or angiography. If the patients do not have evidence of peritonitis during the hospitalization, anticoagulation with heparin and then with Coumadin is done with close observation.

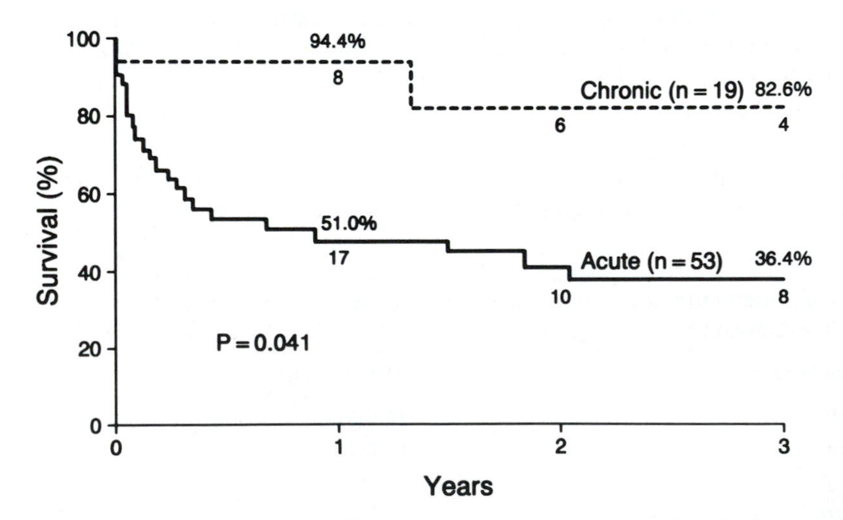

Figure 37–5. Long-term (Kaplan-Meier) survival curves of patients with acute and chronic mesenteric venous thrombosis. *(From Rhee RY, Gloviczki P, Mendonca CT, et al. Mesenteric venous thrombosis: still a lethal disease in the 1990s. J Vasc Surg. 1994;20:688–697.)*

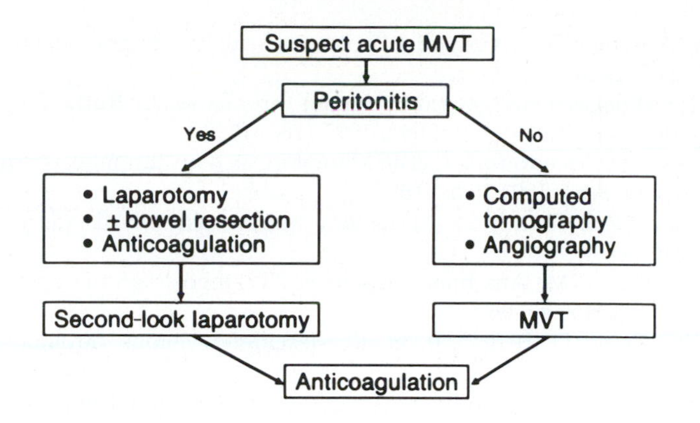

Figure 37–6. Management algorithm for acute mesenteric venous thrombosis (MVT). *(From Rhee RY, Gloviczki P, Mendonca CT, et al. Mesenteric venous thrombosis: still a lethal disease in the 1990s. J Vasc Surg. 1994;20:688–697.)*

CHRONIC MESENTERIC VENOUS THROMBOSIS

Most patients with chronic mesenteric venous thrombosis are asymptomatic or have only vague abdominal pain or distension. A mild leukocytosis was present in 8 (42%) of our 19 patients who were diagnosed as having chronic mesenteric venous thrombosis.[5]

Thrombosis in the mesenteric veins is frequently discovered accidentally during evaluation of other abdominal pathology, such as chronic pancreatitis, portal hypertension, or abdominal malignancy. Computed tomography has a 93% sensitivity to diagnose chronic mesenteric venous thrombosis.[5] Ultrasonography may confirm partially recanalized superior mesenteric vein with low or absent venous flow. Collateral venous circulation is usually adequate in these patients and bowel infarction does not occur. The prognosis is determined by the underlying abdominal disease, and late survival appears to be better than for patients who present with acute mesenteric venous thrombosis (Fig. 37–5).

CONCLUSION

Acute mesenteric venous thrombosis continues to be a lethal disease, with a 30-day mortality of 27% in our experience. Although CT is now easily available as a sensitive diagnostic test, delay in establishing the diagnosis is still frequent. Patient with documented or suspected mesenteric venous thrombosis who have peritonitis should undergo early exploration and resection of the infarcted bowel. Immediate anticoagulation provides the best prognosis. The recurrence rate of acute venous thrombosis is high. Survival of patients with chronic mesenteric venous thrombosis is determined by the underlying disease.

REFERENCES

1. Elliot JW. The operative relief of gangrene of intestine due to occlusion of the mesenteric vessels. *Ann Surg.* 1895;21:9–23.
2. Warren S, Eberhard TP. Messenteric venous thrombosis. *Surg Gynecol Obstet.* 1935;61:102–121.

3. Ottinger LW, Austen WG. A study of 136 patients with mesenteric infarction. *Surg Gynecol Obstet.* 1967;124:251–261.
4. Kazmers A. Intestinal ischemia caused by venous thrombosis. In: Rutherford RB, ed. *Vascular Surgery.* Philadelphia, PA: WB Saunders; 1995:1288–1300.
5. Rhee RY, Gloviczki P, Mendonca CT, et al. Mesenteric venous thrombosis: still a lethal disease in the 1990s. *J Vasc Surg.* 1994;20:688–697.
6. Boley SJ, Kaleya RN, Brandt LJ. Mesenteric venous thrombosis. *Surg Clin North Am.* 1992;72:183–201.
7. Vogelzang RL, Gore RM, Anschnetz SL, et al. Thrombosis of the splanchnic veins: CT diagnoses. *AJR.* 1988;150:93–96.
8. Harward TRS, Green D, Bergan JJ, et al. Mesenteric venous thrombosis. *J Vasc Surg.* 1989;9:328–333.
9. Miller VE, Berland LL. Pulsed Doppler duplex sonography and CT of portal vein thrombosis *AJR.* 1985;145:73–76.
10. Gehl HB, Bohndorf K, Klose KC, et al. Two-dimensional MR angiography in the evaluation of abdominal vein with gradients refocused sequences. *J Comput Assist Tomogr.* 1990;14:619–624.
11. Inahara T. Acute superior mesenteric venous thrombosis: treatment by thrombectomy. *Ann Surg.* 1971;174:956–961.
12. Bergentz SE, Ericsson B, Hedner U, et al. Thrombosis in the superior mesenteric and portal veins: report of a case treated with thrombectomy. *Surgery.* 1974;76:286–290.
13. Bilbao JI, Rodriguez-Cabello J, Longo J, et al. Portal thrombosis: percutaneous transhepatic treatment with urokinase—a case report. *Gastrointest Radiol.* 1989;14:326–328.
14. Robin P, Gurel Y, Lang M, et al. Complete thrombolysis of mesenteric vein occlusion with recombinant tissue-type plasminogen activator. *Lancet.* 1988;1(2):1391.
15. Sack J, Aldrete JS. Primary mesenteric venous thrombosis. *Surg Gynecol Obstet.* 1982;154:205–208.
16. Wilson C, Walker ID, Davidson JF, et al. Mesenteric venous thrombosis and antithrombin III deficiency. *J Clin Pathol.* 1987;40:906–908.
17. Clavien PA, Harder F. Mesenteric venous thrombosis. *Helv Chir Acta.* 1988;55:29–34.
18. Kaleya RN, Boley SJ. Mesenteric venous thrombosis. In: Najarian JS, Delaney JP, eds. *Progress in Gastrointestinal Surgery.* Chicago, IL: Year Book Medical Publishers; 1989:417–425.
19. Harward TRS, Green D, Bergan JJ, et al. Mesenteric venous thrombosis. *J Vasc Surg.* 1989;9:328–333.
20. Levy PJ, Krausz MM, Manny J. The role of second-look procedure in improving survival time for patients with mesenteric venous thrombosis. *Surg Gynecol Obstet.* 1990;170:287–291.
21. Grieshop RJ, Dalsing MC, Cikrit DF, et al. Acute mesenteric venous thrombosis: revisited in a time of diagnostic clarity. *Am Surg.* 1991;57:573–578.

38

Acute Mesenteric Ischemia

Bruce L. Gewertz, MD

Acute mesenteric ischemia usually occurs in patients greater than 70 years of age who suffer from other systemic illnesses, especially gastrointestinal, peripheral vascular, and coronary artery disease. These concomitant factors may color the presentation of the problem and contribute to the frequent delays in diagnosis; such serious comorbidity also decreases the likelihood of successful treatment. In fact, despite increased understanding of the pathophysiology of these syndromes and unquestioned improvements in critical care, the mortality of patients with acute intestinal ischemia remains high.

This chapter reviews the clinical presentations of acute intestinal ischemia, contrasting the differing causes (arterial occlusions, nonocclusive syndromes, and venous thrombosis). The discussion addresses currently accepted therapies as well as special issues that arise during treatment of these syndromes, such as (1) the mechanism of intestinal reperfusion injury; (2) methods to assess bowel viability intraoperatively; and (3) the possible use of fibrinolytic therapy for acute arterial thrombosis.

CLINICAL PRESENTATION

Multiple risk factors identified for acute mesenteric ischemia include valvular heart disease, congestive heart failure, cardiac arrhythmias, dehydration, and recent myocardial infarction.[1–4] Other less common contributing factors include all types of hypercoagulable states (polycythemia rubra vera, myeloid metaplasia, and deficiencies of antithrombin III, protein C, and protein S), collagen vascular diseases (especially lupus erythematosus and scleroderma), and drug abuse (amphetamines and cocaine).[5,6] As noted previously, numerous clinical series have cited peak incidences for acute ischemic syndromes in the seventh and eighth decades of life.[1]

The classic presentation of acute mesenteric ischemia, irrespective of the specific mechanism, is *abdominal pain out of proportion to physical findings.* The pain is usually steady, severe, and midabdominal. If peritoneal signs are elicited, it is likely that intestinal infarction already occurred. Bowel sounds are quiet and variable. Early in the course, ischemic segments with reduced or absent peristalsis may cause functional bowel obstruction, accompanied by high-pitched bowel sounds and evacuation of intraluminal gas distal to the ischemic segment. As ischemia persists or extends, all myoenteric activity ceases and the abdomen is silent to auscultation. Rectal examination rarely yields stool positive for blood early in the disease, although the likelihood of this specific finding is increased by involvement of the right and transverse colon.

The clinician's single greatest tool for the successful diagnosis of an acute mesenteric vascular event is a high index of suspicion about a patient with multiple risk factors. Although many laboratory abnormalities occur with mesenteric ischemia and infarction, most are nonspecific and thus nondiagnostic. These include hemoconcentration, leukocytosis with a significant "left shift," metabolic acidosis, hyperamylasemia, and hyperphosphatemia.[7–9] The search for a specific indicator of intestinal ischemia is further confounded by the fact that most elevations in serum levels occur too late in the process, when infarction has already progressed. More recently, laboratory and clinical investigations have suggested that D(-)-lactate, a by-product of bacterial metabolism, may cross the mucosal barrier early in ischemia and thereby provide an early and relatively specific marker.[10,11] At the current time, this hypothesis has been tested in only a small series of 31 patients with varying intra-abdominal pathology and cannot be considered definitive.

Abdominal roentgenograms are used primarily to exclude other causes of abdominal pain such as urolithiasis, mechanical small-bowel obstruction, perforation of a hollow viscus, or appendicitis with fecalith. As many as 70% of all patients with mesenteric ischemia show at least one of the following nonspecific signs on abdominal films: ileus, ascites, small-bowel dilation, thickening of valvulae conniventes, and separation of small-bowel loops.[1] On occasion, a "gasless" abdomen is seen due to excessive fluid accumulation within the lumen.

Barium studies are contraindicated, but, if performed, they may show evidence of small-bowel dilation and focal mucosal hemorrhage ("thumbprinting") in the right and transverse colon. The considerable disadvantage of intraluminal contrast studies is the potential for interference with arteriography, which is the essential diagnostic study for the syndromes precipitated by arterial insufficiency. In fact, all diagnostic tests except arteriography are flawed by a lack of specificity and reliability.

Successful arteriography requires prior hemodynamic stabilization of the patient, since hypotension alone may cause considerable splanchnic vasoconstriction and preclude an adequate study. Infusion of any vasoactive drug with splanchnic vasoconstrictive properties should be terminated. Both anteroposterior (AP) and lateral views of the aorta are required. The AP view best demonstrates collateral vessels, while lateral aortography better visualizes the origins of major visceral arteries that overlie the aorta in the AP plane.

As noted by Boley and others,[1,7] the mortality from a mesenteric event is directly related to the state of the bowel at the time of diagnosis. The occurrence of bowel infarction greatly increases mortality and morbidity; in some series, infarction is associated with greater than 80% mortality. This fact underscores the importance not only of early diagnosis and treatment of acute ischemia, but also of expeditious arterial reconstructions in patients with chronic ischemic syndromes before acute ischemia supervenes.

ARTERIAL OCCLUSIVE SYNDROMES

Etiology

Arterial embolism accounts for about one-third of all mesenteric vascular catastrophes. Most emboli occur in association with cardiac arrhythmias (especially atrial tachyarrhythmias) or myocardial infarctions.[7] The superior mesenteric artery (SMA) is the site of most embolic occlusions due to its high basal blood flow and near parallel course to the abdominal aorta. As many as 5% of all peripheral emboli lodge in this vessel. The presentation of embolic mesenteric occlusion may be complicated by associated visceral, extremity, or cerebral emboli.

Acute thrombosis of an already compromised vessel lumen occurs in another one-third of the cases.[3] *In situ* thrombosis typically occurs at the origin of the SMA and leads to gut infarction from the proximal jejunum to the midtransverse colon. In most of these cases, patients have previous manifestations of advanced atherosclerosis, including chronic occlusions of the celiac, inferior mesenteric, and internal iliac arteries. Such preexisting lesions are often associated with prodromal symptoms. In fact, more than 50% of all patients who die due to acute SMA thrombosis have a history of postprandial abdominal pain and weight loss consistent with *chronic intestinal ischemia.*

"Intestinal angina" typically occurs 15 to 60 minutes after meals and is more closely correlated with the volume of food consumed rather than any specific type of food. The presentation of chronic ischemia depends on the region of the gut affected. The most common syndromes involve the midgut (jejunum, ileum, and right colon) and reflect vascular insufficiency of the SMA distribution. Ischemia of the foregut (stomach and liver) is much less common and may be irregular in its symptomatology. Patients frequently complain of nonspecific symptoms such as bloating and early satiety; "food fear" and weight loss are often absent.

Diagnosis

Arteriographic signs can generally differentiate embolic occlusions from thrombotic occlusions.[8] Emboli to the SMA usually lodge just proximal or distal to the origin of the middle colic artery and demonstrate the classic meniscus of the long-standing cardiac mural thrombus (Fig. 38–1). The origin of the vessel is usually free of atherosclerotic disease. In contrast, thrombotic occlusions of preexistent proximal SMA lesions are irregular defects usually associated with generalized atherosclerosis of the aorta and extensive collaterals between the celiac and/or superior mesenteric arterial distributions (Fig. 38–2).

Although selective views of the SMA and celiac axis are often necessary for diagnosis, it is also important to visualize the supraceliac aorta, renal arteries, and aortic bifurcation. Multiple emboli occur in a relatively large percentage of patients (15% to 30%), and in instances of thrombotic occlusion the status of the aorta is useful in planning a needed bypass procedure.

If immediately available, deep abdominal imaging with duplex ultrasound can also be considered as an initial diagnostic test. Accuracy is best in relatively thin patients without excessive intraluminal gas. Although such noninvasive imaging techniques can confirm visceral artery occlusion and avoid many of the complications of arteriography, the amount of clinically important information is limited. In particular, it is virtually impossible to distinguish between *in situ* thrombosis and embolization.

Since approximately 85% of all clinically important emboli originate in the heart, it is important to evaluate the patient for arrhythmias (especially atrial flutter or fibrillation) and areas of left ventricular dyskinesia. The added advantage of such investigations is obvious; cardiac morbidity is always a concern in the perioperative period. For more definitive data regarding the origin of emboli, precordial or transesophageal echocardiography can define any residual thrombus in the heart. Of the two studies, transesophageal echocardiography is generally accepted to be more accurate and sensitive. Such tests should be performed prior to patient discharge, but they are unnecessary prior to revascularization and should never delay appropriate therapy. In addition,

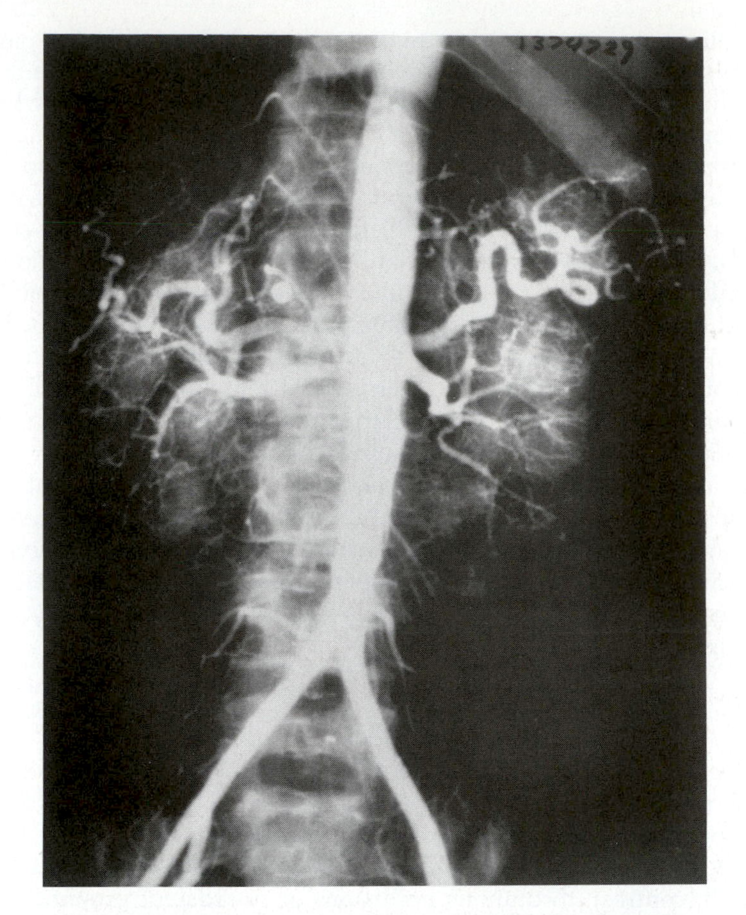

Figure 38–1. Oblique view of the aorta reveals embolic occlusion of the SMA. Note the absence of significant occlusive disease at the origin of the vessel and the abrupt "cutoff" with the meniscus sign.

echocardiography is frequently nondiagnostic (about 40% of the time), even when the nature of the retrieved material is undoubtedly of cardiac origin and all other sources have been excluded. This may reflect complete embolization of all thrombus or the difficulty of adequately imaging the cardiac chambers.

Treatment

All patients with suspected embolic or thrombotic occlusions should undergo urgent laparotomy.[12] Fluid resuscitation and administration of both heparin and antibiotics are indicated prior to surgery. The abdomen is entered through a midline incision, and the bowel inspected. The SMA is identified and exposed just distal to the origin of the middle colic artery by means of an incision in the underside of the small-bowel mesentery (Fig. 38–3). Often, an embolus can be directly extracted from a transverse arteriotomy. If adequate inflow is obtained following the passage of an embolectomy catheter, no additional arterial reconstruction may be required. If complete extraction of the embolic material is not possible, some form of aortomesenteric bypass should be considered.

If thrombosis of an atherosclerotic lesion is evident, it is necessary to ensure adequate inflow through endarterectomy or bypass.[13] Failure to do so frequently results in early rethrombosis. Endarterectomy requires satisfactory exposure of the suprarenal

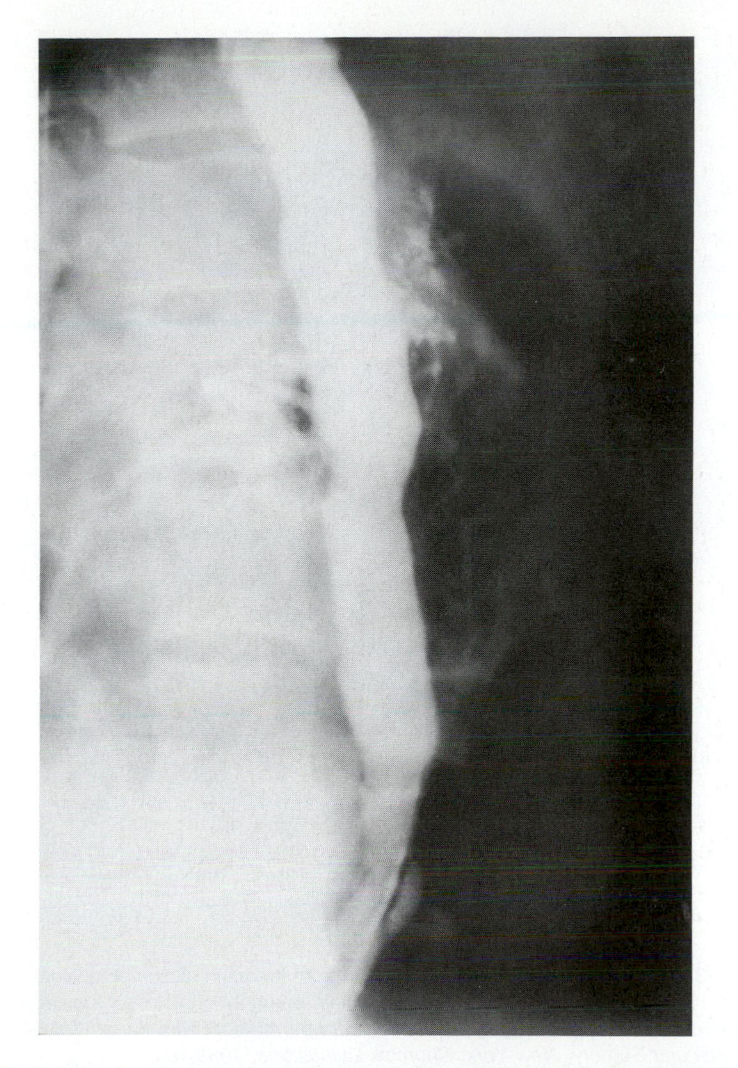

Figure 38–2. Lateral aortogram of a patient presenting with acute intestinal ischemia reveals the absence of all major mesenteric vessels, with occlusions of both the celiac and superior mesenteric arteries.

aorta, usually through medial visceral rotation. This allows total or partial aortic occlusion and facilitates complete removal of the atherosclerotic plaque at the SMA origin. As in all endarterectomies, the distal end point should be visualized and tacked if appropriate.

If bypass is required, the graft can originate in the infrarenal aorta (retrograde bypass) or the supraceliac aorta (antegrade bypass). The latter approach is used most frequently in our practice (Fig. 38–4).) Access to the less diseased supraceliac aorta is not difficult following lateral retraction of the esophagus and division of the diaphragmatic crus. Most important, the path of the antegrade graft, parallel to the anatomic course of the SMA, avoids the kinking and angulation often seen when grafts originate from the distal aorta (Fig. 38–5). Although prosthetic grafts are the preferred conduit in this setting, autologous saphenous vein should be considered if bowel resection is necessary. When considering the two revascularization options, the surgeon should remember that decisions must be individualized and that the most expeditious approach is usually the best in critically ill patients.

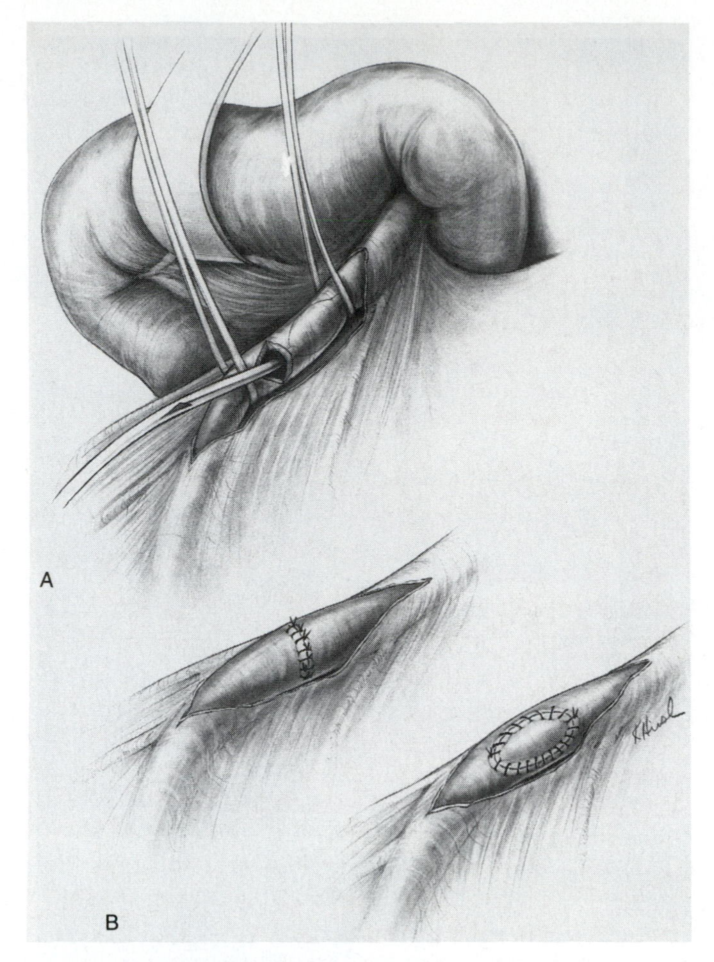

Figure 38–3. (**A**) Exposure of the SMA 5 to 8 cm from its origin allows embolectomy through a transverse incision. (**B**) Arteriotomies can be closed primarily with closely spaced interrupted sutures or with patch angioplasty. *(Reproduced with permission from Zarins CK, Gewertz BL. Atlas of Vascular Surgery. New York: Churchill Livingstone; 1989:105.)*

After revascularization, the intestine is carefully inspected. The proper management of transmural infarcted bowel is resection and, if possible, primary reanastomosis. The most difficult decisions involve determinations of the extent of the resection. A balance must be reached between removing too much intestine, thereby compromising absorptive capacity, and performing an anastomosis to a nonviable intestinal segment. The critical intraoperative assessment of marginally viable intestine is discussed later in this chapter.

NONOCCLUSIVE ARTERIAL INSUFFICIENCY

Etiology

Nonocclusive mesenteric ischemia, which comprises most of the remaining cases of clinically important mesenteric ischemia, affects the SMA distribution almost exclusively. The mechanism is multifactorial but usually involves moderate-to-severe mesenteric

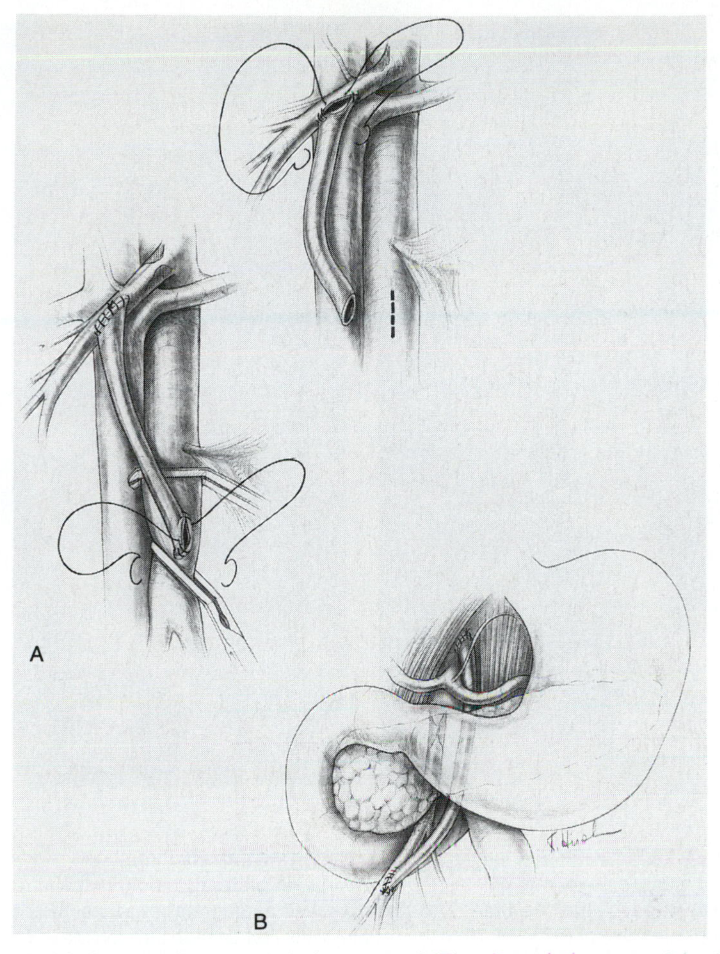

Figure 38–4. (**A**) Retrograde mesenteric bypass and (**B**) antegrade bypass originating in the supraceliac aorta. When performing a retrograde bypass, the surgeon must pull the bypass graft taut to avoid kinking and redundancy. An antegrade bypass usually allows better orientation of the vein or prosthetic graft. *(Reproduced with permission from Zarins CK, Gewertz BL. Atlas of Vascular Surgery. New York: Churchill Livingstone; 1989:107.)*

atherosclerosis, marginal cardiac reserve, and the administration of vasoactive agents, especially digitalis preparations.[4,14–16] Patients at particular risk include those who are dehydrated, who underwent recent cardiac surgery, who have sepsis, or who have another serious illness. In some instances, nonocclusive ischemia can occur after revascularization procedures for acute ischemia or chronic occlusive disease (Fig. 38–6).[17]

The onset is often predated by an acute decrease in cardiac function that simultaneously increases portal pressure and reduces mesenteric perfusion pressure. It is postulated that digitalis impairs the desired vasodilatory response to sudden increases in venous pressure[18]; paradoxic splanchnic vasoconstriction then ensues, with microvascular collapse, formation of microthrombi, and capillary sludging. In cases that occur after arterial revascularization, the presumed mechanism is reflex vasospasm of a "protected" low-pressure capillary bed suddenly exposed to normal perfusion pressures.[17]

The presentation of nonocclusive ischemia may be less dramatic and precipitous than that associated with embolic or thrombotic occlusions. Concurrent illness nearly

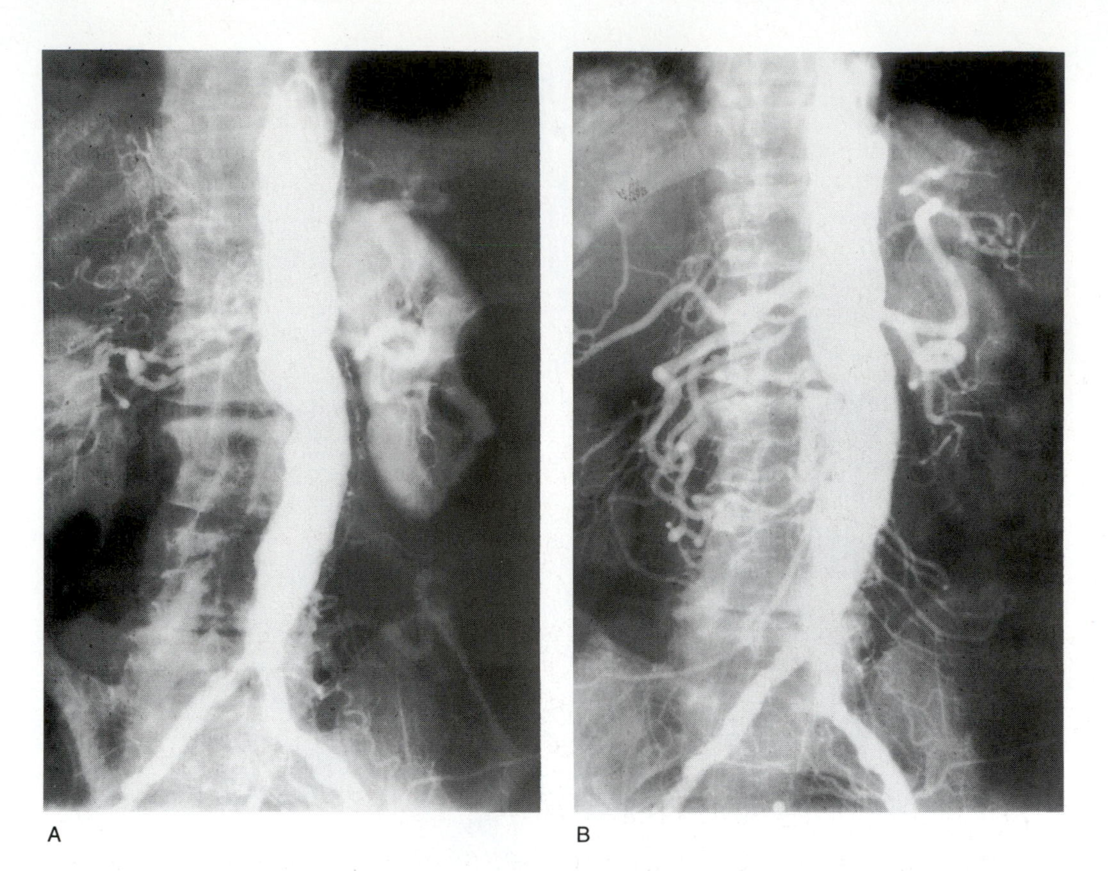

Figure 38–5. (**A**) Preoperative angiogram of a patient with *in situ* thrombosis of the SMA. (**B**) Because of multiple segments of infarcted bowel, a vein graft originating in the infrarenal aorta was used to revascularize the SMA. This postoperative angiogram reveals a patent graft (right of the aorta) with filling of the SMA. Note the collateral flow retrograde through the gastroduodenal artery to opacify the celiac axis.

always complicates the diagnosis. The ischemia rarely involves the entire small bowel and commonly fluctuates in intensity. Nonetheless, once established, especially in critically ill or debilitated patients, nonocclusive ischemia can unquestionably progress to transmural intestinal infarction.

Diagnosis

Selective catheterization of the SMA reveals distinctive arteriographic findings in patients with nonocclusive ischemia. Secondary and tertiary branches of the SMA show narrowing and irregularity, especially at branch points. Sometimes, vessels appear as "strings of sausage," with beading and tubular stenoses. The normal mucosal "blush" is characteristically absent. In most instances, all major mesenteric vessels are patent, and collateral vessels are relatively underdeveloped.

Treatment

Intra-arterial infusion of papaverine or a similar vasodilating drug (alpha-adrenergic antagonists) into the SMA is the primary mode of therapy. Papaverine should be administered at a constant infusion rate of 30 to 60 mg per hour for at least 24 to 48 hours. Swan-Ganz catheter placement with determination of left ventricular filling pressures allows appropriate fluid management and optimization of cardiac output.

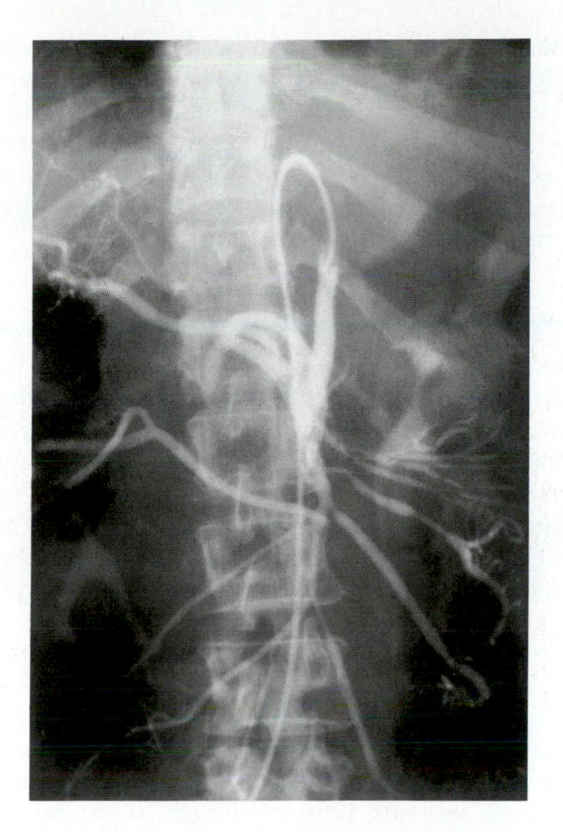

Figure 38–6. Vasospasm following revascularization of an ischemic SMA distribution. Note the constrictions at the branch points and the absence of a mucosal blush.

Broad-spectrum antibiotics are administered and alpha-adrenergic drugs are terminated if possible. Patients requiring vasopressors should receive dopaminergic agents preferably.

Operation may be avoided in patients with nonocclusive ischemia if the diagnosis is clear on the arteriogram and abdominal signs and symptoms totally resolve within 2 to 4 hours of the initiation of papaverine infusions. Selective SMA catheterization allows repeat contrast studies to document improvement and mucosal perfusion. However, irrespective of these findings, it is important to consider operative intervention if pain persists or if leukocytosis progresses.

VENOUS OCCLUSION

Etiology

Venous thrombosis, a relatively uncommon cause of mesenteric vascular compromise, may begin peripherally in the small veins of the mesenteric arcade or centrally in the major trunks of the portal system.[19] Acute major venous occlusion is accompanied by substantial splanchnic fluid sequestration and hemorrhagic intestinal infarction, while subacute thrombosis may be far less symptomatic.[6] Indeed, chronic thrombi in the branches of the superior mesenteric vein or the main trunk may be an incidental finding on computed tomography scans of patients with diverse intra-abdominal pathology, including malignancies and inflammatory bowel disease.

Although patients with extensive mesenteric venous thrombosis may present with constant, diffuse abdominal pain comparable to that of acute arterial occlusion, symptoms may initially be intermittent. About half these patients complain of distension, nausea, and low-grade fever. Many patients suffering from mesenteric venous thrombosis have a history of deep venous thrombosis of the extremities or hematologic evidence of hypercoagulable states. The syndrome may also occur in healthy and athletic people suffering profound dehydration.

Diagnosis

On arteriograms, mesenteric venous thrombosis is characterized by general slowing of arterial blood flow in conjunction with nonopacification of the corresponding mesenteric or portal veins. Often, the specific site of venous occlusion cannot be identified by arterial injections alone. Computed tomography scanning with contrast enhancement can occasionally provide more definitive information about the extent of thrombosis. Abdominal ultrasound can also help, especially if the patient is thin and without gaseous distension. Unfortunately, patients with venous thrombosis usually present with considerable intestinal distension.

Treatment

The operative approach to venous thrombosis involves resection of obviously infarcted bowel; however, infarction usually does not involve the entire length of the small bowel as is seen with acute arterial occlusions. Venous thrombectomy can be considered if thrombosis extends into the larger, more central veins (portal or superior mesenteric), although the likelihood of recurrent thrombosis is relatively high. If thrombectomy is performed, adjunctive treatments should be employed to prevent early postoperative occlusion.[6] These measures include intravenous infusions of heparin and low-molecular-weight dextran, as well as anticoagulation with warfarin for at least 6 months. Fibrinolytic agents have also been used, with anecdotal reports of success.[20]

RELATED ISSUES

Intestinal reperfusion injury invariably accompanies revascularization of ischemic tissue.[21] This process is mediated, in part, by the enzyme xanthine oxidase, which creates oxygen-derived free radicals in the presence of oxygen and hypoxanthine, a by-product of adenosine triphosphate metabolism.[22,23] These free radicals produce considerable local tissue injury by the related mechanisms of lipid peroxidation, membrane disruption, and increased microvascular permeability.[24] Free-radical scavengers, or xanthine oxidase inhibitors, consistently reduce experimental reperfusion injury, although the most compelling data are limited to animal intestinal ischemia–reperfusion models. Interestingly, rat and dog intestines have higher resting levels of xanthine dehydrogenase, the precursor of xanthine oxidase, than those measured in infant or adult humans.[25]

Since the 1980s, research has focused on the role of neutrophils in reperfusion injury.[26] It is well known that these inflammatory mediators are attracted by and produce free radicals. Further, many animal experiments demonstrate decreased tissue injury when ischemic intestine is reperfused with leukopenic blood.[27]

More recent work has centered on the process by which neutrophils roll, adhere, and activate on the endothelium of the microcirculation. It is now well established that these critical processes are mediated by the interaction between neutrophil receptors (especially CD11/CD18) and specific endothelial adhesion molecules (ELAM-1, ICAM-1, and PECAM), which are up-regulated by cytokines produced during ischemia.[28-30] It is believed that these cytokines, especially tumor necrosis factor–alpha and the interleukins-1 and -6, also contribute to distant organ dysfunction in the lung and liver after reperfusion.[31,32] Work in our laboratory demonstrated that the physiologic concentrations of these cytokines produced during ischemia and reperfusion of isolated human intestinal segments will increase the expression of endothelial cell adhesion molecules in cultured endothelial cells.[33]

Strategies have been developed to reduce neutrophil adherence and transendothelial migration by administration of monoclonal antibodies to the endothelial receptors.[34] It is hypothesized that such treatments could be carried out locally, just before revascularization, and provide some attenuation of reperfusion injury. Alternative therapy, though somewhat less effective, would require passage of the initial blood flow through leukocyte filters, paralleling the earlier animal experiments.[35,36]

Intraoperative assessments of intestinal viability may be performed by using a variety of techniques. Clinical judgments are based on the return of normal bowel color, mesenteric arterial pulsations, and peristalsis.[37] Evaluation can be improved by returning the bowel to the abdomen to avoid tension on the mesentery and by irrigating with warm saline. Even with these maneuvers, assessments performed 30 to 60 minutes after revascularization may be confounded by "wishful thinking" or delayed manifestations of reperfusion injury. Hence, simple observation may be supplemented by more objective measures, including detection of pulsatile mural blood flow by intraoperative ultrasound or fluorescein injection followed by inspection with Wood's light. Recent reports suggest that fluorescein is the best initial method, followed by laser velocimetry of the specific bowel segments in question.[38,39]

At times, all efforts to definitively establish long-term viability are unconvincing, yet a decision must be made regarding restoration of intestinal continuity. If any question exists about the viability at the resected margins, exteriorization with cutaneous enterostomies may avoid a "second-look" laparotomy. Otherwise, it is mandatory to re-explore the patient 24 to 36 hours later to confirm the patency of the thrombectomized or bypassed vessels and to assess the status of the revascularized bowel. The decision for repeat laparotomy should be based on the findings at the initial procedure and must not be affected by apparent clinical improvement in the immediate perioperative period.

Fibrinolysis of fresh mesenteric emboli or thrombi has been attempted with limited success.[40,41] This treatment is facilitated by the selective arteriographic studies that are part of the initial diagnostic workup of nearly every one of these patients. Unfortunately, lysis may not occur immediately or completely, delaying operative revascularization. Unlike in the case of nonocclusive ischemia, few clinicians feel comfortable eschewing the direct observation of bowel that has been severely ischemic for any period of time. Finally, in cases of thrombosis of preexistent occlusive lesions, nonoperative therapy with angioplasty is rarely definitive. Orificial lesions nearly always reflect extensive aortic plaque and respond poorly to dilation. Although it could be argued that recent developments, including intraluminal stents, may improve angioplasty results[42] and that minimally invasive procedures may obviate laparotomy, the risks of overlooking any infarcted segment are so great that the complete evaluation of the viscera allowed by formal laparotomy seems the prudent course.

CONCLUSION

The causes and mechanisms of acute mesenteric ischemia are now well understood. Unfortunately, the clinical outcomes of patients with this disease remain poor despite the promulgation of aggressive approaches to diagnosis and treatment. This fact not only reflects the considerable comorbid conditions that frequently initiate or accompany the syndromes, but also indicates an inability to recognize the process early in the course, before intestinal infarction occurs. Definitive diagnosis in this critical time period is essential to further improve survival.

Acknowledgments
The author wishes to acknowledge the outstanding secretarial assistance of Eileen Wayte in the preparation of this manuscript.

REFERENCES

1. Boley SJ, Brandt LJ, Veith FJ. Ischemic disorders of the intestines. *Curr Probl Surg.* 1978;15:46.
2. Mikkelsen WP. Intestinal angina. *Am J Surg.* 1957;94:262.
3. Sachs SM, Morton JH, Schwartz SI. Acute mesenteric ischemia. *Surgery.* 1982;92:646.
4. Gazes PC, Holmes CR, Moseley V, et al. Acute hemorrhage and necrosis of the intestines associated with digitalization. *Circulation.* 1961;23:358.
5. Bernard F, Perdrix JP, Lepape A, et al. Acute intestinal ischemia after voluntary drug poisoning. *Ann Fr Anesth Reanim.* 1991;10(2):158–160.
6. Naitove A, Weismann RE. Primary mesenteric venous thrombosis. *Ann Surg.* 1965;161:516.
7. Boley SJH, Feinstein FR, Sammartano R, et al. New concepts in the management of emboli of the superior mesenteric artery. *Surg Gynecol Obstet.* 1981;153:561.
8. Boley SJ, Sprayegan S, Siegelman SS, et al. Initial results from an aggressive roentgenological and surgical approach to acute mesenteric ischemia. *Surgery.* 1977;82(6):848.
9. Jamieson WG, Marchuk S, Rowsom J, et al. The early diagnosis of massive acute intestinal ischemia. Br J Surg. 1982;69(suppl):S52.
10. Murray MJ, Gonze MD, Nowak LR, et al. Serum D(-)-lactate levels as an aid to diagnosing acute intestinal ischemia. *Am J Surg.* 1994;167(6):575–578.
11. Murray MJ, Barbose JJ, Cobb CF. Serum D(-)-lactate levels as a predictor of acute intestinal ischemia in a rat model. *J Surg Res.* 1993;54(5):507–509.
12. Ottinger LW. The surgical management of acute occlusion of the superior mesenteric artery. *Ann Surg.* 1978;188:721.
13. Zarins CK, Gewertz BL. *Atlas of Vascular Surgery.* New York: Churchill Livingstone; 1989.
14. Ferrer MI, Bradley SE, Wheeler HO, et al. The effect of digoxin in the splanchnic circulation in ventricular failure. *Circulation.* 1965;32:524.
15. Mason DT, Braunwald E, Karsh RB, et al. Studies on digitalis: effects of ouabain on forearm vascular resistance and venous tone in normal subjects and in patients in heart failure. *J Clin Invest.* 1964;43:532.
16. Mikkelsen E, Andersson KE, Pedersen OL. Effects of digoxin on isolated human mesenteric vessels. *Acta Pharmacol Toxicol.* 1979;45:25.
17. Gewertz BL, Zarins CK. Postoperative vasospasm after antegrade mesenteric revascularization. *J Vasc Surg.* 1991;14:382–385.
18. Kim EH, Gewertz BL. Chronic digitalis administration alters mesenteric vascular reactivity. *J Vasc Surg.* 1987;5(2):382.
19. Grendell JH, Ockner RK. Mesenteric venous thrombosis. *Gastroenterology.* 1982;82:358.
20. Demertzis S, Ringe B, Gulba D, et al. Treatment of portal vein thrombosis by thrombectomy and regional thrombolysis. *Surgery.* 1994;115(3):389–393.

21. Parks DA, Granger DN. Contributions of ischemia and reperfusion to mucosal lesion formation. *Am J Physiol.* 1986;250(13):G749–G753.
22. Parks DA, Granger DN. Ischemia-induced vascular changes: role of xanthine oxidase and hydroxyl radicals. *Am J Physiol.* 1983;245(8):G285–G289.
23. Perry MA, Wadhwa S, Parks DA, et al. Role of oxygen radicals in ischemia-induced lesions in the cat stomach. *Gastroenterology.* 1986;90:362–367.
24. DelMaestro RF, Bjork J, Arfors KE. Increase in microvascular permeability induced by enzymatically generated free radicals. II. Role of superoxide anion radical, hydrogen peroxide and hydroxyl radical. *Microvasc Res.* 1981;22:255–270.
25. Granger DN, Hollwarth ME, Parks DA. Ischemia–reperfusion injury: role of oxygen-derived free radicals. *Acta Physiol Scand Suppl.* 1986;548:47–64.
26. Hernandez LA, Grisham MB, Twohig B, et al. Role of neutrophils in ischemia–reperfusion injury. *Am J Physiol.* 1987;253:H699–H708.
27. Sisley A, Harig J, Gewertz BL. Neutrophil depletion attenuates human intestinal reperfusion injury. *J Surg Res.* 1994;57(1):192–196.
28. Harlan JM, Killen PD, Senecal FM, et al. The role of neutrophil membrane glycoprotein GP-150 in neutrophil adherence to endothelium *in vitro. Blood.* 1985;66(1):167–178.
29. Arfors KE, Lundberg C, Lindbom L, et al. A monoclonal antibody to the membrane glycoprotein complex Cdw18 inhibits PMN accumulation and plasma leakage *in vivo. Blood.* 1987;69:338–340.
30. Diener AM, Beatty PG, Ochs HD, et al. The role of neutrophil membrane glycoprotein 150 in neutrophil-mediated endothelial cell injury *in vitro. J Immunol.* 1985;135:537–543.
31. Stephens KE, Ishizaka A, Larrick JW, et al. Tumor necrosis factor causes increased pulmonary permeability and edema. *Am Rev Respir Dis.* 1988;137:1364–1370.
32. Caty MG, Guice KS, Oldham KT, et al. Evidence for tumor necrosis factor–induced pulmonary microvascular injury after intestinal ischemia–reperfusion injury. *Ann Surg.* 1990;212(6):694–700.
33. Wyble C, Desai T, Gewertz BL. Cytokines released from reperfused human intestine upregulates ELAM-1 (Part 1). *FASEB J.* 1995;9(3):203.
34. Luscinskas FW, Brock AF, Gimbrone MA, et al. Endothelial-leukocyte adhesion molecule-1–dependent and leukocyte (CD11/CD18)–dependent mechanism contribute to polymorphonuclear leukocyte adhesion to cytokine-activated human vascular endothelium. *J Immunol.* 1989;142:2257–2263.
35. Clark ET, Gewertz BL. Intermittent ischemia accentuates intestinal reperfusion injury. *J Vasc Surg.* 1991;13:601–606.
36. dela Ossa JC, Malago M, Gewertz BL. Reduction of intestinal reperfusion injury requires near total neutrophil depletion. *FASEB J.* 1991;5(6):7914.
37. Bulkley GB, Zuidema GD, Hamilton SR, et al. Intraoperative determination of small intestinal viability following ischemic injury. *Ann Surg.* 1981;193:628.
38. Horgan PG, Gorey TF. Operative assessment of intestinal viability. *Surg Clin North Am.* 1992;72(1):143–155.
39. Galandiuk S, Fazio VW, Petras RE. Fluorescein endoscopy: a technique for noninvasive assessment of intestinal ischemia. *Dis Colon Rectum.* 1988;31:848.
40. Rodde A, Peiffert B, Bazin C, et al. Intra-arterial fibrinolysis of superior mesenteric artery embolism. *J Radiol.* 1991;72(4):239–242.
41. Boyer L, Delorme JM, Alexandre M, et al. Local fibrinolysis for superior mesenteric artery thromboembolism. *Cardiovasc Intervent Radiol.* 1994;17(4):214–216.
42. Simonetti G, Lupattelli L, Urigo F, et al. Interventional radiology in the treatment of acute and chronic mesenteric ischemia. *Radiol (Torino) Med.* 1992;84(1–2):98–105.

VII

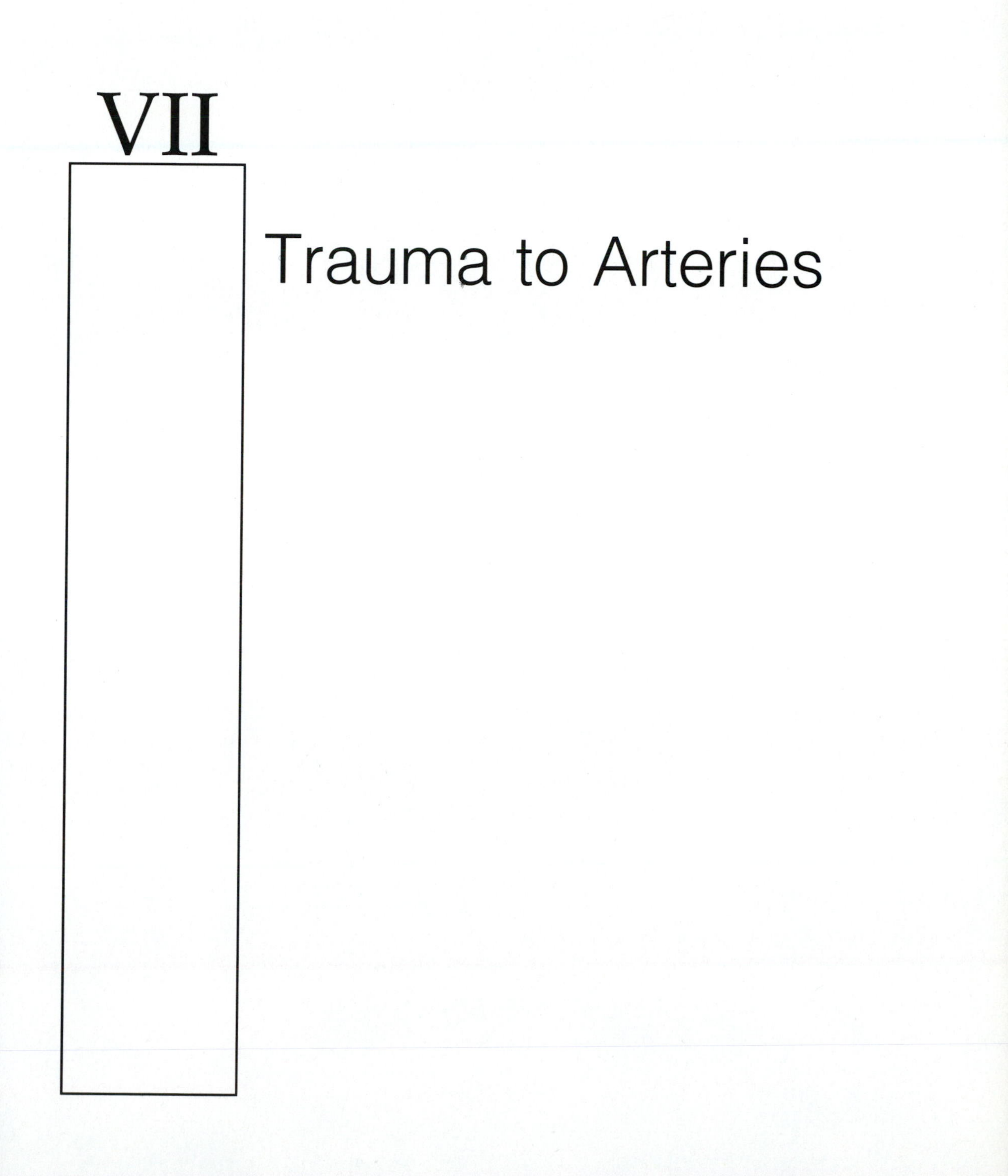

Trauma to Arteries

39

Brachiocephalic Artery Injury

Aires A.B. Barros D'Sa, MD, FRCS

The great vessels of the aortic arch and their major branches traverse the superior mediastinum, thoracic outlet, and neck, and injuries to these vessels constitute one of the most challenging acute problems confronting the vascular surgeon today. These injuries accounted for 12% of all vascular trauma in one large series.[1] The majority are penetrating injuries, and most of the casualties are young males in urban communities wherein a subculture of drugs and gang warfare thrives. Penetrating brachiocephalic arterial injuries are also witnessed amidst civil populations, such as those in Northern Ireland, who have endured indiscriminate assault by terrorists using sophisticated weaponry.[2–5] The distribution of arterial injuries in patients who survived such assault and patients who sustained arterial injuries caused by other mechanisms is shown in Table 39–1.

In metropolitan conurbations, patients who sustain injuries of these vessels are often fortunate enough to be taken to well-equipped trauma centers staffed by specialist surgical personnel. Hemorrhage from brachiocephalic arteries and branches, associated frequently with injury to adjacent vital structures, accounts not only for the high mortality at the scene or in transit, but also for the severe hypotensive shock of patients on admission. When patients survive to be treated, surgical experience and expertise are required for immediate resuscitation, recognition of the true extent and complexity of the trauma, and prompt operative intervention for access, control, and repair of the cervicomediastinal vessels.

ANATOMIC ACCESS AND INCISIONAL APPROACHES

The key to surgical success is rapid exposure, control of hemorrhage, and appropriate arterial reconstruction. While much debate surrounds the use of thoracotomy in gaining access to vascular injuries of the chest, valuable time may be lost in securing direct control of injured great vessels. A median sternotomy (i.e., a midline split of the sternum) offers a simple and swift approach to the innominate artery and the origins of its right common carotid and right subclavian branches, as well as to the left common carotid artery (Fig. 39–1). This approach also permits excellent access to the superior vena cava, the innominate veins, the pulmonary artery, and the heart, enabling expeditious control of a difficult situation. Access to the left subclavian artery for control of

TABLE 39–1. INCIDENCE AND OUTCOME OF BRACHIOCEPHALIC ARTERY INJURIES (ASSOCIATED TRAUMA TO OTHER STRUCTURES, PARTICULARLY IN PENETRATING WOUNDS)

Artery	Penetrating[a]					Blunt/Indirect[a]					Iatrogenic[a]				
	No.	*S*	*NS*	*ND*	*D*	*No.*	*S*	*NS*	*ND*	*D*	*No.*	*S*	*NS*	*ND*	*D*
Innominate	3	3	—	—	2	1	1	—	—	1	—	—	—	—	—
Subclavian	8	8	—	—	3	5	3	2	—	—	5	2	3	—	—
Common carotid	10	9	1	2	1	2	1	1	1	0	5	1	4	1	—
Internal carotid	11	11	—	3	3	8	1	7	6	1	3	3	—	—	—
External carotid	10	10	—	1	2	3	1	2	—	1	1	—	1	—	—
Vertebral	2	1	1	—	—	3	1	2	—	1	2	—	2[b]	—	—
Total	44	42	2	6	11	22	8	14	7	4	16	6	10	1	—

[a] No. = number of injuries; S = surgery; NS = no surgery; ND = neurologic deficit; D = number of deaths.

[b] Balloon occlusion in one case.

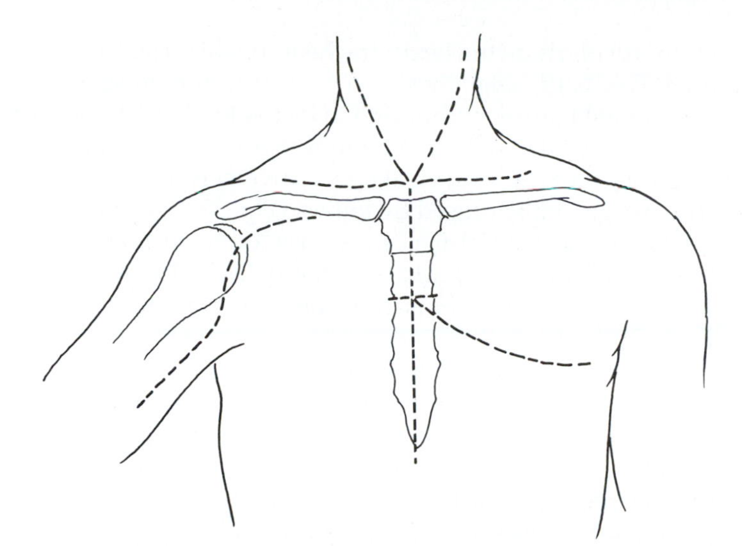

Figure 39–1. Incisional approaches: A median sternotomy provides access to the great vessels of the aortic arch. Extension upward into supraclavicular or oblique cervical incisions permits exposure of the subclavian and carotid arteries, respectively. A left, third intercostal space, anterior thoracotomy—alone or as part of the "trapdoor" approach—provides access to the left subclavian artery. A gentle S-shaped deltopectoral groove incision will expose the axillary artery if required.

bleeding may be gained through a left anterior thoracotomy through the third intercostal space. By adding a left supraclavicular incision, freeing the clavicular insertions of the sternocleidomastoid and strap muscles, and dividing the left midclavicle, the surgeon can create a "trapdoor" approach to the subclavian (Fig. 39–1).[6]

For further access to vessels in the neck, the upper end of the median sternotomy incision can be extended as required (Fig. 39–1). A supraclavicular incision will expose the middle and distal parts of either subclavian artery, combined if necessary with excision of the medial third or half of the clavicle. Similarly, a standard oblique incision along the medial border of the sternocleidomastoid affords exposure to the common, internal, and external carotid arteries. Access to the distal internal carotid artery approaching the base of the skull is facilitated by division of the digastric muscle and the styloid process, and occasionally by mandibular subluxation or mandibulotomy. In patients requiring such access, nasotracheal rather than orotracheal intubation allows the jaws to close, providing more room at the upper angle of the carotid triangle. The first part of the vertebral artery is exposed through a standard supraclavicular incision; the incision for access to the carotid will lead to the second part, which lies distal to the transverse process of the sixth cervical vertebra.

Practical experience in all these anatomic approaches is essential and might be gained—with permission and by adhering to proper guidelines—from cadavers. Familiarity with these incisions will instill confidence in the surgeon when a quick and aggressive approach offers the best chance of patient survival.

INTRATHORACIC ARTERIAL INJURIES

Etiology and Mechanism of Injury

The mortality rate among patients who sustain penetrating trauma of large-caliber arteries and venous trunks in the superior mediastinum, thoracic outlet, and root of the neck is high,[7–9] particularly as the heart, tracheobronchial tree, lungs, or esophagus may also be injured. Few battle casualties or victims of terrorism survive high-velocity missile, bomb, or shrapnel injuries of this kind to be treated.[2–5,10] The severity of trauma and the unacceptable time interval before definitive treatment becomes available in a military scenario accounts for a low survival rate. Conversely, in a civilian urban setting, penetrating injuries are generally caused by knives (Fig. 39–2) or low-velocity bullets,[8] and swift transit to sophisticated trauma centers has led to encouraging survival rates for patients with such injuries, particularly since the 1970s.[1,11] These arterial injuries may present as lacerations, vessel defects, or transections, and not uncommonly manifest as arteriovenous fistulas (Fig. 39–2).[12]

Sudden deceleration forces involved in road traffic accidents, mining disasters, airplane crashes, or falls result in traumatic rupture of the isthmus of the aorta, a mechanism that may equally cause partial or total avulsion of the innominate artery,[11] less frequently the left subclavian artery, and least often the left common carotid artery. Partial avulsion of the innominate artery may form a false aneurysm that may rupture at any time. Indirect injury to the subclavian artery may also be associated with rotation of the head in combination with hyperextension of the neck. In road traffic accidents, a deceleration injury may be compounded by direct trauma from the steering wheel, from which considerable energy may be dissipated as the chest wall is crushed. The subclavian arteries may be injured directly by fractures of the clavicle or upper two ribs.

An unusual injury that may follow tracheostomy—namely, a tracheoinnominate artery fistula—is less frequently observed due to improvements in tracheostomy tube design and placement, and avoidance of overinflation of the cuff. Such an injury, thought to be caused by the tip of an improperly positioned tracheostomy tube in association with local sepsis,[13] is probably initiated by the constant pounding of the innominate artery against the inferior concave border of a rigid tube placed far too

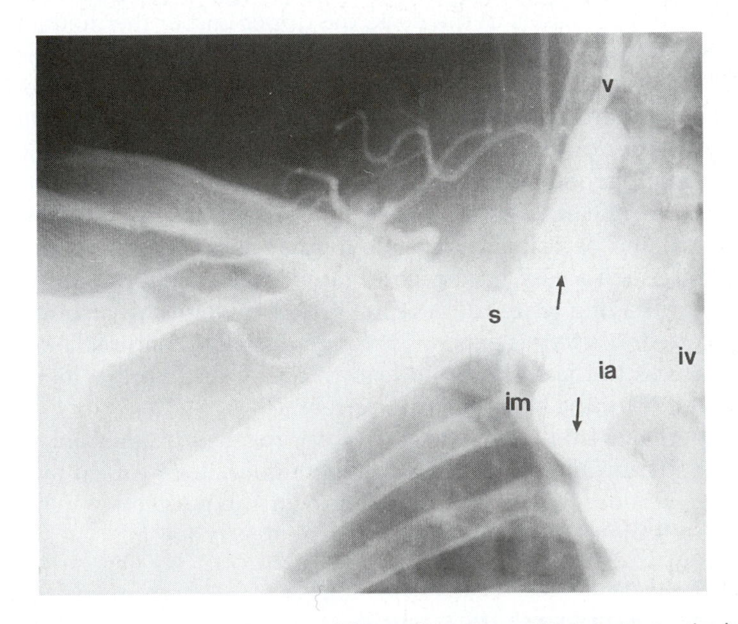

Figure 39–2. A stab wound at the root of the neck creates a fistula between the innominate artery (**ia**) and the innominate vein (**iv**) and produces a confined hematoma tracking upward and downward (*arrows*). The relationship to the right subclavian artery (**s**) and its vertebral (**v**) and internal mammary (**im**) branches is identified. (*Reproduced with permission from Eastcott HHG, ed. Arterial Surgery. Edinburgh, UK: Churchill Livingstone; 1992:388.*)

low within the trachea. It has been suggested that the tracheostomy tube begins to pulsate before the artery perforates.

Clinical Presentation

Penetrating injury of intrathoracic vessels may result in exsanguination externally or into the chest, or a hematoma may be confined at high pressure within the mediastinum. Small entry and exit wounds often belie the gravity of internal injuries. Hemorrhage, shock, sucking neck wounds, and hemoptysis all demand immediate resuscitative measures. These include establishment of an adequate airway, intubation, ventilation, insertion of chest drains, and volume replacement in concert with definitive surgery. Delay for radiologic investigations may lead to fatality.

In cases of blunt arterial injury, the patient may complain of symptoms such as dyspnea, hoarseness, or dysphagia. On examination, there may be a hematoma or surgical emphysema at the root of the neck, pulses in the neck or upper limb may be weak or impalpable, a thrill or a bruit may be present, and there might be evidence of a cranial nerve deficit, Horner's syndrome, or hemispheric ischemia. Injuries of the esophagus and lower trachea are unusual below the level of the clavicle.

Early Management

For patients who present in the resuscitation room with any compromise of the airway, breathing difficulty, or evidence of cerebral hypoxia, immediate endotracheal intubation, inflation of the cuff below the level of a potential tracheal tear or a compressing hematoma, and ventilation will ensure a positive start. As these measures continue, volume replacement, first by the administration of Ringer's lactate through large-caliber intravenous lines, followed by blood as soon as available, will maintain lifesaving organ perfusion. Major loss from a chest drain inserted for hemothorax is a signal for immediate operation. Pericardiocentesis may be indicated for cardiac tamponade, but if it is not at an advanced stage, relief by direct pericardiotomy may be more effective, especially if a median sternotomy is required immediately for attention to injuries of the great vessels.

Radiologic Assessment

Radiologic investigations are acceptable if the patient is stable. In cases of blunt trauma, a chest film may reveal the classic widened mediastinum, possibly along with fractures of the clavicle, the first rib, and even the second rib. In cases of penetrating injury, mediastinal emphysema and hemopneumothorax may be present. The path of a bullet or shrapnel fragment seen on a chest film is not necessarily linear, and speculation as to its presumed track in relation to the entry wound may be misleading.

For the stable patient, angiography and enhanced spiral computed tomography scans will accurately define the arterial injury and assist the surgeon in planning an operation for control and repair. These investigations will also exclude coincidental heart or proximal thoracic aortic trauma, which falls within the expertise of the cardiac surgeon. There should be no delay in operative intervention, as the situation may change precipitately. For example, a high-pressure mediastinal hematoma may rupture into the pleural cavity as a fatal event.

Operative Management

A median sternotomy with the option for intercostal extension laterally or upward in any direction in the neck is ideal for injured arteries in the cervicomediastinal region.[8,9]

Inability to secure swift control of a major bleeding artery is the most common cause of intraoperative mortality. When the patient has a hematoma, firm digital compression is required while adequate exposure is being secured for control. The left innominate vein may be clamped and divided, with impunity, to gain access to life-threatening arterial bleeding beneath. Bleeding from a tear or an avulsion at the origin of the great vessels is controlled by a partially occluding aortic C-clamp. Anomalous origins of the innominate and right subclavian artery should be kept in mind. Lacerations within the innominate and left common carotid arteries are controlled by simple proximal and distal clamping. Cardiac tamponade, if present, may be relieved, and any holes in the heart wall may be sutured. Direct cardiac massage can be performed in cases of incipient arrest.

The value of temporary inlying or externally introduced shunts to maintain cerebral blood flow may be controversial.[8,9,11,12] Nevertheless, they contribute favorably, especially in ensuring maximal perfusion in the hypotensive patient in cases of simultaneous innominate and left common carotid artery injury.[11]

Ligation of both innominate and common carotid arteries generally results in fatal cerebral ischemia. Although ligation of the left subclavian artery is undesirable, it can be undertaken within the chest without serious compromise to upper limb blood flow.

In cases of laceration of these large vessel trunks, lateral suture may be effective, but if a defect exists, prosthetic patch graft angioplasty is preferable. For simple transections, end-to-end anastomosis may be possible in many cases,[12] but in practice, retraction of vessel ends introduces tension, and a prosthetic graft may have to be interposed. Injury at the origin of the innominate artery may necessitate an aortoinnominate bypass from a fresh aortotomy on the ascending aorta. Surgeons experienced in treating this type of injury prefer to leave a contained hematoma at the arch undisturbed and to proceed to an aortoinnominate bypass before finally closing off the defect at the origin of the innominate artery, if necessary by means of a prosthetic patch.[14] A bifurcated graft may be used to restore flow to both innominate and left common carotid arteries, and "jump grafts" taken to the subclavian arteries. In cases of significant contamination, as with concomitant esophageal injury, prosthetic grafts are at risk; therefore, less-than-ideal remote techniques such as axillo–axillary, carotid–carotid, or subclavian–carotid bypasses may have to be employed.

Lacerations in the superior vena cava or innominate veins are usually closed by lateral suture or vein patch angioplasty. Ligation of the innominate veins is acceptable, as in most cases collateral venous circulation prevents the development of symptoms of upper limb venous insufficiency.

Postoperative Care and Outcome

Patients with intrathoracic arterial injuries are admitted to an intensive care unit, where hemodynamic and cardiac function, neck and peripheral pulses, drainage from mediastinal and chest tubes, respiratory status, and neurologic function are monitored. In cases of anastomotic leakage, suspected vessel occlusion, or missed arterial injury, immediate transfemoral aortography should precede reintervention. Antibiotic prophylaxis, especially when prosthetic grafts are used, should be continued for at least 3 days.

In cases of penetrating trauma, the survival rate for patients who undergo definitive vascular repair of the great vessels ranges from 70% to 86%, but it can be as high as 94%.[12] For patients who live to undergo surgery for blunt trauma, the reported survival rate for innominate artery injury is 75%, and for subclavian artery injury, it is as high as 90%[15]; most of the deaths in this group are due to associated nonvascular injuries.

SUBCLAVIAN ARTERY INJURIES

Etiology and Mechanism of Injury

The subclavian artery is infrequently injured simply because it lies relatively well protected by the sternum and clavicles. The incidence of known penetrating subclavian injury on the battlefield is approximately 1%.[16] Injury by knife or bullet in civilian practice (Fig. 39–3) is frequently associated with injury to contiguous structures such as the lung, nerves, or subclavian vein, creating an arteriovenous fistula. The patient may not survive the ensuing torrential hemorrhage externally or into the neck or chest. Cavitational damage from a high-velocity missile injury may not be recognized at initial exploration, and subsequent necrosis of an apparently intact arterial wall may prove fatal.[2] A missed subclavian artery injury may develop into an expanding false aneurysm, causing limb-threatening chronic thromboembolism. Iatrogenic injury to the subclavian artery may occur during catheterization of a subclavian vein.

Direct blunt trauma to the chest wall and clavicle must be severe to produce the sharp bone fragments that injure the underlying subclavian artery.[8] In 60% of all patients with these injuries, varying degrees of damage to the brachial plexus signal a dismal outlook, even after successful vascular repair.[17] Rarely, in cases of deceleration injuries, the left subclavian artery is partially or completely torn at its origin, sometimes in combination with traumatic rupture of the thoracic isthmus.[18]

Clinical Presentation

In most cases of penetrating injury of the subclavian artery, external bleeding is visible at the root of the neck, or it may continue silently into the pleural cavity, accounting for shock that fails to respond to blood transfusion. A cold, pulseless, pallid hand accompanied by paresthesia and arm weakness, a supraclavicular bruit, or an expanding pulsatile hematoma is a feature of blunt subclavian trauma. Traumatic occlusion of the first part of the subclavian proximal to the vertebral artery may give rise to symptoms

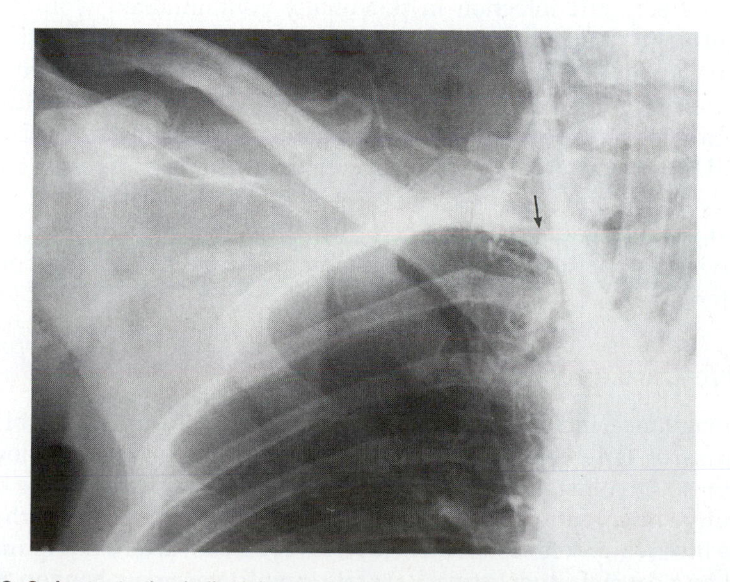

Figure 39–3. A penetrating bullet injury to the root of the neck causes disruption and occlusion (*arrow*) of the first part of the right subclavian artery. (*Reproduced with permission from Eastcott HHG, ed. Arterial Surgery. Edinburgh, UK: Churchill Livingstone; 1992:395.*)

of subclavian steal syndrome. The loss of sensory and motor function consequent upon ischemia may mask the true extent of associated nerve injury. Dyspnea may point to an expanding hematoma at the root of the neck, a large hemothorax, or a hemopneumothorax.

Early Management

All resuscitative measures to secure airway, ventilation, and circulating volume are initiated. Peripheral or central venous lines should not be inserted on the side of the injured subclavian artery. The excellent skeletal protection around the subclavian artery paradoxically represents a physical obstacle to emergency—and even intraoperative—control of bleeding. When the patient is in shock, good clinical acumen and speed of action are essential.

Radiologic Assessment

Radiologic findings such as mediastinal widening or a hemothorax serve to reveal a diagnosis that may have evaded clinical assessment. For the stable patient, transfemoral angiography will delineate the exact site and nature of the injury so that an appropriate incisional approach can be planned.

Operative Management

Thrombosis in continuity following blunt injury is well tolerated in most instances. In some cases of high-velocity bullet and shrapnel wounds, the subclavian, its main branches, and therefore the collateral network are destroyed, and ligation could threaten limb survival. Standard methods of vascular repair include lateral suture or end-to-end anastomosis, the latter being of some merit for contaminated wounds if repair can be achieved without tension. Although polytetrafluoroethylene grafts were used successfully in subclavian artery repair in large civilian series,[19] alertness must be maintained to detect graft infection in potentially contaminated wounds. Even if a permanent neurologic deficit due to brachial plexus injury appears likely, the subclavian artery should be repaired because in a rearterialized extremity, amputation will eventually be performed at a lower level. Adequate tissue cover for this delicate artery is often difficult to achieve, especially in cases of major penetrating injuries. Contaminated wounds should be left open for delayed primary closure. In cases of raised compartment pressure, fasciotomies may be necessary to safeguard the viability of muscles and nerves. Sympathetic blockade is not particularly helpful in influencing outcome. Internal fixation of clavicular fractures, although difficult, will prevent reinjury of a repaired subclavian artery.

Postoperative Care and Outcome

Postoperative vigilance, including ultrasound monitoring of upper limb blood flow, is essential if signs of failure of arterial repair, bleeding, or graft infection are to be detected. In these circumstances, transfemoral angiography is of value in deciding whether operative intervention is indicated. In cases of secondary hemorrhage, arterial ligation can be lifesaving. A few patients with left subclavian artery injury may continue to be troubled by a thoracic duct fistula. Late false aneurysms may develop and demand surgical correction. A mortality rate of 10% among patients with blunt subclavian artery injuries is caused predominantly by other critical associated injuries.[15]

ARTERIAL INJURIES IN THE NECK

Penetrating trauma accounts for most cervical arterial injuries principally involving the common carotid, and the left side is particularly vulnerable to right-handed assailants. Penetrating vascular injuries of the neck represent approximately 5% of all vascular trauma, whether it occurs in wartime, as a consequence of terrorist violence, or in civilian practice. Associated injuries to the larynx, trachea, pharynx, and upper esophagus are common (Fig. 39–4). Penetrating iatrogenic injuries of the carotid artery are rare and may occur during radical neck dissection for malignancy, during tonsillectomy, or during percutaneous cannulation for central venous pressure monitoring. In the latter procedure, the vertebral artery is also vulnerable to arteriovenous fistula formation.

Blunt carotid artery trauma accounts for a small proportion of cervical arterial injuries. Such trauma may be caused (1) indirectly by a blow to the face or head, which causes sudden rotation and hyperextension of the head and neck; (2) by a direct blow to the vessel as a component of fractures of the skull base; or (3) classically when a

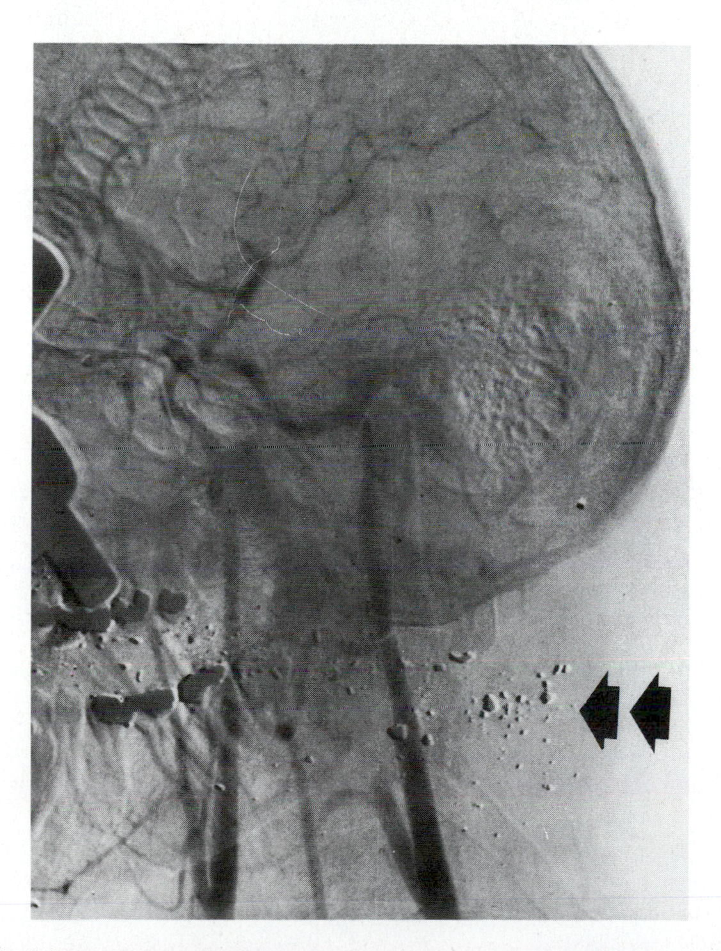

Figure 39–4. A penetrating high-velocity missile injury of the neck, its path traced by fragments traversing the mandible, the mouth, and the maxilla. Pharyngeal hemorrhage (*arrows*) necessitated immediate endotracheal intubation with a cuffed tube. Arch angiography revealed a transected external carotid artery as the source of bleeding. (*Reproduced with permission from Barros D'Sa AAB. A decade of missile-induced vascular trauma. Ann R Coll Surg Engl. 1981;64:40.*)

child falls forward on a pencil held in the mouth. In cases of rotation–hyperextension injury, the ipsilateral distal internal carotid artery is stretched across the bodies of the first and second cervical vertebrae and the transverse process of the third cervical vertebra, sometimes also pinching the contralateral vessel between the mandibular angle and the atlas. Blunt injury, usually involving the carotid bifurcation or the distal internal carotid artery, may take the form of one or more intimal fractures, mural thrombus, dissection, or complete occlusion (Fig. 39–5), and pseudoaneurysm formation may complicate the picture. Gradual mural thrombosis and progressive stenosis may lead to recurrent thromboembolic transient ischemic attacks, followed by completed stroke in some cases. Signs of neurologic impairment may not become apparent for some time, by which stage operative reconstruction is impossible. When a deficit does occur, the tendency is to suspect intracranial rather than cervical causes. The configuration of the unique anastomotic network represented by the circle of Willis varies widely, and frequently it may be congenitally defective or incomplete, thereby limiting the capacity for compensation when flow has been arrested in cases of carotid trauma. Death is usually a sequela of massive cerebral edema rather than of hemorrhagic infarction.[20,21]

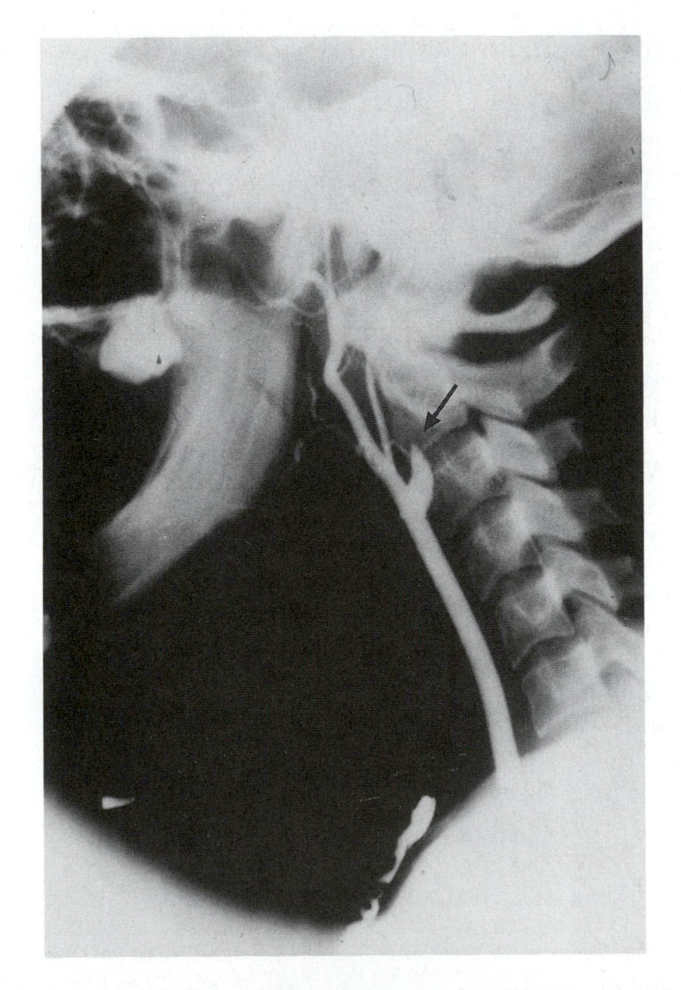

Figure 39–5. A hyperextension injury of the neck causes intimal fracture (*arrow*), dissection, and occlusion of the internal carotid artery. (*Reproduced with permission from Eastcott HHG, ed. Arterial Surgery. Edinburgh, UK: Churchill Livingstone; 1992:392.*)

CAROTID ARTERY INJURY

Clinical Presentation

Not every penetrating wound is deep enough to cause carotid artery injury. Signs of such injury are bleeding through the neck wound, and sometimes an expanding pulsatile hematoma, hoarseness, stridor, a thrill, and a bruit. Concomitant damage to the jugular vein may result in a caroticojugular fistula and machinery murmur (Fig. 39–6). Associated laryngotracheal injury places the respiratory tract in danger from extravasated blood at high pressure. Bruises and abrasions from direct blunt trauma may be apparent, but rotation–hyperextension injury leaves little external evidence.

The duration, extent, and progress of a neurologic deficit are of great importance in management. In the absence of a closed head injury, a neurologic deficit may be presumed to be associated with carotid artery trauma, especially if the patient is fully conscious.

Early Management

Coexisting carotid and tracheal injury demands that the physician immediately institute endotracheal intubation and inflation of the cuff (Fig. 39–7), taking care not to disturb the cervical spine if its stability is in question. The opportunity may be taken to inspect the vocal cords to exclude nerve injury. An ensured airway and ventilation will arrest cerebral hypoxia, minimizing cerebral edema and its sequelae. Control of external bleeding by direct pressure is possible in most instances. Rapid volume replacement to maintain cerebral perfusion may counteract the effects of earlier cerebral hypoxia. Chest drains may have to be inserted to relieve hemopneumothorax. A nasogastric tube may predispose the patient to mediastinitis by penetrating unsuspected injuries of the upper respiratory and alimentary tracts that can be missed on endoscopic and contrast studies.

Investigation and Assessment

The neck can be divided into three convenient zones to facilitate assessment and selection of patients for angiography and surgery. Zone I lies topographically behind and inferior to the clavicle and anterior chest wall and therefore includes the main brachiocephalic vessels and their branches. Zone II covers most of the neck between the clavicle below and the angle of the mandible above and includes the common carotid artery approximately as far up as the bifurcation and the first and second parts of the vertebral artery. Zone III lies between the angle of the mandible and the base of the skull and includes the internal carotid artery and the third part of the vertebral artery.

Urgent operative intervention is obviously necessary in cases of hemorrhage.[22] Wounds that fail to convincingly penetrate deeper than the platysma do not require exploration. For deeper injuries, exploration was routine in the past[23] and is still recommended.[24] A more selective approach is zone II injuries of the carotid artery in patients who are stable, both hemodynamically and neurologically, was recently advocated.[25–28] The rationale behind this approach is multifactorial: (1) a high incidence of negative explorations took place in the past; (2) injuries, such as intimal fracture in either the carotid artery or the vertebral artery, were missed at operation; and (3) delay in exploration does not necessarily induce a higher complication rate. A policy of selective exploration of penetrating neck injury may be sharpened if supported by good angiographic delineation of the carotid system.

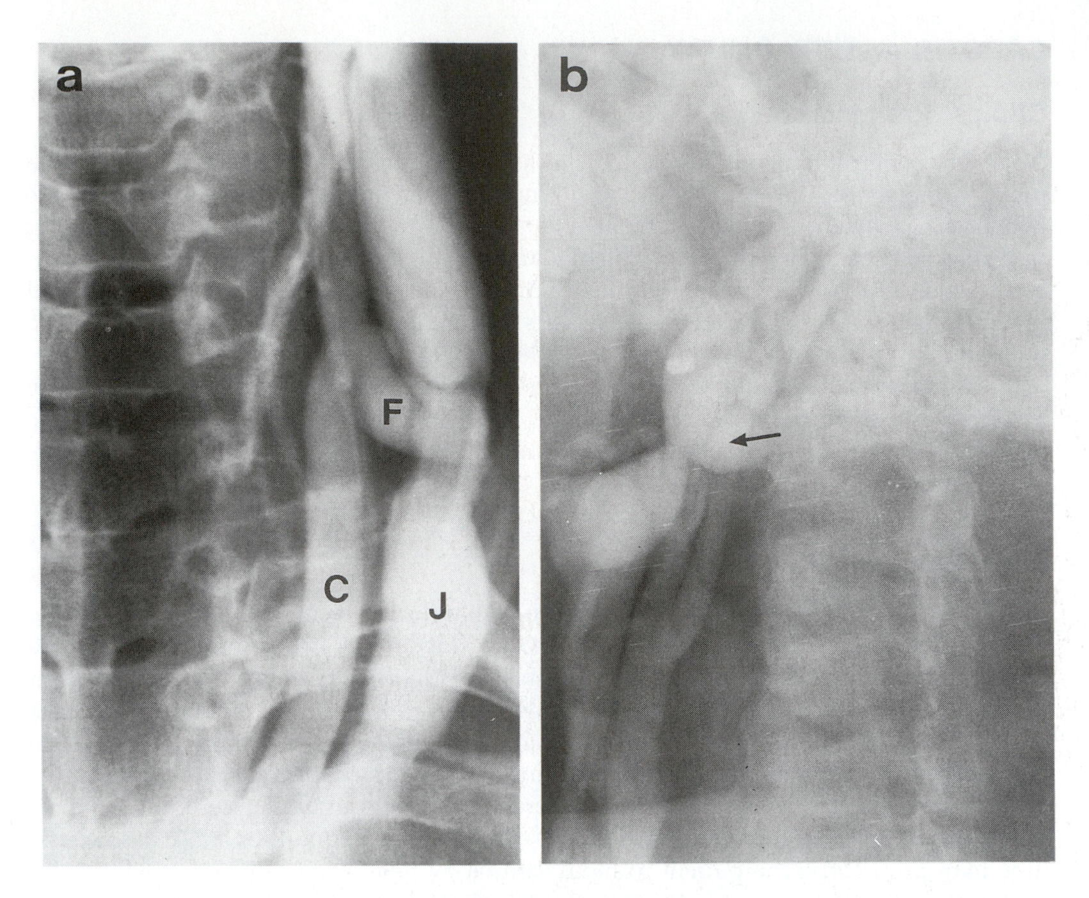

Figure 39–6. Caroticojugular fistulae. (**a**) Low-velocity injury: a proximal fistula (F) between the common carotid artery (C) and the internal jugular vein (J). (**b**) Shell fragment injury: a distal fistula (*arrow*) between the internal carotid artery and the jugular vein. (*Reproduced with permission from Eastcott HHG, ed. Arterial Surgery. Edinburgh, UK: Churchill Livingstone; 1992:392.*)

In general, angiography is of value for zone I and zone III carotid injuries as long as the patient is stable hemodynamically. In cases of penetrating injuries within zone II, preoperative angiography in the stable patient may not be essential, but it is undoubtedly helpful in that the vascular surgeon will know exactly what to expect at operation. When the carotid triangle has been breached by a missile, angiography will reassure the surgeon that the carotid system is intact (Fig. 39–8). Likewise, in cases of blunt trauma, early angiography will define a carotid artery injury while the condition is still remediable. On the whole, angiography improves the accuracy of clinical assessment and reduces the incidence of missed vascular injury.

The practice of withholding exploration of a penetrating neck injury imposes a responsibility of rigorous and prolonged vigilance and a constant state of readiness to intervene at short notice, with its attendant economic implications. Routine neck exploration seems to be both cost-effective and achievable, with minimal complications and no mortality.[29] For patients with developing neurologic signs, a computed tomography scan is of little value in excluding cerebral infarction; if the decision to repair a carotid artery is deferred until a scan is conclusive that action may come too late.

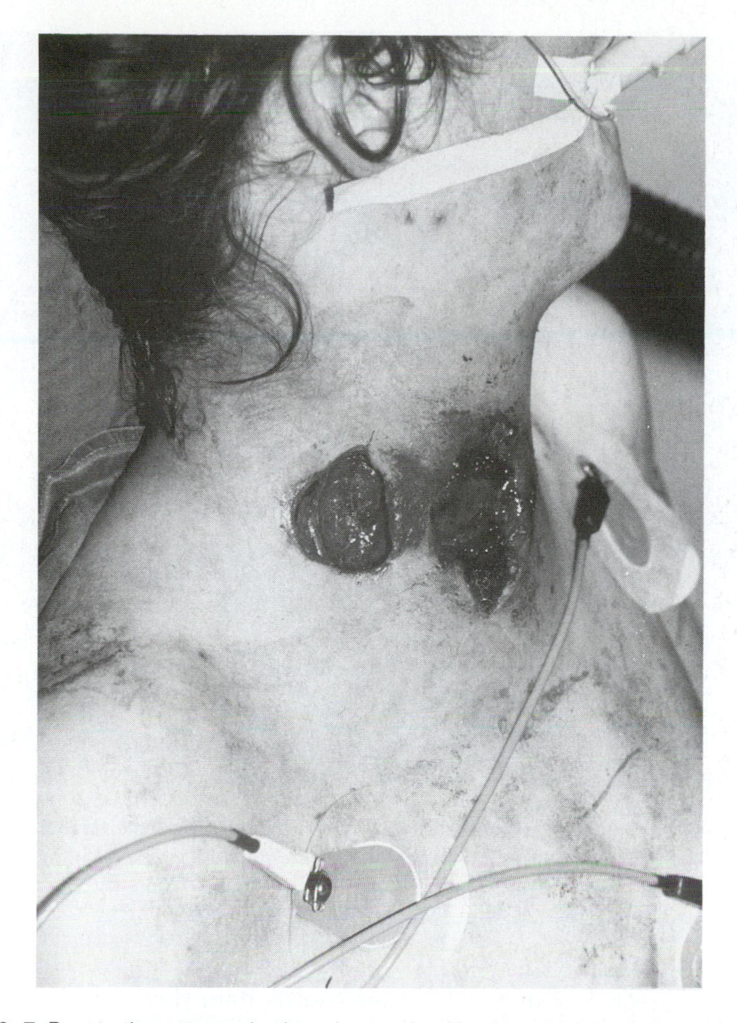

Figure 39–7. Penetrating entry and exit neck wounds with a hematoma and probable tracheal injury. The vital first measure was to insert an endotracheal tube and inflate the cuff beyond the assumed site of injury to prevent blood from entering the lungs. (*Reproduced with permission from Eastcott HHG, ed. Arterial Surgery. Edinburgh, UK: Churchill Livingstone; 1992:390.*)

Operative Management

The selection of patients for carotid artery repair based on the presence or absence of neurologic deficit is surrounded by controversy. The decision to repair a carotid artery in the neurologically intact patient presents no difficulty.[30,31] In one large series,[32] the outcome of carotid artery repair was observed in three groups of patients divided on the basis of the degree of the preoperative neurologic deficit—namely, none, mild, and severe. Among the patients with severe deficits, the mortality rate was prohibitively high, as has been observed by other authors.[20,32–34] This high rate is thought to be caused by hemorrhage into soft infarcted cerebral tissue; however, hemorrhage of some degree always occurs within infarcted tissue regardless of restoration of arterial flow. The true effect of anticoagulatory measures in these situations remains to be elucidated.

The previously held view that ligation was preferable to repair for all patients with neurologic deficits, so as to avert mortality,[35] has been superseded by evidence

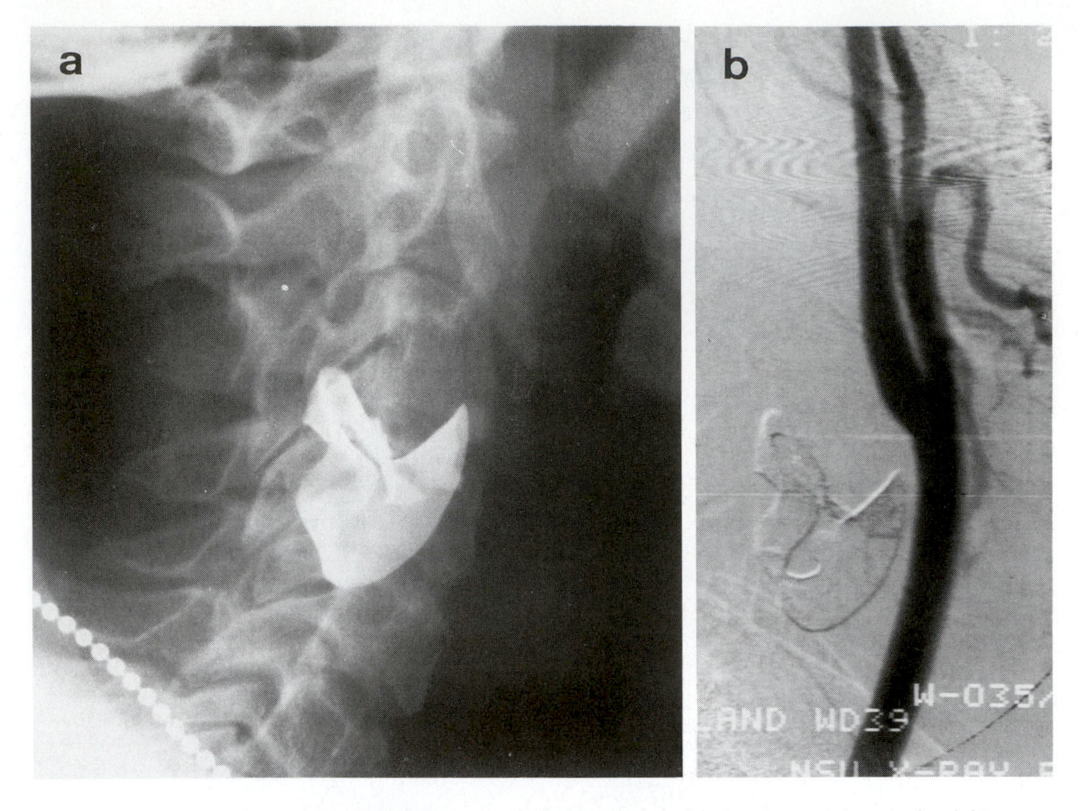

Figure 39–8. (**a**) Fragment of shrapnel lodged in the right carotid triangle very close to the right carotid system. (**b**) This angiogram shows the carotid system to be intact.

that primary vascular repair yields better results than those of ligation. Obviously, ligation might be justifiable in a patient with established neurologic deficit and complete thrombotic occlusion of the entire carotid. The consensus now firmly favors carotid reconstruction in cases of both blunt and penetrating injuries as long as antegrade flow is present.[20,30,31,36,37]

Systemic administration of heparin is acceptable in the patient with an isolated carotid injury, even when signs of cerebral ischemia are present. Consideration may be given to a nimodipine infusion as a means of countering cerebral arterial spasm. Through an oblique cervical incision, hematoma is evacuated and digital arterial control is secured. The risk of air embolism through an injured internal jugular vein calls for immediate head-down tilt to a level below that of the heart and control of the open vessel in preparation for repair. In cases of severe trauma, ligation is acceptable as long as the opposite internal jugular in intact. Distal clot from an injured carotid must be removed by balloon catheter prior to repair or insertion of a shunt. Evidence of backflow, preferably pulsatile, from the internal carotid artery suggests satisfactory cerebral perfusion, especially if it can be recorded above 60 to 70 mm Hg.[38] The presence of an inlying shunt, however, instills confidence and allows time for unhurried repair.

Lateral suture is acceptable for puncture wounds of the carotid artery, but vein patch repair prevents constriction. A short irreparable segment should be excised, and in some cases, end-to-end anastomosis may be possible without tension. In instances when graft interposition is necessary, a segment of proximal long saphenous vein of suitable caliber is harvested and slipped over an intraluminal shunt before it is inserted, to be removed later during completion of the second anastomosis (Fig. 39–9). An alternative to vein graft replacement of a damaged proximal internal carotid artery is to divide an intact proximal external carotid artery at a suitable level, detach it from its branches, and anastomose it obliquely end to end to the distal undamaged internal carotid artery.

In cases of blunt vascular trauma, an extensive segment of artery may have to be replaced by vein graft. Great care must be taken to preserve the cranial nerves that converge upward along with the internal carotid artery. In patients with zone III injuries in particular, a shunt not only ensures continued cerebral blood flow, but also acts as a stent, facilitating precise anastomoses to avoid stenosis. When a distal internal carotid artery stump is too short to permit anastomosis, an extracranial–intracranial bypass procedure might be considered after ligation of both ends of the internal carotid artery.[39] A completion angiogram is recommended to confirm the quality of carotid artery repair and to reveal the state of its intracranial ramifications. A drain is usually necessary, especially when the respiratory or gastrointestinal tract has been injured.

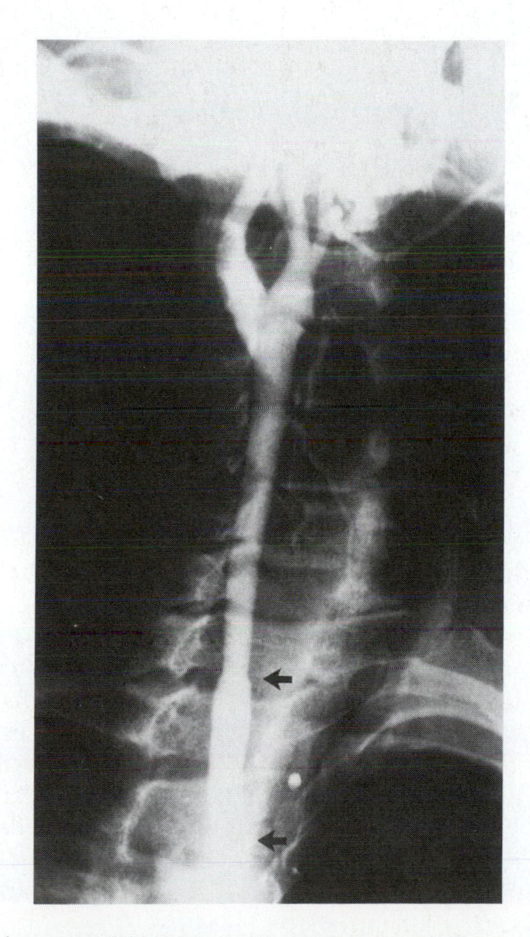

Figure 39–9. A sniper caused this high-velocity injury to the root of the neck; the left common carotid artery, which was severed, was reconstructed by using an interposition vein graft (*between arrows*). (*Reproduced with permission from Carter DC, Polk HC, eds. International Medical Reviews: Surgery. Vol. 1. Trauma. London, UK: Butterworth; 1981:300.*)

Postoperative Care and Outcome

The patient is usually nursed propped up, hemodynamic and neurologic functions are monitored, and wound drainage is checked. Discharge from a pharyngeal or an esophageal fistula may put the carotid repair at risk. Adequate cerebral perfusion must be ensured by volume and blood replacement. Any suspicion of neurologic deterioration must be investigated: While postoperative duplex ultrasound imaging may not be tolerated, transfemoral arch and carotid aortography will easily exclude thrombotic occlusion and identify a possible source of thromboembolism. If indicated, reoperation for thrombectomy and revision of the repair must be immediate, followed once more by angiography to ensure a satisfactory result.

The reported mortality rate among patients with carotid injuries sustained in the battlefield is 15% but decreases to 6% when deaths from other causes are excluded.[35] The mortality rate of patients with zone II penetrating injuries is about 5%,[28] whereas for patients with zone III injuries, it is 8.6%; the majority of the latter deaths are caused

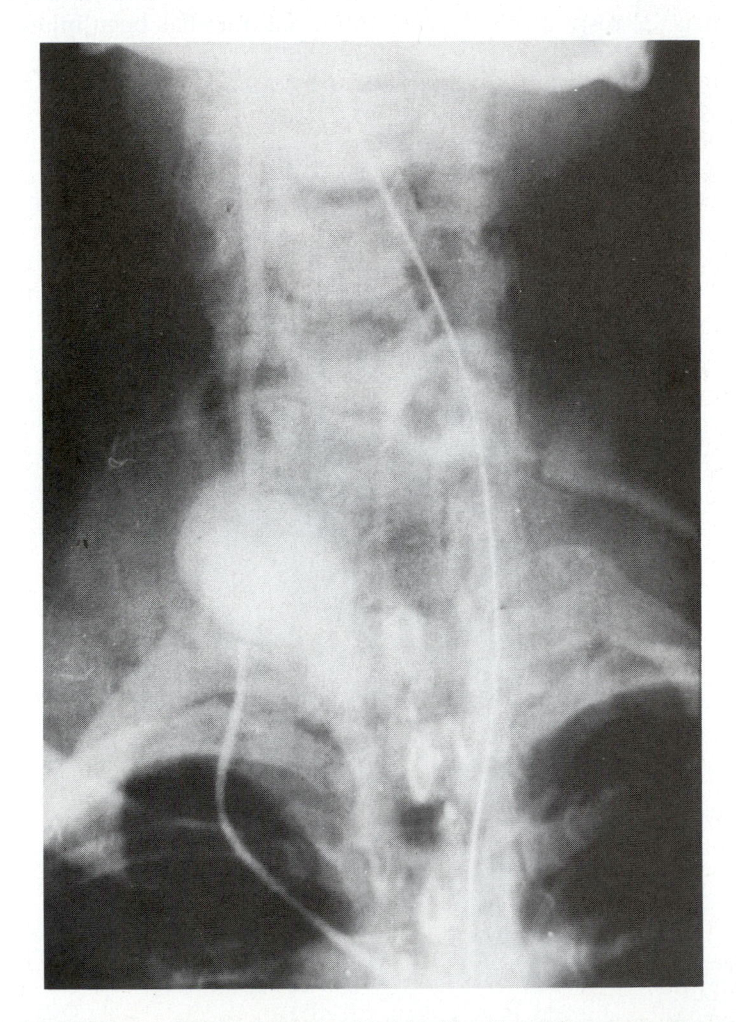

Figure 39–10. A forgotten direct blunt injury to the right side of the neck caused a false aneurysm of the first part of the right vertebral artery. The false aneurysm ruptured 1 year later. Note the tracheostomy and displacement of the nasogastric tube. (*Reproduced with permission from Eastcott HHG, ed. Arterial Surgery. Edinburgh, UK: Churchill Livingstone; 1992:394.*)

by neurologic complications.[40] For patients with blunt injury, the mortality is much higher at 10%, rising to 25% when comatose patients are included.[37,41]

VERTEBRAL ARTERY INJURIES

Injuries to the vertebral artery are rare and are usually caused by penetrating trauma.[42] In clinical terms, injuries of these vessels are generally much less significant than those of the carotid artery. The protected course of the vertebral artery in the neck often shields it from direct injury, except in its first part as it courses upward and posteriorly to enter the foramen in the transverse process of the sixth cervical vertebra. Bleeding, an unusual presentation, may occur in cases of posterolateral neck wounds; if the bleeding continues despite pressure on the carotid artery, the vertebral artery was probably injured. The usual injuries include thrombotic occlusion, false aneurysm, and arteriovenous fistula. Coexisting injuries to adjacent nerves may be expected. An undiagnosed vertebral artery injury may form a false aneurysm that gradually enlarges before it eventually ruptures with serious consequences (Fig. 39–10). Fracture of a cervical transverse process is potentially injurious to the vertebral artery. The third part of the vertebral artery, which lies beyond the scope of the vascular surgeon, may be injured, sometimes with fatal results, during a fistfight or a boxing match.

It is worth remembering that aplasia of the vertebral artery occurs occasionally, more commonly on the left side, and that ligation of a solitary vertebral artery could lead to midbrain necrosis. For this reason, preoperative angiography is essential not only to define the site and nature of the injury so that the operative exposure can be planned, but also to establish the existence of a patent contralateral vertebral artery.

Exposure of the vertebral artery through the neck is difficult but manageable. Ligation of the artery within its bony canal may be necessary on either side of the injury. Although direct repair may be technically feasible,[43] ligation is acceptable if it is known that the patient has a normal contralateral vertebral artery and an intact circle of Willis. Alternatively, a radiologist may be able to insert an occluding balloon, most appropriately in cases of a vertebral arteriovenous fistula, thereby averting a difficult operative intervention.

REFERENCES

1. Mattox KL, Feliciano DV, Burch J, et al. Five thousand seven hundred sixty cardiovascular injuries in 4,459 patients. *Ann Surg.* 1989;209:698–707.
2. Barros D'Sa AAB. A decade of missile-induced vascular trauma. *Ann R Coll Surg Engl.* 1981;64:37–44.
3. Barros D'Sa AAB. Arterial injuries. In: Eastcott HHG, ed. *Arterial Surgery.* Edinburgh, UK: Churchill Livingstone; 1992:355–411.
4. Barros D'Sa AAB. Twenty five years of vascular trauma in Northern Ireland. *BMJ.* 1995;310:1–2.
5. Johnston GW, Barros D'Sa AAB. Injuries of civil hostilities. In: Carter DC, Polk HC, eds. *International Medical Reviews: Surgery.* Vol. 1. *Trauma.* London, UK: Butterworth; 1981:284–301.
6. Bricker DL, Noon GP, Beall AC, et al. Vascular injuries of the thoracic outlet. *J Trauma.* 1970;10:1–15.
7. Reul GJ, Beall AC, Jordon GL, et al. The early operative management of injuries to the great vessels. *Surgery.* 1973;74:862–873.

8. Flint LM, Snyder WH, Perry MO, et al. Management of major vascular injuries in the base of the neck. *Arch Surg.* 1973;106:407–413.
9. Hewitt RL, Smith AD, Becker ML, et al. Penetrating vascular injuries of the thoracic outlet. *Surgery.* 1974;76:715–722.
10. Rich NM, Baugh JH, Hughes CW. Acute arterial injuries in Vietnam: 1000 cases. *J Trauma.* 1970;10:359–369.
11. Graham JM, Feliciano DV, Mattox KL, et al. Innominate vascular injury. *J Trauma.* 1982;22:647–655.
12. Lim LT, Saletta JD, Flanigan DP. Subclavian and innominate artery trauma. A five year experience with 17 patients. *Surgery.* 1979;86:890–897.
13. Silen W, Spieker D. Fatal hemorrhage from the innominate artery after tracheostomy. *Ann Surg.* 1965;162:1005–1012.
14. Johnson RH, Wall MJ, Mattox KL. Innominate artery trauma, a thirty year experience. *J Vasc Surg.* 1993;17:134–140.
15. Posner MC, Deitrick J, McGrath P. Non-penetrating vascular injury to the subclavian artery. *J Vasc Surg.* 1988;8:611–617.
16. Rich NM, Hobson RW, Jarstfer BS, et al. Subclavian artery trauma. *J Trauma.* 1973;13:485–496.
17. Brawley RK, Murray GF, Crisler C. Management of wounds of the innominate, subclavian and axillary vessels. *Surg Gynecol Obstet.* 1970;131:1130–1140.
18. Mitchell RL, Enright LP. The surgical management of acute and chronic injuries of the thoracic aorta. *Surg Gynecol Obstet.* 1983;157:1–4.
19. Feliciano D, Mattox KL, Graham J, et al. Five-year experience with PTFE grafts in vascular wounds. *J Trauma.* 1985;25:71–82.
20. Bradley EL. Management of penetrating carotid injuries: an alternative approach. *J Trauma.* 1973;13:748–753.
21. Legerwood AM, Mullins RJ, Lucas CE. Primary repair versus ligation for carotid artery injuries. *Arch Surg.* 1980;115:488–493.
22. Monson DO, Saletta JD, Freeark RJ. Carotid–vertebral trauma. *J Trauma.* 1969;9:987–999.
23. Fogelman MJ, Stewart RD. Penetrating wounds of the neck. *Am J Surg.* 1956;91:581–593.
24. Roon AJ, Christensen M. Evaluation of the treatment of penetrating cervical injuries. *J Trauma.* 1979;19:391–397.
25. Casbares HV. Selective surgical management of penetrating neck trauma: 15-year experience in a community hospital. *Am J Surg.* 1982;48:355–358.
26. Rao PM, Bhatti MFK, Gaudino J, et al. Penetrating injuries of the neck: criteria for exploration. *J Trauma.* 1983;23:47–49.
27. Golueke PJ, Goldstein AS, Scalfani SJA, et al. Routine versus selective exploration for penetrating neck injuries: a randomized prospective study. *J Trauma.* 1984;24:1010–1014.
28. Noyes LD, McSwain NE, Markowitz TP. Panendoscopy with arteriography versus mandatory exploration of penetrating wounds of the neck. *Ann Surg.* 1986;104:21–31.
29. Meyer JP, Barrett JA, Schuler JJ, et al. Mandatory vs. selective exploration for penetrating neck trauma. *Arch Surg.* 1987;122:592–597.
30. DiVicenti FC, Weber BB. Traumatic carotid artery injuries in civilian practice. *Ann Surg.* 1974;74:277–280.
31. Liekweg WG, Greenfield LJ. Management of penetrating carotid artery injury. *Ann Surg.* 1978;188:587–592.
32. Thal ER, Snyder WH, Hays RJ, et al. Management of carotid artery injuries. *Surgery.* 1974;76:955–962.
33. Yamada S, Kindt GW, Youmans JR. Carotid artery occlusion due to non-penetrating injury. *J Trauma.* 1967;7:333–342.
34. Unger SW, Tucker WS, Mrdeza MA, et al. Carotid arterial trauma. *Surgery.* 1980;87:477–487.
35. Cohen A, Brief D, Mathewson C. Carotid artery injuries: an analysis of 85 cases. *Am J Surg.* 1970;120:210–214.
36. McCormick TM, Burch BH. Routine angiographic evaluation of neck and extremity injuries. *J Trauma.* 1979;19:384–387.
37. Perry MO, Snyder WH, Thal ER. Carotid artery injuries caused by blunt trauma. *Ann Surg.* 1980;192:74–77.

38. Ehrenfeld WK, Stoney RJ, Wylie EJ. Relation of carotid stump pressure to safety of carotid artery ligation. *Surgery.* 1983;93:299.
39. Gewertz B, Samson D, Ditmore QM, et al. Management of penetrating injuries of the internal carotid artery at the base of the skull using extracranial–intracranial bypass. *J Trauma.* 1980;20:365–369.
40. Scalfani SJ, Panetta T, Goldstein AS, et al. Management of arterial injuries caused by penetration of zone III of the neck. *J Trauma.* 1985;25:871–881.
41. Fabian TC, George SM, Croce MA, et al. Carotid artery trauma. Management based on mechanism of injury. *J Trauma.* 1990;30:953–963.
42. Reid JS, Weigelt JA. Forty-three cases of vertebral artery trauma. *J Trauma.* 1988;28:1007–1012.
43. Brink BJ, Meier D, Fry WJ. Operative exposure and management of lesions in the vertebral artery. *J Cardiovasc Surg (Torino).* 1979;20:435–436.

40

Popliteal and Infrapopliteal Arterial Trauma

Joseph H. Frankhouse, MD, Albert E. Yellin, MD, FACS, and Fred A. Weaver, MD, FACS

Popliteal and infrapopliteal arterial trauma maximally challenges the operative and clinical decision-making skills of the vascular surgeon. Although the perigenicular blood vessels sustain only 10% of all vascular trauma, injuries to these vessels account for 65% of all post-traumatic amputations.[1] Proper treatment requires a thorough understanding of the etiologic mechanisms of injury, diagnostic techniques, operative management, adjunctive therapy, and rehabilitation. Advances in each of these areas has resulted in a marked reduction in the number of amputations and has increased the patient's likelihood of regaining a fully functional limb after popliteal or infrapopliteal arterial injury. In our experience with more than 200 popliteal artery (PA) injuries treated during a 20-year period, the amputation rate decreased from 20% to approximately 3%.[2,3] Rarely does an amputation occur as a result of a failed vascular repair. The ultimate functional outcome of the leg depends not on the adequacy of the arterial repair, but on the resolution of the neurologic, orthopedic, and soft tissue injuries that frequently accompany the vascular injury.

HISTORICAL PERSPECTIVE

In terms of time frame, advances in the treatment of arterial trauma have paralleled the major 20th century wars. During the two world wars, because of the fear of infection and fatal delayed hemorrhage, surgeons uniformly treated arterial injuries by ligation. The classic report in 1946 by DeBakey and Simeone[4] documented that this practice resulted in an overall amputation rate of 50% for extremity injuries, but a strikingly higher rate of 73% for PA trauma. During the Korean War, the techniques of vascular repair were introduced, and most arterial injuries were repaired; the result was a lowering of the amputation rate for PA trauma to 32%.[5] Further experience with PA repair during the Vietnam War failed to improve upon the limb salvage rate.[6]

The results of treating civilian vascular injuries have not paralleled those for military vascular trauma: Amputation rates resulting from popliteal and infrapopliteal injuries continue to decline in civilian settings. Limb loss is most frequent following blunt trauma, shotgun wounds, and injuries to all three tibial vessels. Although in some series no major amputations resulted,[7] as recently as 1993 extremity loss occurred in as many as 62% of the cases of blunt traumatic injury.[8] Better results follow the treatment of penetrating injuries: Amputations occur in less than 5% of all cases. Refinements in the diagnostic methods, operative techniques, and adjunctive measures have evolved and contributed to improved extremity salvage rates.

ANATOMY

The origin of the PA lies at the tendinous hiatus of the adductor magnus muscle. It courses behind the distal femur and proximal tibia, extending several centimeters below the knee joint. Although the termination of the PA is frequently referred to as the *trifurcation,* this pattern is uncommon. Usually, the PA bifurcates into the anterior tibial artery (ATA) and the tibioperoneal trunk (TPT) an average distance of 5.8 cm below the tibial plateau.[9] The ATA travels distally in the anterior compartment, accompanied by the deep peroneal nerve. The TPT gives rise to the posterior tibial artery (PTA) and the peroneal artery, both of which lie in the deep posterior compartment. The popliteal vein lies medial to the PA. The tibial nerve continues alongside the artery distally within the deep posterior compartment. This proximate relationship of neurovascular and bony structures accounts for the frequency with which associated injuries are encountered.

The location of the PA renders it uniquely prone to injury during knee dislocation or distal femur and proximal tibia fractures. Superiorly, as the artery enters the popliteal fossa, it is anchored to the femur by the tendon of the adductor magnus. The fibrous arch of the soleus and the interosseus membrane tether it inferiorly. This anatomic arrangement leaves the PA vulnerable to any genicular displacement or laceration by bone fragments.

MECHANISMS OF INJURY

Unlike the military experience, in which the majority of extremity vascular injuries were due to high-velocity missiles, the civilian vascular trauma experience involves a variety of blunt and low-velocity penetrating mechanisms. The relative proportion of blunt trauma versus penetrating trauma reflects the environment. Urban trauma centers report higher percentages of penetrating trauma, whereas in rural settings more blunt injuries are seen.

Penetrating Trauma

Penetrating trauma involves injuries caused by stab wounds, low-velocity handguns, high-velocity rifles, and shotguns. Iatrogenic injuries have also been reported, often associated with penetration of the posterior knee capsule during arthroscopic meniscectomy.[10] The kinetic energy of stabs and most handgun missiles is of insufficient magnitude to produce a significant degree of injury to the surrounding tissue. Therefore, limb salvage rates approach 100% following these injuries. High-velocity rifle missiles and close-range shotgun wounds produce larger vascular injuries and much greater adjacent soft and bony tissue destruction, thereby causing the majority of the morbidity from penetrating PA trauma.

Blunt Trauma

The mechanism of blunt traumatic injuries is highly variable. Typically, there is more extensive injury to skeletal, neural, soft tissue, and vascular structures. Motor vehicle, motorcycle, and automobile accidents, rather than pedestrian accidents, produce the majority of blunt arterial injuries. Industrial accidents, including falls, crush injuries, and avulsion injuries, compose most of the rest. In automobile accidents, the knee and proximal tibia of the passenger commonly come into contact with the instrument panel; the result is posterior dislocation and/or tibial plateau fracture. Pedestrians and motorcycle accident victims often suffer perigenicular crush injuries from contact with automobile bumpers.

Knee dislocation, widely recognized as a causative factor in PA trauma, is associated with a 32% incidence of PA injury.[11] Historically, it was thought that only posterior dislocations of the knee could injure the artery, but it was subsequently shown that injury can occur with dislocation in any direction.[12] Anterior displacement of the knee stretches the PA, commonly resulting in thrombosis from contusion or disruption of the intima. Posterior dislocation characteristically produces a clean, sharp intimal fracture or transection of the artery.[12]

Considerable force must be delivered to the perigenicular area to cause dislocation or fracture. Such injury often causes sufficient soft tissue edema to compress or occlude genicular collateral vessels. Edema and hemorrhage combined with concomitant compartmental hypertension further jeopardize lower extremity perfusion after blunt popliteal or infrapopliteal arterial interruption.

PROGNOSIS OF EXTREMITY SALVAGE

The prognosis of popliteal and infrapopliteal vascular trauma more typically depends on the degree of soft tissue, orthopedic, and nerve damage incurred. Most important, the residual neurologic impairment frequently determines the ultimate functional status of the limb.

Many experts contend that the speed with which arterial continuity is re-established determines the success of extremity salvage. Experimental dog studies demonstrated that in cases in which femoral arterial and collateral blood flow was completely disrupted, extremity salvage rates of 90% occurred when arterial continuity was restored within 6 hours but dropped to 50% when the time of ischemia extended to 12 to 18 hours.[13] Myonecrosis commonly occurs when the total of ischemia time exceeds 6 to 8 hours. Although ischemia time is important, the time delay between injury and revascularization is not uniformly associated with amputation. Frequently, patients with the most severely injured limbs—with the worst soft tissue, bony, and nerve injuries—are taken to the operating room most rapidly.[3] Invariably, these injuries have the worst prognosis. An evaluation of 100 cases of blunt PA injury and 109 cases of penetrating PA injury treated at the Los Angeles County and University of Southern California Medical Center (LAC+USCMC) demonstrated no difference in time to revascularization between patients who underwent amputation and those who did not.[2,3] Functional limb salvage can occur following periods of ischemia in excess of 20 hours.[2,14] Therefore, a lengthy ischemia time should not preclude attempts at revascularization. Nonetheless, unnecessary delay must be avoided, and the preoperative assessment should be performed expeditiously in order to optimize limb salvage.

Restoration of blood flow to the lower extremity following popliteal trauma is not the sole determinant successful limb salvage. Attempts have been made to identify the limbs that are at highest risk for amputation preoperatively and to determine whether primary amputation is preferable. The Mangled Extremity Severity Score is one such attempt.[15] To further identify patients at highest risk of limb loss, we analyzed the 209 cases of PA injury treated at LAC+USCMC. Only severe soft tissue injury and deep soft tissue infection correlated with eventual amputation.[2,3] Since these factors cannot be accurately determined preoperatively, most such evaluation systems fail to reliably differentiate the patient who can regain a functional leg from the patient who will ultimately undergo amputation. Therefore, we opt to aggressively revascularize and treat all patients. We believe that the decision for amputation is best arrived at with the patient and family after maximum attempts at limb salvage have been made, and with input from orthopedists, plastic surgeons, and physiatrists.

Our experience allowed us to identify certain injury characteristics and treatment modalities that seem to predict a successful or an unsuccessful outcome. These factors in patients with blunt or penetrating PA trauma are outlined in Table 40–1.

DIAGNOSTIC CONSIDERATIONS

During World War II and the Korean War, all penetrating wounds with clinical ischemia or near a major vascular structure were routinely explored. This basic philosophy also became the accepted practice in the civilian trauma setting. Routine exploration was advocated in order to avoid missing an occult vascular injury. Surgeons were concerned that missed injuries could result in delayed hemorrhage, embolization, or thrombosis. Although few arterial injuries were missed, an unacceptably large number of unnecessary operations resulted. In the 1970s, routine screening arteriography replaced exploration, but it was not until 1978 that the validity of contrast arteriography was documented to be reliable in excluding penetrating vascular injury.[16] This diagnostic advance eliminated negative surgical explorations and identified clinically occult injuries in as many as 20% of the cases.[17]

In the 1980s, the concept of routine screening arteriography for all patients with penetrating extremity trauma was challenged as excessively broad, with too many negative arteriograms. Moreover, the incidence of false-negative and false-positive arteriograms, although low, is real, with reports as high as 2%.[17] Angiography is expensive, costing as much as $1,500 per study. Furthermore, complications such as nephrotoxicity, allergic reactions, arterial injury, and hematoma can result. Finally, referring a patient to the radiology suite to obtain an arteriogram delays definitive operative repair by 2 to 3 hours in most hospitals.

Based on our experience at LAC+USCMC, a diagnostic algorithm evolved for the management of patients with popliteal or infrapopliteal vascular trauma, regardless of the mechanism (Fig. 40–1). Patients with hard, or obvious, signs of vascular injury include those with arterial hemorrhages; an expanding or pulsatile hematoma; or a cool, ischemic, pulseless foot. This group of patients is best managed by immediate surgery, during which arteriography can be performed if necessary. Referral to the radiology suite for preoperative arteriography in these patients results in a critical delay.

The majority of patients present with less obvious or clinically occult signs of vascular trauma. A prospective study at LAC+USCMC stratified penetrating injuries according to the risk of needing operative intervention and concluded that only a pulse deficit or a Doppler ankle–brachial index (ABI) less than 1.00 predicted a significant injury.[18] Proximity, neurologic deficit, bruit, and fracture were not statistically correlated with arterial injury. Therefore, in the absence of hard signs, either a pulse deficit or an

TABLE 40–1. RISK FACTORS ASSOCIATED WITH AMPUTATION AT LOS ANGELES COUNTY AND UNIVERSITY OF SOUTHERN CALIFORNIA MEDICAL CENTER

	Penetrating Trauma		Blunt Trauma	
Risk Factor	*No. of Patients*	*Amputations (%)*	*No. of Patients*	*Amputations (%)*
Preoperative				
Mechanism of injury[a]				
SGW	20	6 (30)[b]	N/A	
GSW, SW	86	1 (1)		
Soft tissue injury				
Minimal–moderate	94	0 (0)[b]	69	2 (3)[b]
Severe	15	7 (47)	31	13 (42)
Preoperative ischemia				
No	49	2 (4)	36	0 (0)[b]
Yes	60	5 (8)	64	15 (23)
Preoperative compartmental syndrome				
No	91	6 (7)	83	13 (16)
Yes	18	1 (6)	17	2 (12)
Preoperative delay > 6 hr				
No	42	2 (5)	24	5 (21)
Yes	67	5 (7)	40	10 (25)
Preoperative delay > 12 hr				
No	72	6 (8)	50	13 (26)
Yes	37	1 (3)	14	2 (14)
Operative				
Arterial repair				
Primary	74	1 (1)[b]	49	3 (6)[b]
Vein graft	35	6 (17)	51	12 (24)
Intraoperative systemic heparinization				
No	7	1 (14)	29	9 (31)[b]
Yes	102	6 (6)	71	6 (8)
Popliteal vein injury				
No	59	2 (3)	71	9 (13)
Yes	50	5 (10)	29	6 (21)
Vein repair				
None	59	2 (3)	71	9 (13)
Repaired	40	4 (10)	23	4 (17)
Ligated	10	1 (10)	6	2 (33)
Postoperative				
Deep soft tissue infection				
No	99	2 (2)[b]	83	6 (7)[b]
Yes	10	5 (50)	17	9 (53)
Delayed fasciotomy				
No	105	4 (4)[b]	96	14 (15)
Yes	4	3 (75)	4	1 (25)

[a] SGW = shotgun wound; GSW = gunshot wound; SW = stab wound.
[b] $P < 0.05$.

ABI less than 1.00 is an indication for formal arteriography to exclude a lesion requiring surgery. An exception noted from previous studies is shotgun injuries, which can cause a vascular injury in the presence of normal pulses and an ABI greater than or equal to 1.00.[17] In the absence of these predictive findings, the patient may be safely observed. Obviously, concomitant head, chest, or abdominal injuries requiring emergency surgery

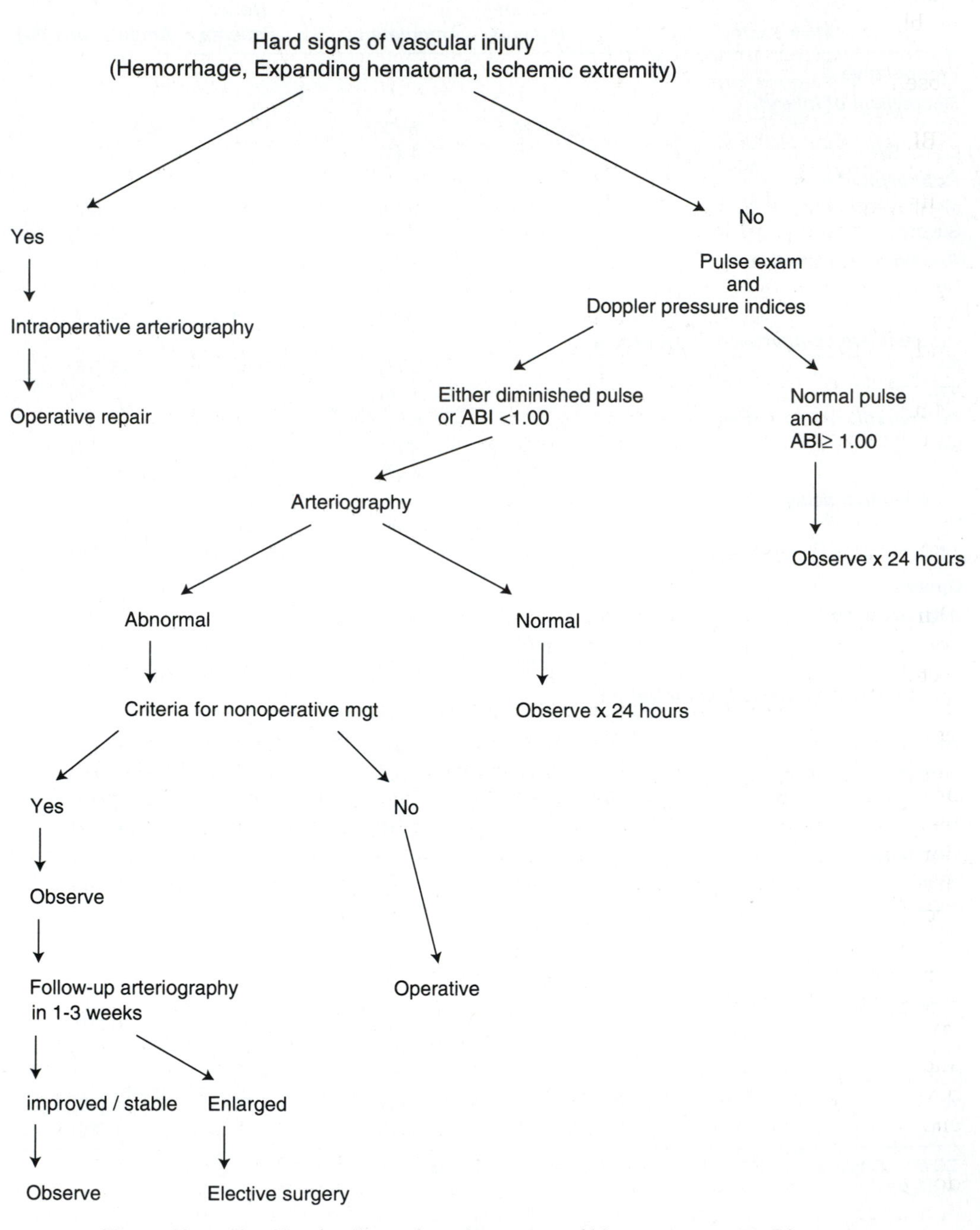

Figure 40–1. Algorithm for diagnosis and treatment of blunt or penetrating PA trauma.

may preclude formal angiography. In this group of patients, intraoperative arteriography is preferable for identifying injuries that need vascular repair.

In cases of blunt arterial trauma, prospective data from LAC+USCMC indicated that a pulse deficit correlated with an injury requiring surgery.[12,19] Because of the nature of blunt injuries, an ABI is frequently not obtainable, but a careful pulse evaluation suffices to determine which patients to refer for arteriography and which to safely observe. However, among our patients for whom an ABI could be obtained, those with arterial injury had a decreased ABI compared with that of those without injury. An ABI less than 1.00 was 100% sensitive in predicting arterial injury but had a low specificity.[19] Prospective studies may further clarify the value of the ABI for patients with blunt vascular trauma. Patients who do not undergo screening arteriography are kept in the hospital for a 24-hour observation period.

Screening potential vascular injuries with duplex ultrasonography has been suggested.[20–22] This technique is an attractive alternative to contrast arteriography due to its noninvasive nature and low cost, but controversy exists in regard to its sensitivity and practicality.[23] This diagnostic modality requires a high level of technical expertise, particularly when there are associated musculoskeletal injuries, and it is rarely available 24 hours a day. Currently, this tool should be used only under investigational guidelines, but it may have potential in the diagnosis of arterial trauma.

NONOPERATIVE MANAGEMENT

Our diagnostic algorithm is predicated on accepting the fact that by not performing routine arteriography a small number of clinically occult arterial injuries will go undetected. The major issue is whether these injuries progress or resolve. To validate the concept of selective arteriography, the physician must understand the natural history of minimal or nonocclusive arterial injuries. It was previously thought that any lesion detected on an arteriogram, no matter how small, could eventually lead to thrombosis or delayed hemorrhage and disastrous medical and medicolegal consequences. This theory led surgeons to attempt to identify and repair all injuries. More recent observations that iatrogenic arterial trauma caused by the devices used in endovascular procedures usually healed without complication prompted prospective studies of clinically occult, arteriographically demonstrated lesions.[24,25] These studies led to specific criteria for the selective management of nonocclusive arterial injuries. Nonoperative treatment is recommended if the following criteria are met: (1) low-velocity injury; (2) minimal arterial wall disruption—less than 5 mm for intimal defects or pseudoaneurysms; (3) adherent or downstream protrusion of intimal flaps; (4) intact distal circulation; and (5) no active hemorrhage.[24] In cases when diminished contrast density is evident beyond the intimal flap, consideration should be given to operative repair. This phenomenon may be observed with intimal flaps causing physiologically diminished distal flow despite the criteria. Serial arteriography or duplex scanning should be used to document stability or healing of the injury, or the need for subsequent surgical intervention. Although some surgeons are reluctant to accept the concept of nonoperative treatment of these injuries, their concerns are increasingly at odds with the growing body of literature regarding the natural history and safety of these nonoperatively managed lesions.[26,27] Although an occasional intimal defect or a small pseudoaneurysm has enlarged, no serious sequelae have occurred, and all such lesions have been repaired electively. Fears of serious complications such as false aneurysm rupture, dissection, arteriovenous fistula, and delayed thrombosis have not been realized in the follow-up of more than 100 patients managed nonoperatively on the basis of the aforementioned criteria.

OPERATIVE MANAGEMENT

Once the decision to perform a vascular repair is made, the lesion should be repaired as expeditiously as possible. Multitrauma victims may have head, chest, and abdominal injuries that take precedence over extremity revascularization. These priorities must be considered by the treating physicians.

Combined Skeletal and Vascular Injuries

Controversy exists regarding the sequence of bone fixation and arterial repair in patients with combined skeletal and vascular trauma. We have not seen any correlation between amputation risk and magnitude of skeletal trauma; therefore, we believe that almost all ischemic limbs warrant re-establishment of blood flow prior to bone fixation. Rare exceptions may exist in cases of nonischemic limbs in which (1) the severity and instability of the fracture are considerable; (2) orthopedic manipulation would likely disrupt the arterial repair; and (3) external fixation can be applied in 30 to 60 minutes. In such instances, some physicians advocate using temporary intraluminal vascular shunts to maintain perfusion during orthopedic stabilization.[28] We rarely find such shunts necessary. The fear that disruption of the arterial repair will occur during orthopedic stabilization is largely unfounded. However, after the orthopedic procedure is completed but prior to wound closure, the vascular surgeon must examine the vessels and confirm the integrity of the repair and the presence of pulses.

External fixation is the most appropriate method of achieving bony stabilization in patients with combined vascular and skeletal trauma. Plaster casts often provide inadequate stabilization, mask or cause the development of compartmental hypertension, and prevent good wound care. Internal fixation has been popularized for closed fractures; however, these time-consuming procedures require extensive muscle dissection, which can destroy collateral circulation. The rapidity with which external fixators can be applied without the need for dissection makes external fixation the procedure of choice.

Techniques of Arterial Repair

Popliteal artery repair can be achieved by means of the medial approach or the posterior approach (Fig. 40–2). For patients in whom the injury is localized in the popliteal fossa, the posterior approach provides better exposure. This requires placing the patient in the prone position and can be done safely despite skeletal trauma. The medial approach is best suited for the majority of injuries and allows for proximal or distal extension of the incision. This approach permits surgical correction of coexisting injuries to the distal superficial femoral artery, popliteal trifurcation, and PTA. Blood loss can be reduced by placing a sterile pneumatic tourniquet on the thigh and inflating it during the dissection and at appropriate times during the repair. The entire contralateral leg should be prepared into the operative field in the event that a saphenous vein bypass or interposition graft is needed. Theoretically, all veins in the injured extremity should be preserved, including the superficial veins, since the deep venous system is often occluded or compromised. If both legs suffered trauma, upper extremities can be used to harvest cephalic vein.

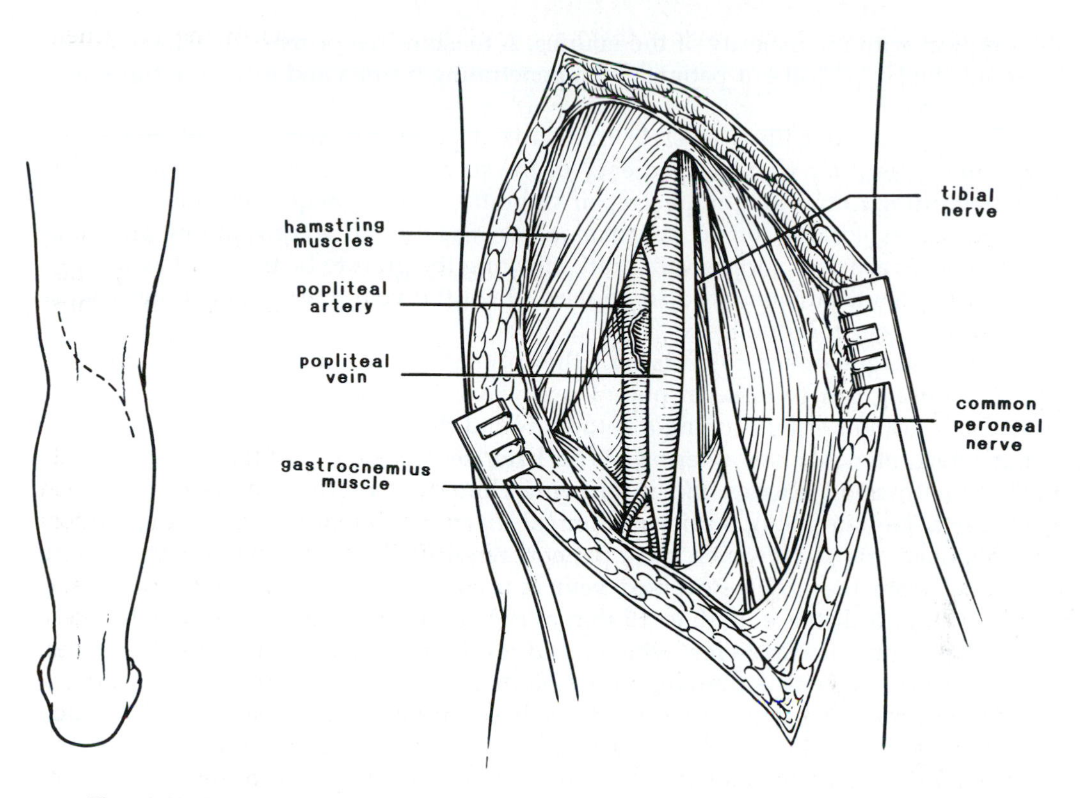

Figure 40–2. Posterior approach for localized PA trauma. *(Reprinted from Trauma Surgery: Techniques in Thoracic, Abdominal, and Vascular Surgery (1994) by Arthur Donovan, M.D.; Mosby–Year Book, 259.)*

Once the injured PA is exposed, all traumatized arteries should be debrided. The extent of injury can extend beyond that which grossly appears contused. This possibility is of particular concern in cases of blunt trauma and high-velocity missile injuries due to the associated concussive forces of these injuries. Any portion of artery with buckled or disrupted intima should be debrided. If any doubt exists, debridement beyond the grossly injured artery is recommended.

Following removal of local thrombus and adequate debridement of injured artery, as long as there is brisk forward bleeding and back bleeding, there is no need for passing Fogarty embolectomy catheters. If blood flow appears reduced, gentle irrigation will frequently dislodge thrombus. If this fails, Fogarty catheters may be passed proximally and distally. However, care must be taken not to overinflate the Fogarty balloon during withdrawal. Otherwise, the endothelial surface will be damaged and rendered thrombogenic, and the risk of vasospasm will increase.

The subject of primary reanastomosis versus liberal use of autologous vein graft remains controversial. Lim and associates[14] contend that the extensive mobilization of the artery required to achieve approximation of the ends mandates the sacrifice of valuable genicular collateral pathways. Our experience, as well as that of others,[2,3,29] shows that the majority of injuries can be repaired primarily and that there is an increased rate of amputation when vein grafts are required. The increased frequency of limb loss with vein interposition reflects the severity of the underlying trauma that necessitated the graft, not an inherent property of the graft. The genicular collateral vessels are unlikely to be important in a nonatherosclerotic, acutely traumatized artery, as is typical with the majority of the injuries. A tension-free primary anastomosis was accomplished in 68% of our patients with penetrating trauma and in 49% of those with blunt trauma.[2,3]

For the patient with a severely traumatized popliteal fossa or with major soft tissue injury, and for whom expediency of the surgery is important, we rely on vein bypass grafting rather than in-line repair or grafts. This technique obviates a difficult and tedious exploration of the vascular injury. Superficial femoral inflow and tibial target arteries are used for the vein graft, allowing the graft to be tunneled away from the injury. This technique can also be used when the vein graft would otherwise be exposed due to soft tissue loss.

The technique of anastomosis for either primary repair, interposition grafting, or bypass grafting can be done in one of two ways: The anastomosis may be done in trifurcated fashion or by running a suture around the posterior half of the vessel and using interrupted sutures anteriorly. The latter technique is routinely employed in patients with small arteries and in growing children. Contralateral saphenous vein from the ankle may be of sufficient luminal diameter to match a small popliteal or infrapopliteal artery. However, most patients require a larger caliber saphenous vein harvested from the groin. Reversed vein is used. The artery and vein are usually spatulated for a distance of 10 to 15 mm at each end, to avoid size mismatch and to prevent anastomotic narrowing, which could result in delayed thrombosis. Anastomoses are completed with a running 5-0 to 7-0 monofilament suture, depending on the size of the vessels. When the injury extends beyond the origin of the ATA, this vessel is ligated, and the distal end of the graft is anastomosed to the TPT. Completion arteriography should be done to detect the adequacy of the anastomosis, to check for distal unrecognized injuries or retained thrombus, and to demonstrate runoff to the foot. Any abnormality should be corrected immediately, while the patient is still in the operating room.

Choice of Graft Material

Restoring arterial continuity with a tension-free primary anastomosis is ideal. When this is not possible, two conduits, autologous vein and polytetrafluoroethylene (PTFE), are commonly used for interposition or bypass grafting. Experience has been gained by using PTFE grafts as the conduit of choice in trauma and elective vascular surgery.[30–32] However, because of the problems of PTFE crossing the knee joint, the consensus is that PTFE is significantly inferior to autologous vein in terms of patency. Autologous vein can be harvested from multiple sites, depending on availability: opposite leg, lesser saphenous, or arm vein. In most instances, only several centimeters of graft are required.

Certain situations may preclude the use of autologous vein. Polytetrafluoroethylene may be a reasonable alternative for the hemodynamically unstable patient for whom the added time for vein harvest is deemed unsafe. However, as previously stated, rapid revascularization may be possible by utilizing a vein bypass without entering the popliteal space. Other patients may have no usable vein due to previous intravenous drug abuse or may have inadequate veins due to stenoses, aneurysmal dilatations, or size less than 4 mm. Invariably, there is a short segment of lesser saphenous vein available. In extremities with large contaminated wounds or in the face of potentially exposed graft, PTFE has shown superiority to autologous vein in some clinical and animal studies.[31,32] If, in the surgeon's judgment, PTFE is necessary, the diameter of the graft should be at least 6 mm, since smaller grafts result in unacceptably high rates of thombosis.[31]

Popliteal Vein Injury

The management of popliteal venous trauma has sparked debate since Rich et al[33] first reported that during the Vietnam War popliteal venous ligation resulted in a higher amputation rate than that associated with venous repair. It has been suggested that venous repair improves the patency of the arterial repair and minimizes the long-term sequelae of venous hypertension. Because of the anatomic proximity of the PA and the popliteal vein, injury to both vessels occurs in one-third of the patients. Animal studies have demonstrated substantially reduced blood flow in the femoral artery after femoral vein ligation.[34] This reduced flow could predispose the arterial repair to thrombosis. Acute venous hypertension resulting from popliteal vein ligation that resolved with venous repair has also been reported.[35] A 10-year follow-up study of Vietnam veterans who underwent popliteal vein ligation revealed significant edema in 51% of the patients who underwent ligation, compared with 13% of those who underwent vein repair.[36] Conversely, postoperative venograms have documented that more than 50% of all venous repairs thrombose within 1 week and that thrombosis is not necessarily associated with clinically evident edema.[37] Historically, venous ligation has been associated with more severe injuries, which perhaps accounts for the increased morbidity. Recent data, including our own, fail to provide convincing evidence that vein ligation increases the risk of amputation or edema.[3,38,39]

It has been argued that because most venous repairs thrombose, there is an increased risk of pulmonary embolus and clinical thrombophlebitis. However, this phenomenon has not been observed clinically, even when a venous repair does thrombose. The goal of venous repair is to maintain early patency in order to augment venous return during the early postoperative period while collateral venous channels develop. It is well recognized that thrombosis of venous repairs commonly occurs after 24 hours, is usually asymptomatic, and has the potential for recanalization.[35] Despite the ongoing debate regarding the merit of venous repair, we attempt repair in any patient whose condition is not unduly compromised. Lateral venorrhaphy, vein patch angioplasty, primary repair, and vein interposition grafting are all acceptable techniques. Conversely, in a critically ill patient, when the operating time has been lengthy, or when local factors make it difficult to effect a simple tension-free repair, we do not hesitate to ligate the popliteal vein. The patient's leg is then kept elevated postoperatively and wrapped in an elastic bandage.

Compartmental Syndrome and the Use of Fasciotomy

Compartmental hypertension is a frequent occurrence before, during, and after surgery. Muscles of the lower leg can become markedly edematous due to the trauma as well as to reperfusion syndrome following ischemia. Intracompartmental hemorrhage can also lead to this condition. The preoperative diagnosis of compartmental hypertension is primarily clinical, but it can be obscured by an associated neurologic injury. A tense compartment is the hallmark sign, typically associated with hypesthesia or pain with passive stretch. If any question remains about the existence of this syndrome, one of several commercially available needle catheter pressure transducers can be used to determine the pressure within the compartments. Fasciotomy should be considered when pressures exceed 30 mm Hg and is definitely indicated for pressures in excess of 40 mm Hg. If this condition is left untreated, venous return and arterial flow will be impaired, which can result in thrombosis of the vascular repair, myonecrosis, and permanent loss of neurological function. The morbidity can range from footdrop due to a deep peroneal nerve deficit, to loss of all muscles and amputation.

Much of the credit for improved limb salvage rates goes to the liberal use of intraoperative prophylactic fasciotomy. Several authors recommend performing four-compartment fasciotomy prophylactically in the setting of certain risk factors.[7,14] The factors that predispose a patient to postoperative compartmental hypertension are prolonged ischemia (>6 hours), vein injury, fractures, major soft tissue injury, and arterial laceration with intracompartmental bleeding.[14] Whether to perform fasciotomy prior to or following revascularization is debatable. It has been suggested that fasciotomy precede arterial repair in order to enhance collateral flow and possibly prevent myonecrosis pending revascularization.[14] Alternatively, and more typically, the decision is made after restoration of arterial continuity. Tense compartments, alone or in combination with one of the previously mentioned risk factors, indicate the need for decompression. The surgeon should have a low threshold for performing fasciotomy; therefore, there should rarely be the need for delayed postoperative fasciotomy. We found that the myonecrosis invariably associated with delayed treatment of compartmental hypertension increases the risk of invasive wound sepsis and amputation.[2]

The most effective, least time-consuming technique for performing four-compartment fasciotomy is that popularized by Mubarak and Owen.[40] This procedure utilizes an anterolateral incision to gain access to the anterior and lateral compartments. A posteromedial incision enables decompression of the superficial and deep posterior compartments. To prevent the skin from acting as a tourniquet and to ensure that the fascia has been opened the length of the leg, we modify the procedure by extending the skin incisions the length of the fasciotomy, thus creating a dermotomy–fasciotomy (DF) (Fig. 40–3).[41]

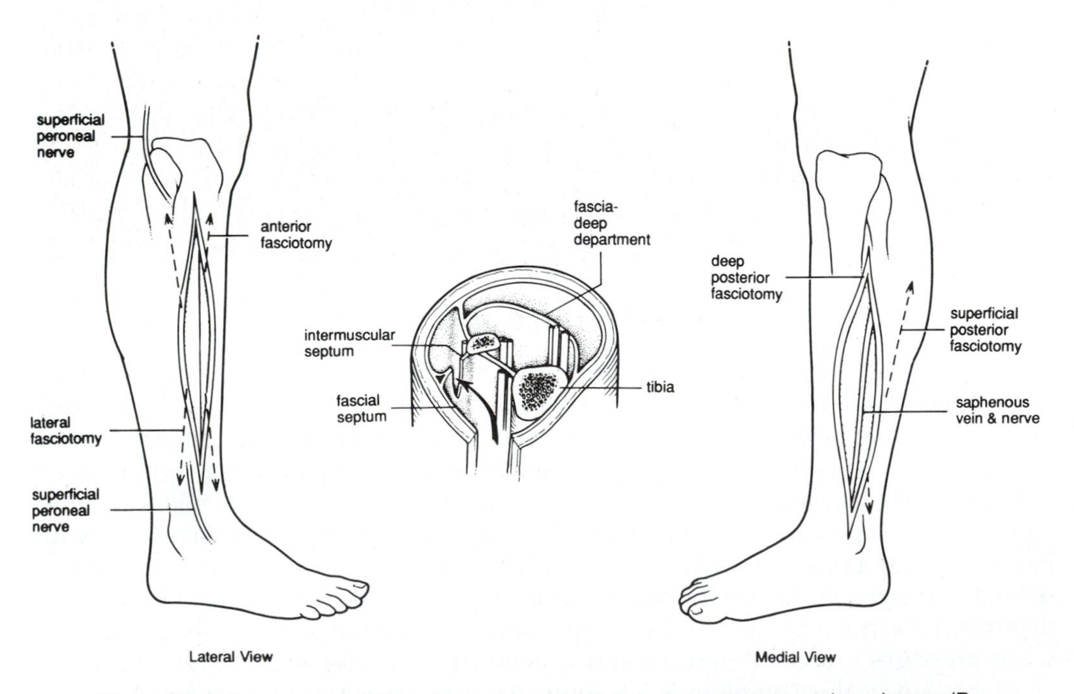

Figure 40–3. Dermotomy and four-compartment fasciotomy for compartmental syndrome. *(Reprinted from Trauma Surgery: Techniques in Thoracic, Abdominal, and Vascular Surgery (1994) by Arthur Donovan, M.D.; Mosby–Year Book Inc., 261.)*

Prevention of Limb Sepsis

Following DF, the patient is often left with large wounds and bulging muscle, which, when left open, can become a septic source. At LAC+USCMC, a wound complication rate of 51% occurred when DF incisions were closed secondarily; this rate was reduced to 5% when wounds were skin grafted at the initial operation.[41] The most effective method for closing the DF wounds entails primary closure of the anterolateral incision and immediate skin grafting of the posteromedial wound. Rarely can the surgeon safely reapproximate both dermotomy incisions primarily. A few extreme cases require skin grafting to both.

Among the most ominous factors we found to be associated with eventual limb loss are the presence of severe soft tissue injury and invasive wound sepsis.[2] The latter is usually preventable. Small-vessel thrombosis and infection of devitalized tissue in these high-risk patients may be prevented by expeditious vascular reconstruction and aggressive soft tissue debridement.[2] Since the institution of this policy of aggressive debridement in 1980, our infection rate fell from 25% to 9%, with no amputations related to limb sepsis.[2] The desire to preserve tissue of questionable viability in order to cover the vascular repair or to maintain function of the extremity should be discouraged. Large soft tissue defects can be covered by local rotational and free muscle flaps. When the viability of the remaining muscle is questionable, wounds should be left open, and plans made for both a "second-look" procedure and repeat debridement within 24 to 48 hours. All patients with persistent, unexplained sepsis should undergo wound re-exploration. In extreme situations, porcine skin grafts can be used to cover the arterial repair.[42] The combination of aggressive debridement, primary skin coverage, and broad-spectrum antibiotics is paramount in the prevention of deep wound sepsis, which is the most common cause of amputation in these severely injured extremities.

Adjunctive Measures

Patients without contraindications to anticoagulation—namely, concurrent intracranial, intrathoracic, or intra-abdominal injuries—benefit from early systemic heparinization.[3,14,43] It is thought that anticoagulation prevents collateral, distal arteriolar, and venous thrombosis, thereby preserving any remaining circulation. Once small-vessel thrombosis occurs, it is impossible to remove or flush out the clots. Therefore, early intraoperative anticoagulation may help prevent irreversible muscle ischemia while the vascular reconstruction is completed. In a series of 100 blunt injuries treated at our institution, heparinization was one of several variables associated with a decline in the amputation rate from 31% to 9%.[2] Heparin is given as a bolus at 10 U/kg of body weight as soon as the injured vessels are isolated. Heparin may be repeated as necessary and is usually reversed with protamine at the conclusion of the case. The routine intraoperative use of heparin in more than 200 cases of penetrating and blunt injuries was not associated with hemorrhagic complications. Intraoperative bleeding can be minimized by performing the vascular repair and debridement with the assistance of a tourniquet. When comorbid conditions preclude the use of anticoagulation, patients may derive some benefit from the regional use of heparin or from the antithrombotic, antiplatelet effects of dextran.

Severe muscle edema due to reperfusion following ischemia is well recognized. The underlying mechanism is the generation of oxygen-derived free radicals, which increase vascular permeability. Mannitol, 25 g administered intravenously immediately prior to reperfusion, reportedly reduces the need for fasciotomy.[7] The theoretical foundation for the use of mannitol is that it inactivates oxygen-derived free radicals and is a potent osmotic diuretic. These two actions serve to limit compartmental pressure. On the basis of its low toxicity and apparent benefit, mannitol should be used routinely.

SPECIAL CONSIDERATIONS REGARDING INFRAPOPLITEAL ARTERIAL INJURIES

The optimal management of infrapopliteal, or shank, arterial trauma is not as clearly defined as it is for PA injuries. Infrapopliteal trauma comprises only 5% of all reported civilian vascular injuries.[44] Because of the relative infrequency of these injuries, literature is not abundant, and uniform protocols for diagnosis and treatment do not exist.

The parallel blood supply of the infrapopliteal arteries affords natural protection against ischemia. Therefore, preoperative ischemia is not nearly as common as in cases of popliteal trauma. Accordingly, severe crush injuries, shotgun wounds, and multiple gunshot wounds are more likely to compromise blood flow by injuring more than one of the infrapopliteal vessels. However, the number of patent arteries to the foot necessary to maintain viability and prevent symptoms is unclear. The issue is central to management decisions when one, two, or all three shank arteries are injured. The clinical decision is when to repair, ligate, embolize, or observe. In the absence of clinical ischemia, injuries to a single shank artery are often unrecognized or deliberately not treated. Some patients return with delayed complications of pseudoaneurysm, arteriovenous fistula, or claudication. The incidence of late complications from undiagnosed injuries has never been documented but may be higher than previously realized. Experience has shown that delayed arterial repair for missed injuries or delayed presentation is considerably more difficult and is associated with a higher amputation rate.[45] Hence, as with PA injuries, early diagnosis and treatment should be routine.

Diagnostic Considerations

Our diagnostic algorithm for infrapopliteal arterial injury is similar to that for PA injury. Rapid revascularization is required in patients presenting with acute ischemic symptoms. A careful pulse examination and Doppler pressure indices will determine which patients need arteriography. Peroneal artery injuries frequently do not affect the pulse. Patients with single ATA or PTA injuries may present with normal pulses due to plantar collateral flow. Suspicion should be raised if manual compression of one tibial vessel results in loss of pulse in the other. Unlike in the case of PA injury, arteriography is especially useful for determining which arteries are affected, the level at which they are affected, and whether there is runoff to the foot. When the patient has a clearly ischemic extremity, hemorrhage, an expanding hematoma, or preoperative compartmental syndrome, this information can be obtained from an intraoperative arteriogram as opposed to a formal angiogram.

The loss of one infrapopliteal artery is well tolerated.[44,46,47] An exception is an injury at the level of the TPT. Some authors have suggested that this principle may pertain to low-velocity penetrating injuries but not to blunt trauma.[45] Authors who advocate restoring flow to all three arteries quote the World War II and Korean War experience with high-velocity missile wounds, in which the amputation rate was 14% after single tibial vessel ligation and 70% following ligation of two vessels.[45] However, these amputation rates do not seem to apply to civilian trauma. The majority of surgeons treating civilian trauma believe that two of three patent shank arteries will maintain limb viability. In our experience, limb loss has not been observed after single artery loss, regardless of the mechanism of injury. Therapeutic angiographic embolization can be done for injured single tibial vessels. Indications include extravasation, a pseudoaneurysm, or an arteriovenous fistula. To prevent late complications, the surgeon must exercise good clinical judgment when deciding which injuries merit embolization and which require operative ligation.

Regardless of the mechanism, when two of three tibial vessels or the TPT is injured, reconstruction is necessary. Preoperative arteriography will identify the level of the target vessels. Patients who sustain injury to all three tibial vessels uniformly present with ischemia and should be operated on without delay. The previously described principles of nonoperative management of nonocclusive injuries apply regardless of the number of injured arteries.

Operative Repair

The operative preparation for infrapopliteal arterial reconstruction is identical to that for PA reconstruction. The contralateral extremity is prepared for possible saphenous vein harvest. The posterior tibial and peroneal arteries are best approached medially, and a more distal incision is made than that used for PA repair. The ATA may be exposed with an anterior longitudinal incision. Primary repair is ideal if a tension-free anastomosis is possible, but this situation is infrequent. Autogenous vein interposition or bypass grafting is the preferred method of reconstruction. In cases of severe soft tissue defects, the bypass graft should be routed through uninjured areas. Ligation or embolization of either the ATA or the PTA is permissible as long as the peroneal artery is patent. In cases of three-vessel injuries, most surgeons recommend revascularization of at least two arteries, provided that the patient's condition permits the procedure. Ligation of isolated tibial vein injuries, compared with popliteal vein ligation, has minimal morbidity. As in the case of PA trauma, heparinization, aggressive debridement, liberal use of fasciotomy, use of mannitol, and completion arteriography are the identified measures that can optimize limb salvage.

Infrapopliteal Arterial Spasm

Spasm of the distal uninjured infrapopliteal and even smaller collateral arteries is common in infragenicular arterial trauma. Contusion or stretch and ischemia can produce more arterial vasoconstriction in the normal muscular vessels of young trauma patients than in the arteriosclerotic vessels of elderly patients undergoing distal bypass procedures. Mechanical dilation with metal sounds or Fogarty catheters can injure the endothelium or increase the spasm. Hydrostatic dilation may temporarily relieve the spasm, but it can injure the endothelium. Commonly, intra-arterial papaverine is used to relieve the spasm. Shah et al[45] described the use of a femoral artery infusion of dextran, papaverine, and heparin that was continued for 12 to 24 hours postoperatively. We have had success infusing tolazoline, a competitive alpha-adrenergic blocking agent. An infant feeding tube is introduced into the superficial femoral artery by means of a transected side branch, exiting the skin from a separate site, thus allowing continuous tolazoline infusion for 24 to 48 hours postoperatively.[48] Nitropaste application to the affected foot and oral nifedipine may also relieve the spasm, improve pedal microcirculation, and therefore merit consideration.

POSTOPERATIVE MANAGEMENT

Postoperative management of the patient can be equally important in preventing the morbidity of popliteal and infrapopliteal arterial trauma. Successful functional limb salvage frequently requires a teamwork approach from vascular, orthopedic, and plastic surgeons as well as rehabilitation specialists.

In the immediate postoperative period, meticulous attention must be paid to changes in the pedal pulses. Loss of a pulse is an operative emergency and is attributed to thrombosis of the repair until proven otherwise. This phenomenon occurs in as many as 10% of the cases. Half of these are due to distal small-vessel thrombosis, and the remainder are due to technical factors related to the anastomosis. Hence, Fogarty catheter thrombectomy, revision of the anastomoses, and local heparin infusion will salvage half the limbs, if done promptly. Local urokinase infusion has met with limited success. Clot lysis with this technique should be apparent within 1 hour, or the procedure should be abandoned due to concern about hemorrhage. Compartmental hypertension due to failure to perform a fasciotomy or due to an inadequate fasciotomy can lead to thrombosis.

Crush injuries and compartmental syndrome are often associated with postoperative rhabdomyolysis. Patients exhibiting such risk factors should undergo postoperative mannitol diuresis in addition to intraoperative mannitol. This treatment, along with aggressive intravenous hydration and alkalinization of the urine, may prevent myoglobinuria from leading to renal failure.

Postoperative transient leg edema is common, usually mild, and often unrelated to known venous injuries. Edema is reported as a complication, regardless of whether the popliteal vein was ligated, repaired, or uninjured. This condition can be minimized by extremity elevation, compressive stockings, and sequential compression devices. It is thought that as collateral venous channels develop, the edema resolves.

In view of the potential for popliteal venous thrombosis and subsequent pulmonary embolism, noninvasive color-flow duplex studies should be done postoperatively in veins of all edematous limbs and in patients with venous repairs. Despite the fact that early thrombosis of venous repairs is common, often asymptomatic, and capable of recanalization,[35,37] attempts to prevent early thrombosis are warranted. Pneumatic sequential compression devices are effective in reducing the incidence of postoperative venous thrombosis. They can be applied to the uninjured extremity but usually not to the injured extremity. Recently, sequential foot compression devices became available and are used as deep venous thrombosis prophylaxis in patients undergoing knee and hip arthroplasty.[49,50] These devices may be of benefit in this group of vascular trauma patients. There is also a small experimental experience using low-molecular-weight dextran administered perioperatively when vein repair is performed.[2] Dextran infusion is continued for 3 to 5 days postoperatively or until the patient is ambulatory. Routine surveillance of the venous repair is done by Doppler or duplex examination at 3 to 4 days and is repeated at 10 to 14 days postoperatively. If thrombus is present, anticoagulation therapy is initiated with heparin and is continued on an outpatient basis with coumadin for 6 to 12 weeks.

Careful surveillance must be done for muscle viability, hematoma, and limb sepsis. Failure to identify these changes can lead to limb loss or mortality due to systemic sepsis. When there is any suspicion that these problems exist, an immediate return to the operating room is warranted. Re-exploration is guided by clinical assessment and may be required as soon as 24 hours and as long as 5 to 7 days postoperatively. The zone of injury, not readily apparent initially, may declare itself only during this later period, particularly in cases of blunt trauma. Rising serum creatine kinase levels may provide an additional clue to the presence of retained nonviable muscle. Plans for repeat wound exploration and debridement should be made when any muscle of marginal viability remains. In these situations, delayed skin grafting can be performed after repeated aggressive debridement. If serial debridement results in a defect with exposed bone or artery, delayed muscle rotation or a free muscle transfer can be done.

As experience is gained with limb reimplantation, microsurgical tissue transfer, nerve grafts, bone grafting, and newer forms of skeletal fixation, almost all limbs can be restored to some useful function. The majority of patients, particularly blunt trauma victims, require multiple orthopedic procedures and a protracted course of rehabilitation. Persistent nerve palsy is the primary determinant of a functional limb. Orthoses and remedial operations can assist the patient in regaining function. Severely injured limbs may require as much as 1 year of rehabilitation before the ultimate outcome can be determined. In rare cases, despite a successful vascular and osteocutaneous reconstruction, the patient may eventually benefit from amputation of an insensate, functionless limb. An aggressive multidisciplinary approach to the rehabilitation of these patients provides hope to the victims of these debilitating injuries and the physicians who treat them.

REFERENCES

1. Peck JJ, Eastman AB, Bergan JJ, et al. Popliteal vascular trauma: a community experience. *Arch Surg.* 1990;125:1339–1344.
2. Wagner WH, Yellin AE, Weaver FA, et al. Acute treatment of penetrating popliteal artery trauma: the importance of soft tissue injury. *Ann Vasc Surg.* 1994;8(6):557–565.
3. Wagner WH, Calkins ER, Weaver FA, et al. Blunt popliteal artery trauma: one hundred consecutive injuries. *J Vasc Surg.* 1988;7(5):736–748.
4. DeBakey ME, Simeone FA. Battle injuries of the arteries in World War II: an analysis of 2,471 cases. *Ann Surg.* 1946;123(4):534–571.
5. Hughes CW. Arterial repair during the Korean War. *Ann Surg.* 1958;147(4):555–561.
6. Rich NM, Baugh JH, Hughes CW. Acute arterial injuries in Vietnam: 1,000 cases. *J Trauma.* 1970;10(5):359–369.
7. Shah DM, Naraynsingh V, Leather RP, et al. Advances in the management of acute popliteal vascular blunt injuries. *J Trauma.* 1985;25(8):793–797.
8. van Wijngaarden M, Omert L, Rodriquez A, et al. Management of blunt vascular trauma to the extremities. *Surg Gynecol Obstet.* 1993;177:41–48.
9. Snyder WH. Popliteal and shank arterial injury. *Surg Clin North Am.* 1988;68(4):787–806.
10. Jeffries JT, Gainor BJ, Allen WC, et al. Injury to the popliteal artery as a complication of arthroscopic surgery: a report of two cases. *J Bone Joint Surg.* 1987;69A(5):783–785.
11. Green NE, Allen BL. Vascular injuries associated with dislocation of the knee. *J Bone Joint Surg.* 1977;59A(2):236–239.
12. Treiman GS, Yellin AE, Weaver FA, et al. Examination of the patient with a knee dislocation: the case for selective arteriography. *Arch Surg.* 1992;127:1056–1063.
13. Miller HH, Welch CS. Quantitative studies on the time factor in arterial injuries. *Ann Surg.* 1949;130(3):428–440.
14. Lim LT, Michuda MS, Flanigan DP, et al. Popliteal artery trauma: 31 consecutive cases without amputation. *Arch Surg.* 1980;115:1307–1313.
15. Johansen K, Daines MH, Howey T, et al. Objective criteria accurately predict amputation following lower extremity trauma. *J Trauma.* 1990;30(5):568–571.
16. Snyder WH, Thal ER, Bridges RA, et al. The validity of normal arteriography in penetrating trauma. *Arch Surg.* 1978;113:424–428.
17. Weaver FA, Yellin AE, Bauer M, et al. Is arterial proximity a valid indication for arteriography in penetrating extremity trauma? A prospective analysis. *Arch Surg.* 1990;125:1256–1260.
18. Schwartz MR, Weaver FA, Bauer M, et al. Refining the indications for arteriography in penetrating extremity trauma: a prospective analysis. *J Vasc Surg.* 1993;17(1):116–124.

19. Applebaum R, Yellin AE, Weaver FA, et al. Role of routine arteriography in blunt lower-extremity trauma. *Am J Surg.* 1990;160:221–225.
20. Fry WR, Smith S, Sayers DV, et al. The success of duplex ultrasonographic scanning in diagnosis of extremity vascular proximity trauma. *Arch Surg.* 1993;128:1368–1372.
21. Bynoe RP, Miles WS, Bell RM, et al. Noninvasive diagnosis of vascular trauma by duplex ultrasonography. *J Vasc Surg.* 1991;14:346–352.
22. Schwartz M, Weaver FA, Yellin AE, et al. The utility of color flow Doppler examination in penetrating extremity arterial trauma. *Am Surg.* 1993;59:375–378.
23. Weaver FA, Yellin AE. Letter to the editor. *Arch Surg.* 1994;129:669.
24. Stain SC, Yellin AE, Weaver FA, et al. Selective management of nonocclusive arterial injuries. *Arch Surg.* 1989;124:1136–1141.
25. Frykberg ER, Vines FS, Alexander RH. The natural history of clinically occult arterial injuries: a prospective evaluation. *J Trauma.* 1989;29(5):577–583.
26. Perry MO. Complication of missed arterial injuries. *J Vasc Surg.* 1993;17:399–407.
27. Weaver FA, Yellin AE. Letter to the editor. *J Vasc Surg.* 1993;18:1077–1078.
28. Eger M, Golcman L, Goldstein A, et al. The use of a temporary shunt in the management of arterial vascular injuries. *Surg Gynecol Obstet.* 1971;132:67–70.
29. Downs AR, MacDonald P. Popliteal artery injuries: civilian experience with sixty-three patients during a twenty-four year period (1960 through 1984). *J Vasc Surg.* 1986;4:55–62.
30. Veith FJ, Gupta SK, Ascer E, et al. Six-year prospective multicenter randomized comparison of autologous saphenous vein and expanded polytetrafluoroethylene grafts in infrainguinal arterial reconstructions. *J Vasc Surg.* 1986;3:104–114.
31. Feliciano DV, Mattox KL, Graham JM, et al. Five-year experience with PTFE grafts in vascular wounds. *J Trauma.* 1985;25(1):71–82.
32. Shah PM, Ito K, Clauss RH, et al. Expanded microporous polytetrafluoroethylene (PTFE) grafts in contaminated wounds: experimental and clinic study. *J Trauma.* 1983;(23) 12:1030–1033.
33. Rich NM, Jarstfer BS, Geer TM. Popliteal artery repair failure: causes and possible prevention. *J Cardiovasc Surg (Torino).* 1974;15:340–345.
34. Barcia PJ, Nelson TG, Whelan TJ. Importance of venous occlusion in arterial repair failure: an experimental study. *Ann Surg.* 1972;175(2):223–227.
35. Rich NM, Hobson RW, Collins GG, et al. The effect of acute popliteal venous interruption. *Ann Surg.* 1975;183(4):365–368.
36. Rich NM. Principles and indications for primary venous repair. *Surgery.* 1982;91(5):492–495.
37. Meyer J, Walsh J, Schuler J, et al. The early fate of venous repair after civilian vascular trauma: a clinical, hemodynamic and venographic assessment. *Ann Surg.* 1987;206(4):458–464.
38. Mullins R, Lucas C, Ledgerwood A. The natural history following venous ligation for civilian injuries. *J Trauma.* 1980;20(9):737–743.
39. Timberlake G, O'Connell R, Kerstein M. Venous injury: to repair or ligate, the dilemma. *J Vasc Surg.* 1986;4:553–558.
40. Mubarak S, Owen C. Double-incision fasciotomy of the leg for decompression in compartment syndromes. *J Bone Joint Surg.* 1977;59A(2):184–187.
41. Johnson S, Weaver FA, Yellin AE, et al. Clinical results of decompressive dermotomy–fasciotomy. *Am J Surg.* 1992;164:286–290.
42. Ledgerwood A, Lucas C. Massive thigh injuries with vascular disruption: role of porcine skin grafting of exposed arterial vein grafts. *Arch Surg.* 1973;107:201–207.
43. Snyder W. Vascular injuries near the knee: an updated series and overview of the problem. *Surgery.* 1982;91(5):502–506.
44. Keeley S, Snyder W, Weigelt J. Arterial injuries below the knee: fifty-one patients with 82 injuries. *J Trauma.* 1983;23(4):285–292.
45. Shah DM, Corson JD, Karmody AM, et al. Optimal management of tibial arterial trauma. *J Trauma.* 1988;28(2):228–234.
46. Ballard J, Bunt TJ, Malone J. Management of small artery vascular trauma. *Am J Surg.* 1992;164:316–319.
47. Holleman J, Killebrew L. Tibial artery injuries. *Am J Surg.* 1982;144:362–364.

48. Peck J, Fitzgibbons T, Gaspar M. Devastating distal arterial trauma and continuous intraarterial infusion of tolazoline. *Am J Surg.* 1983;145:562–566.
49. Wilson NV, Das Sk, Kakkar VV. Thrombo-embolic prophylaxis in total knee replacement. *J Bone Joint Surg.* 1992;74B:50–52.
50. Fordyce MJF, Ling RSM. A venous foot pump reduces thrombosis after total hip replacement. *J Bone Joint Surg.* 1992;74B:45–49.

41

Trauma to the Aorta and Its Major Branches

Kenneth L. Mattox, MD, Matthew J. Wall, Jr., MD, and Asher Hirshberg, MD

HISTORICAL PERSPECTIVE

It is appropriate that injury to the aorta be included in a textbook that is the outgrowth of a symposium dedicated to Michael E. DeBakey, M.D. DeBakey's classic paper on vascular injuries during World War II cites complications associated with injury and ligation of major vessels.[1] He has written classic papers on injuries to the subclavian vessels, abdominal aorta, iliac arteries, and thoracic aorta as well. His writings address both acute and chronic injury. DeBakey established many general principles of vascular trauma. Those most applicable include attention to detail, simplicity in arteriography, the judicious use of local heparinization, elective intravascular stenting, the adaptive use of synthetic prostheses, and expeditious surgery.

NATURAL HISTORY

Injury to the aorta and its major branches is basically a product of the 20th century and urban violence. Although sporadic cases of aortic, innominate, subclavian, and iliac aneurysms have been described not only in the private sector throughout history, but also in the military literature, most were case history anomalies. DeBakey's classic review of vascular surgery during World War II reported 3 aortic, 21 subclavian, 2 renal, 44 iliac, and 0 innominate injuries.[1] DeBakey coauthored the 1989 review from the Ben Taub General Hospital, which reported 393 aortic, 39 innominate artery, 94 subclavian artery, and 232 iliac artery injuries, representing 19% of all cases of vascular trauma among the 5,760 cardiovascular injuries reported at that time.[2] In the 20th century, more than 92% of the reported military vascular injuries are in the extremities, whereas more than 65% of the vascular injuries in the urban centers are truncal. This variance from the military experience relates to the wounding agent, the transport time, and the availability of organized trauma centers.

ETIOLOGY

Aortic branch artery injuries may be secondary to penetrating or blunt trauma, or they may be iatrogenic. Blunt injuries occur predominantly in the chest, while penetrating trauma is seen more often in the abdominal aorta and its major branches. Iatrogenic injuries are occurring with increasing frequency secondary to the use of large central venous access lines, intra-aortic manipulations, and percutaneous endoscopic surgery. Iatrogenic injuries occurring during orthopedic and neurosurgical procedures, as well as during some vascular, thoracic, and abdominal surgeries, were reported in the past. This contrasting etiologic breakdown is presented in the classic epidemiologic review from the Ben Taub General Hospital (Table 41–1). Recent seat-belt, passive automobile restraint, and gun control legislation has not reduced the incidence or the locations of injuries to the aorta and its major branches.

CHANGING PATHOPHYSIOLOGIC CONCEPTS

From the 1960s to the 1980s, physicians and paramedics were trained to administer aggressive fluid resuscitation in the ambulance, emergency department, and operating room when treating patients with injury to the aorta or its major branches. Emergency medical service protocols and the treatment of shock were based on algorithms and paradigms developed from "controlled" hemorrhagic shock models. In practice, attempts at intravascular volume restoration and elevation of blood pressure often resulted in either the patient's demise prior to arrival at the hospital or secondary irreversible hypotension and/or significant coagulopathy and respiratory insufficiency. Various measures were used preoperatively to elevate the blood pressure, including vasoactive drugs, application of military antishock trousers, infusion of large volumes of balanced salt solutions, and infusion of hypertonic saline solutions.[3–8] Since the 1980s, experience

TABLE 41–1. CAUSES OF AORTIC AND MAJOR BRANCH INJURIES AMONG 5,760 CARDIOVASCULAR INJURIES REPORTED BY MATTOX ET AL IN 1989

	Cause[a]						
Anatomic Component	***GSW***	***SW***	***BT***	***SGW***	***Iat***	***Unk***	***Total***
Ascending aorta	15	12	3	3	0	0	33
Aortic arch	13	7	1	1	—	—	22
Innominate artery	20	8	7	2	2	—	39
Subclavian arteries	61	30	2	1	—	—	94
Descending thoracic aorta	25	5	59	—	—	—	89
Abdominal aorta	180	40	5	17	2	5	249
Mesenteric arteries	136	45	14	7	—	14	216
Renal arteries	53	22	18	1	—	4	98
Iliac arteries	172	30	11	11	2	6	232
Total	675	199	120	43	6	29	1,072

[a] GSW = gunshot wound; SW = stab wound; BT = blunt trauma; SGW = shotgun wound; Iat = iatrogenic; Unk = unknown.
Adapted from Mattox KL, Feliciano DV, Beall AC, et al. Five thousand seven hundred sixty cardiovascular injuries in 4459 patients: epidemiologic evolution, 1958–1966. *Ann Surg.* 1989;209:698–705.

with patients with uncontrolled hemorrhagic shock, presenting at a variety of institutions, as well as studies involving a lacerated aorta swing model at Letterman Army Institute for Research, led clinical investigators to limit crystalloid fluid resuscitation until operative control was achieved in patients with truncal injury.[5,9] Attempts to elevate blood pressure by using vasoactive drugs and military antishock trousers for patients with potential aortic and major branch vessel injuries also did not demonstrate survival advantages. Currently, the principle of waiting to control hypotension until operative control is accomplished in patients with leaking abdominal aortic aneurysms or acute dissecting thoracic aortic aneurysms, especially in the descending thoracic aorta, is universally taught and practiced. Likewise, for the patient with thoracic aortic injury who has a stable blood pressure between 70 and 90 mm Hg, limiting aggressive resuscitation until the time of operative control is now believed to be the most appropriate practice guideline.

EVALUATION

Patients with aortic or major branch vessel injury virtually always present at the hospital with signs of major trauma and/or hypotension. The initial evaluation includes obtaining a medical history, a physical examination, a chest x-ray, the hematocrit, and arterial blood gas levels to assess an aortic injury and/or to determine the need for more urgent intervention. Aortography, computed tomography (CT) scanning, and transesophageal echocardiography are helpful in evaluating blunt injury to the thoracic aorta and its branches. Imaging for penetrating trauma is rarely helpful.

The decision to operate depends on a number of factors. The aortic injury in a patient presenting with penetrating abdominal trauma is usually found incidentally at the time of exploration. For penetrating wounds of the thoracic outlet, operation is based on arteriographic findings that demonstrate the injury and guide the choice of incision. For blunt injury to the thorax, arteriographic findings and on rare occasion transesophageal echocardiographic findings are the determinants for surgery. For blunt injury to the abdominal aorta, the decision to operate is based on clinical findings indicating other abdominal injuries requiring surgical intervention, and the abdominal aortic injury is discovered incidentally at surgery.

Regardless of the factors that indicate the necessity for urgent surgery, the decision is made in the emergency department or the angiography suite. Minimal laboratory and imaging evaluations are required. A urinalysis is performed to determine concomitant urologic injury. A complete blood cell count, an electrolyte determination, a sequential multiple analyzer computer–20 study, clotting studies, and drug screens may be interesting and subsequently used in court, but rarely do any of these tests alter or affect treatment, including an operation. A chest x-ray, an arterial blood gas level determination, and blood typing and cross matching are valuable tests in the emergency department. Angiography is helpful in determining approaches, including the choice of incisions for thoracic outlet injury, but it is not acutely helpful in cases of penetrating aortic, mesenteric, renal, or iliac artery injury. Aortography is helpful in making the diagnosis of blunt thoracic aortic injury, and transesophageal echocardiography is beginning to be used as a gross screening technique for selective patients with thoracic aortic injury.

INCISIONS

Four basic incisions, with some minor variations, serve the surgeon well for patients with aortic or aortic branch injury. For injury to the ascending aorta, aortic arch, and innominate artery, as well as suspected proximal intrathoracic left carotid injury, the incision of choice is a median sternotomy. For thoracic outlet injury, the incision is tailored to the surgeon's experience and the location of the suspected injury. Subclavian artery injuries historically have been approached through a wide variety of incisions. The principles of anticipated proximal and distal control should govern the choice of incision for subclavian injuries. In general, right subclavian arterial injury is approached by means of a median sternotomy with a right supraclavicular extension. Left subclavian artery injuries and occasionally injuries to the left intrathoracic carotid artery are approached through a median sternotomy with a left neck extension. Extrathoracic subclavian artery injuries are approached by means of a third intercostal space incision to achieve proximal tourniquet control of the intrathoracic subclavian artery. A left supraclavicular incision and resection of the medial one-third of the clavicle expose the artery for repair. Descending thoracic aortic injuries are approached through a posterolateral thoracotomy, while abdominal aortic and abdominal aortic branch arteries are repaired by means of a long midline abdominal incision. The "trapdoor" and "thoracoabdominal" incisions are *not* standard for approaches to aortic or major branch artery injury. Virtually all abdominal vascular injuries are approached by a midline laparotomy.

OPERATIVE PRINCIPLES

At surgery, patients with aortic or major branch injury have either a large, contained, pulsatile hematoma or extensive exsanguinating hemorrhage. The midline aorta is often deep to associated injuries and in a relatively inaccessible site. The first priority is control of the bleeding, and the second is control of contamination from an adjacent enteric injury. Proximal and distal control is achieved in all locations outside the field of the hematoma, unless the patient is experiencing fatal exsanguinating hemorrhage. In this situation, control might be achieved at the site of the injury with the aid of intraluminal balloon occlusion. In the chest, this control requires meticulous dissection and may consume more time than the actual aortic or branch artery repair. Proximal control in the abdomen is aided by digital occlusion of the aorta at the hiatus or by use of a retrograde femoral aortic occlusion balloon (Fig. 41–1). Exposure of the abdominal aorta is aided by medial rotation of the viscera. This exposure for trauma is an adaptation of control and exposure techniques proposed by DeBakey in 1952 for thoracoabdominal aneurysms.

ASCENDING AORTIC INJURY

Injury to the ascending thoracic aorta is almost universally fatal prior to the patient's arrival at a hospital, although patients with penetrating or blunt injuries occasionally arrive alive with signs of pericardial tamponade or exsanguinating hemorrhage.[10,11] The ascending aortic injury is often a "surprise" found upon either emergency center thoracotomy or arteriography. Simple puncture wounds may be managed by simple lateral aortorrhaphy, but complex blunt tears require cardiopulmonary bypass for reconstruction. The overall mortality rate for blunt and penetrating ascending aortic injuries seen in patients arriving alive in the hospital exceeds 50%.

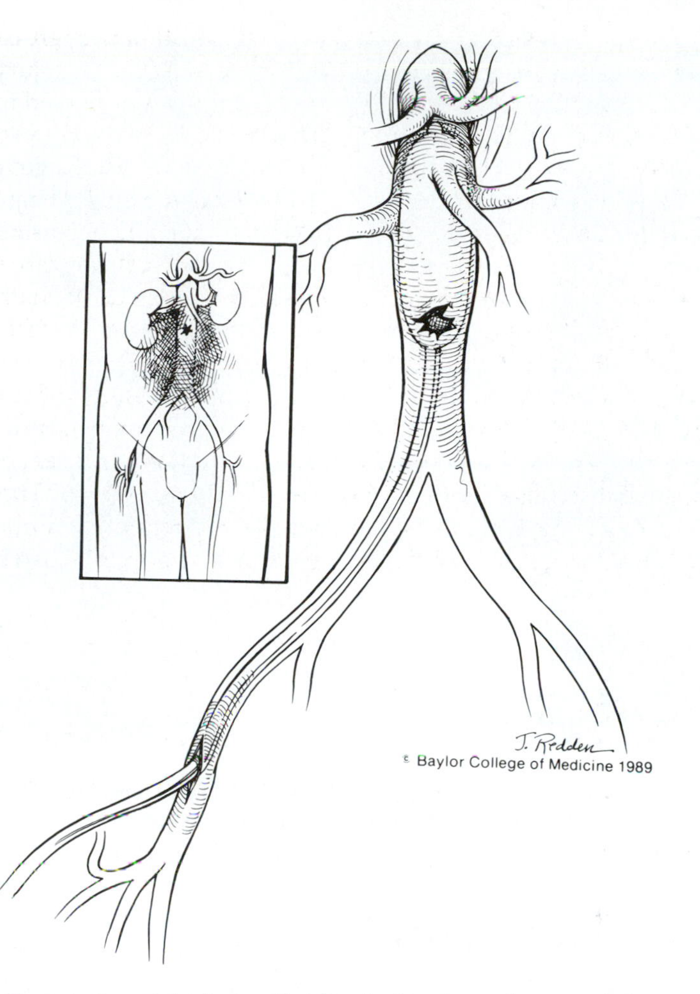

Figure 41–1. Control of an abdominal aortic injury by transfemoral retrograde insertion of an occluding balloon.

AORTIC ARCH–INNOMINATE ARTERY INJURY

Except for an occasional penetrating wound to the aortic arch (which has "sealed off" by the time the patient reaches an emergency center), most injuries in the area of the aortic arch occur at the junction of the arch and the innominate artery, with a "rolling up" of the intima to a position about 1 cm up the innominate artery. This type of injury rarely ruptures within the first few hours following the initial trauma, and patients can usually be transported to a higher level facility without much difficulty. The initial chest x-ray reveals an upper mediastinal hematoma, with the trachea in the midline and lack of obliteration of the aortic knob contour (Fig. 41–2). The diagnosis is made by aortography, and the surgical approach is through a median sternotomy. Insertion of a bypass graft from the ascending aorta to the mid-to-distal innominate artery is performed *without the use of heparin, hypothermia, or shunts* (Fig. 41–3). After the bypass, the area of injury is repaired by arch aortorrhaphy. The in-hospital mortality rate from this type of injury is less than 10%; mortality results from associated injuries, not the aortic arch–innominate artery injury.[12,13]

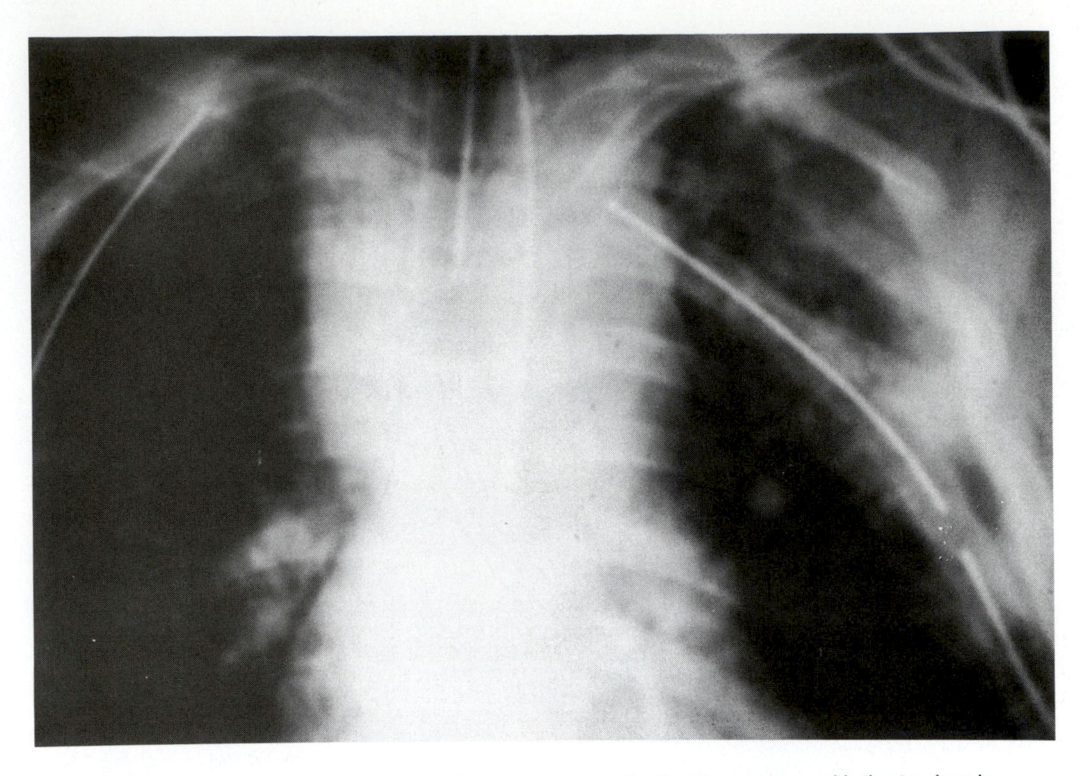

Figure 41–2. Plain chest x-ray revealing an upper mediastinal hematoma, with the trachea in the midline. Subsequent aortography revealed an aortic arch–innominate artery injury.

SUBCLAVIAN ARTERY INJURY

Subclavian artery injuries can be classified, by location, as cervical zone 1, upper extremity, thoracic outlet, or chest injuries.[14,15] The subclavian artery occupies locations in each of these areas. Preoperative arteriography provides a road map for appropriate incision and operative management. Cervical extension of a median sternotomy is indicated for right-sided subclavian artery injuries, and a supraclavicular incision combined with a third intercostal space anterolateral incision is the approach for most left-sided subclavian artery injuries. Care must be taken to protect the phrenic nerve. Documentation of preoperative concomitant injury to the brachial plexus is desirable. Repair is usually accomplished by lateral arteriorrhaphy or Dacron graft interposition; rarely can end-to-end anastomosis be accomplished. Excluding patients who are moribund on admission, the mortality following this injury is less than 5%.

DESCENDING THORACIC AORTIC INJURY

Injury to the descending thoracic aorta may be produced by penetrating, blunt, or iatrogenic trauma.[2,15–17] Penetrating injuries carry a mortality of greater than 50%, as most patients die from exsanguinating hemorrhage prior to arrival at the hospital. In the United States, more than 8,000 persons per year sustain blunt injury; the worldwide incidence is unknown. Eighty-five percent of all patients with this type of injury die prior to arrival at the hospital, and the 48-hour mortality rate for patients who do not undergo surgery is 1% per hour. Fifty percent of these patients have no external sign

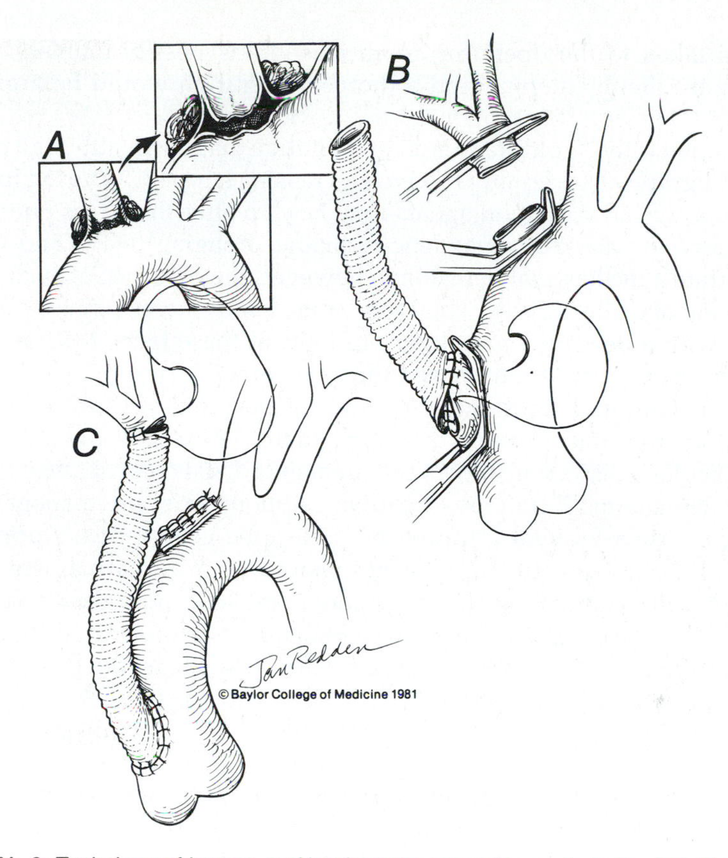

Figure 41–3. Technique of bypass grafting from the ascending aorta to the distal innominate artery for injury to the proximal innominate artery. (**A**) Detail of injury. (**B**) Clamp application and proximal suture line. (**C**) Completion of distal anastomosis and oversew of aortic arch.

of trauma. Clues to elicit suspicion of such an injury are obtained from historical data obtained from paramedics and the patient, physical examination of the patient, and clues seen on the initial chest x-ray that are often described as a "funny-looking mediastinum" but actually represent one or more of the following:

- Widening of the mediastinum greater than 8 cm
- Depression of the left main-stem bronchus greater than 140 degrees
- Presence of a hematoma in the left pleural area
- Fracture of the left first and/or second rib
- Fracture of the sternum and/or clavicle
- Massive left hemothorax
- Fracture dislocation of the thoracic spine
- Loss of the aortopulmonary window on lateral x-ray
- Anterior displacement of the trachea on the lateral chest x-ray
- Deviation of the nasogastric tube to the right in the esophagus
- Deviation of the trachea to the right
- Calcium "layering" in the aortic knob
- Loss of the aortic knob contour
- Loss of the paraspinal pleural stripe

Although none of these signs are diagnostic, any of them should lead the clinician to obtain additional, more diagnostic imaging studies. When imaging confirms an injury, the patient is taken to the operating room as soon as possible, unless concomitant injuries are more life-threatening and a thoracic operation would be a greater threat to life.[18]

Aortorrhaphy is the "gold standard" of definitive diagnosis, although transesophageal echocardiography has recently received increasing support.[19] During imaging studies, the use of afterload reduction agents may help to alter the stress on the aorta and any false aneurysm wall. Both magnetic resonance imaging (MRI) and CT scanning may demonstrate a mediastinal hematoma; however, the presence of such a hematoma is *not* diagnostic of an aortic tear. Therefore, it is usually necessary to follow the MRI and CT scan with a definitive aortogram. In light of these facts, MRI and CT should not be used for evaluation of an injured thoracic aorta.

With the patient in a right lateral recumbent position, a fourth intercostal space posterolateral thoracotomy reveals the aortic injury. Aided by one-lung anesthesia, slow and meticulous dissection allows proximal and distal control away from the area of maximum hematoma. Numerous treatment options exist for management of this injury, including three standard approaches using the clamp–repair principle (Table 41–2).[15,20–25] All these adjunctive approaches should be in the armamentarium of the surgeon. The specific choice for a particular patient must be individualized according to the injury and the conditions encountered. Mortality rates averaging 15% and paraplegia rates ranging from 2% to 25% continue to be reported. Much debate focuses on attempts to prevent or decrease the incidence of paraplegia. The length of cross-clamping time, the use of specific shunting techniques, monitoring techniques, management of cerebrospinal fluid levels, and the use of pharmacologic agents have all been overstated and over-rated in the literature and courtrooms as main and contributing causes. Undoubtedly, patients with longer cross-clamping times have more complex injuries. Theoretically, a spinal canal compartmental syndrome may contribute to ischemic changes in the tenuous and single anterior spinal artery (Fig. 41–4). Furthermore, the use of routine cardiopulmonary bypass, insertion of a cannula for centrifugal pumps and shunts, and systemic heparinization are *not* without complications. The choice of a particular standard technique of repair does not necessarily infer legal liability if paraplegia occurs. In truth, an extremely long list of potential and complex conditions have been postulated to contribute to the occurrence of paraplegia (Table 41–3).

TABLE 41–2. THERAPEUTIC APPROACHES TO THE MANAGEMENT OF TRAUMATIC THORACIC AORTIC INJURY

Aneurysm wrapping (historic interest only)
Insertion of stainless steel wire (historic interest only)
Exclusion and bypass grafting
Nonoperative and/or purposeful delayed operation
Observation alone
Pharmacologic treatment
Clamp and reconstruction (direct repair with and/or without an interposition graft)
Pharmacologic control of proximal hypertension
Temporary bypass shunts
Pump-assisted bypass
Traditional cardiopulmonary bypass (with total body heparinization)
Centrifugal pump (without heparinization)

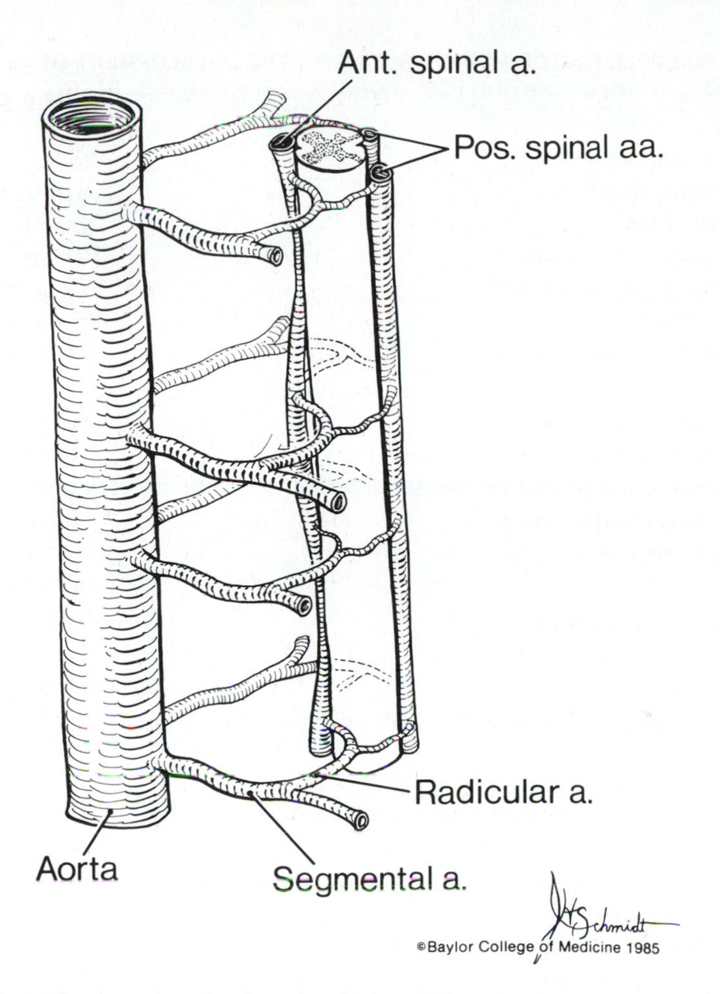

Figure 41–4. Blood supply to the thoracic spinal cord. Note the tenuous and variable anterior radicular and anterior spinal arteries.

ABDOMINAL AORTIC INJURY

Acute injury to the abdominal aorta and its major branches is not usually discovered until an urgent laparotomy is performed for other penetrating or blunt trauma to the abdomen. Chronic false aneurysms and arteriovenous fistulas from these arteries may be diagnosed with special imaging studies. Acutely, a laparotomy is performed through a liberal midline incision, and rapid assessment of the injury reveals a midline hematoma in either the upper abdomen or the midabdomen. Blind groping into the middle of the contained hematoma should be avoided. Once the intra-abdominal bleeding is controlled, the surgeon must take time to make necessary preparations to optimize exposure and repair of aortic or branch arteries. He or she must ensure the availability of autotransfusion equipment, adequate units of bank blood, additional help, and vascular instruments and grafts. Exposure of the suprarenal abdominal aorta is enhanced by a medial rotation of the viscera (Mattox maneuver), behind the kidneys, from the left side (Fig. 41–5).[26] Although retrograde transfemoral aortic occluding balloons are currently being investigated, aortic cross-clamping is a time-honored maneuver used as an adjunct to resuscitation and as a means of reducing massive arterial

TABLE 41–3. POSSIBLE FACTORS CONTRIBUTING TO THE DEVELOPMENT OF PARALYSIS FOLLOWING OPERATION FOR THORACIC GREAT VESSEL INJURY

Injury Factors

Direct segmental artery injury
Direct radicular artery injury
Direct spinal artery injury
Spinal cord contusion or concussion
Spinal canal compartmental syndrome
Severity of aortic injury
Specific anatomic location of aortic injury

Patient Factors

Location of arteriae radicularis magma (?)
Continuity of anterior spinal artery
Caliber of individual segmental radicular arteries
Congenital narrowing of spinal canal (?)
Increased blood supply

Operative Factors

Required occlusion of segmental arteries
Pharmacologic agents required (?)
Declamping hypotension (?)
Required cross-clamping times (in combination with anatomic and injury factors cited in this table)
Length of required interposition grafting or required exclusion
Level of systolic (or mean) proximal aortic blood pressure (?)
Level of distal aortic mean blood pressure (?)
"Flow" in the aorta distal to the clamp

Postoperative Factors

Progressive swelling of the spinal cord
Spinal canal compartmental syndrome
Delayed or secondary occlusion of injured or contused segmental, radicular, or spinal arteries
Pharmacologically induced spasm of spinal cord nutrient arteries

hemorrhage. The aorta may be clamped at various locations in the four manners described:

1. The supradiaphragmatic descending aorta is cross-clamped through a left thoracotomy. Used mainly as one of the steps in a resuscitative thoracotomy, it is also a technique for controlling the aorta prior to laparotomy.
2. The supraceliac aorta may be clamped at the diaphragmatic hiatus through the lesser sac. The peritoneum over the esophagus is opened, and the esophagus is encircled and reflected (with blunt dissection of the left diaphragmatic crus to the left of the esophagus). The same site may also be approached through medial rotation of the left-sided abdominal viscera (Mattox maneuver).
3. The suprarenal aorta is clamped or compressed directly through an opening in the lesser sac.
4. The intrarenal aorta is clamped beneath the left renal vein by reflection of the small bowel to the right, division of the ligament of Treitz, and opening of the posterior parietal peritoneum between the duodenum and the inferior mesenteric vein.

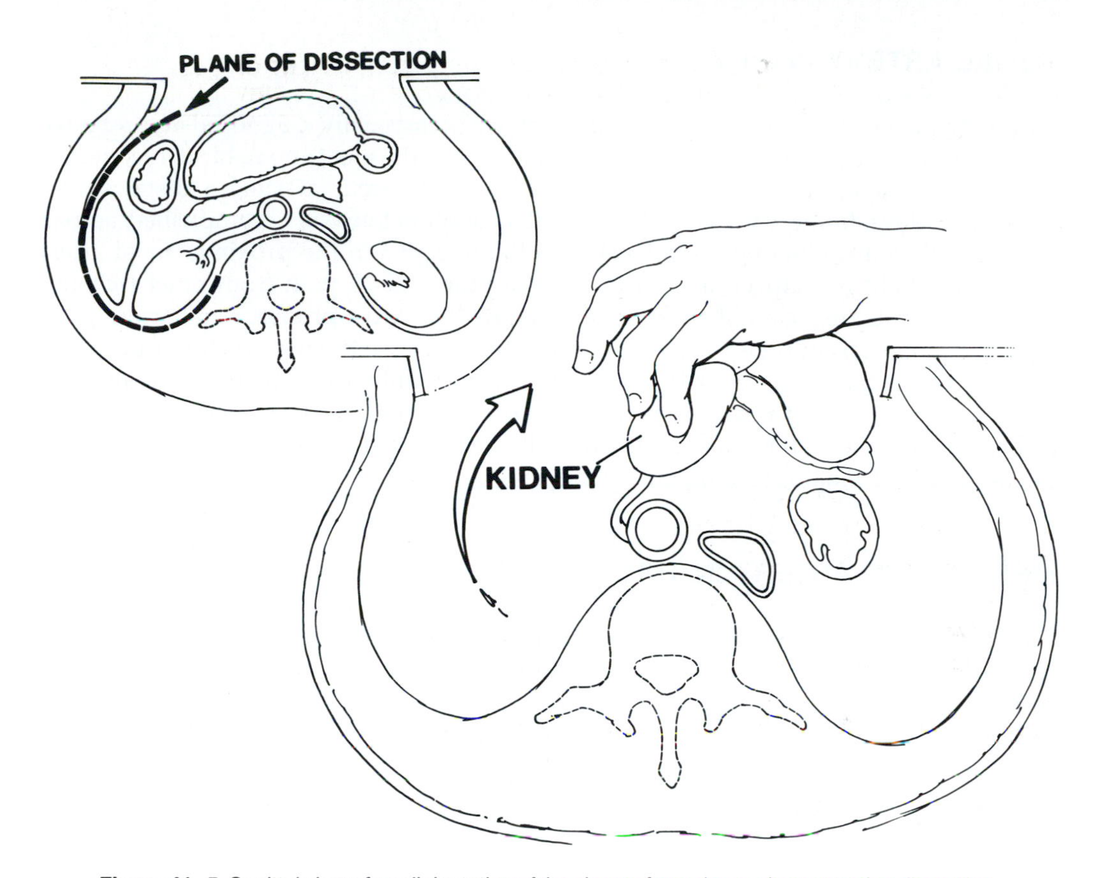

Figure 41–5. Sagittal view of medial rotation of the viscera from above, demonstrating dissection behind the left kidney.

Two major problems with aortic clamping are not mentioned in the literature but are openly acknowledged by trauma and vascular surgeons. First, clamping the aorta through the lesser sac is not quick and easy, especially when the surgeon encounters a pool of blood. Meticulous dissection is impossible, and iatrogenic injury (to adjacent structures) is a realistic concern. The second problem is the physiologic effects of clamping. The procedure improves the "numbers" on the monitoring screen, while increasing visceral and peripheral ischemia, which further contributes to the patient's already borderline physiologic reserves. Consequently, aortic clamping should be used judiciously, not routinely or simply on reflex. Furthermore, manual compression of the aorta at the diaphragmatic hiatus is less likely to cause iatrogenic damage than blunt dissection and clamping are, and it achieves the same effect.

Aortic injuries rarely occur as isolated events. The surgeon should contain concomitant visceral spillage as quickly as possible, while reducing the rate of hemorrhage through the aortic or branch artery. Once exposed, the aorta can be repaired by lateral aortorrhaphy in approximately 50% of the cases. The size of the aorta does not lend itself to the use of autogenous conduits; therefore, insertion of a Dacron synthetic conduit should *not* be avoided. Furthermore, a late-appearing graft infection following trauma to the abdominal aorta has not been reported in the literature. Following proximal and distal control, reconstruction of the injured aorta follows standard vascular principles, except for patients who have undergone exposure through a Mattox maneuver. For these patients, reconstruction is most easily accomplished from the left side of the operating room table. Perioperative mortality rates for this injury exceed 50%.

RENAL ARTERY INJURY

Although penetrating injury to the renal arteries is occasionally diagnosed and repaired successfully, blunt injury to the proximal renal artery is the most amenable to reconstruction.[27] Most penetrating injuries to the renal arteries occur at such a distal site or have such devastating concomitant injury that nephrectomy is accomplished as part of "damage-control" surgery. Patients with blunt injury to the proximal renal artery may have slight hematuria or no urologic symptoms. Back pain from renal ischemia may be present. Suspicion of such an injury should lead to a prompt renal arteriogram and an equally prompt renal artery reconstruction because the window of opportunity for repair is usually less than 4 hours (if not 2 hours), unless adequate collateralization is present. The injured renal artery is approached in the same manner as for a renal artery reconstruction for renal artery stenosis. Reconstruction is accomplished by any of the standard renal artery repair techniques.

MESENTERIC ARTERY INJURY

Mesenteric arterial injury is uncommon.[28,29] The proximal inferior mesenteric artery and the distal branches of the superior mesenteric artery can be ligated with impunity following injury. If the superior and inferior mesenteric arteries are intact, ligation of the celiac axis can be tolerated in approximately 50% of the patients. Ligation of the superior mesenteric artery is *not* tolerated, and revascularization at the initial operation is indicated. Rarely, a temporary intraluminal or bridging shunt can be inserted as part of damage-control surgery, with secondary reconstructive surgery at a later date. Following acute ligation and/or reconstruction of the celiac axis or the superior mesenteric artery, a "second-look" operation 8 to 24 hours later is a wise consideration.

ILIAC ARTERY INJURY

Blunt injury to branches of the iliac arteries often accompanies pelvic fractures and might be controlled with embolization by the interventional radiologists. Penetrating injury to the major iliac arteries carries a mortality approaching 35%.[30] Often, a hematoma expanding deep in the pelvis is difficult to control and expose. Initially, digital (or sponge-stick) compression allows for more precise dissection, rotation of the viscera up and out of the abdomen, and then precise placement of vascular clamps. Reconstruction may be accomplished by standard vascular reconstruction, although in damage-control surgery, ligation is performed to control hemorrhage in the acidotic, coagulopathic, and hypothermic dying patient. When ligation is chosen, the viability of the leg on the side of the iliac artery ligation should be evaluated in the operating room. If the leg is determined to be nonviable, a femoral artery–to–femoral artery bypass can be accomplished through groin incisions while attempts at rewarming are applied to the upper body and the abdomen. In such instances, the surgeon should also consider a fasciotomy.

CONCLUSION

Injuries to the aorta and its major branches are among the most challenging situations confronting trauma and vascular surgeons. In addition to his many other contributions,

DeBakey significantly added to the understanding of trauma care, vascular trauma, and adjunctive management of trauma complications. His contributions to this literature began in the 1930s and continued through the 1990s. This chapter focused on a practical and systematic approach to these complex injuries.

REFERENCES

1. Simeone FA. Battle injuries of arteries in World War II: an analysis of 2,471 cases. *Ann Surg.* 1946;123:5334.
2. Mattox KL, Feliciano DV, Beall AC, et al. Five thousand seven hundred sixty cardiovascular injuries in 4459 patients: epidemiologic evolution, 1958–1966. *Ann Surg.* 1989;209:698–705.
3. Pepe PE, Wyatt CH, Bickell WH, et al. The relationship between total prehospital time and outcome in hypotensive victims of penetrating injuries. *Ann Emerg Med.* 1987;16:293–297.
4. Mattox KL, Bickell W, Pepe P, et al. Prospective MAST study in 911 patients. *J Trauma.* 1989;29:1104–1112.
5. Bickell WH, Shaftan GW, Mattox KL. Intravenous fluid administration and uncontrolled hemorrhage. *J Trauma.* 1989;29:409.
6. Martin RR, Bickell WH, Pepe PE, et al. Prospective evaluation of preoperative fluid resuscitation in hypotensive patients with penetrating truncal injury: a preliminary report. *J Trauma.* 1992;33:354–362.
7. Mattox KL, Maningas PA, Moore EE, et al. Prehospital hypertonic saline/dextran infusion for post-traumatic hypotension. *Ann Surg.* 1991;213:482–491.
8. Bickell WH, Wall MJ, Pepe PE, et al. Immediate versus delayed fluid resuscitation for hypotensive patients with penetrating torso injuries. *N Engl J Med.* 1994;331:1105–1109.
9. Bickell WH, Bruttig SP, Millnamow GA, et al. The detrimental effects of intravenous crystalloid after aortotomy in swine. *Surgery.* 1991;110:529–536.
10. Reyes LH, Rubio PA, Korompai FL, et al. Successful treatment of transection of aortic arch and innominate artery. *Ann Thorac Surg.* 1975;19:468–471.
11. Mavroudis C, Roon AJ, Baker CC, et al. Management of acute cervicothoracic vascular injuries. *J Thorac Cardiovasc Surg.* 1980;80:342–349.
12. Graham JM, Feliciano DV, Mattox KL. Innominate vascular injury. *J Trauma.* 1982;22:647.
13. Johnston RH Jr, Wall MJ Jr, Mattox KL. Innominate artery trauma: a thirty-year experience. *J Vasc Surg.* 1993;17(1):134–140.
14. Graham JM, Feliciano DV, Mattox KL, et al. Management of subclavian vascular injuries. *J Trauma.* 1980;20:537.
15. Mattox KL. Approaches to trauma involving the major vessels of the thorax. *Surg Clin North Am.* 1989;69:77.
16. Childs D, Wilkes RG. Puncture of the ascending aorta—a complication of subclavian venous cannulation. *Anesthesia.* 1986;41:331–332.
17. Pate JW, Cole FH, Walker WA, et al. Penetrating injuries of the aortic arch and its branches. *Ann Thorac Surg.* 1993;55:586–592.
18. Fisher RG, Oria RA, Mattox KL, et al. Conservative management of aortic lacerations due to blunt trauma. *J Trauma.* 1990;30:1562–1566.
19. Kearney PA, Smith DW, Johnson SB, et al. Use of transesophageal echocardiography in the evaluation of traumatic aortic injury. *J Trauma.* 1993;34:696–703.
20. Fabian TC, Walker WA. Acute traumatic rupture of the aortic isthmus: repair with cardiopulmonary bypass. *Ann Thorac Surg.* 1995;59:90–99.
21. von Oppell UO, Dunne TT, De Groot MK, et al. Traumatic aortic rupture: twenty-year metaanalysis of mortality and risk of paraplegia. *Ann Thorac Surg.* 1994;58:585–593.
22. Cowley RA, Turney SZ, Hankins JR, et al. Rupture of thoracic aorta due to blunt trauma: a 15 year experience. *J Thorac Cardiovasc Surg.* 1990;100:652–661.
23. Hilgenberg AD, Logan KL, Akins CW, et al. Blunt injuries of the thoracic aorta. *Ann Thorac Surg.* 1992;53:233–239.

24. Read RA, Moore EE, Moore FA, et al. Partial left heart bypass for thoracic aorta repair. *Arch Surg.* 1993;128:746–752.
25. Mattox KL. Fact and fiction about management of aortic transection [Editorial]. *Ann Thorac Surg.* 1989;48:1–2.
26. Mattox KL, McCollum WB, Beall AC Jr, et al. Management of penetrating injuries of the suprarenal aorta. *J Trauma.* 1975;15:808–815.
27. Brown MF, Graham JM, Mattox KL, et al. Renal vascular trauma. *Am J Surg.* 1980;140:802–806.
28. Graham JM, Mattox KL, Beall AC Jr, et al. Injuries to the visceral arteries. *Surgery.* 1978;84:835–839.
29. Accola KD, Feliciano DV, Mattox KL, et al. Management of injuries to the superior mesenteric artery. *J Trauma.* 1986;26:313–317.
30. Burch JM, Richardson RJ, Martin RR, et al. Penetrating iliac vascular injuries: recent experience with 233 consecutive patients. *J Trauma.* 1990;30:1450–1459.

42

The Widened Mediastinum

Mark W. Sebastian, MD, and Walter G. Wolfe, MD

The initial stabilization, evaluation, and management of the trauma victim suffering suspected injury to the mediastinum and its vascular structures is the same as that used for any trauma victim. The ABCs of resuscitation come into play with injuries to this area: Ensurance of an effective airway and assessment and ensurance of breathing and adequate circulation are performed in sequence, with control of external hemorrhage and establishment of large-bore peripheral intravenous access.[1] The patient's medical history relevant to the chest and the mechanism of injury help the physician to further categorize the patient according to his or her relative risk for mediastinal injury. For motor vehicle accident victims, the speed and deceleration of the vehicle, the use of restaints, the injuries to other parties, and the condition of the vehicle are useful and critical components of the initial assessment. For penetrating injury victims, the nature of the weapon or device involved is key, although the reliability of scene reports varies greatly. For any injury, the physiologic state of the victim at the scene, the patient's response to scene stabilization and resuscitation, the length of time at the scene, and transport data contribute to early triage and the level of suspicion of life-threatening mediastinal injury.

ANATOMIC CONSIDERATIONS

The mediastinum is an anatomic area of the thorax defined by the thoracic inlet superiorly, the diaphragm inferiorly, the sternum anteriorly, the vertebral column posteriorly, and the parietal pleura laterally. Classic descriptions of the mediastinum divided this area further into superior, anterior, middle, and posterior subdivisions utilizing a transverse plane from the sternal angle to the fourth intercostal space to separate the superior subdivision and then utilizing the pericardial sac as the middle mediastinum. Currently, the convention is to divide the mediastinum into anterosuperior, middle, and posterior subdivisions. The anterosuperior subdivision contains the thymus, aortic arch and great vessels, great veins, lymphatics, and fatty areolar tissue. The middle mediastinum contains the heart, pericardium, phrenic nerves, tracheal bifurcation, hila of each lung, and lymph nodes. The posterior mediastinum contains the esophagus, vagus nerves, sympathetic chain, thoracic duct, descending aorta, azygous and hemi-azygous venous systems, paravertebral lymphatics, and fatty areolar tissue.

The issue in evaluating the widened mediastinum revolves around not only the patient's medical history and physical examination, but also the location of the widened area on plain film, the quality of the film, the position of the patient, and the depth of inspiration at exposure.

INITIAL ASSESSMENT

As with any trauma patient, the assessment begins with complete exposure of the patient and a search for visible signs of injury and points of ongoing hemorrhage. Visible signs may provide useful clues to the underlying injury. The respiratory rate, pattern of respirations, chest wall motion, and ventilatory effectiveness are all assessed in the primary survey. The presence of flail chest or splinting suggests fractures that could have associated mediastinal injury, while the location of penetrating injury to the base of the neck or in the area between the nipples extending inferiorly to the subxyphoid area increases the possibility of injury to mediastinal structures. Palpation and auscultation of the chest follow, with areas of tenderness, instability, crepitation, and decreased or deranged breath sounds identified.

Radiologic examination with a standard 100-cm anteroposterior plain chest radiograph is part of all trauma resuscitation protocols. In the patient with blunt or penetrating chest injury, spinal immobilization must be maintained until cervical spinal injury is ruled out. Rib fractures and clavicular, thoracic spine, and scapular injuries are readily identified on an adequate film. Further, first and second rib and scapular fractures suggest severe chest injury and should prompt vigilance and evaluation for severe mediastinal injury. Haziness of one hemithorax on a supine film suggests hemothorax, and another radiograph in the erect position must include a nasogastric tube, if not contraindicated by facial fractures, to evaluate for possible deceleration aortic injury and aortic transection. With the presence of a widened mediastinum, a deviated nasogastric tube, an apical pleural cap, left hemothorax, a shift of the trachea to the right of the T-4 spinous process, a depressed left main-stem bronchus more than 40 degrees below the horizontal, or an axial transverse chest injury, the patient should undergo aortography.[2]

Attempts to standardize the most commonly cited radiologic findings have centered around mediastinal widening. Mediastinal widening is the most sensitive and specific finding suggestive of mediastinal great vessel or aortic injury. A recent series from the University of Wisconsin evaluated mediastinal widening found on radiographs of 16 patients with subsequently documented aortic and great vessel injury.[3] These films were compared with 50 radiographs obtained from normal volunteers. The volunteers were varied as far as position and depth of inspiration. A statistically significant difference in mediastinal width was found among inspiratory–supine, expiratory–supine, and upright–inspiratory techniques. A widening to 9 cm of the superior mediastinum in an upright position and in the inspiratory phase was judged the most reliable finding and the most reliable type of x-ray. In summary, the absence of abnormalities on an erect, inspiratory x-ray has a greater negative predictive value than the positive predictive value of the presence of abnormalities.[4] Despite this finding, a negative chest x-ray does not completely rule out the possibility of aortic or great vessel injury. It is estimated for blunt trauma and deceleration injury that a possible 1.7% of patients may have aortic or brachiocephalic arterial rupture with no mediastinal abnormality or clinical finding.[5]

ADDITIONAL STUDIES

Transesophageal echocardiography (TEE), contrast-enhanced computed tomography (CT) scanning, and magnetic resonance imaging (MRI) can also make the diagnosis of great vessel injury and have been advocated when x-ray studies are suboptimal or when optimal x-rays yield equivocal findings. Transesophageal echocardiography was studied in a recent review of 22 thoracic trauma patients and 20 brain dead patients.[6] The specificity for TEE was 75%, and the sensitivity was 100%. Three criteria for identification of mediastinal hematoma were identified:

1. Increased distance between the probe and the aortic wall of 3 mm
2. Double contour of the aortic wall
3. Visualization of the ultrasound signal between the aortic wall and the visceral pleura

A recent series demonstrated a potential role for CT scanning in the case of the hemodynamically stable patient with equivocally abnormal mediastinal contours on plain chest x-ray.[7] In a series of 90 patients, 16 (18%) had CT scans demonstrating evidence of mediastinal blood or great vessel contour abnormality. Of these 16 patients, 4 had injury to the great vessels.

Magnetic resonance imaging can be an alternative for the hemodynamically stable patient allergic to contrast agents. The advantages of MRI include direct multiplanar imaging and an ability to visualize the entire thoracic and abdominal aorta. The disadvantages include a relative scarcity of the technology compared with the availability of CT scanning and arteriography, a high-strength magnetic field, a small-sized imaging chamber, and a relatively long imaging time.

Even though these three imaging modalities—TEE, CT, and MRI—are cited frequently in the literature, arteriography remains the "gold standard" for specificity and sensitivity of vascular injury to the mediastinum.[4,8] Further, beyond diagnosis, arteriography is critical in planning the operative strategy.

Indications for surgery in patients with mediastinal injury include injuries to the heart or major vessels with hemorrhage from blunt or penetrating trauma, cardiac tamponade, and angiographically demonstrated injury to the great vessels. Full arch aortograms should be obtained to demonstrate the aortic root; the innominate, left subclavian, left carotid, and vertebral arteries; and the diaphragmatic hiatus.

AORTIC INJURY

Thoracic aortic injuries account for 15% to 20% of all fatalities from motor vehicle accidents and are a result of rapid deceleration upon impact, which causes injury at the junction of mobile and fixed portions of the aorta. There is disruption of the intima and elastic media, with adventitial containment of the bleeding, leading to a false aneurysm. Typically, the areas potentially prone to this type of injury are (1) just distal to the aortic valve; (2) distal to the left subclavian artery at the ligamentum arteriosum; and (3) at the diaphragmatic hiatus. Disruption at the aortic root is nearly universally fatal. In the majority of trauma victims surviving aortic disruption, the tear is located in the descending arch. Diaphragmatic injuries are rare. Pseudoaneurysm or free rupture may ensue. There is an 80% fatality rate at the scene, and of the patients who survive to be transported from the scene, 50% die within the first 24 hours after injury if no treatment is instituted. Ultimately, 90% of the patients die within 3 months without treatment. This important topic is addressed in more detail in Chapter 41.

Penetrating aortic injuries are usually repaired by direct pledgeted suturing, patch aortoplasty, or interposition graft placement, depending on the location and extent of the injury. The use of complete cardiopulmonary bypass requiring full heparinization has been shown to increase morbidity and mortality in patients who have other injuries, especially cerebral and vascular injuries.

MYOCARDIAL CONTUSION

The dilemma of myocardial contusion centers around a lack of standardized definition and diagnostic criteria. Some series claim an incidence of myocardial contusion as high as 75% among patients sustaining major chest trauma. When the incidence of clinically significant complications attributable to myocardial contusion is studied, the incidence falls to 10% of all chest trauma patients.[9] The standardization of diagnostic tests is also difficult because of the lack of accepted diagnostic criteria. Electrocardiogram (EKG) findings are nonspecific and involve ST-T segment changes; atrial, supraventricular, and ventricular dysrhythmia; and nodal dysfunction. Dysrhythmia, especially ventricular, is the most standard criterion for admission and monitoring. Various centers rely on the determination of the creatine phosphokinase (CPK) myocardial band (MB) fraction to confirm the diagnosis. Elevation of the CPK-MB fraction to greater than 5% of the total, or a total plasma CPK concentration of more than 100 IU/mL is considered diagnostic at some centers.[4] Documented dysrhythmia is treated aggressively, but no benefit to prophylactic antiarrhythmic administration has been demonstrated. Although technetium scanning and echocardiography have been used in some centers, the consensus in the literature centers around treating documented arrhythmias and the requirement of as little as 8 hours of monitoring for the stable, otherwise uninjured, patient with no dysrhythmias.

PERICARDIAL TAMPONADE

Both blunt and penetrating injuries to the heart can result in pericardial tamponade. In the acute setting, as little as 150 mL of blood can compromise hemodynamics. For this reason, tamponade can be immediately life-threatening. Blunt injury to the heart is difficult to assess for the reasons cited previously. However, autopsy series cite 10% evidence of myocardial damage, and 5% of all deaths due to blunt trauma are attributable to cardiac damage.[9] For myocardial injury to be sustained in cases of blunt trauma, the heart must be maximally distended (end diastole) when the blow is delivered. The likely area of injury is the right ventricle or the right atrium, especially the right atrial appendage. Although any area of the heart can potentially rupture, especially in combination with a sternal fracture, only a small injury resulting in a slow leak could result in tamponade instead of sudden death. Penetrating injury to the heart is a much more common cause of pericardial tamponade. As with other organs, the size of the injury is related to the ballistic characteristics of the missile or the size of the blade. High-velocity, large-caliber wounds are usually fatal. Likewise, stab wounds larger than 2 or 3 cm that penetrate a cardiac chamber are frequently fatal.[4] Smaller stab wounds, wounds only partially penetrating the myocardium, and tamponade resulting from iatrogenic injury such as cardiac catheterization, central venous catheterization, or pericardiocentesis have a better prognosis.

The diagnosis of pericardial tamponade should be suspected in any patient with penetrating injury to the central chest or base of the neck, or in any patient who sustained a blunt injury to the chest, is hypotensive, and has no evidence of hemorrhage in the thorax, abdomen, or pelvis. The absence of both chest radiographic findings and EKG changes does not rule out tamponade. The physical signs of Beck's triad: distant heart tones, jugular venous distension, and decreased pulse pressure are inconsistently seen. A pericardial friction rub is a useful but nonspecific finding. If the diagnosis is suspected, central monitoring can be helpful, and central venous pressures of 14 to 16 cm of water in the resuscitated patient suggest tamponade. In a series of penetrating wounds to the mediastinum, 47 patients underwent surgical intervention.[10] Of the 47 patients, 40 (85.1%) had pericardial tamponade. When measured, central venous pressure was elevated to 15 cm of water or greater in 28 (87.5%) of 32 patients with tamponade. In contrast, Beck's triad was noted in 48% of the patients with tamponade.

The most useful noninvasive test is echocardiography. If this test is readily available, it can make the diagnosis with certainty and can be used to aid therapeutic intervention, as aspiration can be done under direct vision. If echocardiography is not available and the diagnosis is suspected, pericardiocentesis may be performed by inserting a needle into the subxyphoid space and advancing it at a 45-degree angle toward the left nipple. An EKG electrode attached to the needle helps to identify epicardial contact.[11] Even the aspiration of 30 mL of unclotted blood is diagnostic and can lead to hemodynamic improvement. The aspiration of nonclotting blood from the pericardium is an indication for thoracotomy. However, pericardiocentesis can lead to ventricular puncture, and laceration of a coronary artery has been reported. Instead, some centers prefer to perform a subxyphoid pericardial window while the patient is under general anesthesia, with wide surgical preparation and the intention to proceed to sternotomy if the pericardial window yields blood.[11] This approach allows for diagnostic certainty, full pericardial decompression, and a controlled surgical setting in which immediate and definitive therapy can be instituted.

EMERGENCY DEPARTMENT PROCEDURES

The combination of a penetrating central chest injury and an emergency room presentation *in extremis* is an indication for left anterolateral thoracotomy with opening of the pericardium longitudinally and preservation of the left phrenic nerve. Penetrating cardiac injury is controlled with digital pressure while access by means of a right atriotomy with purse string and Foley catheter placement is used for high-volume infusion and restoration of circulating volume.[1] When volume is restored, repair is accomplished with nonabsorbable pledgeted monofilament sutures. Teflon or pericardium may be used as a pledget. After definitive repair, the pericardium is left open and mediastinal drains are placed. Survival ranges from 50% to 90% for patients with penetrating cardiac injury who arrive with measurable blood pressure.

Major mediastinal vessel injuries are often fatal, due to both the large caliber of the vessels and a lack of surrounding structures capable of tamponading the injury. Tube thoracostomy reveals significant hemothorax and ongoing hemorrhage. This situation is a surgical emergency requiring emergency department thoracotomy or emergent transfer to the operating room. For patients with major chest injury who remain hemodynamically stable after tube thoracostomy, the constellation of medical history, physical examination, and plain radiography is used to determine the likelihood of mediastinal vessel injury and the need for arteriography. Major vascular injuries of the mediastinum are rarely completely occlusive, so examination of the extremities may not yield pulse deficits in the presence of significant injury. However, the finding of a pulse deficit or asymmetry between the two upper extremities or the upper and lower extremities is strongly predictive of major injury. Simple lacerations are the most common injuries to both the arteries and the veins of the mediastinum. The vessels are rarely completely severed, so there is no retraction and thrombosis, and consequently hemorrhage can be much more severe. Intimal flap occlusion as a consequence of trauma is common, as is the development of arteriovenous fistulas after penetrating injury. Blunt injury may result in intimal disruption with sparing of the muscular and adventitial layers, leading to thrombosis, dissection, or pseudoaneurysm formation with delayed rupture and exsanguination. Chronic problems include pseudoaneurysm and distal embolization.

GREAT VESSEL INJURY

In cases of great vessel injury, physical examination findings depend on the affected artery. Subclavian artery injuries often present with absent or diminished distal pulses. Proximal carotid injuries may lead to audible bruits, and brachiocephalic, vertebral, and internal mammary arteries produce no specific clinical symptoms or signs.

Plain radiography is of limited but well-defined utility in the diagnosis of major vessel injury to the mediastinum. The most common finding of widened mediastinum is seen with brachiocephalic artery laceration and varies from 30% to 100% in series.[12] This finding may also occur with carotid or aortic injuries. The clinical history, physical examination, and plain film radiographs are best used to suggest which mediastinal great vessels were at risk of injury. Most penetrating injuries are the result of direct penetration of the vessel. It has been shown in the literature that only structures within a 5-cm radius of the projected wound path are at risk of direct injury.[13] It is important to note that high-velocity gunshot wounds cause cavitary blast injury and may involve considerably more tissue damage than the entrance wound suggests. For a patient with a gunshot entrance wound but no exit wound, plain radiography should also be used in a search for the retained missile. Bullet embolus complicates 0.33% of all gunshot-related vascular injuries.[14] This search is of more than academic interest, as the missile can enter either the arterial system or the venous system. Arterial embolization can affect any area or organ, but there is a predilection for the left leg. A missile in the venous system can migrate through the right ventricle into the pulmonary circulation and result in pulmonary embolism. Because of morbidity associated with infection and ischemia, removal of bullet emboli is recommended. This can be accomplished either surgically or by means of an interventional radiology approach using an intravascular basket or snares.

As with suspected aortic injury, arteriography is critical to the management of suspected vascular injury to the great vessels of the mediastinum in a hemodynamically stable patient with central chest injury. Six considerations in the performance of the arteriogram maximize its diagnostic accuracy and utility for therapeutic intervention:

1. Adequate monitoring should be in place while the patient is in the angiography suite.
2. The entrance and exit wounds should be marked with radiopaque markers.

3. Contrast injection should be far enough away from the suspected injury to minimize artifact.
4. Biplanar views of the artery should be obtained.
5. A minimum of 15 to 20 cm of normal artery must be visualized proximal and distal to the injury.
6. Early and delayed views should be obtained to detect the presence of an arteriovenous fistula or a pseudoaneurysm.

Properly performed arteriography has a high sensitivity, a high specificity, and a positive predictive value. However, a suboptimal study in the setting of high clinical suspicion should be followed by repeat arteriography or surgical exploration.

OPERATIVE STRATEGY

Penetrating wounds to the ascending aorta, innominate artery, and right subclavian artery are best approached by median sternotomy. The surgical preparation should always allow for extrathoracic extension of the incision, and the legs should also be prepared, both for saphenous vein harvesting and femoral artery access. Left common carotid artery injuries can also be approached by median sternotomy. Left subclavian and descending thoracic aorta injuries are best approached by left thoracotomy. This is true for the subclavian artery due to its posterior takeoff from the aortic arch. More distal exposure of the left subclavian artery is accomplished through a "trapdoor" incision, which divides the sternum superiorly and continues along the superior border of the left clavicle. If an emergency department thoracotomy is undertaken, exposure can be optimized by carrying the incision to the right side of the chest. It should be emphasized that a right thorax injury in the hypotensive patient should be initially approached by left thoracotomy for volume infusion prior to any attempt to gain vascular control in the right hemithorax. The major complication of aortic and great vessel repair is paraplegia resulting from cross-clamping of the aorta in the chest; paraplegia rates of 8% are standard in the literature, despite maximization of distal perfusion and minimization of the segment cross-clamped, avoidance of hypovolemia, and rapid vascular repair. Vascular repair involves primary repair of the vessel whenever possible. However, tissue damage may require graft interposition. Proximal innominate or left common carotid injuries can be treated by oversewing of the vessel and aortotomy with graft restoration of vessel continuity.[15] If the distal innominate is injured, a bifurcated graft may be used and sewn to the right subclavian and common carotid arteries.[15] Isolated brachiocephalic vein injuries may be primarily repaired, but they can be ligated if necessary. In a large series of penetrating injuries to the neck and superior mediastinum, direct venous repair was attempted for isolated injury, and ligation was performed when complex repairs were required. Of the 55 incidences of ligation, 14 brachiocephalic confluences, 9 proximal subclavian veins, and 1 superior vena cava was ligated. No venous stasis problems were seen in any patient in the 2- to 26-month follow-up period.[16]

CONCLUSION

The treatment of traumatic injury to the heart and great vessels in the mediastinum centers around a high index of suspicion. For the stable patient, a proper physical examination and plain x-rays are useful screening tools. An upright inspiratory chest x-ray is the most useful screening examination for mediastinal vascular injury, and 9-cm widening is the most sensitive and specific finding for vascular injury that is seen on plain film. However, definitive studies in the patient at risk for these potentially morbid and fatal injuries are crucial. Arteriography remains the "gold standard" in the literature for diagnosis and planning of the operative strategy.

REFERENCES

1. Committee on Trauma. *Advanced trauma life support manual.* Chicago, IL: American College of Surgeons; 1989.
2. Marsh D, Sturm J. Traumatic aortic rupture: roentgenographic indications for angiography. *Ann Thorac Surg.* 1976; 21(4):337.
3. Lee F, Katzberg R, Gutierrez O, et al. Reevaluation of plain radiographic findings in the diagnosis of aortic rupture: the role of inspiration and positioning on mediastinal width. *J Emerg Med.* 1993;11(3):289.
4. Groskin S. Injuries from blunt and penetrating chest trauma. In: *Radiological, Clinical and Biomechanical Aspects of Chest Trauma.* Berlin, Germany: Springer-Verlag; 1991.
5. Woodring J. The normal mediastinum in blunt traumatic rupture of the aorta and brachiocephalic arteries. *J Emerg Med.* 1990;8(4):467.
6. LeBret F, Ruel P, Rosier H, et al. Diagnosis of traumatic mediastinal hematoma with transesophageal echocardiography. *Chest.* 1994;105(2):373.
7. Richardson P, Mirvis S, Scorpio R, et al. Value of CT in determining the need for angiography when findings of mediastinal hemorrhage on chest radiographs are equivocal. *AJR.* 1991;156(2):273.
8. Kram H, Appel P, Wohlmuth D, et al. Diagnosis of traumatic thoracic aortic rupture: a 10 year retrospective analysis. *Ann Thorac Surg.* 1989;47(2):282.
9. Demuth W, Baue A, Odom J. Contusions of the heart. *J Trauma.* 1967;7:443.
10. Peper W, Obeid F, Horst H, et al. Penetrating injuries of the mediastinum. *Am Surg.* 1986;52(7):359.
11. Davis J. Trauma: definitive care phase: chest injuries. In: Greenfield LI, Mulholland MW, Oldham KT, Zelenock GB, ed., *Surgery: Scientific Principles and Practice.* Philadelphia, PA: JB Lippincott; 1993:278–291.
12. Fisher R, Ben-Merachem Y. Penetrating injuries of the thoracic aorta and brachiocephalic arteries: angiographic findings in 18 cases. *AJR.* 1989;149:607.
13. Rose S, Moore E. Angiography in patients with arterial trauma: correlation between angiographic abnormalities, operative findings and clinical outcome. *AJR.* 1989;149:613.
14. Buckels J, Holburn C, Bonser R, et al. Multiple pulmonary missile emboli. *Injury.* 1986;17:129.
15. Hood D, Yellin A, Weaver F. Vascular trauma. In: Dean R, Yao J, Brewster D, eds. *Current Diagnosis and Treatment in Vascular Surgery.* Norwalk, CT: Appleton & Lange; 1995:405–428.
16. Robbs J, Reddy E. Management options for penetrating injuries to the great veins of the neck and superior mediastinum. *Surg Gynecol Obstet.* 1987;165(4):323.

VIII

Miscellaneous Conditions

43

Arterial Lesions Associated with Radiation Therapy

George Andros, MD, and Christopher M. Rose, MD

In 1988, more than 490,000 patients received radiation therapy in the United States.[1] By 1994, that number exceeded 550,000.[2] The occurrence of arterial occlusive lesions following radiation therapy has also increased in numbers since the 1970s, as has an understanding of their relationship to radiation therapy. Nevertheless, the number of vascular lesions remains minuscule in comparison to the number of patients receiving radiotherapy. From 1975 to 1995, we treated 31 patients who developed arterial lesions within the x-ray portal following therapeutic doses of external radiation.[3] Divided among carotid, subclavian and axillary, and aortoiliofemoral distributions, these cases compose the clinical background of this chapter.

HISTORICAL OVERVIEW OF RADIOTHERAPY

Tissue injury produced by ionizing radiation was observed by Gassman[4] within 4 years of the discovery of x-rays by Roentgen. This injury involved intimal thickening and medial vacuolization in small arteries adjacent to radiation-induced skin ulcers. Later, Wolbach[5] observed endothelial cell proliferation and medial fibrosis of arteries in patients with radiation dermatitis. These findings were corroborated by Warren and Friedman.[6] In the last half of the 20th century, an increasing stream of publications describing significant vascular damage have established that the vascular lesions were delayed and slowly evolving. The significance of these lesions was magnified by the development of radiation therapy, beginning in 1922 with the successful treatment of six cases of carcinoma of the larynx by Regaud et al.[7] Confronting the limitations of inherent radioresistance and/or deep-seated lesions, physicians delivered inordinate doses to the overlying normal tissues. However, by the late 1930s, supervoltage radiation (ionizing radiation with photon energies greater than 500,000 electron volts [eV]) could be delivered with resonant transformer-derived photons. After World War II, megavoltage radiation (energies greater than 1 million electron volts [MeV]) delivered by cobalt 60, or betatrons, which accelerated electrons utilizing the cyclotron principle, became clinically applicable. Unfortunately, the cobalt- 60-derived radiation had penetration limits and field edges that could not be sharply columnated. The betatrons were heavy and fragile, and the ability to deliver multiple fields coincident upon the volume was somewhat limited.

In the mid 1950s, engineers and physicists at Varian Associates in the United States and at General Electric Limited in the United Kingdom more or less simultaneously developed linear accelerators (LINACs) that used microwave energy to accelerate electrons down an evacuated waveguide to impact upon a tungsten target and produce photons with energies between 5 and 35 MeV. These LINACs were compact enough to be gantry mounted; thus, radiation could be delivered in any axial orientation. In the 1980s, the Scandatronics Corporation commercialized a compact ellipse-shaped cyclotron that allowed the use of gantry-mounted electron therapy with energies as high as 55 MeV or the use of photons derived from these electrons with similar high energies. Currently in commercial development, with the expectation of availability by 1999, proton and neutron accelerators promise greater biologic damage per unit physician ionization and improved dose distribution.

The revolution in computer imaging and technology control has allowed for more precise targeting of tumors within the body. Computer-controlled multiple-leaf columnators now shape the radiation beam to conform precisely to the irregular shape of tumors or modify the beam strength to distribute high doses to the regions around the tumors. Material scientists produced a number of thermal labile plastics, which are used to immobilize patients and thus provide more setup reliability. These new technologies have led to the development of a number of new techniques termed *conformal radiation*. Conformal techniques may allow an approximately 20% increase in the dose delivered to deep-seated tumors with a concomitant 20% to 50% decrease in the dose to surrounding tissues. However, small portions of immediately adjacent normal tissues are receiving similar or slightly higher doses than those previously delivered. Whether this will increase late normal-tissue damage as the result of an increase in cured patients or an abrogation of "partial tolerance" of portions of organs to withstand higher doses is the object of much of the currently ongoing clinical radiation therapy research.

This information is of clinical relevance because of the need for accurate record keeping about patients who develop vascular lesions associated with radiation therapy. Documentation of the underlying tumor, its stage, and its grade, as well as specific parameters of the radiation therapy, should become an integral part of the patient's clinical record. Only in this way, with the correlation of vascular lesions and radiation therapy techniques, will the biology of the former be better understood and the methodology of the latter be improved. The numbers of patients receiving radiation therapy will certainly continue to grow in the future as a part of the burgeoning of less-invasive treatment strategies. An understanding of radiotherapy side effects and complications depends on accurate documentation and dialogue between vascular surgeons and radiation therapy specialists.

VASCULAR LESIONS

Radiation vasculopathy is both time and dose dependent. The larger the dose, the greater the effect; the longer the time after exposure, the more severe the lesion. In human tissues, the effect of varying the dose is generally not obvious since cancer therapy requires the use of maximum-tolerance doses. These doses are delivered in most instances by using external beams of electromagnetic radiation, but vascular lesions have also been described following brachytherapy with intracavitary and interstitial implantation[8] and with radioisotopes,[9] as might be the case with iodine 131 therapy for hyperthyroidism and carcinoma of the thyroid. It is important to note that radiation does not produce pathognomonic lesions in mammalian organs or tissues; blood vessels are no exception. The combination of vascular lesions within therapeutic portals and associated lesions in adjacent tissues is often characteristic enough to be recognized as radiation induced.[8]

Clinically significant arterial lesions occur most commonly in large arteries. Paradoxically, of all vessels, these seem to be the least affected by ionizing radiation because of the differential radiation sensitivity of the cellular components of the vascular wall.[10] Large-vessel endothelial cells may suffer extensive damage, but the strong support supplied by the elastic membranes, media, and adventitia prevents collapse. Obstructive platelet aggregation at the site of injury usually does not occur because of an adequate lumen. This also applies to large veins.[11] The most commonly occurring lesion following radiation therapy is myoproliferation.[8] Compared with arteriosclerosis, the appearance of lipid-laden macrophages and cholesterol crystals is less common. Intimal deposit of histiocytes, collagen, and fibrin is succeeded ultimately by fibrosis, late stenosis, and ultimately thrombotic occlusion. The most dramatic late complication of radiation vasculopathy is pseudoaneurysm formation leading to rupture and frequently exsanguinating hemorrhage. Microscopic examination of the involved segment reveals focal or segmental transmural necrosis of the arterial wall with exudates of neutrophils in the adventitia and media and variable degrees of thrombosis. The elastic lamellae are focally disrupted. These lesions occur most frequently in patients who are subjected to both surgery and radiotherapy for carcinomas of the head and neck, juxtaesophageal aorta, or genitalia.[8] In the older literature, these lesions were also noted to occur with high-dose, less well columnated radiotherapy or in patients treated with radioimplants. It should be emphasized that arterial rupture following radiation therapy is multifactorial.

Important radiation lesions have also been described in capillaries and sinusoids, the smallest segments of the vascular tree and those most sensitive to ionizing radiation.[8] This is because endothelial cells, which are the most radiosensitive portion of vascular structures, represent the most important element of the vascular wall. Moreover, although endothelial cells divide slowly, they are highly radiosensitive. This accounts for the occurrence of radiation pneumonitis and radiation nephropathy. Dermatologists ascribe the characteristic telangiectasia of radiodermatitis to the asymmetric capillaries and sinusoids in the upper dermis that develop in the post-treatment period.[8]

As with capillaries, small- and medium-sized arterial lesions are also common. The microscopic appearance of these lesions ranges from early epitheliolysis to delayed fibrinoid necrosis and late hyaline fibrosis. Delayed lesions in medium-sized arteries are common and include the collection of foam cells in the subendothelial space and occasional cholesterol clefts. These delayed changes have led to the misconception that radiation damage is indistinguishable from spontaneous arteriosclerosis and therefore not a specific entity.

Hemodynamic and morphologic parameters, in both patients and investigational animal studies, have documented the importance of dosage to the arterial response and the staging of the vascular lesion. In addition, the relationship of progressively worsening lesions with time has been approximated in experimental animals and only incompletely described in clinical settings. This is only partially explained by differential radiosensitivity.

CLINICAL SYNDROMES

It is axiomatic that radiation-affected vessels must lie within the field of treatment. Radiation-induced vasculopathy resembles arteriosclerosis in that it is segmental in distribution. However, radiation arteritis lesions characteristically occur in atypical sites. Extracranial cerebrovascular lesions of the carotid arteries occur as a result of both causes, but in cases of radiation arteritis the bifurcation may be entirely spared and subjacent vertebral arteries are often narrowed at sites other than their origins. Both types of vascular lesions are associated with the arteriosclerotic risk factors (e.g., hypertension and hyperlipidemia), and both are associated with clinical syndromes (Fig. 43–1). Irradiation of mediastinal malignancies such as carcinoma of the breast, lung, and thyroid; thymoma; and high-grade lymphoma may produce lesions of the coronary arteries, the aorta, and the innominate artery. Radiation penumonitis lesions have also been described.

The most commonly irradiated lesions that produce carotid and vertebral artery injury include carcinomas of the head and neck, oropharynx, and thyroid plus salivary gland tumors and high-grade lymphomas. Axillary–subclavian artery lesions following radiation therapy occur most commonly after treatment of carcinoma of the breast in

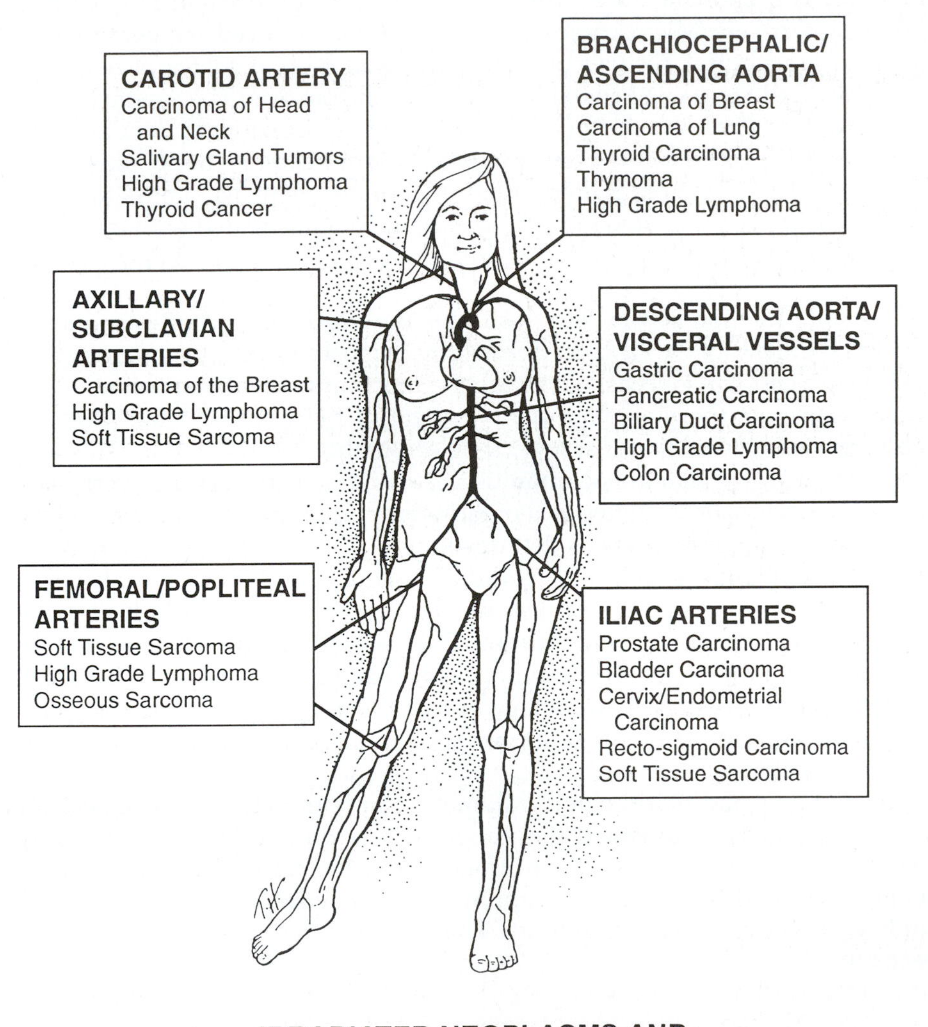

Figure 43–1. Irradiated neoplasms, and arteries at risk of delayed complications.

women, but these lesions have also been observed following treatment of high-grade lymphomas and soft tissue sarcomas. Irradiation for carcinoma of the stomach, pancreas, and bile ducts; colon lymphoma; and high-grade lymphoma accounts for the majority of lesions in the superior mesenteric, celiac, and renal arteries, as well as in the mid- and distal abdominal aorta. The distribution is often unusual for arteriosclerosis, occurs in younger patients, and tends to set these lesions apart from those occurring solely due to arteriosclerotic causes. Pelvic irradiation—both for female and male genitourinary carcinomas such as carcinoma of the cervix, endometrium, bladder, or prostate, and for rectosigmoid carcinoma and soft tissue sarcomas—contributes to the occurrence of external iliac and common femoral arterial occlusions. Finally, treatment of sarcomas of the long bone, soft tissue sarcomas, and lymphomas may result in late femoral and popliteal lesions. In all the clinical syndromes, venous occlusive lesions are rare, and nerve injuries are rarer still.

PERSONAL EXPERIENCE

From 1975 to 1995, 31 of our patients (10 males and 21 females, varying in age from 52 to 78 years [mean, 68 years]) were treated for arterial lesions following radiotherapy. All patients received between 5,000 and 8,000 rads of external ortho-, super-, or megavoltage therapy through one or more portals. In recent years, patients receiving LINAC therapy have also been encountered. Accurate treatment protocols were available for 14 of the 31 patients, and those whose protocols were unavailable often presented with prior ortho- or supervoltage treatment. In many cases, there was evidence of radiodermatitis and cutaneous tattooing of x-ray portals. All vascular lesions consisted of arterial ulceration, stenosis, and/or occlusion. No occurrence of aneurysm or arterial rupture was observed in this series.[3]

Carotid Artery Lesions

Radiotherapy for squamous carcinoma of the head and neck was given to 8 of the 11 patients who subsequently developed carotid artery lesions. Symptoms developed from 1 to 37 years after therapy. In 8 patients, the presenting complaint was transient ischemic attack or stroke. Carotid endarterectomy and saphenous vein patch angioplasty (six) and greater saphenous interposition graft (two) were the most common procedures. Bypass grafts from the subclavian artery to the carotid artery were performed in 2 patients, and a right-to-left carotid–carotid saphenous vein bypass graft was performed in 1. Two patients with concomitant contralateral carotid lesions were treated, and both were heavy smokers; four additional subjacent vertebral stenoses were observed within the x-ray portal. Characteristic of radiation lesions in general, atypical locations were noted: a critical common carotid artery stenosis proximal to the bifurcation and external carotid stenoses. In 3 of the 11 patients, intramural thrombus was present and ulceration was noted.

Subclavian–Axillary Lesions

Symptomatic subclavian–axillary artery stenoses or occlusion was noted in nine radiated women. All had undergone mastectomy, ranging from simple mastectomy to radical mastectomy, for breast cancer. On average, ischemic symptoms developed 7 years following radiation therapy. Effort fatigue and painful ulceration suggested chronic occlusive disease in the majority of the patients, although two had ulcerated stenotic lesions with evidence of thrombus in the base of the ulceration. One elderly woman declined revascularization because her symptoms were in her nondominant hand. There were no instances of severe edema to suggest venous occlusion, nor was there clinical evidence of nerve injury following radiation therapy.

Lesions of the Abdominal Aorta and Its Branches

The disparate group of 11 patients with lesions of the abdominal aorta or its branches included 5 patients with limb-threatening ischemia and 4 with claudication, both of which were caused by aortoiliac occlusive disease. One patient (treated for carcinoma of the prostate) developed a left iliac occlusion that was treated with a common iliac–to–common femoral bypass. Two years later, a similar lesion developed on the right and was treated in a like manner. One patient presented with significant renal artery stenosis and arterial hypertension and was treated with a renal artery bypass, and another underwent a multiple visceral bypass for arterial hypertension and short-distance claudication. Both patients presented late following radiation therapy (17 and 25 years, respectively). One patient who developed bilateral pedal gangrene approximately 40 years after radiation for carcinoma of the uterus underwent axillobifemoral bypass grafting. This patient also had irradiation cystitis and proctitis. In another patient, a superficial femoral artery occlusion occurred 35 years after femur irradiation for Ewing's sarcoma; a greater saphenous vein femoropopliteal bypass graft (using the ipsilateral vein) has effectively relieved his rest pain for 11 years.

The overall results of revascularization of postirradiation vascular lesions approximates the results obtainable for arteriosclerotic lesions. There were no strokes, graft disruptions, or failures of graft incorporation. There also was no limb loss, and all patients obtained relief of arterial hypertension for renovascular lesions and claudication for revascularization of the infrarenal aorta and its runoff. There were, however, delayed complications that ultimately contributed to 2 deaths. One patient, having undergone carotid saphenous vein interposition grafting for common carotid artery stenosis, required a myofascial free flap so that the operative site could be adequately covered. In addition to radiation, he had undergone a radical neck dissection for carcinoma of the tongue. Seven months later, he sustained a completed stroke with hemiparesis contralateral to the grafted carotid artery. The status of the graft at the time of death was unknown. In the only patient requiring a prosthetic extra-anatomic bypass, gastroenterologic complications led to the patient's death 2 months postbypass from necrotizing radiation rectoproctitis. A rectosigmoidectomy was performed together with a colostomy, and the patient died in acute renal failure following this procedure. *In situ* aortic reconstruction was contraindicated because of peritonitis. There were no deaths and no amputations.

CONCLUSION

The precise relationship between radiation therapy and subsequent arterial lesions remains the focus of investigation. The vascular defects observed within an irradiated field may resemble those seen in nonirradiated arteriosclerotic arteries, or they may be atypical in location and/or appearance.[12] Radiation therapy may be a unique causative factor. It may contribute in synergy with an arteriosclerotic diathesis, or there may be a noncausal association. Coincidental factors in postirradiation patients may contribute to the development of these arterial lesions. For example, all but two of the patients in our series were habitual smokers. Some investigators have implicated arteriosclerotic risk factors such as elevated serum cholesterol levels and hyperlipidemia,[13,14] and hypertension[15] as contributors to the development of arterial lesions in clinical or experimental studies.

We observed radiation arteritis lesions in patients whose treatment ranged from orthovoltage therapy in the 1940s to contemporary LINAC treatment. The precise incidence for each type of therapy is unknown in general and is also unknown for any given family of neoplasms. In a retrospective study of 910 patients surviving at least 5 years after undergoing cervical irradiation for Hodgkin's disease, Elerding et al[16] investigated the incidence of carotid lesions. Not only was there an increased risk of stroke in this group of patients, but in a prospective study of 118 patients, a high incidence of carotid lesions was detected and attributed to the irradiation. The findings of Moritz et al[17] are also consistent with this hypothesis. Thirty percent of their patients who received therapeutic doses of external irradiation for head and neck cancer had a significant carotid artery lesion, compared with 6% of a control group. Ten percent of the irradiated patients had symptomatic lesions when the group was studied 28 months after high-dose therapy. This finding prompted some investigators[16,17] to recommend routine postoperative duplex screening of carotid arteries when these vessels lie within irradiated fields so that carotid lesions can be detected before they become symptomatic or proceed to total occlusion in 5-year survivors of radiotherapy. Not all researchers, however, agree with this recommendation.[18]

As partial mastectomy plus radiotherapy becomes the dominant therapeutic strategy for many types of breast cancer,[19] lesions of the axillary and subclavian arteries will assume greater importance. Often, the first symptom that the patient experiences from a late-appearing arterial lesion is acute ischemia due to occlusion or embolization.

Several operative methods and principles were applied in the management of our patients. We believe that the application of these methods and principles, led to our low mortality and morbidity. Dissection of the carotid arteries is frequently difficult because of induration of the skin and the brawny nature of the artery. This dissection must be done sharply, with minimal disturbance to the carotid bifurcation and the occlusion-bearing portion of the vessel. Often, the carotid artery is rigid and fibrotic, and the cleavage plane between the arterial wall and the thickened intima and media is difficult to establish. For this reason, we routinely perform autogenous patching with greater saphenous vein, preferably harvested from the groin. If adequate primary coverage is not possible, concomitant or delayed myocutaneous free-flap construction is a useful strategy. Prosthetic material, either for patching or for bypass grafting, should be avoided because of the risk of nonincorporation and/or infection. All axillary and subclavian lesions were bypassed with autogenous vein, either from the contralateral arm, the leg, or the saphenous system. As an inflow site, either the carotid or the proximal subclavian artery was used, and tunnels were made beneath the clavicle under direct vision. In patients undergoing aortofemoral or iliofemoral bypass, we liberally used ureteral catheters and found them to be a useful adjunct to identify and protect the ureters intraoperatively within the fibrotic retroperitoneun. Once again, orthotopic tunnels were used, and only one extra-anatomic bypass was performed because of a "hostile" abdomen. Although extra-anatomic bypass has been recommended,[20] in our experience it has not been necessary, and we have seen no instances of failure of graft incorporation or delayed disincorporation. The ultimate autogenous orthotopic revascularization, percutaneous transluminal balloon angioplasty, has also been a successful treatment for radiation-induced arterial stenoses.[21]

A growing amount of literature about arterial lesions associated with radiation therapy can be anticipated as the number of patients undergoing this form of treatment increases. For example, contemporary treatment protocols differ from earlier ones in that previously all the dose to the tumor was delivered from either one field or one field per day. As a result, the adjacent arteries within the field received 10% to 50% more radiation than the daily tumor dose. This was the case when cardiovascular complications of radiotherapy for Hodgkin's disease were studied: The probability of coronary artery disease was higher with treatment of one field per day than when both fields were treated daily. It is anticipated that with multiple-field treatment, the incidence of these complications will decrease; however, multiple-field treatment will involve different and varied beam orientations. Consequently, the relationship of the radiation therapy to the late-occurring arterial lesion will become even more problematic because there will be no telltale overlying skin changes or tattoos. The surgeon caring for these patients would be wise to maintain accurate records, not only of the operative procedure, but also of the characteristics of the radiotherapy administered because consultation with radiation oncologists will become increasingly important. Often the patients undergoing radiotherapy are younger than the average arteriosclerotic patient and develop their lesions many decades after radiotherapy. For all intents and purposes, all are cured of their underlying neoplasms. Whether long-term screening of carotid, subclavian, and aortic runoff lesions will be useful or practical is a subject for continuing discussion.

REFERENCES

1. Owen J. Facilities survey of the patterns of care survey of the American College of Radiology. *Int J Radiat Oncol Biol Phys.* 1992.
2. Owen J. (in press).
3. Andros G, Schneider PA, Harris RW, et al. Management of arterial occlusive disease following radiation therapy. *Cardiovasc Surg.* (in press).
4. Gassman A. Zur histologie der Roentgenulcera. *Fortschr Rontgenstrahlen.* 1899;2:199.
5. Wolbach SB. The pathological histology of chronic x-ray dermatitis and early x-ray carcinomas. *J Med Res.* 1909;21:415–429.
6. Warren S, Friedman NB. Pathology and pathologic diagnosis of radiation lesions in the gastrointestinal tract. *Am J Pathol.* 1942;18:499.
7. Regaerd, Coutard, Hautant.
8. Fajardo LF, Berthrong M. Vascular lesions following radiation (Part 1). *Pathol Annu.* 1988;23:297–330.
9. Fee WE, Goffinet DR, Guthaner D, et al. Safety of ^{125}iodine and ^{192}iridium implants to the canine carotid artery: preliminary report. *Laryngoscope.* 1985;95:317.
10. Johnson L, Longenecker JP, Fajardo LF. Differential radiation response of cultured endothelial cells and smooth myocytes. *Anal Quant Cytol.* 1982;4:188.
11. Fajardo LF. *Pathology of Radiation Injury.* New York, NY: Masson; 1982.
12. Bergentz SE, Bergqvist D. Radiation-induced vascular injuries. In: *Iatrogenic Vascular Injuries.* New York, NY: Springer-Verlag; 1989:63–75.
13. Silverberg GD, Britt RH, Goffinet DR. Radiation-induced carotid artery disease. *Cancer.* 1978;41:130–137.
14. Amromin GD, Gildenhorn HL, Solomon RD, et al. The synergism of x-irradiation and cholesterol-fat feeding on the development of coronary artery lesions. *J Atheroscler Res.* 1964;4:325–334.
15. Asscher AW, Wilson C, Anson S. Sensitisation of blood-vessels to hypertensive damage by x-irradiation. *Lancet.* 1961;11:580–583.
16. Elerding SC, Fernandez RN, Grotta JC, et al. Carotid artery disease following external cervical irradiation. *Ann Surg.* 1981;194:609–615.

17. Moritz MW, Higgins RF, Jacobs JR. Duplex imaging and incidence of carotid radiation injury after high-dose radiotherapy for tumors of the head and neck. *Arch Surg*. 1990;125:1181–1183.
18. Lopez M, El-Bayar H, Hye RJ, et al. Carotid artery disease in patients with head and neck carcinoma. *Am Surg*. 1990;56:778–781.
19. Harris JR, Hellman S, Kinne DW. Special report: limited surgery and radiotherapy for early breast cancer. *N Engl J Med*. 1985;21:1365–1368.
20. Phillips GR III, Peer RM, Upson JF, et al. Late complications of revascularization for radiation-induced arterial disease. *J Vasc Surg*. 1992;16:921–925.
21. Guthaner DF, Schmitz L. Percutaneous transluminal angioplasty of radiation-induced arterial stenoses. *Radiology*. 1982;144:77–78.

44

Vascular Malformations

Effective Treatment with Absolute Ethanol

Robert L. Vogelzang, MD, and Wayne F. Yakes, MD

SCOPE OF THE PROBLEM

Vascular malformations are extremely challenging lesions. The clinical presentations of these congenital abnormalities are protean and range from asymptomatic birthmarks to life-threatening congestive heart failure or exsanguinating hemorrhage. These abnormalities are rare; most clinicians see only a few in a lifetime of practice. Thus, patients afflicted with these disorders often seek help from many different physicians and undergo repetitive examination, diagnosis, and frequent failed attempts at "definitive" therapy that lead to exacerbation of symptoms, lesion recurrences, and disability.[1]

Vascular anomalies were first treated by surgeons. The early surgical paradigm of proximal arterial ligation of arterial feeders proved futile when the phenomenon of neovascular recruitment rapidly reconstituted arterial inflow to the arteriovenous malformation (AVM) and as microfistulous connections became macrofistulous feeders. Complete extirpation of an AVM nidus proved very difficult and very hazardous in that massive hemorrhage often occurred. Partial resections could cause an initial good clinical response, but with time the patient's symptoms usually recurred or worsened (Fig. 44–1). With time, it became apparent to vascular surgeons that, as stated by D. E. Szilagyi, M.D., and coworkers,[2] " . . . with few exceptions, their cure by surgical means is impossible. We had intuitively thought that the only answer of a surgeon to the problem of disfiguring, often noisome and occasionally disabling blemishes and masses, prone to cause bleeding, pain, or other unpleasantness, was to attack them with vigor and with the determination of eradicating them." The results of this attempt at radical treatment were disappointing. In Szilagyi and coworkers' series of 82 patients, only 18 were believed to be operable, and of those, 10 were improved, 2 were the same, and 6 were worse at follow-up.[2]

As the discipline of interventional radiology developed, embolization of these lesions with particulate matter became widely used in an attempt to completely destroy the lesion, or to control flow (and therefore symptoms), or as a preoperative maneuver to reduce blood loss and allow complete removal.[3–5] With time, however, it was found that complete destruction, or "cure," of an AVM with particulate embolotherapy was rare. Despite the use of smaller particles and marked improvement in catheter delivery systems, the use of mechanical occlusive agents was ultimately a disappointment for

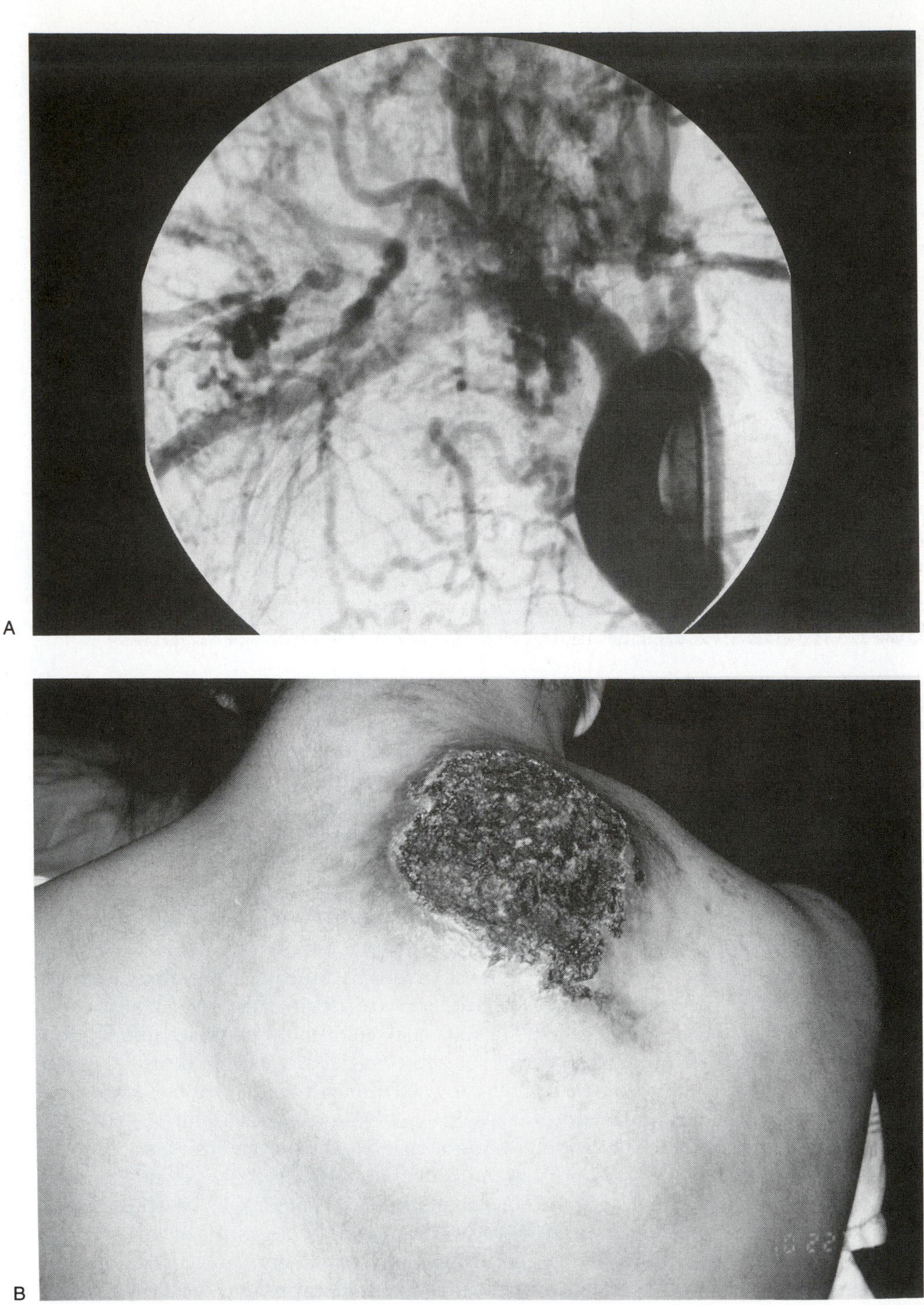

Figure 44–1. A 20-year-old woman had a massive AVM of the posterior upper thorax and occiput. (**A**) Arch arteriogram demonstrating the extensive AVM, which is fed by branches of the subclavian, vertebral, axillary, and carotid arteries. (**B**) The ulcerated area overlying an extensive mass on the posterior trunk. Surgical debridement of this area was performed.

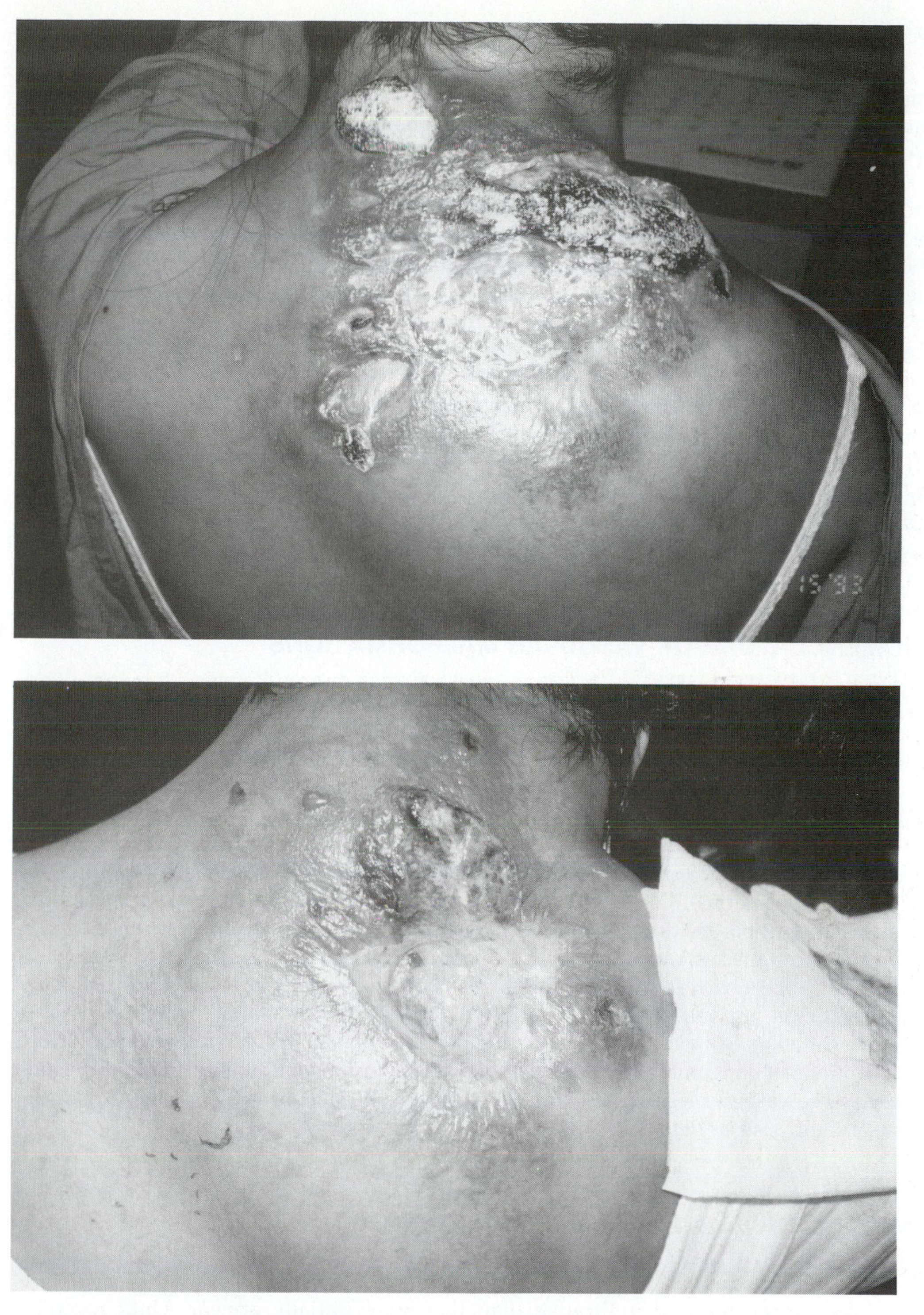

Figure 44–1. *(continued)* (**C**) Three months after surgical excision, there was marked exacerbation of the lesion with extensive ulceration and tissue breakdown. (**D**) After four sessions of ethanol embolotherapy, the lesion had healed significantly.

us and others. The majority of AVMs recurred after embolization just as they did after surgery: by neovascular recruitment with reconstitution of arterial inflow into the AVM nidus.

Liquid agents such as tissue glues, alcohol, and sodium tetradecyl sulfate (Sotradecol) were used sparingly as vascular occlusive agents by interventional radiologists for a number of years; these agents were used in the liver, bronchial arteries, and kidneys.[6,7] Sodium tetradecyl sulfate was also commonly used to treat superficial venous varicosities with good results. The action of liquid embolic agents appeared to be mediated by a more potent and destructive mechanism than the simple vascular occlusion provided by particles, but intravascular liquids were believed to be far too hazardous for general use. However, in 1986, Yakes et al[8] described curative treatment of an extremity AVM with absolute alcohol. Since then, it has become increasingly apparent that ethanol embolotherapy for vascular malformations can be curative, even for complex AVMs (Figs. 44–2 and 44–3). In this chapter, we discuss the use of alcohol to treat a variety of high-flow and low-flow vascular lesions. We believe that alcohol offers significant promise for the patients afflicted with these disorders and now believe it to be the agent of choice for vascular malformation therapy.[1,9]

NOMENCLATURE OF VASCULAR MALFORMATIONS

Until recently, classification of vascular malformations was confusing. Authors and workers used inaccurate or ill-defined terms, such as *cavernous hemangioma, venous angioma, cirsoid aneurysm, congenital arteriovenous fistula,* and many others. The lack of a standard nomenclature caused much diagnostic inaccuracy and confusion, but the recent classification system of Mulliken and Young[10] clarified the field considerably. In this chapter, we use their system for dividing vascular malformations into high-flow lesions (AVMs and arteriovenous fistulas) and low-flow lesions (venous, lymphatic, and mixed malformations). The term *hemangioma* should be used only for lesions in children that become apparent during the first month of life, rapidly proliferate, then slowly involute spontaneously to almost complete resolution at a young age (4 to 7 years old). For adults, the term *hemangioma* should *not* be used since the lesions are not truly hemangiomas but rather venous malformations. Port-wine stains (which were previously called *capillary hemangiomas*) should be called *capillary malformations.* In addition, descriptions of congenital syndromes often include inappropriate terminology to characterize the vascular lesions associated with them. Whenever possible, these descriptions should also be replaced with the more accurate terms just noted.

IMAGING OF VASCULAR MALFORMATIONS

Imaging of vascular malformations is vitally important since these lesions are by definition more extensive and infiltrative than they may initially appear. Until recently, arteriography and venography were the sole methods of assessment, and although the information obtained from these techniques remains initially important (we never treat a lesion without careful selective and superselective arteriography or venography), cross-sectional imaging has assumed pre-eminence in the identification, characterization, and localization of vascular malformations. Two modalities in particular, color-flow Doppler ultrasound and magnetic resonance imaging (MRI), now play a dominant role in imaging of these lesions.

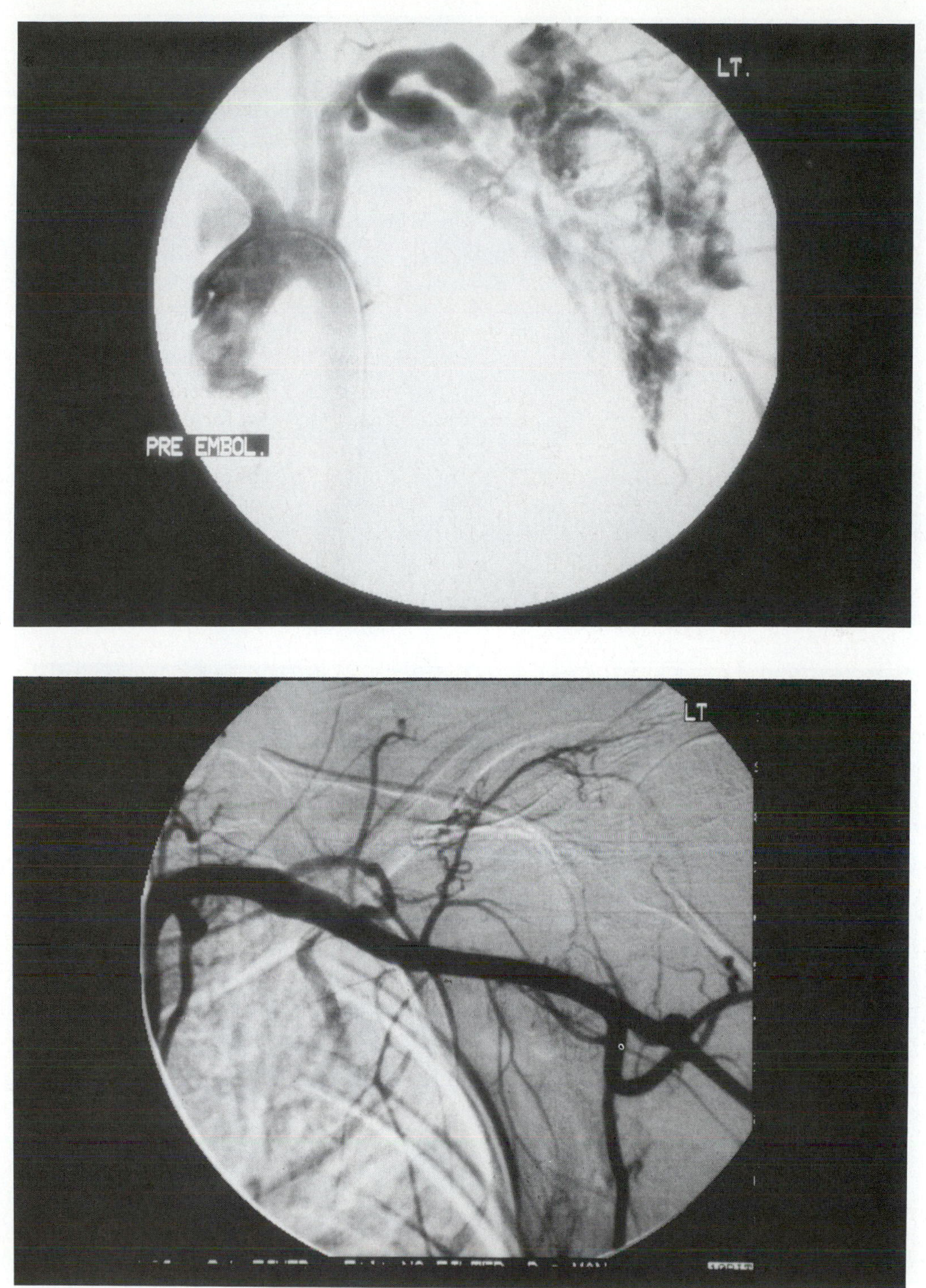

Figure 44–2. (**A**) Arteriogram of a 23-year-old woman with an extensive AVM of the left shoulder. The lesion is being fed from branches of the left subclavian and axillary arteries. (**B**) Two years after curative ethanol embolotherapy, a left subclavian arteriogram reveals a normal appearance.

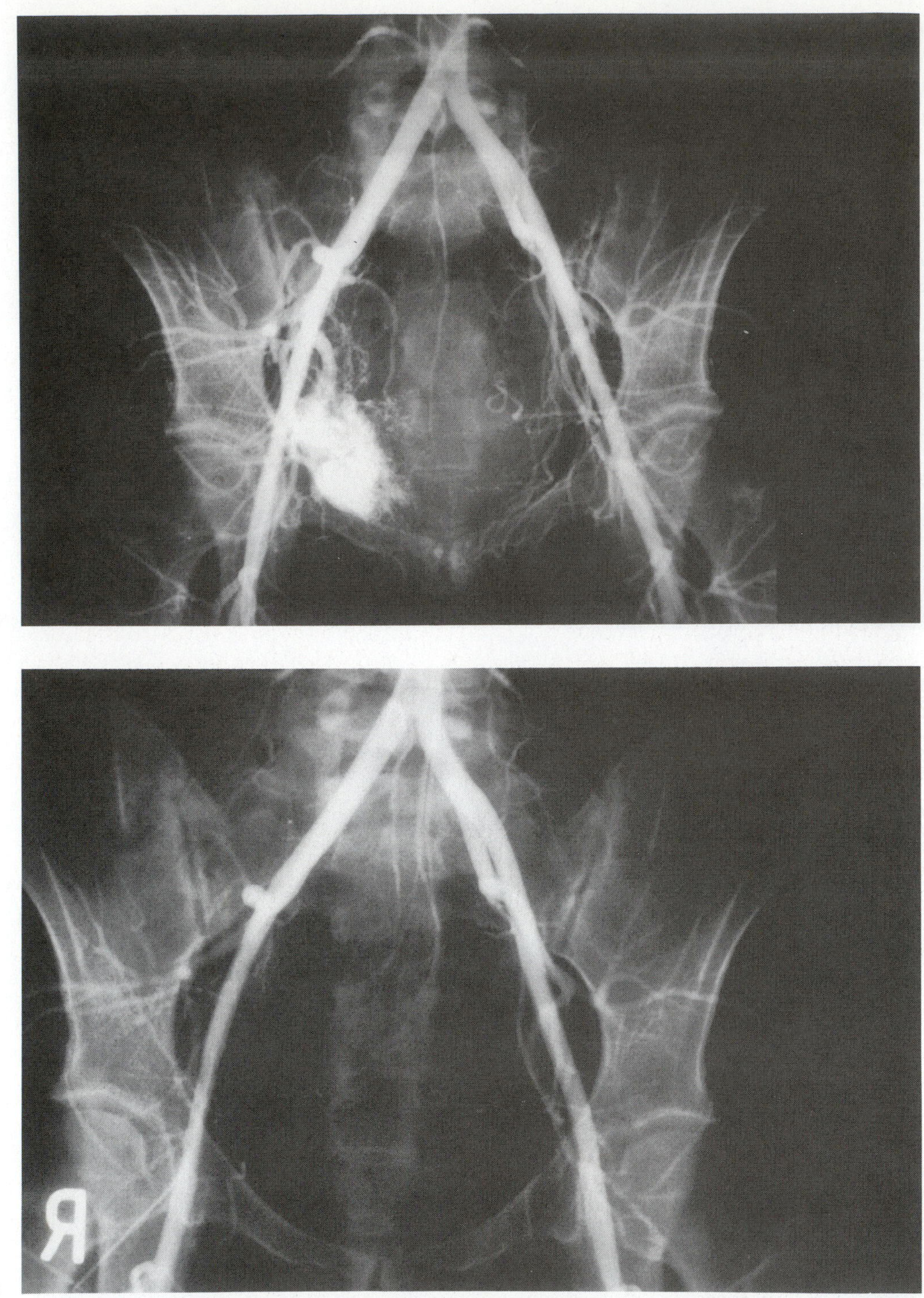

Figure 44–3. (**A**) Pelvic arteriogram of a 24-year-old female with a large right pelvic AVM. Ligation of the anterior division of the right internal iliac artery had been performed 3 months prior but had not modified the symptoms or the flow. (**B**) Pelvic arteriogram 5 years after ethanol embolotherapy. The right internal iliac artery is intact; however, there is no longer filling of the pelvic malformation.

Magnetic Resonance Imaging

In our experience, MRI is *the* definitive tool for cross-sectional imaging of vascular malformations. Rak et al[11] identified and characterized the MRI appearance of malformations, including venous malformations, AVMs, and arteriovenous fistulas, and showed that MRI was essential in separating vascular lesions into high-flow and low-flow types. The predominant distinction between venous malformations and arteriovenous fistulas and malformations can be seen on T2-weighted MRIs. On these sequences, venous malformations are of high signal intensity ("bright") (Fig. 44–4). Conversely, arteriovenous fistulas and AVMs demonstrate little or no signal due to the phenomenon known as *flow void*. In addition, MRI shows involvement of neural, subcutaneous, and/or muscular structures due to its superior tissue differentiation. The multiplanar imaging capabilities of MRI also allow localization and characterization of complex lesions, whether truncal or extremity in location.

Compared with computed tomography (CT) (which we used in the past), MRI is superior in virtually all aspects. Except for specific situations, we have abandoned the use of CT in the workup and evaluation of vascular malformations.

Color-flow Doppler Ultrasound

Color-flow Doppler ultrasound is also useful for identifying both high-flow and low-flow vascular lesions. We also found this technique essential in guiding direct puncture of malformations by permitting accurate localization of the nidus. Follow-up examination is commonly used to document the decreased vascular flow rates and thromboses that occur after successful therapy.

ETHANOL AS A VASCULAR OCCLUSIVE AGENT

Ethanol is a powerful sclerosing agent that denatures blood proteins and destroys vascular endothelial cells by dehydration and denudation. These changes (which essentially cause tissue necrosis and death) occur rapidly and cause thrombosis of the malformation. In malformations, these changes are desirable and account for the curative effects of this therapy. However, clearly the use of ethanol in a normal vascular structure is to be eschewed, as introduction into vessels supplying structures such as nerves, muscles, or connective tissue will result in necrosis of that tissue. Ethanol treatment of vascular malformations thus requires significant experience with the agent, as well as extreme caution and a complete understanding of the pathophysiology of the vascular malformation being treated. It should be stressed that some of the most challenging and complex cases seen by vascular specialists involve patients with vascular malformations. We believe that these abnormalities should be treated only at medical centers where such patients are seen regularly. In an average practice (even a busy one), only a handful of vascular malformations are ever seen during the course of a career, and in these cases the injudicious or inappropriate use of alcohol is most hazardous since the agent necessary to produce a cure can also produce severe complications.

Safe Use of Ethanol in Vascular Malformations

Technical intraprocedural requirements for the use of ethanol include the following: (1) superselective catheter placement or direct deposition of ethanol within the nidus of the vascular lesion; (2) avoidance of alcohol injection into normal vessels; (3) use of

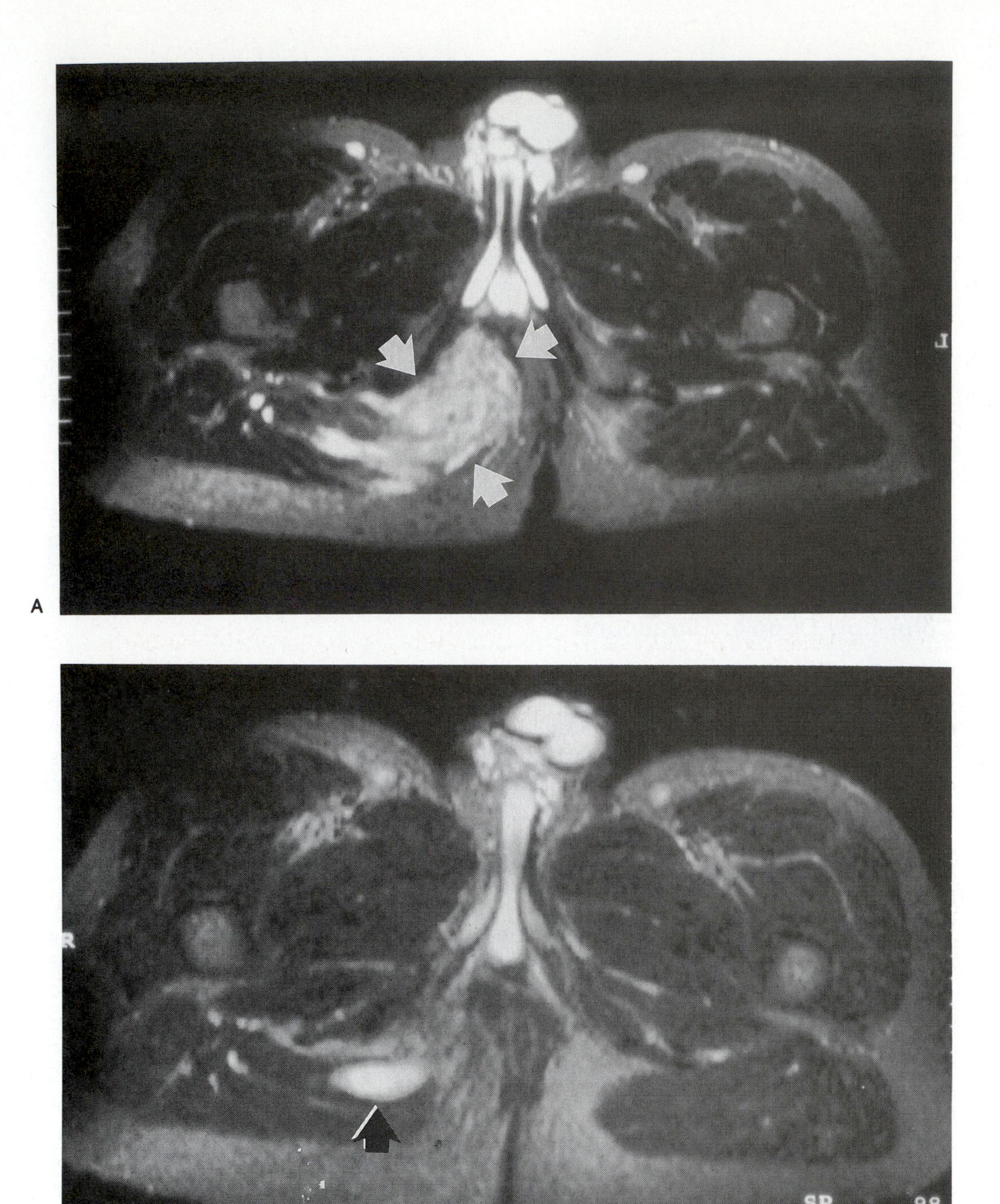

Figure 44–4. A 28-year-old man had a painful gluteal and ischiorectal fossa venous malformation. Two atttempts at surgical removal resulted in massive bleeding. (**A**) T2-weighted MRI demonstrating the bright venous malformation (*arrows*). The lesion was treated with percutaneous ethanol injections (five sessions). (**B**) Follow-up MRI, 6 weeks after the final injection, shows a small residual venous malformation (*arrow*), but the patient's pain has disappeared.

general anesthesia with appropriate intraprocedural monitoring; (4) good immediate postoperative care, including the appropriate use of medications to reduce side effects; and (5) careful clinical follow-up with appropriate retreatment when necessary to produce the maximum benefit. Each of these issues is discussed in greater detail next.

1. *Superselective catheterization and deposition of alcohol directly into the vascular malformation.* This essential and vital principle underlies the safe and effective use of ethanol. As we stated earlier, absolute alcohol destroys tissues, which is the desired effect in vascular malformations but is a toxic and morbid one when normal tissues are involved. Only when alcohol can be accurately placed into the lesion will consistent and reproducible results be obtained. The necessity for superselective catheterization of these lesions requires the physician to have significant experience in recognition of the nidi of vascular malformations. In our estimation, this is the most important element of treatment of vascular malformations. Arteriovenous malformations are extremely complex, and their architecture can be confusing. On this point there is no equivocation: Determination of the angioarchitecture of a vascular malformation should be left to an experienced interventional radiologist who recognizes not only many of the pitfalls of lesion detection, but also where the lesion should be treated to produce a cure. Even for the experienced interventionalist, recognition of the nidus of the lesion can be difficult and require all his or her diagnostic skills. Once the nidus is recognized, however, access to the area can be planned and usually achieved by either superselective catheterization or direct puncture so that the appropriate amount of alcohol can be used to destroy the nidus. In our experience, it is common to spend 3 to 4 hours evaluating a lesion with multiple angiographic or venographic injections before catheterization or puncture of the vascular malformation can be performed and result in a benefit without toxicity.

Many tools and techniques can be used to catheterize and treat these lesions, including real-time ultrasound, coaxial microcatheters, inflow and/or outflow occlusion (to increase the dwell time of the ethanol in the vascular malformation), and extensive use of digital subtraction arteriography.

2. *Avoidance of injection of normal vessels. Only* by careful catheterization of the vascular nidus can normal vessels be avoided. Thus, the operator must be aware of regional anatomy as well as the vascular supply to adjacent normal structures, which might lie in the area being treated and whose inadvertent embolization may cause problems. Such knowledge is particularly necessary to reduce neural complications; for this reason, we consider MRI to be helpful in preoperative staging of these lesions since it accurately depicts the relationship between the lesion and normal structures.

Part of the process of ethanol therapy is a rigorous and frequently lengthy intraoperative use of test injections of contrast material, during which a number of parameters are manipulated. These variables include injection rates, injection volumes, and application of occluding tourniquets or direct digital compression to control the flow rate of ethanol through the lesion. In general, we try to keep ethanol in contact with the nidus for a minimum of 10 minutes by controlling outflow and/or inflow vessels. Thus, extensive test injections of contrast material tell the interventionalist whether normal vessels will be filled and what the pressure–volume relationships should be to either allow filling or avoid filling of the normal vessels.

3. *Use of general anesthesia with careful physiologic monitoring.* In our early experience, we did not use general anesthesia but opted for heavy conscious sedation. We found this approach unsatisfactory for two reasons: First, the use of ethanol is painful, and inadvertent movement of the patient during the injection frequently causes problems

with withdrawal of a perfectly placed catheter or needle, thus increasing the likelihood of complications. Second, the cardiovascular condition cannot be monitored. Ethanol therapy has been associated with some cardiovascular events, including cardiovascular collapse and pulmonary embolism, among others.[1,7,12] Alcohol may also cause pulmonary vasospasm and/or some cardiac effects, particularly when given in larger volumes. We found that general anesthesia with careful cardiovascular monitoring, including Swan-Ganz catheterization and measurement of cardiopulmonary parameters, is vital for management of these patients, particularly at the time of injection of ethanol. We can state unequivocally that such support is mandatory for appropriate outcomes. In addition, the complexity of procedural performance in these cases demands that the operating interventionalist be able to concentrate fully on the case at hand, without concern for stabilization and monitoring of the patient's vital signs and overall status.

4. *Postoperative follow-up and medication.* Ethanol embolotherapy is almost inevitably accompanied by edema and some degree of thrombosis, both expected events. Some of the most common problems that we have seen include edema with production of adjacent ischemia and/or neuropathy. Aggressive management of this expected edematous process demands the use of Decadron intraoperatively, as well as oral corticosteroids postoperatively for 5 to 7 days. Other medications used include Toradol, aspirin, and heparin to prevent thrombosis of adjacent nontarget structures.

Other issues of postoperative importance include careful monitoring for skin complications. Occasionally, skin loss may necessitate grafting, although this is not generally the case. Also important is appropriate pain management with narcotics and/or transcutaneous electronic nerve stimulation, which we found to be very useful in dealing with the considerable postoperative pain.

5. *Careful clinical follow-up and reintervention.* Frequent and careful follow-up of these patients is mandatory. The patient must be observed for complications and the lesion imaged at frequent intervals with MRI and/or color-flow Doppler ultrasound. Angiographic or venographic follow-up may also be necessary.

Because of the time needed for treatment and the limitations on the total volume of alcohol for use during any one procedure (generally 30 to 50 mL), only a segment or a portion of an extensive lesion can be treated in 1 session. In our experience, the average malformation (arteriovenous *or* venous) requires 4 to 5 sessions, and we have treated some patients with extensive vascular malformations as many as 25 or 30 times to achieve appropriate results. Only a coordinated and dedicated team of specialists consisting of interventional radiologists, vascular surgeons, plastic surgeons, and pain specialists can handle these patients in an appropriate manner.

The application of the aforementioned principles permits treatment of specific types of vascular lesions. In the next sections, we discuss how alcohol can be used effectively and safely in various malformations.

Ethanol Treatment of Venous Malformations

Venous malformations are congenital lesions that present with a variety of abnormalities ranging from relatively focal, contained vascular lesions to infiltrating vascular abnormalities with multiple venous channels. Venous malformations generally present with pain as a predominant symptom, although they may cause tissue ulceration or induce changes in adjacent bones. Cosmetic deformities, particularly with head and neck venous malformations, are also important issues. In the extremities, venous malformations usually produce pain and frequently induce swelling of an extremity; venous ulcerations may also appear.[10]

The arteriogram inevitably demonstrates normal size and flow in the arteries; there may be minimal contrast pooling within the abnormal venous structures on late-phase films. For this reason, arteriography is generally a poor tool for identifying venous malformations. In our experience, the procedure of choice for identification of venous malformations is MRI, which shows the lesions to be very bright on T2-weighted studies. Other mandatory workup includes closed system venography and/or direct-puncture venography, which better demonstrates the size and volume of the venous malformation. Color-flow Doppler ultrasound is also useful.

The treatment of venous malformations epitomizes the successes that we achieved with ethanol sclerotherapy in that the majority of lesions can be successfully extirpated with alcohol. Venous malformations are inevitably best treated by direct percutaneous puncture to directly access the abnormal venous elements. The venous malformation is carefully evaluated at the time of therapy for total volume and through the aforementioned methods of flow occlusion and compression. The volume of contrast needed to fill the lesion is assessed repeatedly. During this assessment, avoidance of flow into normal veins is paramount; once the appropriate volume and pressure relationships are achieved, the desired volume of ethanol is injected (Fig. 44–5). Postoperative complications are generally minimal, although we have seen neuropathy and skin ulceration.[13]

We believe that the majority of venous malformations can be cured or considerably reduced in size (to an asymptomatic level) by the use of ethanol therapy. We use follow-up MRI frequently; it inevitably demonstrates absent signal in an area that previously showed intense signal on T2-weighted studies. This appearance documents the destruction and complete thrombosis of the venous malformation (Figs. 44–4 and 44–5).

Ethanol Treatment of Arteriovenous Malformations

Arteriovenous malformations are congenital lesions in which abnormal primitive communications exist between artery and vein. The central and significant feature of an AVM is the presence of a primitive vascular nidus that rapidly empties into dilated tortuous outflow veins without the presence of a normal capillary bed. The symptoms associated with AVMs include high-output cardiac failure, disfigurement, pain, neuropathy, exsanguinating hemorrhage, and venous hypertension, particularly when the malformation is located in a limb. In these patients, ulceration related to venous hypertension is a chronic and troubling issue and is often the symptom that leads to contact with a physician. Mulliken and Young[10] characterized the effects of AVMs as predominantly related to vascular shunting through the malformation. These effects include (1) increased flow in the inflow artery, with dilatation, thickening, and tortuosity; (2) parasitic flow through the fistula, which causes reversal of normal flow in the distal arterial segment; (3) lowering of distal arterial pressure with production of ischemia in the structure supplied; (4) an increase in peripheral venous pressure, which accentuates the peripheral arterial ischemia and precipitates pain, ulceration, edema, and gangrene; and (5) increased cardiac output with subsequent development of heart failure. These five effects usually mandate the ultimate treatment of AVMs, although we have seen relatively asymptomatic AVMs in patients as old as 65 years.

Treatment requires superselective catheterization or direct puncture of the nidus to prevent complications of inadvertent nontarget embolization. Inflow or outflow occlusion is generally required to produce vascular stasis. Another important principle is the use of staged or multiple procedures. However, when appropriately utilized, alcohol ablation of AVMs can be curative. The use of ethanol led us to conclude that

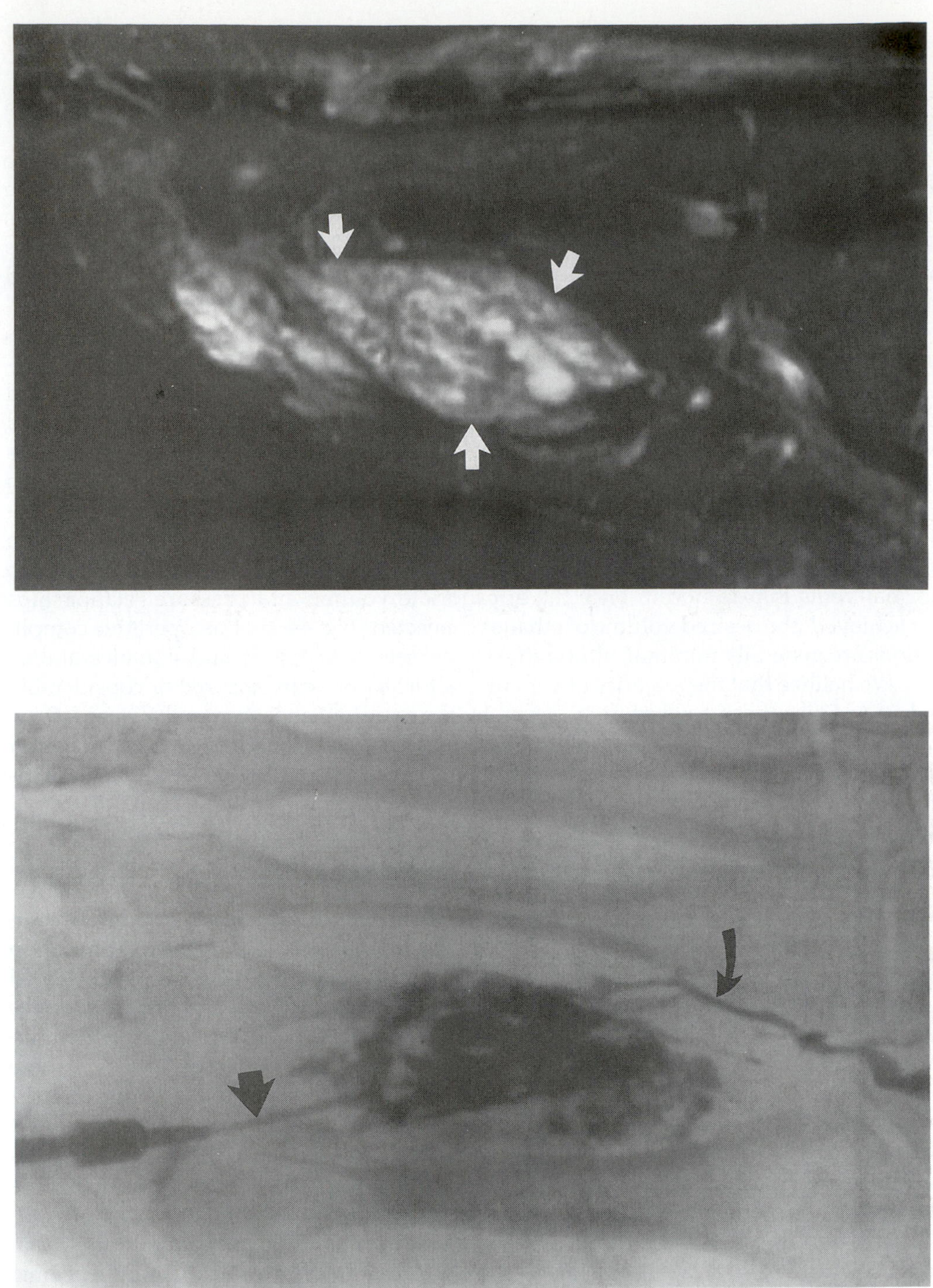

Figure 44–5. A 30-year-old woman had a painful venous malformation of the right foot that was operated on five times and continued to recur. (A) Sagittal T2-weighted MRI of the foot shows a bright venous malformation on the dorsum (*arrows*). (B) Intraoperative test injection technique showing the needle (*arrow*) in the lesion.

C

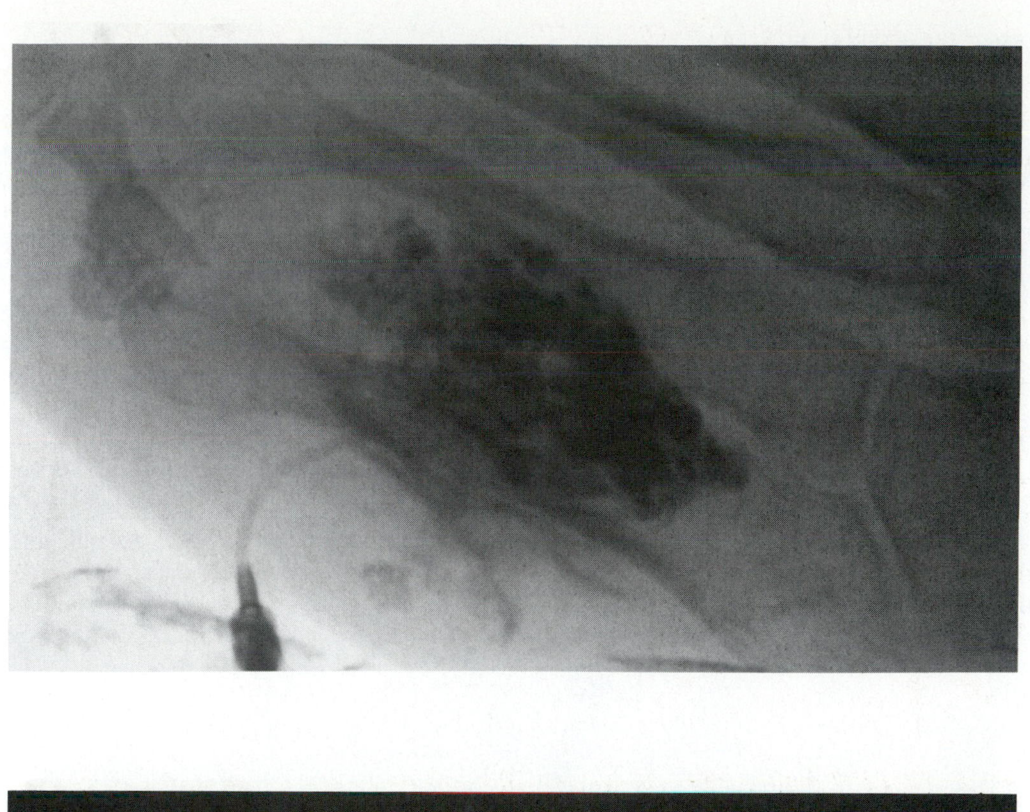

D

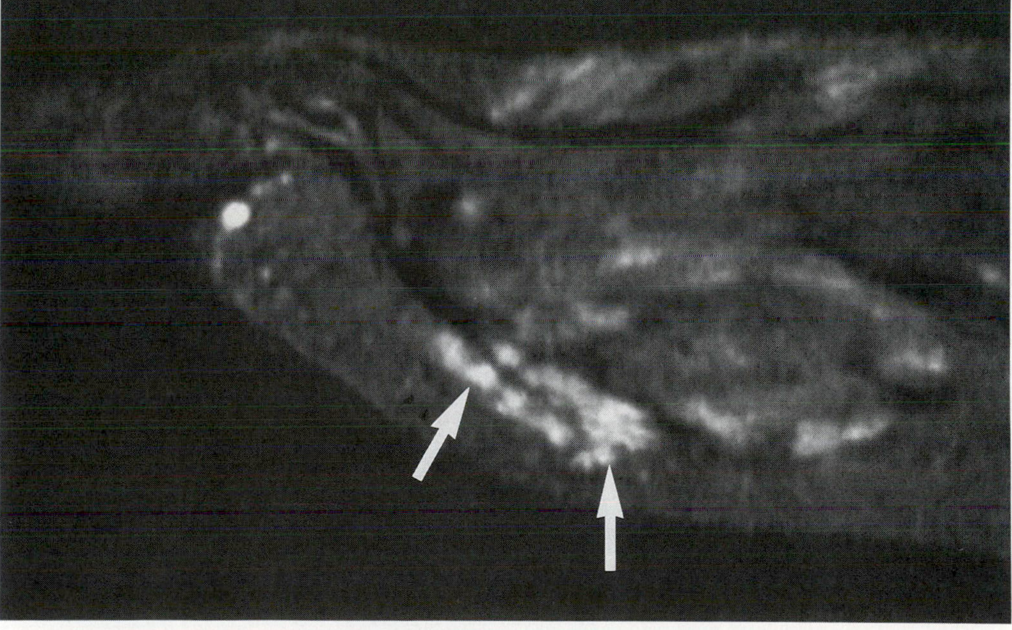

Figure 44–5. (*continued*) On this test injection, an outflow vein (*curved arrow*) filled, and manual pressure was reapplied to achieve filling of the lesion only (**C**). Following this test injection, 4 mL of ethanol was injected without complication, and the patient's pain promptly disappeared. (**D**) Follow-up MRI 6 months after treatment shows the disappearance of signal in the lesion. A small focal venous malformation persists (*arrows*), but since the patient was asymptomatic, further treatment was deferred until symptoms recur.

the possibility of cure even in complex or large lesions can now be legitimately discussed with many patients (Figs. 44–2 and 44–3). Although cure is not always possible in every patient, ethanol therapy can often reduce flow in and the size of the lesion to a point where symptoms are not present, a limb is saved, or cardiac output is reduced to reasonable levels, thus avoiding the long-term problems associated with high output through such fistulous lesions (Fig. 44–6).

On the other hand, the use of alcohol in AVMs raises the stakes considerably as far as complications are concerned. These high-flow lesions can be difficult to localize and/or catheterize, and the risk of nontarget embolization remains relatively high. Neural ischemia is our most feared complication, but we have also observed pulmonary embolism during treatment of large fistulous AVMs. Currently, our combined complication rate for AVM therapy is 15%. The majority of these complications are self-limited and reversible, although permanent neural ischemia and neuropathy have certainly been observed. Despite these potential problems, we remain extremely encouraged

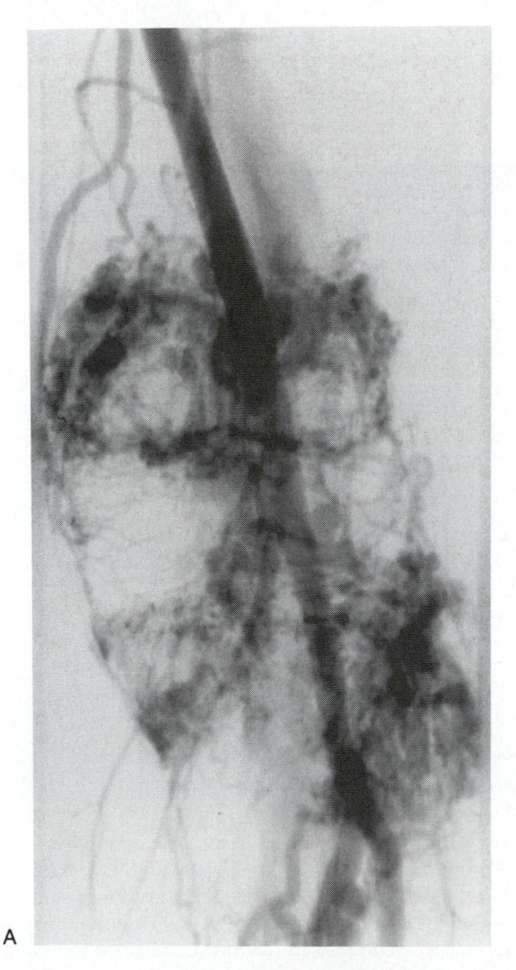

Figure 44–6. A 17-year-old male presented with a massive AVM of the left lower extremity. This lesion involved the distal thigh, calf, and foot. (**A**) Arteriogram of the knee before treatment shows extensive involvement of the entire area. During a 4-year period, 12 separate treatments with alcohol were performed by using a combination of intra-arterial therapy, direct puncture, and venous occlusion.

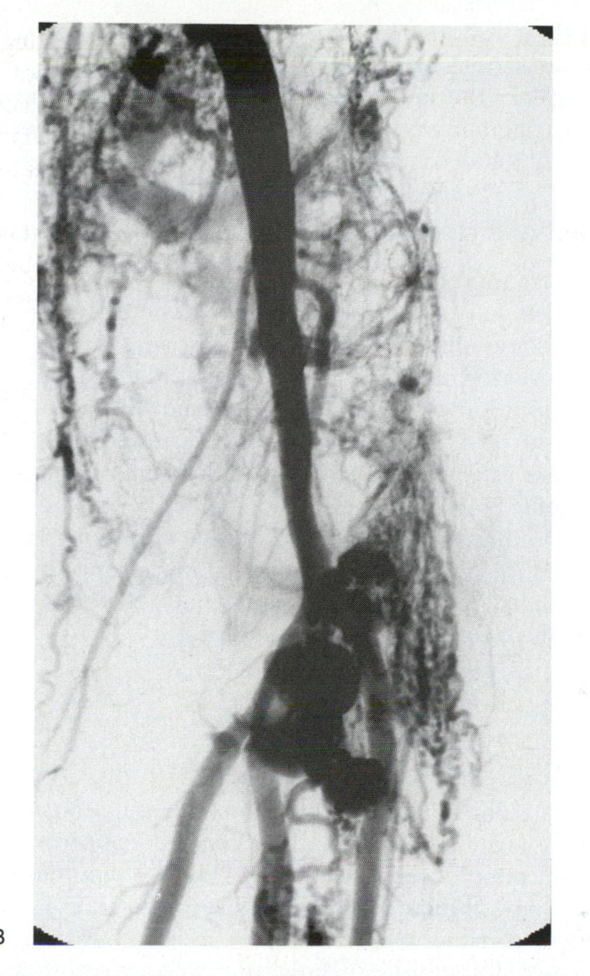

Figure 44–6. (*continued*) (**B**) Follow-up arteriogram of the knee shows marked diminution of the AVM. Pain and chronic swelling of the extremity have disappeared. Treatment of focal areas will continue.

about the use of ethanol and believe it to be the only agent that should be used in AVMs.[1,9] We believe strongly that conventional occlusive embolic agents such as polyvinyl alcohol particles, Gelfoam pledgets, glue, and coils should *never* be used because of the inevitable recruitment of collateral and neovascular vessels that either exacerbates symptoms or makes appropriate treatment with ethanol more difficult by limiting access to major vascular channels.

Ethanol Treatment of Pediatric Hemangiomas

Pediatric hemangiomas are self-limited lesions, thus they usually do not require treatment. On the other hand, therapy may be warranted when rare problems such as congestive heart failure or Kasabach-Merritt syndrome occur. Kasabach-Merritt syndrome is a consumptive coagulopathy secondary to platelet trapping that produces systemic bleeding complications. In general, corticosteroids will treat this problem, but we have seen some situations in which corticosteroids were not effective and direct alcohol injection into the malformation was necessary to stabilize the patient. In other anatomic sites, pediatric hemangiomas may cause compression on vital structures such as the airway, and these lesions may cause visual disturbances when located in and around the eye. In such cases, the need for treatment and alleviation of symptoms must be balanced against the knowledge that the lesion will inevitably involute. In these cases of pediatric hemangioma, treatment with ethanol is performed in a similar manner to treatment of venous malformations.

Ethanol Treatment of Arteriovenous Fistulas

Congenital and post-traumatic arteriovenous fistulas are interesting lesions. For the most part, large fistulas that occur traumatically can be treated readily by surgery or embolization, but in some situations chronic arteriovenous fistulas can be confused with AVMs on both arteriograms and MRIs because the multiple inflow arteries can simulate an AVM. In addition, these lesions may mimic AVMs in terms of complications and deficits. Treatment of arteriovenous fistulas is unlike that of the other lesions mentioned in that cure *can* be accomplished with agents besides ethanol, including balloons, glue, and coils. However, these lesions must be treated by closing the fistula directly and not the feeding vessels because we have seen a number of situations in which incomplete closure by surgical ligation or inappropriate embolization causes recanalizations and recurrences. In some circumstances, ethanol can also be successfully used for the management of arteriovenous fistulas.[14]

CONCLUSION

Alcohol therapy of vascular malformations is a challenging but ultimately rewarding pursuit. Since the 1980s, we have learned much about the appropriate imaging workup and pathologic classification of these lesions. We believe that many venous malformations and AVMs can now be cured with the use of alcohol sclerotherapy. In other lesions, alcohol offers considerable promise of lesion control and improvement of symptoms. Alcohol embolotherapy can, however, produce significant morbidity; therefore, we strongly advise that these lesions be treated by an interventionalist with significant knowledge and skill. We believe that ethanol ablation of vascular malformations is now the preferred technique for the management of these extremely complex and challenging lesions.

REFERENCES

1. Yakes WF, Parker SH. Diagnosis and management of vascular anomalies. In: Castaneda-Zuniga WR, Tadavarthy SM, eds. *Interventional Radiology*. Vol. 1. Baltimore, MD: Williams & Wilkins; 1992:152–189.
2. Szilagyi DE, Smith RF, Elliott JD, et al. Congenital arteriovenous anomalies of the limbs. *Arch Surg*. 1976;111:423–429.
3. Gomes AS, Mali WP, Oppenheim WL. Embolization therapy in the management of congenital arteriovenous malformations. *Radiology*. 1982;144:41–49.
4. Kaufman SL, Kumar AAJ, Roland JMA. Transcatheter embolotherapy in the management of congenital arteriovenous malformations. *Radiology*. 1980;137:21–29.
5. Doppman JL, Pevsner P. Embolization of arteriovenous malformations by direct percutaneous puncture. *AJR*. 1983;140:773–778.
6. Klimberg I, Hunter P, Hawkins IF, et al. Preoperative angioinfarction of localized renal cell carcinoma using absolute ethanol. *J Urol* (*Paris*). 1985;133:21–24.

7. Sarin SK, Sethi KK, Nanda R. Pulmonary hemodynamic changes after intravariceal sclerotherapy with absolute alcohol. *Gastrointest Endosc.* 1988;34:403–406.
8. Yakes WF, Peosner PH, Reed MD, et al. Serial embolizations of an extremity arteriovenous malformation with alcohol via direct percutaneous puncture. *AJR.* 1986;146:1038–1040.
9. Yakes WF, Gibson MD, Parker SH, et al. Alcohol embolotherapy of vascular malformations. *Semin Interv Radiol.* 1989;6:146–161.
10. Mulliken JB, Young AE, eds. *Vascular Birthmarks: Hemangiomas and Malformations.* Philadelphia, PA: WB Saunders, 1988.
11. Rak KM, Yakes WF, Ray RL, et al. Imaging of symptomatic peripheral vascular malformations. *AJR.* 1992;159:107–112.
12. Parikh SS, Amarapurkar DN, Dhawan PS, et al. Development of pleural effusion after sclerotherapy with absolute alcohol. *Gastrointest Endosc.* 1993;39:404–405.
13. Yakes WF. Extremity venous malformations: diagnosis and management. *Semin Interv Radiol.* 1994;11:332–339.
14. Yakes WF, Leuthke JM, Merland JJ. Ethanol embolization of arteriovenous fistulas: a primary mode of therapy. *J Vasc Interv Radiol.* 1990;1:89–96.

45

Management of Axillofemoral Graft Failure

Enrique Criado, MD, and Blair A. Keagy, MD

Axillofemoral bypass has been used since its inception as an alternative to reconstructions based on aortic inflow. It is most often employed in patients with failed conventional aortofemoral grafts, in patients considered at high risk for aortic surgery, and in patients with infections or other contraindications to the use of the aorta as an inflow source. The 5-year patency rates for axillobifemoral bypass reported during the last 10 years range from 45% to 80% and are generally lower for axillounifemoral bypasses.[1] Although the 5-year survival of patients undergoing axillofemoral grafting is generally less than 50%,[1] remedial procedures are required in a substantial number of patients to maintain graft patency. In our experience, during 11 years we managed 37 patients with thrombosed or infected axillofemoral grafts, and we performed 88 new axillofemoral bypasses.[2] One-fourth of the patients with failed grafts were referred to us from other institutions. The majority of axillofemoral bypasses are performed for critical ischemia or following failure of conventional anatomic aortoiliac bypasses.[3] Therefore, subsequent thrombosis or removal of an axillofemoral graft generally leads to limb-threatening lower extremity ischemia requiring revascularization. For this reason, and because of the comorbid processes frequently present in these patients, axillofemoral graft failure poses a great challenge to the vascular surgeon.

MECHANISMS OF AXILLOFEMORAL BYPASS FAILURE

The treatment of failed axillofemoral bypasses requires a thorough understanding of the multiple factors that may influence the patency of these grafts. As with any other vascular bypass procedure for aortoiliac reconstruction, the long-term results of axillofemoral grafting are primarily determined by the adequacy of inflow, the quality of runoff vessels and their subsequent progression of occlusive disease, and the technical performance of the procedure. Despite angiographic and surgical exploration of the failed axillofemoral graft, the cause of early or late graft failure cannot be determined in about one-third of the cases.[2,4] Interestingly, we found no relationship between the cause of graft failure and postreconstruction patency in our review of this problem.[2]

In a report including data about 28 thrombosed axillofemoral grafts, poor runoff was identified in more than 50% of the cases of early failure, and progression of distal disease was noted in more than one-third of the cases of late failure.[4] With regard to the quality of the runoff, superficial femoral artery occlusion, prior to axillofemoral bypass, appears to be associated with lower long-term patency rates, according to several retrospective reports.[1,5] In our experience, when graft infections were not included, 30% of all axillofemoral graft thromboses were due to outflow disease.[2] In addition, myointimal hyperplasia involving the distal anastomosis was found in 10% to 14% of the cases of late failure.[2,4]

Progression of inflow disease at the subclavian or axillary artery level is unusual and accounted for about 10% of all axillofemoral graft failures, both in our experience and in that of others.[2,4] Less commonly, undetected subclavian inflow stenosis is present prior to axillofemoral grafting and can lead to early thrombosis or hemodynamic failure.

Subcutaneous grafts are more vulnerable to infection than intracavitary or deep-seated grafts are. Furthermore, a significant number of axillofemoral reconstructions are performed when infected aortic grafts need to be removed, making recurrent infection in the new graft much more likely. Therefore, infection is a common mechanism of failure for axillofemoral grafts. In our series, 9 (24%) of 37 axillofemoral graft failures were due to infection[2]; however, our experience does not reflect the true incidence of infection for this type of graft because the majority of our patients with infected grafts were referred to us from other institutions.

Occasionally, hypercoagulable states and low cardiac output can be responsible for axillofemoral graft failure. These possibilities should be considered in the differential diagnosis.

The early and long-term patency of an axillofemoral graft is also influenced by the specific technical aspects of its performance. In this regard, several factors appear to be important. The axillary artery anastomosis must be as proximal as possible, medial to the pectoralis minor muscle. It is advisable to divide this muscle during the procedure. The graft tunnel is directed laterally following the middle or posterior axillary line, under the pectoralis major muscle and the external oblique fascia. If the graft is placed too distal in the axillary artery, it may be prone to undue anastomotic tension during arm abduction. This may result in anastomotic pseudoaneurysms or even acute disruption. If the graft is tunneled too anteriorly, it may be subjected to excessive kinking during flexion of the torso. External graft compression is always a concern with subcutaneously routed grafts, and a significant decrease in the ankle–brachial index (ABI) and the pulse-wave amplitude was documented in cases of axillofemoral bypass when body-weight compression of the graft occurred for a few minutes.[6] The use of externally ring-supported grafts appears to offer some protection from thrombosis due to external compression.[7]

The type of graft material, polytetrafluoroethylene or Dacron, did not appear to influence the results in retrospectively analyzed clinical series of axillofemoral bypass. However, graft materials for this procedure have not been compared in a randomized prospective fashion.

Outflow tract resistance and flow rate through the graft also influence long-term patency. In this regard, compared with axillounifemoral bypasses, axillobifemoral bypasses have significantly higher flow rates.[8] This higher rate is probably related to the lower resistance in the graft, which flows into two outflow tracts. The higher patency rates of axillobifemoral grafts found in most series, compared with the patency of axillounifemoral grafts, may be attributed in part to their hemodynamic difference, and it seems advisable that axillobifemoral grafts should be constructed whenever possible.

A variety of geometric designs for the distal anastomoses in bifemoral and unifemoral grafts have been advocated by different authors. However, it is difficult, if not impossible, to attribute better results to any particular configuration. Nevertheless, one important detail in the design of the outflow anastomoses is avoidance of competitive flow in parallel vessels. To prevent this problem, whenever there is a continuous flow channel from the aorta to the femoral artery through the common and external iliac arteries, the surgeon should interrupt this flow by ligating the common femoral or external iliac artery. If the common iliac artery is totally occluded, an end-to-side anastomosis should be constructed to the iliofemoral segment to preserve retrograde pelvic perfusion.

The use of axillofemoral grafting for the treatment of acute vascular occlusion has a deleterious effect on its results. When compared with elective procedures performed for chronic symptoms, axillofemoral bypass for acute vascular occlusion not only has a significantly higher mortality and morbidity, but also has lower graft patency and limb salvage rates.[9]

Finally, the operative mortality associated with axillofemoral bypass has to be considered as the ultimate mechanism of failure of the procedure. Axillofemoral bypass is commonly misperceived as a low-mortality operation, while on the contrary, because of the poor status of the patients undergoing the procedure, axillofemoral bypass carries a mortality rate similar to or higher than that of elective aortic surgery.[3] In situations where the operation is used to bypass aortic infections or to treat acute ischemia, the mortality may be as high as 25%.[2,3,9]

MANAGEMENT OF THE THROMBOSED AXILLOFEMORAL GRAFT

When facing the patient with a thrombosed axillofemoral graft, the surgeon has to determine whether revascularization is necessary based on limb viability and severity of symptoms, and must select a treatment strategy based on the patient's surgical risk.

Occasionally, there is no need for revascularization after axillofemoral graft thrombosis because of minimal symptoms, as it may occur in those patients in whom the initial indication for bypass was claudication or to allow healing of an ischemic ulcer. Unfortunately, the majority of patients with axillofemoral graft thromboses present with limb-threatening ischemia or recurrent rest pain and require revascularization. In our experience, 8 (89%) of 9 patients who did not undergo a remedial procedure following axillofemoral graft thrombosis required a major amputation.[2]

The success of remedial procedures for axillofemoral graft thrombosis is limited. A review of our experience revealed that only 28% of axillofemoral grafts remained patent at 2 years after a remedial procedure, with an amputation rate of 36% at 30 months. However, we found striking differences in the results depending on the type of remedial procedure performed (Table 45–1).[2] We did 43 operations to treat axillofemoral graft thrombosis; one-third were done electively, while two-thirds were done emergently or urgently. Overall, we had a 13% operative mortality among all patients with thrombosed axillofemoral bypasses, including those who had primary amputations without revascularization. The mortality rate for patients undergoing remedial procedures was 6%.[2]

Twenty-one patients who were treated with graft thrombectomy alone had the following indications: acute ischemia in 16 patients, chronic rest pain in 3, and tissue necrosis in 2. The results of isolated graft thrombectomy were poor, with a 2-year graft patency rate of 10%. Thirteen graft thromboses were treated with thrombectomy and

TABLE 45–1. REMEDIAL PROCEDURES FOR FAILED AXILLOFEMORAL GRAFTS

Thrombectomy and Graft Revision
Revision of distal anastomosis
Short distal graft extension
Additional outflow bypass
Revision of proximal anastomosis

New Aortoiliac Reconstruction
Aortofemoral or ileofemoral bypass
Thoracofemoral bypass
Ipsilateral or contralateral axillofemoral bypass
Femorofemoral bypass
Obturator bypass (for infection)

graft revision, including seven distal anastomotic revisions or short graft extensions, four new femoropopliteal bypasses to provide outflow, and two revisions of the proximal anastomosis. The results of graft thrombectomy with simultaneous revision were also disappointing, with a 2-year graft patency rate of 16%. Finally, in 9 patients the thrombosed axillofemoral bypass was abandoned, and an alternative new reconstruction was performed. Bypass from the descending thoracic aorta to the femoral arteries was done in six cases, a standard aortobifemoral bypass in one, a contralateral axillofemoral bypass in one, and a femorofemoral bypass in one. The 2-year graft patency rate following a new alternative reconstruction was 81%, a significantly better rate than that of thrombectomy alone or thrombectomy with graft revision.

We found that the ABI following a remedial procedure for axillofemoral graft thrombosis was predictive of graft outcome.[2] Among 11 grafts in patients with postoperative ABIs less than 0.5, none remained patent at 6 months. On the other hand, six patients with postoperative ABIs greater than 0.9 maintained patent grafts for at least 1 year. Eighteen patients with postoperative ABIs between 0.5 and 0.9 had a 54% 2-year graft patency, a rate significantly different from that of both other groups.

Because the results of graft thrombectomy for axillofemoral graft thrombosis are poor, at the time of graft thrombectomy every effort should be made to identify the cause of thrombosis and to correct it if possible. In many patients the cause of graft thrombosis cannot be found, and in others thrombosis recurs despite graft revisions at the time of thrombectomy. Therefore, a new alternative bypass seems advisable whenever possible. This is specially true for patients with recurrent axillofemoral graft thrombosis. Axillofemoral graft thrombectomy, with or without revision, should be reserved for patients with limited life expectancies and for emergency situations as a temporary measure to maintain limb viability while the cause of graft failure is investigated and a definitive procedure is planned.

A variety of secondary alternative aortoiliac reconstructions can be used after an axillofemoral bypass failure, depending on the individual situation of the patient. Contralateral axillofemoral bypass or femorofemoral bypass may be indicated in the unusual situation where the cause of axillofemoral graft failure is the axillary inflow and the contralateral axillary or femoral artery is an adequate source of inflow. An axillopopliteal bypass can be considered when the groin vessels cannot provide adequate outflow. Ascer et al[10] reported a 40% 3-year graft patency rate with 55 axillopopliteal bypasses. Rescue of a failed axillofemoral bypass with direct aortic reconstruction may be indicated in the patient who has not undergone a previous aortic procedure, if the general status of the patient does not contraindicate the reconstruction. Commonly, patients with axillofemoral bypasses performed as a primary aortoiliac reconstruction who were previously considered at "very high risk" for aortic surgery are found suitable candidates for aortic surgery when carefully re-evaluated at the time of their axillofemoral graft thrombosis. This approach was successful in 13 patients with failed axillofemoral bypasses reported by Gayle et al[11] and provided a 100% graft patency rate at 2 years. When the infrarenal aorta or other new extra-anatomic bypasses are not viable or appropriate options, the use of a bypass from the descending thoracic aorta to the femoral arteries may be an excellent choice. We used a thoracofemoral bypass in 6 patients, following axillofemoral graft thombosis, without any operative deaths. Five of six grafts remained patent at 2 years after surgery.

The use of thrombolytic therapy in acute axillofemoral graft thrombosis is a reasonable, although expensive, alternative. However, following successful thrombolysis, the cause of graft thrombosis, if identifiable, must be corrected by using one of the aforementioned surgical options. Otherwise, thrombolysis alone of prosthetic grafts is typically followed by early rethrombosis.

MANAGEMENT OF THE INFECTED AXILLOBIFEMORAL GRAFT

Because of the superficial route of an axillobifemoral bypass graft, the diagnosis of infection is relatively easy. There may be palpable fluid around the graft, and tissue overlying the conduit is often thickened with associated cellulitis. Drainage from the incision sites may be present in the groin or the infraclavicular region. In addition, computed tomography scanning may document the presence of fluid around the prosthesis, and a gallium scan may provide confirmatory evidence of the infection.[12]

Different authors have recommended various treatment options to deal with the problem of axillobifemoral graft infection. Consideration may be given to eradicating the local infection and covering the original graft with a muscle flap. This approach has been used to treat graft infections in various locations, including the infraclavicular region.[13] The pectoralis muscle is available for coverage of the graft, but this form of treatment is potentially successful only if the infection is confined to either the axilla or the groin and the graft in its tunnel is well incorporated by surrounding tissue.

If the situation is believed to be secondary to a biofilm infection, the old graft may be removed and a new prosthetic conduit placed in the same location as the excised graft.[14] This procedure is technically easy to perform, although there is a risk of recurrent infection.

One author reported treating graft infection with cadaveric venous homografts.[15] This approach may have some merit, but the complexity of this undertaking makes its general acceptance unlikely. In addition, a recurrent infection in the presence of a tissue graft may be associated with sudden and massive hemorrhage.

In most instances, graft removal is necessary. If the entire prosthesis is involved with the infectious process, it is important not only to remove all foreign material from the anastomotic sites in the axilla and the groin, but also to remove the body of the graft. The most desirable situation is when the extremities remain viable after graft removal. All wounds are allowed to heal before consideration is given to placing a new prosthesis.

If limb viability depends on a patent graft, a route outside the previous graft sites is chosen. Generally, this involves exposure of the superficial femoral and/or profunda femoris arteries at a location lower in the thigh. The source of inflow may be the abdominal aorta or the iliac artery with an associated tunnel through the obdurator foramen. Another alternative is the use of the thoracic aorta as a source of inflow, with placement of the graft lateral to the previous tunnel and groin incision.

Eighty-eight axillofemoral grafts were performed at the University of North Carolina between 1982 and 1993. Of the nine patients treated for axillofemoral graft infections during this period (Fig. 45–1), the majority were transferred from other institutions. Two of these patients underwent graft excision with no attempt at revascularization. Both required amputation, and one perioperative death resulted.[2] Seven of the nine infected patients underwent associated revascularization of the lower extremities, requiring a total of nine procedures. Revascularization operations included femorofemoral bypass, new axillofemoral graft, axillofemoral graft revision, and obdurator bypass. One patient underwent bypass from the descending aorta to the popliteal artery. There was one perioperative death, and three of the remaining six patients required major amputation, all because of recurrent infection of the revised or new graft.[2] A similar poor outcome associated with recurrent graft infection was reported by other authors.[16] All three of the patients without recurrent graft infection had patent grafts at 14 to 24 months after operation.

CONCLUSION

In general, axillofemoral or axillobifemoral bypass procedures have not been extremely durable. The superficial location of the graft predisposes the graft to compression, and the length of the relatively small-caliber prosthesis may promote thrombosis. Axillofemoral bypass is most often used in the patient with a previously failed or infected abdominal aortic graft, or in those in extremely poor health who cannot tolerate a more extensive operation.

Younger patients who are in good health and who have had an axillofemoral bypass performed in association with an abdominal aortic graft infection should have this bypass converted to a more durable situation after the infection has been eradicated. Our choice is the thoracobifemoral bypass graft.[17]

Patients with axillofemoral graft infection have a particularly poor course, with a high risk of perioperative death or major amputation. Most patients who undergo

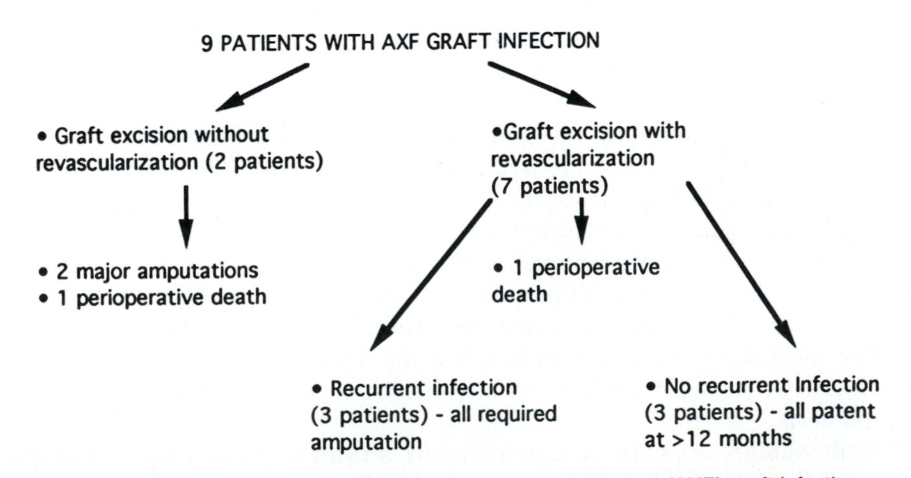

Figure 45–1. Results of treatment of nine patients with axillofemoral (AXF) graft infection.

amputation after management of an infected axillofemoral graft do so because of recurrent graft infection.

Axillofemoral or axillobifemoral bypass is an extra-anatomic bypass procedure that is easy to perform and is associated with a minimal physiologic insult to the patient. The lower patency rates associated with the operation mandate that it be used in specialized circumstances only. Thrombosed or infected grafts are treated following principles and techniques common to all graft complications.

REFERENCES

1. Blaisdel FW. Axillofemoral bypass: long term results. In: Yao J, Pearce W, eds. *Long Term Results in Vascular Surgery*. Norwalk, CT: Appleton & Lange; 1993:395–399.
2. Marston WA, Risley GL, Criado E, et al. Management of failed and infected axillofemoral grafts. *J Vasc Surg*. 1994;20:357–366.
3. Fann JI, Harris EJ, Dalman RL. Extra-anatomic bypass. Basic data underlying clinical decision making. *Ann Vasc Surg*. 1993;7:378–383.
4. Ascer E, Collier P, Gupta SK, et al. Reoperation for polytetrafluoroethylene bypass failure: the importance of distal outflow site and operative technique in determining outcome. *J Vasc Surg*. 1987;5:298–310.
5. Rutherford RB, Patt A, Pearce WH. Extra-anatomic bypass: a closer view. *J Vasc Surg*. 1987;6:437–446.
6. Cavallaro A, Sciacca V, diMarzo L, et al. The effect of body weight compression on axillofemoral bypass patency. *J Cardiovasc Surg (Torino)*. 1988;29:476–479.
7. Harris EJ, Taylor LM, McConnell DB, et al. Clinical results of axillobifemoral bypass using externally supported polytetrafluoroethylene. *J Vasc Surg*. 1990;12:416–421.
8. Lo Gerfo FW, Johnson WC, Corson JD, et al. A comparison of the late patency rates of axillobilateral femoral and axillounilateral femoral grafts. *Surgery*. 1977;81:33–40.
9. Agee JM, Kron IL, Flanagan T, et al. The risk of axillofemoral bypass grafting for acute vascular occlusion. *J Vasc Surg*. 1991;14:190–194.
10. Ascer E, Veith FJ, Gupta S. Axillopopliteal bypass grafting: indications, late results, and determinants of long term patency. *J Vasc Surg*. 1989;10:285–291.
11. Gayle RG, Gandhi RH, Katz D, et al. Rescue of failing axillofemoral grafts with direct aortic reconstruction. *J Vasc Surg*. 1993;17:240–241.
12. Banzio E, Quirce R, Serrano J, et al. Ga-67 citrate scan in vascular graft infection. *Ann Nucl Med*. 1992;6(4):235–239.
13. Meland NB, Arnold PG, Pairolero PC, et al. Muscle-flap coverage for infected peripheral vascular prosthesis. *Plast Reconstr Surg*. 1994;93(5):1005–1011.
14. Towne JB, Seabrook GR, Bandyk D, et al. In-situ replacement of arterial prosthesis infected by bacterial biofilms: long-term follow-up. *J Vasc Surg*. 1994;19(2):226–233.
15. Snyder SO, Wheeler JR, Gregory RT, et al. Freshly harvested cadaveric venous homografts as arterial conduits in infected fields. *Surgery*. 1987;101(3):283–291.
16. Yeager RA, Moneta GL, Taylor LM, et al. Improving survival and limb salvage in patients with aortic graft infections. *Am J Surg*. 1990;159(5):466–469.
17. Criado E, Keagy B. Use of the descending thoracic aorta as an inflow source in aortoiliac reconstruction: indications and long-term results. *Ann Vasc Surg*. 1994;8:38–42.

Index

Page numbers followed by *t* and *f* refer to tables and figures, respectively.

Page numbers followed by *t* and *f* refer to tables and figures, respectively.

Page numbers followed by *t* and *f* refer to tables and figures, respectively.

Page numbers followed by *t* and *f* refer to tables and figures, respectively.

Page numbers followed by *t* and *f* refer to tables and figures, respectively.

Page numbers followed by *t* and *f* refer to tables and figures, respectively.

Page numbers followed by *t* and *f* refer to tables and figures, respectively.